ANATOMY AND PHYSIOLOGY OF
Farm Animals
SIXTH EDITION

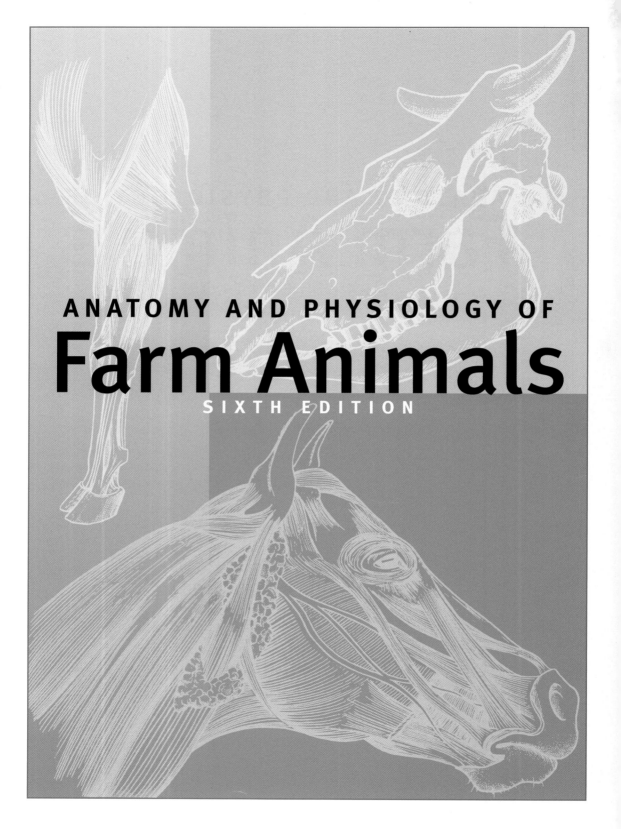

ANATOMY AND PHYSIOLOGY OF
Farm Animals
SIXTH EDITION

R. D. Frandson, BS, DVM, MS

Professor Emeritus, Department of Anatomy and Neurobiology
College of Veterinary Medicine and Biomedical Sciences
Colorado State University
Fort Collins, Colorado

W. Lee Wilke, DVM, PhD

Associate Professor, Department of Biomedical Sciences
College of Veterinary Medicine and Biomedical Sciences
Colorado State University
Fort Collins, Colorado

Anna Dee Fails, DVM, PhD

Assistant Professor, Department of Biomedical Sciences
College of Veterinary Medicine and Biomedical Sciences
Colorado State University
Fort Collins, Colorado

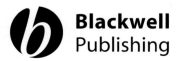

Blackwell
Publishing

Blackwell Publishing Professional
2121 State Avenue, Ames, Iowa 50014, USA

Orders:	1-800-862-6657
Office:	1-515-292-0140
Fax:	1-515-292-3348
Web site:	www.blackwellprofessional.com

Blackwell Publishing Ltd
9600 Garsington Road, Oxford OX4 2DQ, UK
Tel.: +44 (0)1865 776868

Blackwell Publishing Asia
550 Swanston Street, Carlton, Victoria 3053, Australia
Tel.: +61 (0)3 8359 1011

First Edition, 1965
Second Edition, 1974
Third Edition, 1981
Fourth Edition, 1986
Fifth Edition, 1992

Library of Congress Cataloging-in-Publication Data

Frandson, R. D.
    Anatomy and physiology of farm animals / R.D. Frandson, W. Lee Wilke, Anna Dee Fails.—
6th ed.
        p. cm.
    Includes bibliographical references (p.) and index.
    ISBN-13: 978-0-7817-3358-8
    ISBN-10: 0-7817-3358-8
    1. Veterinary anatomy. 2. Veterinary physiology. I. Wilke, W. Lee. II. Fails, Anna
Dee. III. Title

SF761 .F8 2003
636.089'2—dc21

2002029860

The last digit is the print number: 9 8 7 6 5 4 3

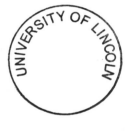

PREFACE

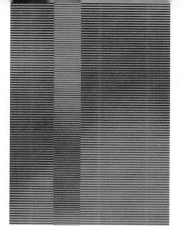

The first edition of *Anatomy and Physiology of Farm Animals* combined accuracy with simplicity and clarity of expression and gained considerable acceptance among veterinary and veterinary technician students as well as those majoring in the animal sciences and vocational agriculture. Later editions were revised to increase the value of the book to first-year veterinary students. Now in its sixth edition, this text maintains a strong reputation by achieving a balance in both depth and scope of its subject.

Summary of Key Features

This edition includes a number of new or updated features that further enhance the appeal of the text.

Extensive New Art Program. The art program in this book has undergone a major revision: approximately 100 new, original line drawings have been added, and many outdated illustrations from the fifth edition have been replaced with newer figures.

Cellular and Molecular Mechanisms. This edition has an increased emphasis on the cellular and molecular mechanisms in physiological processes. While this is in keeping with current trends in physiology and medicine, attempts are made to illustrate the relationships between these mechanisms and phenomena that can be observed in intact animals. Where controversial subjects are discussed, the generally accepted view is given in greatest detail.

Species Orientation. As in the first five editions, general principles of anatomy and physiology are discussed as they apply to farm animals. Important species differences are described, with the most attention given to the horse and the cow. The sheep, goat, and hog are described where important and relevant species differences exist. When the goat is not mentioned specifically, it may be assumed that the goat is similar to the sheep.

Clinical Extracts. Clinical Extracts, material especially useful in a clinical setting, are highlighted in blue throughout the text. These extracts help students understand the practical value of anatomy and physiology.

Nomina Anatomica Veterinaria. Every effort has been made to bring the anatomical nomenclature used in this text into accordance with the fourth edition of the Nomina Anatomica Veterinaria. Exceptions are made only when a different term is in such common usage as to argue for an older name.

Glossary and Terminology. Because abbreviations may be confusing and difficult to remember, a glossary of commonly used abbreviations is included in the appendix. Technical terms are used throughout the book, but most terms not found in an ordinary college dictionary are defined within the text.

Addition to Authorship

This edition welcomes **W. Lee Wilke** and **Anna Dee Fails.** Drs. Wilke and Fails provide the input of a veterinary physiologist and anatomist, respectively. Both hold PhD and DVM degrees and teach at Colorado State University in Fort Collins, Colorado. These authors have shown considerable energy and enthusiasm toward revision of this text.

Fort Collins, Colorado
R.D. Frandson

ACKNOWLEDGMENTS

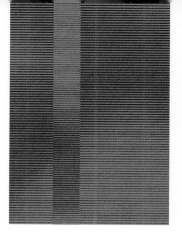

Acknowledgment of all sources of information and assistance in the evolution of this book from its first edition in 1964 to this, the sixth edition, is impossible. However, I would like to thank specifically the following colleagues and friends for their many and varied contributions.

Dr. Y. Z. Abdelbaki, Dr. T. H. Belling Jr., Miss Elsie Bergland, Mr. J. M. Bradley, Dr. H. E. Bredeck, Dr. P. A. Brooks, Dr. R. W. Davis, Dr. G. P. Epling, Mr. John Foss, Dr. R. A. Kainer, Dr. Neil May, Dr. D. Will, Mr. C. MacLeod, Mr. K. Nakamoto, and Dr. H. Meyer.

Artists: Mrs. D. Dietemann, Mr. D. Giddings, Miss M. Haff, Miss R. Haff, Mrs. D. Jeffry, Mrs. W. Musslewhite, Mrs. S. Nuss, Mr. Chris Pasquini, and Mrs. B. Sparks.

The many publishers who loaned illustrations and tables.

I offer a special acknowledgment to the following contributors:

Dr. Elmer H. Whitten for contributions in physiology to the second and third editions.

Dr. Charles W. Miller for the section in the fourth edition on the use of ultrasound.

Dr. Gordon C. Solomon for his extensive assistance in revising, correcting, editing, and proofreading the fourth edition.

Dr. Thomas Spurgeon for his valuable assistance in revising the fifth edition and particularly for rewriting the sections on muscles and cell biology.

Dr. Anna Fails and Dr. Lee Wilke for rewriting the fifth edition as coauthors of this sixth edition.

Ms. Michele Graham for her original artwork for this sixth edition.

R. D. Frandson

CONTENTS

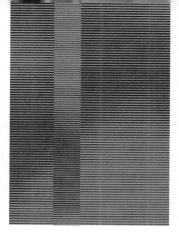

INTRODUCTION TO ANATOMY AND PHYSIOLOGY

The term *anatomy* has come to refer to the science that deals with the form and structure of all organisms. Literally the word means *to cut apart;* it was used by early anatomists when speaking of complete dissection of a cadaver.

In contrast to anatomy, which deals primarily with structure, *physiology* is the study of the integrated functions of the body and the functions of all its parts (systems, organs, tissues, cells, and cell components), including biophysical and biochemical processes.

When anatomy and physiology courses are taught separately, the approach to the laboratory portion of each course is considerably different. Study in a typical *gross anatomy* laboratory is based primarily on dissection of animal cadavers. These usually have been preserved by embalming, and one or more parts of the vascular system have been injected with a colored material to facilitate identification of the vessels. Careful dissection coupled with close observation gives the student a concept of the shape, texture, location, and relations of structures visible to the unaided eye that can be gained in no other way. Similarly, the use of the microscope with properly prepared tissue sections on slides is essential for understanding structures that are so small they cannot be seen without optical or electron microscopic assistance.

In the physiology laboratory the student studies the response of whole animals, isolated organs, or individual cells to changes in their environment (both internal and external).

Changes may be induced by almost any agent or manipulation, for example, -drugs, changes in temperature or altitude, surgical modifications (such as neutering), and changes in diet. Monitoring of the responses may be as simple as monitoring changes in body weight or as complex as measuring the electrical potential across the cell membrane of a single cell.

Anatomists and physiologists working in research use some of the same techniques that are used in teaching laboratories but with considerable refinement. Both types of scientists use equipment and methods developed in the physical sciences, particularly chemistry and physics. The anatomist applies the principles of physics to use of microscopes and applies knowledge of chemistry in the staining of various parts of cells and tissues. The combination of chemistry and microscopic anatomy is known as **histochemistry.**

Although anatomy and physiology are commonly pursued as more or less independent disciplines, they are both facets of the study of the animal body. A thorough knowledge of structure imparts much information about its function. However, a mere description of structure without describing function would be of little practical value. Conversely, it is impossible to gain a thorough understanding of function without a basic knowledge of structure.

The science of anatomy has become so extensive that it is now divided into many specialized branches. In fact, *Dorland's Medical*

Dictionary defines 30 subdivisions of anatomy. This text chiefly describes **gross (macroscopic) anatomy.** This is the study of the form and relations (relative positions) of the structures of the body that can be seen with the unaided eye. **Comparative anatomy** is a study of the structures of various species of animals, with particular emphasis on those characteristics that aid in classification. **Embryology** is the study of developmental anatomy, covering the period from conception (fertilization of the egg) to birth. Another large branch of anatomy consists of the study of tissues and cells that can be seen only with the aid of a microscope. This is known as **microscopic anatomy,** or **histology.**

The most recent development in the study of anatomy is **ultrastructural cytology,** which deals with portions of cells and tissues as they are visualized with the aid of the electron microscope. The term *fine structure* is used frequently in reference to structures seen in electron micrographs (photographs made with the electron microscope).

Our approach to the study of anatomy will be chiefly by systems—*systematic anatomy.* To name the study, the suffix -ology, which means *branch of knowledge or science,* is added to the root word referring to the system. Table 1–1 indicates the commonly accepted systems, the name of the study of those systems, and the chief structures involved in each system.

Physiology has also become so extensive in scope that many areas of specialization are rec-

Table 1-1. Nomenclature for Systematic Anatomy		
System	*Name of Study*	*Chief Structures*
Skeletal system	Osteology	Bones
Articular system	Arthrology	Joints
Muscular system	Myology	Muscles
Digestive system	Splanchnology	Stomach and Intestines
Respiratory system	Splanchnology	Lungs and airways
Urinary system	Splanchnology	Kidneys and urinary bladder
Reproductive system	Splanchnology	Ovaries and testes
Endocrine system	Endocrinology	Ductless glands
Nervous system	Neurology	Brain, spinal cord, and nerves
Circulatory system	Cardiology	Heart and vessels
Sensory system	Esthesiology	Eye and ear

Plate 1: Tissue Types

(Numbers 1, 3, 7, 10, and 12 are from Bacha & Wood, *Color Atlas of Veterinary Histology*, Lea & Febiger, 1990; Numbers 6 and 11 are from Banks, *Applied Veterinary Histology*, 2nd Edition, Williams & Wilkins, 1986; Numbers 2, 4, 5, 8, and 9 are courtesy of Sandra Pitcaithley, DVM.)

1. Simple cuboidal epithelium lining the collecting tubules of the bovine kidney.
2. Simple columnar epithelium of the colonic mucosa.
3. Psuedostratified columnar epithelium characteristic of respiratory epithelium. Note ciliated surface.
4. Stratified squamous epithelium, non-keratinized.
5. Transitional epithelium of the urinary bladder.
6. Dense, regular connective tissue in a longitudinal section of tendon.
7. Areolar (loose) connective tissue from mesentery. Note the fine elastic fibers and thicker collagen fibers. A capillary runs from top to bottom in this view. Most cells outside the capillary are fibroblasts.
8. Adipose (fat) tissue.
9. Hyaline cartilage.
10. Bone in cross section. Osteocytes reside in small lacunae in the concentric circles of the haversian system.
11. Skeletal muscle in longitudinal section.
12. Smooth muscle in the wall of a medium-sized artery. The lumen of the artery is at the top of the micrograph; muscle cells lie just beneath the endothelium of the vessels. Darker pink is the elastic tunica adventitia outside the muscle.

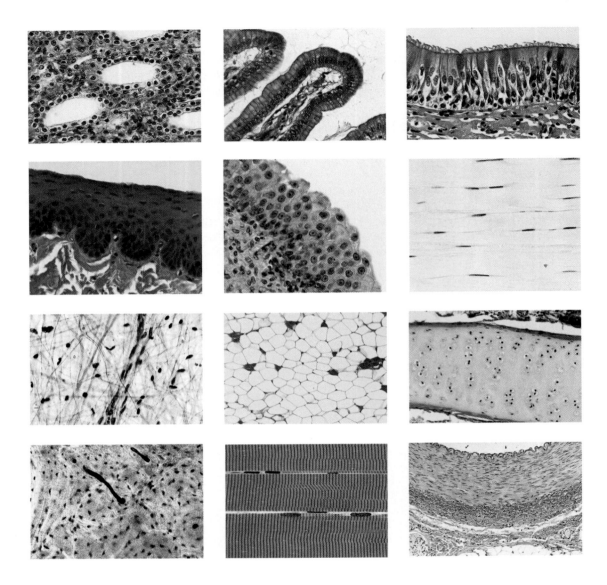

Plate II: Types of Blood Cells

(Numbers 3 and 5–8 are from Bacha & Wood, *Color Atlas of Veterinary Histology*, Lea & Febiger, 1990; Numbers 1 and 2 are courtesy of Sandra Pitcaithley, DVM; Number 4 is from Schalm OW, Jain NC, Carroll EJ: *Veterinary Hematology*, 3rd edition, Philadelphia, Lea & Febiger, 1986.)

1. Canine red blood cells (erythrocytes). Small, dark-staining, enucleate platelets can be seen.
2. Canine neutrophil.
3. Equine basophil (left) and neutrophil (right). Small platelets and red blood cells are also seen.
4. Equine eosinophil (left) and basophil (right).
5. Bovine eosinophil.
6. From left to right: Neutrophil, monocyte, and lymphocyte.
7. From left to right: two lymphocytes and a monocyte.
8. Low power micrograph of feline blood showing a variety of blood cell types. 1: red blood cell; 2: eosinophil; 3: lymphocyte; 4: monocyte; 5: neutrophil; 6: platelets.

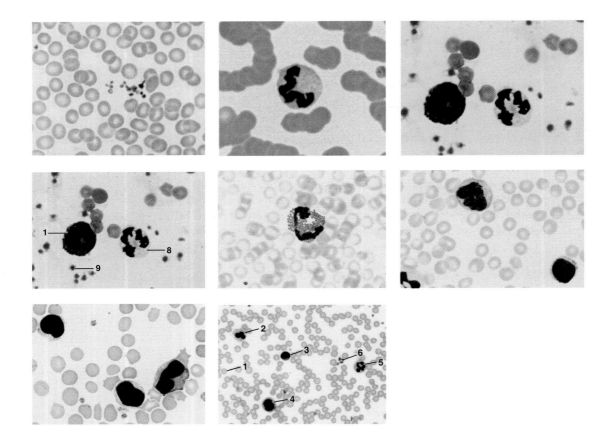

ognized. Like anatomy, these may be based on body systems (e.g., neurophysiology, gastrointestinal physiology, cardiovascular physiology, respiratory physiology, endocrine physiology, and reproductive physiology) or the level of biological organization (cell physiology and organismal physiology). All of these subdivisions become the parts of such overall areas of study as applied physiology, comparative physiology, pathophysiology, medical physiology, and mammalian physiology. We will be concerned with these systems and studies as they relate specifically to farm animals.

Descriptive Terms Useful in the Study of Anatomy

When giving geographic locations, we make use of certain arbitrary frames of reference known as meridians of latitude and longitude. However, since an animal is rarely oriented exactly with a line on the earth's surface, our frames of reference must be in relation to the animal itself and must apply regardless of the position or direction of the animal (Fig. 1–1). Many terms of direction differ significantly between human and domestic animal anatomy, because of the orientation of bipedal versus quadrupedal stance. Although use of common terminology between bipedal and quadrupedal species usually leads to confusion, the terms *anterior, posterior, superior,* and *inferior* are frequently used to describe the eye and aspects of dental anatomy of both human beings and domestic animals (see Chapter 12).

Cranial is a directional term meaning toward the head. The shoulder is cranial to the hip; it is closer to the head than is the hip.

Caudal means toward the tail. The rump is caudal to the loin.

Rostral and *caudal* are directional terms used in reference to features of the head to mean toward the nose (rostral) or toward the tail (caudal).

The *median plane* is an imaginary plane passing through the body so as to divide the body into right and left halves. A beef carcass is split into two halves on the median plane.

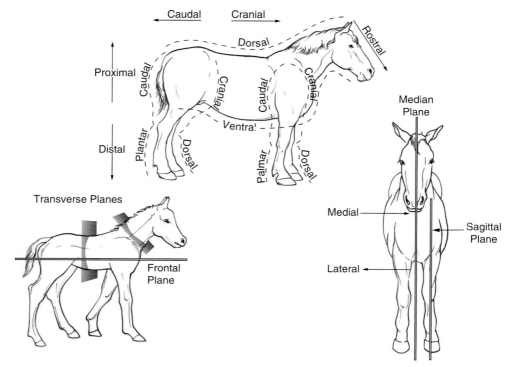

Figure 1-1. Directional terms and planes of the animal body.

A *sagittal plane* is any plane parallel to the median plane. The median plane is sometimes called the *midsagittal plane.*

A *transverse plane* is at right angles to the median plane and divides the body into cranial and caudal segments. A cross-section of the body would be made on a transverse plane. The cinch of a saddle defines a transverse plane through the thorax of a horse.

A *horizontal plane* is at right angles to both the median plane and transverse planes. The horizontal plane divides the body into dorsal (upper) and ventral (lower) segments. If a cow walks into a lake until the water comes above the chest, the surface of the water is in a horizontal plane in relation to the cow.

In addition to the planes of reference, other descriptive terms are valuable in defining an area we wish to discuss.

Medial is an adjective meaning close to or toward the median plane. The heart is medial to the lungs; it is closer to the median plane than are the lungs. The chestnut is on the medial aspect (inside) of a horse's limb; it is on the side closest to the median plane.

Lateral is the antonym of medial; it means away from the median plane. The ribs are lateral to the lungs, that is, farther from the median plane.

Dorsal means toward or beyond the backbone or vertebral column. The kidneys are dorsal to the intestines; they are closer to the vertebral column. Dorsum is the noun referring to the dorsal portion or back. A saddle is placed on the dorsum of a horse.

Ventral means away from the vertebral column or toward the mid abdominal wall. The udder is the most ventral part of the body of a cow: the part of the body farthest from the vertebral column.

Deep and *internal* indicate proximity to the center of an anatomical structure. The humerus (arm bone) is deep to all other structures in the arm.

Superficial and *external* refer to proximity to the surface of the body. Hair is superficial to all other structures of the body.

Proximal means relatively close to a given part, usually the vertebral column, body, or center of gravity. Proximal is generally used in reference to an extremity or limb. The carpus or knee is proximal to the foot.

Distal means farther from the vertebral column, and like proximal, it is generally used in reference to portions of an extremity. The hoof is distal to the carpus or knee.

The suffix *-ad* is used to form an adverb from any of the above-named directional terms, indicating movement in the direction of or toward, as in *dorsad, ventrad, caudad,* and *craniad,* that is, respectively, toward the dorsum, toward the belly, toward the tail, and toward the head.

In describing the thoracic limb (forelimb) distal to (below) the carpus, *palmar* refers to the flexor or caudal surface. *Dorsal* is used in this region to refer to the opposite (cranial) side. In describing the pelvic limb (hindlimb) distal to the hock, *plantar* refers to the caudal surface, and dorsal here too refers to the side directly opposite (the cranial side).

Prone refers to a position in which the dorsal aspect of the body or any extremity is uppermost. *Pronation* refers to the act of turning toward a prone position.

Supine refers to the position in which the ventral aspect of the body or palmar or plantar aspect of an extremity is uppermost. *Supination* refers to the act of turning toward a supine position.

Microscopic Anatomy: Animal Cells and Tissues

All living things, both plants and animals, are constructed of small units called *cells.* The simplest animals, such as the ameba, consist of a single cell that is capable of performing all functions commonly associated with life. These functions include growth (increase in size), metabolism (use of food), response to stimuli (such as moving toward light), contraction (shortening in one direction), and reproduction (development of new individuals of the same species).

A typical cell consists of three main parts, the *cytoplasm,* the *nucleus,* and the *cell membrane* (Fig. 1–2). Detailed structure of the individual cell is described in Chapter 2. Tissues are discussed in this chapter.

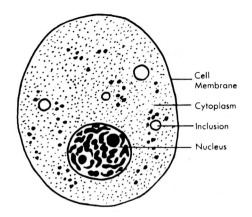

Figure 1-2. A cell as seen with a light microscope.

In complex animals, certain cells specialize in one or more of the functions of the animal body. A group of specialized cells is a **tissue.** For example, cells that specialize in conducting impulses make up nerve tissue. Cells that specialize in holding structures together make up **connective tissue.** Various tissues are associated in functional groups called **organs.** The stomach is an organ that functions in digestion of food. A group of organs that participate in a common enterprise make up a **system.** The stomach, liver, pancreas, and intestines are all part of the digestive system.

The primary types of tissues include (1) **epithelial tissues,** which cover the surface of the body, line body cavities, and form glands; (2) **connective tissues,** which support and bind other tissues together and from which, in the case of bone marrow, the formed elements of the blood are derived; (3) **muscle tissues,** which specialize in contracting; and (4) **nervous tissues,** which conduct impulses from one part of the body to another.

Epithelial Tissues

In general the epithelial tissues are classified as **simple** (composed of a single layer) or **stratified** (many-layered). Each of these types is further subdivided according to the shape of the individual cells within it (Fig. 1–3). Simple epithelium includes squamous (platelike) cells, cuboidal (cubic) cells, columnar (cylindrical) cells, and pseudostratified columnar cells.

Simple squamous epithelium consists of thin, platelike cells. They are much expanded in two directions but have little thickness. The edges are joined somewhat like mosaic tile covering a floor. A layer of simple squamous epithelium has little tensile strength and is found only as a covering layer for stronger tissues. Simple squamous epithelium is found where a smooth surface is required to reduce friction. The coverings of viscera and the linings of body cavities and blood vessels are all composed of simple squamous epithelium.

Cuboidal epithelial cells are approximately equal in all dimensions. They are found in some ducts and in passageways in the kidneys. The active tissue of many glands is composed of cuboidal cells.

Columnar epithelial cells are cylindrical. They are arranged somewhat like the cells in a honeycomb. Some columnar cells have whiplike projections called **cilia** extending from the free extremity. The cells lining the trachea (windpipe) are of this type. The cilia wave in such a manner as to move any foreign material in the trachea toward the mouth, where it can be coughed out or swallowed.

Pseudostratified columnar epithelium is composed of columnar cells. However, they vary in length, giving the appearance of more than one layer or stratum. This type of epithelium is found in the upper respiratory tract, where the lining cells are ciliated.

Stratified epithelium consists of more than one layer of epithelial cells and includes stratified squamous, stratified columnar, and transitional epithelia.

Stratified squamous epithelium forms the outer layer of the skin and the lining of the first part of the digestive tract as far as the stomach. In ruminants, stratified squamous epithelium also lines the forestomach (rumen, reticulum, and omasum). Stratified squamous epithelium is the thickest and toughest of the epithelia, consisting of many layers of cells. From deep to superficial, these layers include the **basal layer** (**stratum basale**), the **parabasal layer** (**stratum spinosum**), **intermediate layer** (**stratum granulosum**), and **superficial layer** (**stratum corneum**). The deepest layer, the stratum basale, contains the actively growing and multiplying cells. These cells are somewhat cuboidal, but as

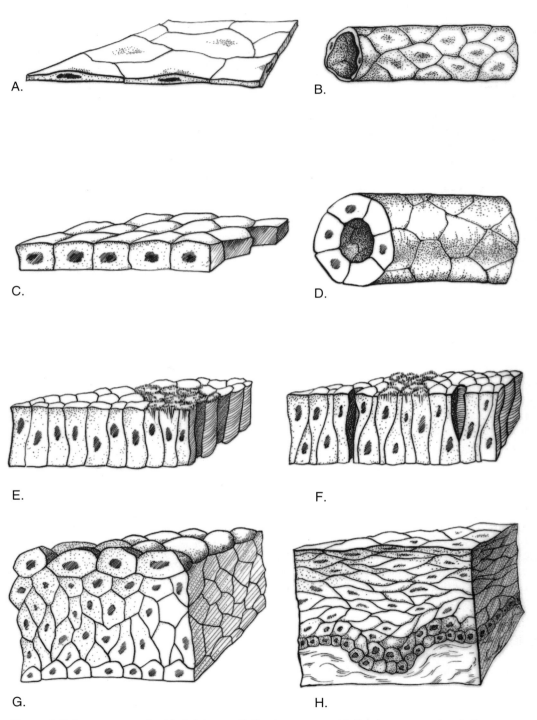

Figure 1-3. Primary types of epithelial tissues. *A)* Simple squamous. *B)* Simple squamous in tubular arrangement. *C)* Simple cuboidal. *D)* Simple cuboidal arranged as a duct. *E)* Simple columnar. *F)* Pseudostratified columnar with cilia. *G)* Transitional. *H)* Stratified squamous.

they are pushed toward the surface, away from the blood supply of the underlying tissues, they become flattened, tough, and lifeless and are constantly in the process of peeling off. This layer of cornified (keratinized) dead cells becomes very thick in areas subjected to friction. Calluses are formed in this manner.

Stratified columnar epithelium is composed of more than one layer of columnar cells and is found lining part of the pharynx and salivary ducts.

Transitional epithelium lines the portions of the urinary system that are subjected to stretching. These areas include the urinary bladder and ureters. Transitional epithelium can pile up many cells thick when the bladder is small and empty and stretch out to a single layer when completely filled.

Glandular epithelial cells are specialized for secretion or excretion. *Secretion* is the release from the gland cell of a substance that has been synthesized by the cell and that usually affects other cells in other parts of the body. *Excretion* is the expulsion of waste products.

Glands may be classified either as *endocrine glands* (glands without ducts, which empty their secretory products directly into the blood stream) or as *exocrine glands* (glands that empty their secretory products on an epithelial surface, usually by means of ducts).

The endocrine glands are an important part of the control mechanisms of the body, because they produce special chemicals known as *hormones.* The endocrine glands are discussed in Chapter 12. Hormones carried to all parts of the body by the blood constitute the humoral control of the body. Humoral control and nervous control are the two mechanisms maintaining *homeokinesis,* also called *homeostasis,* a relatively stable but constantly changing state of the body. Humoral responses to stimuli from the environment (both external and internal) are slower and longer acting than responses generated by way of the nervous system. The nervous system is described in some detail in Chapters 9 and 10.

Collectively, the endocrine glands constitute the *endocrine system,* which is studied in *endocrinology.* However, exocrine glands are scattered throughout many systems and are discussed along with the systems to which they be-

long, such as the digestive, urogenital, and respiratory systems.

According to their morphologic classification (Fig. 1–4), a gland is *simple* if the duct does not branch and compound if it does. If the secretory portion forms a tubelike structure, it is called *tubular;* if the secretory portion resembles a grape or hollow ball, it is called *alveolar* or *acinar* (the terms are used interchangeably). A combination of tubular and alveolar secretory structures produces a *tubuloalveolar gland.*

Compound glands often are subdivided grossly into *lobes,* which in turn may be further subdivided into *lobules.* Hence the connective tissue partitions (called *septa*) are classified as interlobar septa if they separate lobes and as interlobular septa if they separate lobules. Similar terminology may be applied to ducts draining lobes or lobules of glands, that is, interlobar ducts and interlobular ducts, respectively.

Another classification of glands is based on the manner in which their cells elaborate their secretion. By this classification, the most common type is the *merocrine gland.* Merocrine glands pass their secretory products through the cell wall without any appreciable loss of cytoplasm or noticeable damage to the cell membrane. The *holocrine gland* is the least common type. After the cell fills with secretory material, the entire holocrine gland cell discharges to the lumen of the gland to constitute the secretion. Sebaceous glands associated with hair follicles of the skin are the most common holocrine glands. An intermediate form of secretion in which a small amount of cytoplasm and cell membrane is lost with the secretion is sometimes described for the prostate and some sweat glands. Such glands are called *apocrine glands.*

Connective Tissues

Connective tissues, as the name implies, serve to connect other tissues. They give form and strength to many organs and often provide protection and leverage. Connective tissues include elastic tissue, collagenous (white fibrous) tissue, reticular (netlike) tissue, adipose (fat) tissue, cartilage, and bone.

Elastic tissue contains kinked fibers that tend to regain their original shape after being

TYPES OF EXOCRINE GLANDS

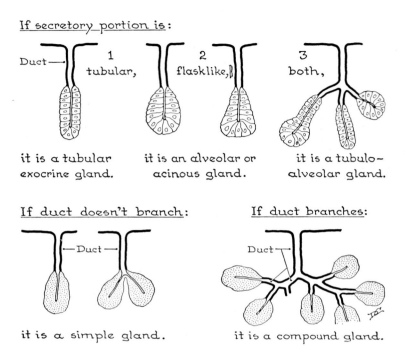

Figure 1-4. Different kinds of secretory units of exocrine glands and comparison of simple and compound glands. (Reprinted with permission from Ham AW, and Cormack DH. *Histology.* 8th ed. Philadelphia: Lippincott Williams & Wilkins, 1979.)

stretched. This tissue is found in the ligamentum nuchae, a strong band that helps to support the head, particularly in horses and cattle. Elastic tissue also is found in the abdominal tunic, in the ligamenta flava of the spinal canal, in elastic arteries, and mixed with other tissues wherever elasticity is needed.

Collagenous (*white fibrous*) *tissue* is found throughout the body in various forms. Individual cells (fibroblasts) produce long proteinaceous fibers of collagen, which have remarkable tensile strength. These fibers may be arranged in regular repeating units, or laid down in a more random, irregular arrangement.

In *dense regular connective tissue* (Fig. 1–5), the fibers are arranged in parallel bundles, forming cords or bands of considerable strength. These are the *tendons,* which connect muscles to bones, and the *ligaments,* which connect bones to bones.

The fibers of *dense irregular connective tis-sue* are arranged in a thick mat with fibers running in all directions. The dermis of the skin, which may be tanned to make leather, consists of dense irregular connective tissue. This forms a strong covering that resists tearing and yet is flexible enough to move with the surface of the body.

Areolar (*loose*) *connective tissue* (Plate I) is found throughout the body wherever protective cushioning and flexibility are needed. For example, blood vessels are surrounded by a sheath of areolar connective tissue, which permits the vessels to move and yet protects them.

Beneath the dermis is a layer of loosely arranged areolar connective tissue fibers that attaches the skin to underlying muscles. This attachment is flexible enough to permit movement of the skin. It also permits the formation of a thick layer of fat between the skin and underlying muscles. Whenever the skin is adherent to bony prominences because of a lack of

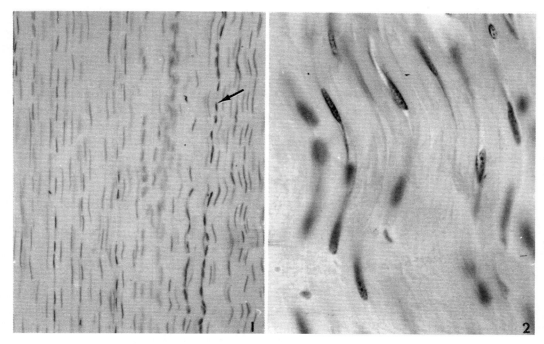

Figure 1-5. Longitudinal section through a tendon showing the histological appearance of dense regular connective tissue. *Left)* notice the line of nuclei (*arrow*), indicating the loose connective tissue surrounding blood vessels and nerves. Hematoxylin and eosin stain, ×226. At higher power (*right*), spindle-shaped fibroblasts can be seen among collagen fibers. Hematoxylin and eosin stain, ×660. (Reprinted with permission from Dellmann, H.D. and Brown, E.M. *Textbook of Veterinary Histology.* 2nd ed. Philadelphia: Lea & Febiger, 1981.)

areolar tissue, the skin will not move, and no layer of fat can form. This feature is seen in beef cattle that have **ties;** in this case, the skin over the back shows large dimples where fat cannot fill in because the skin is adherent to the vertebrae.

Reticular connective tissue consists of fine fibrils and cells. Reticular tissue makes up part of the framework of endocrine and lymphatic organs.

Adipose tissue (fat) forms when connective tissue cells called *adipocytes* store fat as inclusions within the cytoplasm of the cell. As more fat is stored, the cell eventually becomes so filled with fat that the nucleus is pushed to one side of the cell, which, as a result, becomes spherical (Plate I). Most fat in the animal body is white, although it may have a yellow tinge in horses and some breeds of dairy cattle because of carotenoids in the feed.

In contrast to this white fat, a small amount of **brown fat** may be found in domestic mammals, hibernating mammals, rodents, and human infants. The brown fat is found between the scapulae, in the axillae, in the mediastinum, and in association with mesenteries in the abdomen. Brown fat apparently generates heat to protect young mammals and hibernating mammals from extreme cold.

Cartilage is a special type of connective tissue that is firmer than fibrous tissue but not as hard as bone. The nature of cartilage is due to the structure of the intercellular material found between the *chondrocytes* (cartilage cells). The three types of cartilage described are hyaline, elastic, and fibrous.

Hyaline cartilage is the glasslike covering of bones within joints. This type of cartilage forms a smooth surface that reduces friction, so that one bone easily glides over another. The actively growing areas near the ends of long bones also consist of hyaline cartilage. *Elastic cartilage* consists of a mixture of cartilage substance and elastic fibers. This type of cartilage gives shape and rigidity to the external ear. **Fibrocartilage** consists of a mixture of cartilage and collagenous fibers, which forms a semielastic cushion of great strength. The intervertebral discs between the bodies of adjacent vertebrae are composed of fibrocartilage.

Bone is produced by bone-forming cells called **osteoblasts.** These cells produce **osteoid tissue,** which later becomes calcified to form bone. The bone may be arranged in the form of spicules (small spikes) and flat plates, forming a spongelike network called **cancellous bone** or **spongy bone.** Alternatively, it may be laid down in the form of laminated cylinders (**Haversian** or **osteonal systems**), closely packed together to form **compact bone** (Plate I).

Blood. **Blood** consists of a fluid matrix (liquid portion), the plasma, a variety of cells (Plate II), proteins, monosaccharides (simple sugars), products of fat degradation, and other circulating nutrients, wastes, electrolytes, and chemical intermediates of cellular metabolism. It is sometimes considered to be a connective tissue because of the origin of some of its components.

Red blood cells (**RBCs**) are also called **erythrocytes.** In most domestic mammals they are nonnucleated biconcave disks that contain the protein **hemoglobin.** The main function of the RBCs is to carry hemoglobin. Hemoglobin in turn has the primary function of carrying oxygen from the lungs to all tissues of the animal. At the tissue level, oxygen is released to the cells, while carbon dioxide, which is produced by the cells, diffuses into the blood to be carried back to the lungs, where it can be eliminated during breathing. **Anemia** is a reduction in the concentration of functional RBCs in the blood. It can result from a loss of red cells (as in hemorrhage), insufficient RBC production, or inappropriate or premature degradation of the red cells.

White cells (also called **leukocytes**) are one of the body's first lines of defense against infection. They include agranulocytes and granulocytes. **Agranulocytes** are of two kinds: **monocytes,** large cells that engulf and destroy foreign particles, and **lymphocytes,** which usually are smaller and which are associated with immune responses. An excess of agranulocytes tends to be associated with chronic types of diseases.

Granulocytes (**polymorphonuclear leukocytes**) are of three types and are described according to their affinity for different stains. Granules in **neutrophils** stain indifferently; **basophils** have dark-staining granules when stained with common blood stains; and **eosinophils** have red-staining granules. Blood **platelets** (**thrombocytes**) are small, irregularly shaped cellular fragments that are associated with the clotting of the blood. Mammalian platelets lack a nucleus.

Plasma is the fluid part of unclotted blood. Plasma is particularly useful as a substitute for blood in transfusions because the proteins in it give it the same osmotic pressure as blood. Plasma therefore will not escape from blood vessels as readily as a salt solution.

Serum is the supernatant fluid that remains after a clot forms and incorporates the cellular components of blood. It is similar to plasma but lacks most of the clotting factors. Serum is sometimes administered for prevention and treatment of diseases because it contains the antibody fractions of the blood.

Muscle Tissue

The three types of muscle tissue are skeletal, smooth, and cardiac (Plate I; Figs. 1–6). Both skeletal and cardiac muscle cells consist of fibers that under the microscope show characteristic cross-striations, so both are classified as **striated muscle.** Smooth muscle cells lack distinct cross striations.

Each skeletal muscle cell must have its own nerve supply, and when stimulated, the whole fiber contracts. This is the all-or-none law of muscle contraction. However, the force of contraction depends on the state of the fiber at any one moment. For example, is it already fatigued, is it warmed up, is it stretched? Striated skeletal muscle tissue plus some connective tissue makes up the flesh of meat-producing animals.

Smooth muscle cells are spindle-shaped cells that contain one centrally located nucleus per cell. Smooth muscle is found in the walls of the digestive tract, in the walls of blood vessels, and in the walls of urinary and reproductive organs. These cells contract more slowly than skeletal

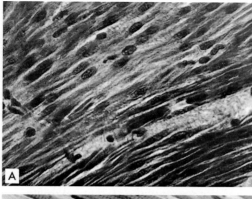

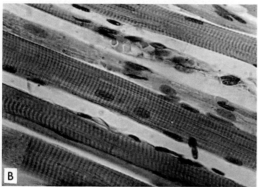

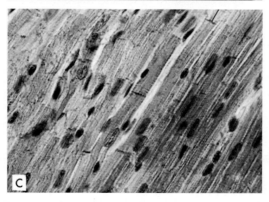

Figure 1-6. Types of muscle tissue. *A)* smooth muscle; *B)* skeletal muscle; *C)* cardiac muscle. (Reprinted with permission from Crouch, J.E. *Functional Human Anatomy.* 4th ed. Philadelphia: Lea & Febiger, 1985.)

muscle and in response to a variety of stimuli, although they are not under voluntary control.

Cardiac muscle is also known as involuntary striated muscle because it is not usually under conscious control, yet it does have cross-striations. The heart muscle is composed of a complex branched arrangement of cardiac muscle cells. Modified muscle cells called *Purkinje*

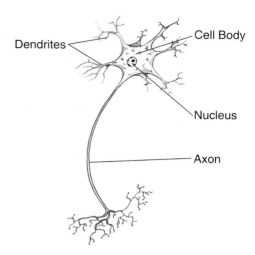

Figure 1-7. A typical motor neuron.

fibers conduct impulses within the heart, much as nerve fibers do in other parts of the body.

Nervous Tissue

The essential cell of nervous tissue is the *neuron* (nerve cell). The neuron consists of a nerve cell body and two or more nerve processes (nerve fibers). The processes are called *axons* if they conduct impulses away from the cell body and *dendrites* if they conduct impulses toward the cell body (Fig. 1–7).

Bundles of axons in the spinal cord are called *tracts,* and those in the periphery are called *nerves.* A nerve fiber may be covered by a *myelin sheath,* a specialized wrapping created by supportive cells called *Schwann cells* in nerves or by *oligodendrocytes* within the brain and spinal cord.

The special connective tissues of nervous tissue are called *neuroglia* and are found only in the central nervous system. Outside the central nervous system, in addition to the Schwann cells, ordinary white fibrous tissue serves as the major protective covering for the nerves.

The General Plan of the Animal Body

All farm animals are vertebrates, and as such they have a vertebral column. The body (with the exception of a few internal organs) exhibits bilateral symmetry. This means that the right and left sides of the body are mirror images of each other. Similar right and left structures are called paired structures, such as a pair of gloves that are similar but not interchangeable. Most unpaired structures are on or near the median plane, and of course, only one of each unpaired structure exists in any given animal. The tongue, trachea, vertebral column, and heart are examples of unpaired structures. The ribs, limbs, eyes, and most muscles are paired structures.

The medial view of the body shows two cavities: a **dorsal cavity** containing the brain and spinal cord and a **ventral cavity** containing most of the viscera (soft structures) of the body. The ventral cavity is subdivided by the diaphragm into the thoracic cavity cranially and the abdominopelvic cavity (which includes the abdominal cavity and the pelvic cavity) caudally.

The **thoracic cavity** contains the **pericardial sac,** which surrounds the heart, and two **pleural sacs,** which surround the two lungs. These sacs are formed by serous membranes, a layer of simple squamous epithelium with underlying connective tissue, moistened with the scant fluid within the cavity of the sac. The simple squamous epithelium lining various body cavities is also called **mesothelium.**

The **abdominal cavity** contains the kidneys, most of the digestive organs, and a variable amount of the internal reproductive organs in both sexes. The **pelvic cavity** contains the terminal part of the digestive system (the rectum) and all of the internal portions of the urogenital system not found in the abdominal cavity. The abdominal and pelvic cavities are continuous with one another; the brim of the pelvis marks the transition from one to the other. The serous membrane that surrounds the abdominal viscera and part of the pelvic viscera is called **peritoneum.**

A transverse section through the abdominal cavity illustrates the general plan of the body as a tube (the digestive tract and its derivatives) within a tube (the body wall) (Fig. 1–8). The region between the two tubes is the ventral

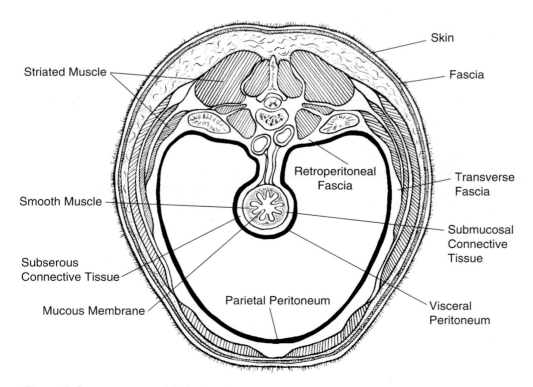

Figure 1-8. Cross-section of the body wall and digestive tract.

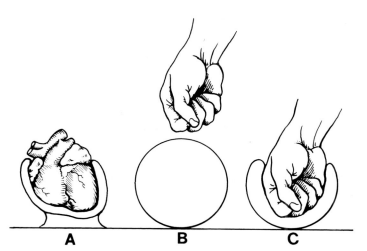

Figure 1-9. *A,* Invagination of serous membrane to form outer (parietal) and inner (visceral) layers. This is similar to a fist pushed into a balloon (*B* and *C*).

body cavity, which is derived from the embryonic **coelom.** Normally there are few air-filled spaces in the animal body except in the respiratory system and the ear. However, for the sake of clarity, many illustrations show a considerable separation between structures that in the animal body are actually in contact.

The layers of the body wall and the layers of the digestive tract show a striking similarity, although in reverse order. Layers of the body wall from outside inward are (1) epithelium (epidermis of the skin), (2) connective tissue (dermis and fascia), (3) muscle (striated), (4) connective tissue (transverse fascia), and (5) mesothelium (parietal peritoneum). The layers of the gut wall from outside inward are (1) mesothelium (visceral peritoneum), (2) connective tissue (subserous connective tissue), (3) muscle (smooth), (4) connective tissue (submucosa), and (5) epithelium (mucous membrane) (Fig. 1–8).

The serous membranes mentioned previously (pericardium, pleura, and peritoneum) are all derivatives of the lining of the celomic cavity of the embryo. Each serous membrane forms a continuous sac that is usually empty except for a small amount of serous (watery) fluid that acts as a lubricant. In other words, no viscera are found in any of the serous sacs, although most viscera are covered by at least one layer of a serous membrane. A simple analogy is that of pushing one's fist into a partially inflated balloon. The fist is never actually within the balloon proper, but still it is surrounded by a portion of the balloon (Fig. 1–9).

The part of the serous membrane covering a viscus is called the **visceral serous membrane** (visceral pericardium, visceral pleura, and visceral peritoneum). The serous membrane lining a body cavity is called the **parietal serous membrane** (parietal pleura and parietal peritoneum). The continuity of each serous sac is maintained by connecting layers of serous membrane that extend from the visceral layer of each serous membrane to the parietal layer of the same serous membrane. The names of these connecting layers of serous membranes are based on the specific areas they connect, and they are discussed in some detail along with the relevant systems.

ANATOMY AND PHYSIOLOGY OF THE CELL

Discovery of living cells would have been difficult, if not impossible, before Zacharias Jansen of the Netherlands invented the compound microscope in 1590. Robert Hooke of England used the term *cell* to describe the cavities he saw in sections of cork. In 1665, Hooke published a description of cork cells based on a study done with his improved compound microscope.

In 1839 Matthias Schleiden, a German botanist, and Theodor Schwann, an animal anatomist, formulated the **cell theory,** which set forth the concept that "the elementary parts of all tissues are formed of cells in an analogous, though very diversified, manner, so that it may be asserted that there is one universal principle of development for the elementary parts of organisms, however different, and that this principle is the formation of cells."

The word cell comes from the Latin *cella* meaning small chamber. In biology, particularly animal biology, the term cell refers more specifically to the individual units of living structure rather than the compartments that may contain them. There actually are no compartments as such in most tissues (with the exception of bone and cartilage), but the living units, cells, are found in groups in which mainly adjacent cells restrain individual cells. As early as 1772, Corti observed the jellylike material in the cell that later was called protoplasm.

Properties of Life

It is difficult to give a satisfactory definition of life. However, the cell is the functional unit of all animal life. It is the unit that makes up all tissues, organs, and systems, which in turn make up the total animal. Therefore, the properties of the cell are equated with those of life. These properties include homeostasis, growth, reproduction, absorption, metabolism, secretion, irritability, conductivity, and contractility. The last two, however, are not properties of all cells. Conductivity is an important functional characteristic of both nerve and muscle cells, while contractility is a property of muscle cells.

Homeostasis is the tendency for living things to attempt to maintain a state of relative stability. At the whole-animal level or at the cellular level, all living things respond to stresses placed upon them by changes in their environment. Their responses are attempts to maintain a state of homeostasis.

Growth is increase in size. Increase in size of a cell or organ beyond normal is called **hypertrophy.** An increase in the size of a structure because of an increase in the number of cells is called **hyperplasia.** A decrease in size from normal is called **atrophy.** Failure of a tissue or organ to develop is called **aplasia,** while incomplete development or defective development of a tissue or organ is called **hypoplasia.**

Reproduction of a cell or of an organism implies the ability to produce more cells or more organisms that are essentially the same as the original. Some fully differentiated cells, for instance nerve cells, do not normally retain the ability to reproduce in the adult.

Cells may be found in solutions whose composition is quite different from that of the fluid within the cells. To maintain intracellular homeostasis in these conditions, the passage of particles and water in and out of the cell must be regulated. **Absorption** is the process of taking dissolved materials or water through the cell membrane into the substance of the cell. This can be a passive process dependent on the forces of diffusion and osmosis, an active process requiring the expenditure of energy from adenosine triphosphate, or the result of electrochemical ionic forces and affinities that require no direct expenditure of energy. All three can occur at the same time across the same cell membrane.

Endocytosis is another means by which extracellular materials may enter a cell. In endocytosis the exterior cell membrane moves to surround extracellular materials in a membrane pocket (Fig. 2–1). This membrane **vesicle** detaches from the inner surface of the cell membrane and moves into the interior of the cell.

If a large amount of particulate material is endocytosed by ameboid movements of a cell, the process is more specifically termed **phagocytosis** (Fig. 2–1), and cells capable of taking in large amounts of material are called phagocytes. This ability is characteristic of some white blood cells, which engulf large particulate matter, tissue debris, or bacteria. After a phagocytic

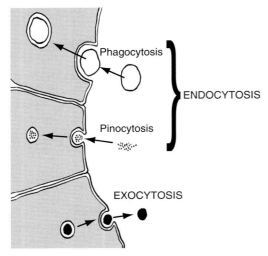

Figure 2-1. Endocytosis (phagocytosis and pinocytosis) and exocytosis.

vesicle enters the substance of a cell, it may fuse with a different type of membrane vesicle, a *lysosome* that was produced within the cell. Lysosomes are specialized membrane vesicles that contain enzymes, also produced within the cell. This fusion permits the lysosomal enzymes to act upon the contents of the phagocytic vesicle in a small, local area that is isolated from the cytosol. Most types of cells are capable of endocytosing small amounts of fluid containing dissolved particles. This type of endocytosis is termed pinocytosis (Fig. 2–1).

Metabolism refers to the sum total of the physical and biochemical reactions occurring in each cell and therefore in the entire animal. Reactions that build and maintain cellular components are called **anabolic,** and those that break down cellular components or constituents are called **catabolic.** The oxidation of carbon compounds to carbon dioxide and water, with the release of energy, is a catabolic reaction.

The secretion of products synthesized by the cell into the extracellular fluid (ECF) that surrounds the cells occurs by **exocytosis** (Fig. 2–1), which is essentially the opposite of endocytosis. Membrane-bound secretory vesicles containing substances synthesized within the cell and packaged by the Golgi apparatus migrate in the cytoplasm to the plasma membrane.

Here the membrane of a secretory vesicle fuses to the exterior cell membrane, an opening appears at the point of fusion, and the contents of the vesicle are released into the extracellular fluid.

Irritability (also called excitability) is the property of being able to react to a stimulus. The reaction must necessarily consist of one of the other properties of protoplasm, such as conduction, contraction, or secretion.

Conductivity is the property of transmitting an electrical impulse from one point in the cell to another. This property is discussed in more detail later in this chapter. Nerve cells and muscle cells are specialized for conductivity and irritability.

Contractility is the ability to shorten in one direction. Muscle cells are specialized for contractions, although many other cells and cell organelles also contain contractile proteins and exhibit limited movement (e.g., cilia).

Chemical Composition of the Cell

Chemical composition of various parts of the cell plays an important role in cellular function. The approximate composition of protoplasm by constituent is water, 85%; protein, 10%; lipid, 2%; inorganic matter, 1.5%; and other substances, including carbohydrates, 1.5%.

Water

Each cell is about 60–65% water. Water is by far the largest constituent of protoplasm, which is largely a colloidal suspension in water. Water acts as a solvent for inorganic substances and enters into many biochemical reactions.

Most body water is within cells, and this fluid volume is called **intracellular fluid.** This fluid volume is about 40% of body weight. The remaining fluid (about 20% of body weight), found outside of cells, is termed **extracellular fluid** (ECF). Most ECF (about 15% of body weight) surrounds cells throughout the body and is termed **interstitial fluid.** Unique interstitial fluids include the cerebrospinal fluid, the fluid in the joints, the fluid in the eyes (aqueous and vitreous humors), and the serous fluid in the visceral spaces (i.e., pericardial, pleural, and peritoneal spaces). Blood plasma, a specific type of extracellular fluid, is about 5% of total body weight. The percentages for the different types of body fluids vary from one animal to another. Factors affecting these percentages include condition (amount of fat), age, state of hydration, and species.

Water is constantly lost from the body, and it must be replenished if the animal is to remain in water balance and not become dehydrated. Most is lost via the urine, but it is also lost in the feces and by evaporation from body surfaces, such as the skin and respiratory passages. Water replacement is almost entirely by drinking, because minimal amounts of water are produced in the bodies of domestic animals as a result of cellular metabolism (metabolic water).

Proteins

After water, proteins are the next largest constituent of protoplasm. **Proteins** are complex high-molecular-weight colloidal molecules consisting primarily of amino acids that are polymerized (joined) into **polypeptide** chains (Fig. 2–2). The union of amino acids within a protein molecule is by way of a peptide linkage, a bond between the amino (NH_2) group of one amino acid and the carboxyl (COOH) group of another amino acid, with the elimination of water. A small chain of amino acids is called a peptide. A polypeptide is a chain of more than 50 amino acids connected by peptide linkages, and a chain that contains more than 100 amino acids is called a protein.

The peptide linkages between amino acids in a protein are somewhat flexible, and this permits the chain to bend into various three-dimensional shapes (Fig. 2–2B). These configurations may become relatively stable, because chemical attractions, or bonds, form between amino acids at various points in the chain. The three-dimensional shape of a protein is an important determinant of its biologic function, because the shape can determine what segments of the protein chain are exposed and available to interact with other molecules.

Amino acids, and thus proteins, contain carbon, hydrogen, oxygen, and nitrogen. Proteins

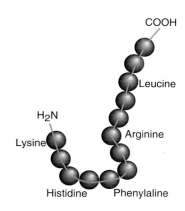

2.a.

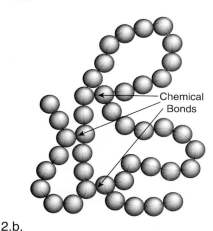

2.b.

Figure 2-2. *A)* A chain of amino acids joined by peptide bonds to form a protein. *B)* A large protein. Each filled circle represents a single amino acid. Chemical bonds between amino acids at distant points in the chain produce the three-dimensional shape of the protein molecule.

may also contain other elements, such as sulfur, phosphorus, or iron. Simple proteins yield only amino acids or their derivatives upon hydrolysis. The simple proteins, and examples of each, are as follows:

1. Albumins (plasma albumin, milk lactalbumin)
2. Globulins (plasma globulins, globulins in plant seeds)
3. Protamines (in sperm cells)
4. Histones (with nucleoproteins in cell nuclei)
5. Albuminoids (collagen and elastin of connective tissue)

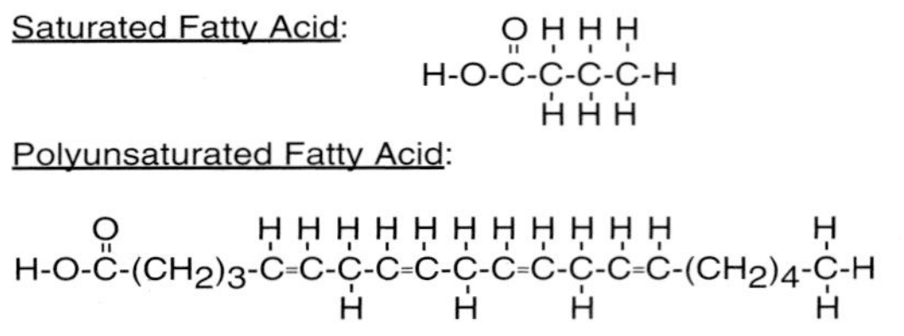

Saturated Fatty Acid:

$$H\text{-}O\text{-}\overset{O}{\underset{}{C}}\text{-}\overset{H}{\underset{H}{C}}\text{-}\overset{H}{\underset{H}{C}}\text{-}\overset{H}{\underset{H}{C}}\text{-}H$$

Polyunsaturated Fatty Acid:

$$H\text{-}O\text{-}\overset{O}{\underset{}{C}}\text{-}(CH_2)_3\text{-}C\text{=}\overset{H}{\underset{H}{C}}\text{-}C\text{=}C\text{-}\overset{H}{\underset{H}{C}}\text{-}C\text{=}C\text{-}\overset{H}{\underset{H}{C}}\text{-}C\text{=}C\text{-}(CH_2)_4\text{-}\overset{H}{\underset{H}{C}}\text{-}H$$

Figure 2-3. Saturated and polyunsaturated fatty acids. The 4-carbon saturated fatty acid is butyric acid, and the 20-carbon fatty acid is arachidonic acid.

Conjugated proteins consist of simple proteins combined with a component that is not a protein or amino acid but that is called a prosthetic group. The conjugated proteins and examples of each are as follows:

1. Glycoproteins: includes mucopolysaccharides and oligosaccharides as the carbohydrate prosthetic group (in connective tissue and salivary mucus)
2. Lipoproteins: prosthetic group is lipid (in blood plasma and egg yolk)
3. Nucleoproteins: nucleic acid prosthetic group (in cell nuclei, chromosomes, and viruses)
4. Chromoproteins: Fe-porphyrin prosthetic group (hemoglobin, cytochromes)
5. Metalloproteins: contain iron, zinc, or copper (blood transferrin, ferritin, carbonic anhydrase)
6. Phosphoproteins: phosphate prosthetic group (casein in milk, vitellin in eggs)

Most proteins can be classified as **structural proteins** or as **reactive proteins.** Structural proteins include these fibrous proteins: **collagens,** which are the major proteins of connective tissue and which represent about 30% of the total protein content of the animal body; **elastins,** which are present in elastic tissues such as the ligamentum nuchae, the abdominal tunic, and some arteries; and **keratins,** which are the proteins of wool, hair, horns, and hoofs. Reactive proteins include **enzymes, protein hormones, histones** associated with nucleic acids in the nucleus of cells, and **contractile proteins** in muscle (actin and myosin). Many varieties of proteins are found in blood plasma. Functions of plasma proteins include the transport of substances such as hormones and lipids in the blood, contributing to the process of blood coagulation, and creating an effective osmotic pressure difference between the plasma and interstitial fluid. Plasma proteins also include antibodies, which are produced by certain blood cells and are part of an overall immune response.

All cell membranes contain proteins, and like plasma proteins, the proteins in cell membranes have a variety of functions. These include serving as membrane receptors for hormones and drugs, contributing to the transport of water and particles into and out of cells, acting as membrane-bound enzymes, and serving as markers to permit the immune system to recognize cells as normal or abnormal body components.

Differences in the sequence of the amino acids of the polypeptide chains of proteins often occur between species. **For example, the serum albumin in the blood plasma of horses is different from that in the plasma of cattle and sheep. In cattle, the protein hormone insulin is slightly different from that in swine. Such variable proteins may still function in a different species, though usually at levels below that of the naturally occurring form of the molecule.** Note: Throughout the text, **clinical extracts** are set in blue type. These are examples of the application of basic anatomy and/or physiology in clinical settings.

Lipids

Lipids (fatty substances) consist primarily of carbon, hydrogen and oxygen, but some also contain minor amounts of phosphorus, nitrogen, and sulfur. Most lipids are nonpolar molecules and thus are insoluble in water. The four primary chemical types of lipids in animals are fatty acids, triglycerides or triacylglycerols, phospholipids, and steroids.

Fatty acids are chains of covalently bound carbon atoms with hydrogens attached (Fig. 2–3). If each carbon atom has four single covalent bonds, the fatty acid is **saturated.** If any carbon atom has fewer than four single bonds, the fatty acid is **unsaturated.** A polyunsaturated fatty acid has multiple carbon atoms with less than four single bonds. Animal tissues tend to have higher amounts of saturated fatty acids than do vegetable oils.

Prostaglandins and *leukotrienes,* derived from fatty acids, are produced by a variety of cells throughout the body. In many cases, these serve as local messengers that permit one cell to affect the function of another nearby. Both prostaglandins and leukotrienes are local messengers in the process of inflammation, and prostaglandins regulate ovarian function in some species.

Triglycerides consist of a glycerol molecule with three fatty acids attached (Fig. 2–4). Also known as neutral fats, triglycerides are the primary form of lipid storage in adipose tissue in animals. Fatty acids must be detached from glycerol before they can undergo further metabolism. This detachment is the function of enzymes known as *lipases.* Because triglycerides are not soluble in water, most are not transported as individual molecules in blood plasma. For transport, they are combined with other lipids and proteins into relatively large particles known as *lipoproteins.* In this form they can be transported from site to site within the body.

The glycerol and fatty acids derived from the breakdown of triglycerides are all sources of energy. Glycerol can serve as a substrate for the *glycolytic pathway* in the cytosol. Fatty acids enter the mitochondria, where they are broken down into two carbon units, which become *acetyl coenzyme A* (*acetyl CoA*). The metabolism of acetyl CoA within the mitochondria ultimately results in the production of the high-energy compound *adenosine triphosphate* (*ATP*). Details about the role of the mitochondria in the production of ATP are described in the section on organelles later in this chapter.

Phospholipids are similar to triglycerides except that a molecule containing a phosphate group has replaced one of the three fatty acids. The replacement of the nonpolar (*hydrophobic*) fatty acid with a nonlipid polar (*hydrophilic*) molecule creates a unique compound with two regions that vary in water solubility. The phosphate-containing region becomes water soluble and the remainder of the phospholipid molecule is water insoluble. This unique characteristic is important in the role of phospholipids in the structure of cell membranes. Cell membranes throughout the body primarily consist of phospholipids.

Steroids are lipids in which the carbon atoms are connected in ring structures. *Cholesterol* is a steroid (Fig. 2–5), and most of the steroids found in animals are derived from cholesterol (e.g., bile salts and various hormones, including several reproductive hormones). Cholesterol itself is an essential constituent of the cell membrane of all animal cells. **Cholesterol can be obtained from dietary sources, but it is also synthesized in the liver of animals, including humans. Inappropriate rates of cholesterol synthesis by the liver are responsible for elevation in serum cholesterol in humans in spite of reductions in dietary intake of cholesterol.**

Waxes are a class of lipids. The waxes synthesized in the animal occur mostly in the epithelial cells of the skin. Here the waxes form a protective coating on the skin or hair as a water repellent and as a barrier against bacteria. Lanolin is wool fat, and cerumen is earwax.

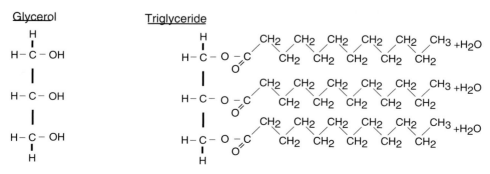

Figure 2-4. Three fatty acids combined with glycerol to form a triglyceride.

Cholesterol:

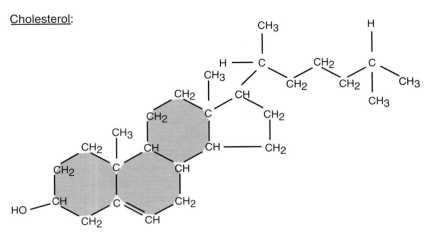

Figure 2-5. Cholesterol. Different biologic steroids are formed by modifying the cholesterol molecule, but the four carbon rings remain intact.

Carbohydrates

Like lipids, **carbohydrates** are composed of carbon, oxygen, and hydrogen. Simple sugars, or **monosaccharides,** are carbohydrates containing three to seven carbon atoms. **Glucose,** with six carbon atoms, is the most prevalent simple sugar in the body. Two simple sugar molecules may be combined to form a **disaccharide.** Some common and important disaccharides are sucrose, or table sugar (glucose + fructose); lactose, or milk sugar (glucose + galactose); and maltose (glucose + glucose).

Multiple molecules of glucose can be linked (polymerized) to form a polysaccharide, **glycogen.** Two major sites of glycogen synthesis are the liver and skeletal muscle. In the liver, the stored glycogen can be broken down to glucose and metabolized by liver cells or secreted as glucose into the blood. In skeletal muscle, glycogen stores are an immediate source of energy, but this glycogen cannot be a source of glucose for release into the blood.

Glucose is a source of cell energy, and the enzymatic pathway that metabolizes glucose to produce energy is **glycolysis.** This pathway can be completed within the cytosol, resulting in the production of ATP and pyruvate. If oxygen is readily available, the pyruvate can enter the mitochondria to be metabolized.

The sugar deoxyribose is found in combination with a base (purine or pyrimidine) and a phosphate, forming **DNA (deoxyribonucleic acid).** DNA is the carrier of all genetic information from generation to generation and from cell to cell and ultimately controls all functions of the cell. DNA is found almost exclusively in the nucleus of the cell. A related substance, **RNA (ribonucleic acid),** includes the sugar ribose combined with a base and a phosphate. RNA is intimately associated with synthesis of all cell proteins.

Even though carbohydrates are a major part of the diet of most animals, the amount of carbohydrates in animal's bodies is relatively small. Carbohydrates make up less than 1% of most cells.

Inorganic Substances

Of the atoms or elements found in protoplasm, more than 99% are hydrogen, carbon, oxygen, and nitrogen contained in the organic compounds described earlier. Protoplasm also has inorganic compounds containing iodine, iron, phosphorus, calcium, chlorine, potassium, sulfur, sodium, magnesium, copper, manganese, zinc, cobalt, chromium, selenium, molybdenum, fluorine, silicon, tin, and vanadium. Of the 24 elements found in the body cells, 20 represent less than 1% of the total amount of elements in living tissue.

An **electrolyte** is any molecular substance that in solution dissociates into its electrically charged components, called *ions*. For example, this occurs when sodium chloride in solution dissociates into Na^+ and Cl^-. The solution can then carry an electrical charge and current.

The major ions found within cells in order of abundance, expressed in milliequivalents per liter of fluid, are potassium (K^+) 140 mEq/L; phosphate (HPO_4^{2-}), 75 mEq/L; magnesium (Mg^{2+}), 60 mEq/L; sodium (Na^+) 10 mEq/L; bicarbonate (HCO_3^-) 10 mEq/L; and chloride (Cl^-) 4 mEq/L.

A *milliequivalent* is one-thousandth of an equivalent. An equivalent weight is the weight in grams that will displace or react with 1 gram–atomic weight of hydrogen ion (H^+ = 1.008 g).

The practical importance of this concept is that laboratory reports and records of measurements of body fluid electrolyte and ion concentrations are often expressed as mEq/L. Another way of expressing measurements is in mg%, or milligrams per 100 milliliters (mg/100 mL). Measurements may also be expressed as milligrams per deciliter (mg/dL); a deciliter is 100 mL, or a tenth of a liter. A liter is 1000 mL, or 1.06 quarts.

Bone contains about 65% inorganic material by volume. Most of this mineral material is in the form of hydroxyapatite crystals with a molecular formula $Ca_{10}(PO_4)_6(OH)_2$. In addition, sodium, magnesium, and iron may be incorporated in the mineral structure.

Acids, Bases, and pH

An *acid* is a compound that is capable of ionizing and releasing a hydrogen ion. The pH of a solution is a measure of the concentration of H^+. However, pH is reported as the *negative* of the *logarithm* to the base 10 of the H^+ concentration in moles, so the greater the H^+ concentration, the more negative, or lower, the pH. H^+ concentrations in normal body fluids are much lower than other electrolytes. A typical H^+ concentration in plasma is 4×10^{-9} moles per liter, or 4 nanomoles per liter, equivalent to a pH of 7.45. A nanomole is one-millionth of a millimole.

A *base* is a compound that is capable of reducing the concentration of hydrogen ions in a solution by combining with them. When bases are added to solutions, the H^+ concentration is reduced, so the pH rises. Chemical *buffer* solutions contain both acids and bases and therefore are capable of either releasing or combining with H^+. This dual ability tends to provide a relatively stable pH.

All body fluids, intracellular and extracellular, contain mixtures of several chemical buffers. These buffers act simultaneously to maintain a relatively stable pH within their respective fluids. This stability is critical for normal metabolic processes and enzymatic reactions.

Microscopic Study of the Cell

Cells range in diameter from about 10 to 100 μm (micrometers). Cells that are actively multiplying range from about 20 to 30 μm in diameter. Table 2.1 lists the relationships among metric units of measurement used for microscopy. (For example, 1 μm is one-thousandth of a millimeter, and there are about 25 mm in 1 inch; thus, approximately 1000 cells, each 25 μm in diameter, could be lined up between the 1- and 2-inch marks of a ruler.) Sizes of cells

Table 2-1. Metric Linear Measurements

Unit	Abbreviation	Relationships
Meter	m	1 m = 10^2 cm, 10^3 mm, 10^6 μm, 10^9 nm, 10^{10} Å
Centimeter	cm	1 cm = 10^{-2} m, 10^1 mm, 10^4 μm, 10^7 nm, 10^8 Å
Micrometer (micron)	μm	1 μm = 10^{-6} m, 10^{-4} cm, 10^{-3} mm, 10^3 nm, 10^4 Å
Nanometer	nm	1 nm = 10^{-9} m, 10^{-7} cm, 10^{-6} mm, 10^{-3} μm, 10 Å
Angstrom	Å	1 Å = 10^{-10} m, 10^{-8} cm, 10^{-7} mm, 10^{-4} μm, 10^{-1} nm

vary considerably from one type of cell to another, but with the exception of the yolks of birds' eggs (which are considered single cells), the distance from the center of the cell to some portion of the cell membrane (surface of the cell) is seldom more than a few micrometers.

The outer cell membrane is thin, 7 to 10 nm. Regardless of its composition, a membrane of this dimension can have little tensile strength; this is another reason cells must be small.

The uniformly small size of cells and the much smaller sizes of structures within the cell have made effective study of cells difficult. As noted earlier, the existence of cells was not confirmed before the microscope was invented. Details of the actual structure of the various parts of cells were not known with any degree of certainty until after the development of the electron microscope. The study of gross anatomy goes back several centuries, but understanding of the finer structure of the animal body awaited more recent technologic developments.

Light Microscopy

Some cells are in tissues that are thin enough to be illuminated from one side and observed with a microscope from the opposite side. This is true of the web of the foot of the frog, the mesentery of the intestine, and a few other tissues. In these instances, living cells can be observed directly, and this technique is useful for the study of blood circulation. Specific cells may also be taken from a living animal and grown on artificial medium by *tissue culture.* These cells may then be studied in the living state, even at high magnifications.

Except for the forgoing situations, cells usually are studied after undergoing some degree of manipulation, so that what is actually seen with the microscope bears little resemblance to the living cell. A typical treatment of tissue before it can be examined with a light microscope includes the following:

1. *Fixation* with an agent, such as an aldehyde, that will cross-link the tissue proteins and prevent further changes in the tissue, such as autolysis and bacterial degradation. Alternatively, tissue may be frozen in liquid nitrogen to prevent such degenerative changes.

2. *Embedding* the tissue in a material that will permit cutting very thin sections. Paraffin is used for producing sections of 5 to 10 μm thickness; sections as thin as 1 to 2 μm can be obtained by embedding in a plastic, such as glycol methacrylate. Since most embedding media are not water soluble, the fixed tissue must be dehydrated and then infiltrated with some material such as xylene, which is miscible with the embedding medium. Frozen tissues need not be embedded.

3. *Sectioning* the tissue into very thin slices so that the sections may be placed on a glass slide. A *microtome* is used for this purpose. It consists of a sharp blade and a mechanism for moving the tissue past the blade and then advancing it a defined distance after each cutting. Frozen tissues are sectioned in a cryostat, which is a microtome housed in a freezer cabinet.

4. *Staining* the section so that different cells or different parts of cells can be differentiated according to color. *Hematoxylin* and *eosin* are stains commonly used together, and this treatment is described as an H & E stain. The hematoxylin tends to stain acidic portions of a cell dark blue or purple (these *basophilic* areas include the cell nucleus, which contains nucleic acids), and the eosin tends to stain the basic portions of a cell pink to red (these *acidophilic* areas include much of the more basic protein within the cell). *Wright's stain,* used to stain blood cells (Plates I and II), stains basophilic areas blue with methylene blue and acidophilic areas red with eosin. Sections can also be treated with a variety of chemical solutions to demonstrate the presence of certain types of chemicals or the activity of enzymes in the tissue or cell, a technique called *histochemistry* (Fig. 2–6). The presence of specific types of molecules can be determined by exposing the section to a solution containing *antibodies* to those molecules. This technique is called *immunocytochemistry.*

5. The last step, of course, is the actual examination of the stained section of tissue on the slide by means of a microscope and light transmitted through the section.

This approach to the study of the animal body has been standard for many years and will

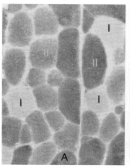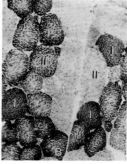

Figure 2-6. Serial sections of horse triceps brachii muscle histochemically stained for enzymatic activity. The same muscle cells (*I* and *II*) are visible in both sections. *A)* Calcium-dependent ATPase activity. *B)* Activity of a mitochondrial oxidative enzyme.

continue to be useful regardless of newer developments. However, some factors should be kept in mind when studying sections or photographs of sections.

The relationship of the tissue sections to the actual tissue is about the same as that of a sack of potato chips to a growing potato. Both the sections and the potato chips have been processed so that actual resemblance to the original structure is limited. Both are seen in two dimensions, length and width, with thickness relatively unimportant for visualization. Recent technological advances such as confocal microscopy and computer reconstruction provide three-dimensional views of cellular and tissue structure.

The light microscope can magnify objects to a maximum of about 1500 times the original size. This is known as the magnification, or power, of the microscope. Resolving power refers to the property of showing two objects as separate structures. The light microscope can resolve (separate) two structures that are as close as approximately 0.2 μm (about 200 nm). This resolving power depends greatly on the wavelength of the light used to observe the tissue and the optical quality of the objective lens of the microscope.

Other developments in light microscopy include phase contrast and fluorescence microscopy. Phase contrast microscopy can be used with unstained and/or living cells, because it depends on differences in refraction of vari-ous parts of a cell for image formation. Fluorescence microscopy is often teamed with immunocytochemistry, in which antibody-labeled cells are identified by causing them to fluoresce upon exposure to light of a specific wavelength.

X-ray diffraction is used to study the structure of inorganic and organic crystals and the molecular structure of biologic substances such as DNA, collagen, and hemoglobin. It consists of passing a beam of x-rays through the substance and recording the diffraction pattern (scattering of the beam) on a photographic emulsion.

Electron Microscopy

Electron microscopes do not use visible light for the delineation of structures as in the light microscope; they use a beam of electrons focused by electromagnetic lenses. The electron beam may pass through a thin specimen in the **transmission electron microscope** or be reflected from the surface of an object and studied with the **scanning electron microscope.** The images, however, are only black and white with the electron microscope. (For an example of a scanning electron micrograph, see Fig. 15–2.)

The scanning electron microscope is a versatile instrument with a magnification range from ×15 to ×10,000 and a resolution in the vicinity of 10 nm. Depth of field with the scanning electron microscope is much greater than with any light microscope. Preparation of specimens for observation with the scanning electron microscope is relatively simple. Nonmetallic biologic material generally is dehydrated and coated with a thin layer of metallic gold before it is placed in the scanning electron microscope.

The transmission electron microscope is capable of much higher magnification (as much as ×1 million), with an effective resolution of 0.1 nm. By the use of photographic enlargement and projection techniques, the magnifications can exceed 1 million and still show good detail. (A typical transmission electron micrograph is shown in Fig. 19–10. Because so much more detail can be seen in a small area, tissue preparation for transmission electron microscopy is much more exacting and time-consuming than for light microscopy.

The best means of fixation is to apply a fixative (commonly glutaraldehyde followed by osmium tetroxide) to the living tissue or biopsy specimen. The time from the living state to immersion in the fixative should not exceed 2 minutes, and the size of tissue should not exceed 1 mm on a side. Osmium tetroxide acts both as a fixative and as a stain. Other heavy metals, including lead, may be used as so-called stains. The term *stain* may be used somewhat loosely, because the areas where the metals concentrate inhibit the passage of electrons, giving an electron-dense appearance that shows up as a dark area in the final photographic print. After fixation, the tissue is dehydrated and infiltrated with plastic and embedded in plastic for sectioning. The sections are cut extremely thin (less than 30 nm), placed on a grid, and examined with the electron microscope.

The picture of the typical cell viewed with the electron microscope still shows most of the structures described by light microscopy but in much greater detail. The typical cell seen in light microscopy consists of a nucleus and cytoplasm surrounded by the cell membrane (Fig. 2–7). The nucleus contains a **nucleolus** and **chromatin material,** which forms into **chromosomes** during cell division. A membrane called the nuclear envelope surrounds the nucleus. The cytoplasm contains a number of structures, or **organelles,** including the endoplasmic reticulum, Golgi apparatus, mitochondria, and inclusions.

The Cell Membrane

Structure of the Membrane

The outer cell membrane, also known as plasma membrane, and other membranes within the cell primarily consist of phospho-

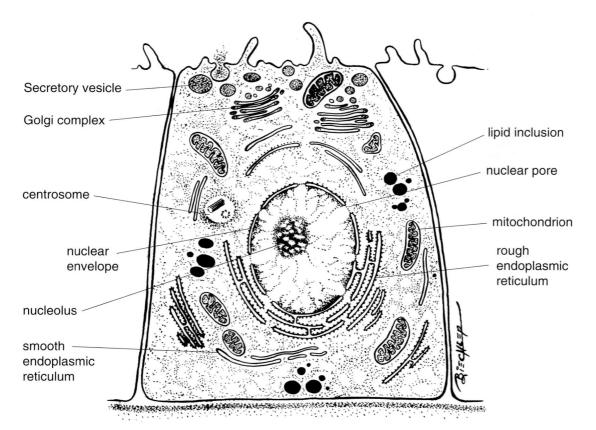

Figure 2-7. The general organization of a cell. The nucleus contains a distinct nucleolus. (Reprinted with permission from Dellmann, H. D., Eurell, J. *Textbook of Veterinary Histology.* 5th ed. Baltimore: Lippincott Williams & Wilkins, 1998.)

lipids, proteins, and cholesterol. According to the fluid mosaic model, the phospholipids are arranged with their polar (hydrophilic) ends facing the protein layers, while their nonpolar (hydrophobic) ends face each other in the center of the membrane (Fig. 2–8). Because of the hydrophobic properties of the phospholipids, the membrane forms a water-impermeable barrier that separates the interior of the cell from the ECF. This barrier protects the cell by preventing the simple diffusion of water and water-soluble particles. Plasma membranes contain varying amounts of cholesterol, which is found between the phospholipid molecules and adjusts the fluidity and flexibility of the membrane.

The protein composition of the outer cell membrane is extremely variable among different types of cells, and this variation has a great deal of influence on functional differences between cells. Some membrane proteins are firmly inserted into the membrane among the phospholipids (Fig. 2–8). These are *integral proteins;* they may be arranged so that they extend completely across the membrane. Proteins that are exposed to both the cytosol inside the cell and the extracellular fluid surrounding the cell are *transmembrane proteins* (Fig. 2–8). Many transmembrane proteins are involved in transport processes to move substances across the cell membrane. In Figure 2–8 a transmembrane protein forms a channel to permit passage across the cell membrane. Proteins may

also be found bound to the surface of the membrane, and such proteins are classified as *peripheral proteins* (Fig. 2–8). Most of these are on the cytosolic surface of the membrane, and they are often found bound to an integral protein.

The functions of cell membrane proteins include (1) transport of substances across the membrane; (2) provision of a site of binding for substances found in extracellular fluid, such as hormones; (3) contribution to the formation of cell-to-cell junctions; (4) provision of enzymes with active sites facing either the cytosol or the extracellular fluid; and (5) identification or recognition of cell type or cell origin by other cells. These functions are discussed in more detail later in this chapter.

Structural modifications of the cell membrane occur largely on the free surface of cells (a surface not adjacent to any other cells). These modifications usually increase the cell surface and presumably function in absorption or secretion. The *striated* or *brush border* seen in light microscopy appears in electron micrographs to consist of uniform fingerlike projections called *microvilli*. Less regular projections, called stereocilia, are irregular branched extensions of the cell cytoplasm that are not motile.

Motile cilia (kinocilia) are complex elongated, fingerlike projections from cell surfaces found in areas where material is moved past the surface, as in the linings of the trachea and the

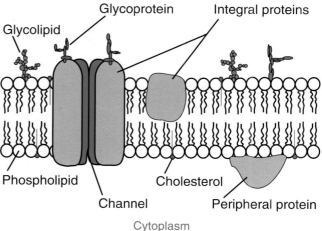

Extracellular medium

Figure 2-8. Fluid mosaic model of the cell membrane. Phospholipids are arranged in a bilayer. (Adapted with permission from Rhoades, R.A. and Tanner G.A. *Medical physiology.* Boston: Little, Brown, 1995.)

uterine tubes. Each cilium is associated with a basal body that resembles a centriole normally seen in the cytoplasm of all cells.

Intercellular Contact and Adhesion

All vertebrates develop from division of a single cell, the fertilized egg. Unicellular animals also develop by division of a single parent cell. When the parent cell of a unicellular animal divides, the resulting daughter cells each go their own separate way, but the daughter cells of the fertilized ovum of a multicellular animal stay together and eventually differentiate into cells making up different tissues.

The ability of multiple individual cells to remain together and function as a tissue or organ depends on local modifications of the outer cell membrane. In some cases, these modifications simply physically connect one cell to another. In other cases, these modifications connect cells and form a passageway for exchanges between them. The cell membrane modifications entail focal accumulations of specific membrane proteins termed **cell adhesion molecules.** The areas of cell membranes involved in intercellular contact and adhesion were named when they were initially examined by light and electron microscopy.

In electron micrographs, **desmosomes** appear as local thickenings of adjacent plasma membranes, with tiny fibrils radiating from the thickening into the cytoplasm of the cell (Fig. 2–9). Desmosomes tightly bind adjacent cells by the interactions between membrane proteins extending out from the surface of the cell membranes. They are seen as a single site or as a more extensive beltlike circle surrounding cells.

Tight junctions appear as an area or zone

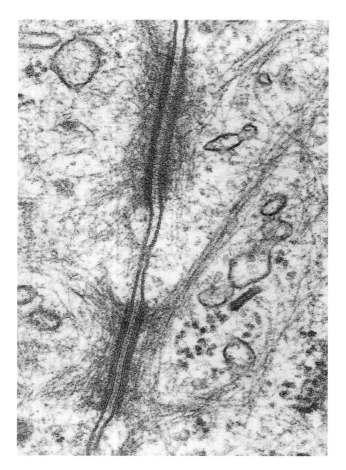

Figure 2-9. Two desmosomes connecting the membranes of two cells. (Reprinted with permission from Dellmann, H. D. and Eurell J. *Textbook of Veterinary Histology.* 5th ed. Baltimore: Lippincott Williams & Wilkins, 1998.)

where the plasma membranes of two adjacent cells immediately adhere to each other. These are often found just below the free surface of epithelial cells. Each tight junction passes completely around the periphery of the cell at the same level. Tight junctions restrict the movement of water or dissolved materials into the space between adjacent cells.

Gap junctions are formed by membrane proteins that extend between adjacent cells to form a passage for exchange of small molecules and ions (Fig.2–10). The exchange of ions permits one cell to affect the electrical activity of the adjacent cell. These types of exchanges have special functional importance in cardiac muscle and certain types of smooth muscle in the gastrointestinal tract.

Transport Across Cell Membranes

The plasma membrane and the membranes of intracellular organelles have an important function in determining what enters and leaves the

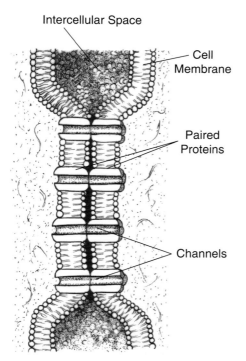

Intercellular Space

Cell Membrane

Paired Proteins

Channels

Figure 2-10. Two cell membranes connected at a gap junction by proteins that extend between them.

cell or its organelles. Our very life and that of animals depend on this ability to control what enters and leaves the cells. It is therefore important to understand and appreciate the processes of membrane transport before discussing the functions of the animal's organs and systems. Transport into and out of cells may occur by simple and facilitated diffusion, osmosis, active transport, endocytosis, or exocytosis. (Endocytosis and exocytosis are described at the beginning of this chapter.)

Simple and Facilitated Diffusion

Diffusion is a passive mechanism. It is simply the distribution of a substance in a solvent medium , usually water, so that it becomes equally concentrated throughout the medium. Diffusion occurs because all molecules and ions have kinetic energy. They collide with each other and bounce away, becoming so dispersed in the solvent that an equal concentration appears throughout. In solutions, diffusion proceeds from a region of greater concentration of particles to a region of lower concentration, so the net diffusion is said to occur down a **concentration gradient.**

Only a few substances, such as oxygen, carbon dioxide, and alcohol, are membrane soluble, that is, capable of diffusing freely through the lipid bilayer of plasma membranes. Such molecules must be lipid soluble. Certain drugs, such as barbiturates, a class of anesthetics, are membrane soluble. If a substance cannot diffuse freely through the lipid bilayer of the cell membrane, its ability to diffuse in or out of a cell depends on some other means of crossing the membrane.

One way lipid-insoluble substances cross the cell membrane is via a transmembrane protein or proteins that form a channel, or passageway, through the membrane (Fig. 2–8). If a channel that permits the passage of a given molecule is present, the membrane is said to be **permeable** to the molecule. The degree of permeability of an individual channel may also be subject to regulation by factors such as the electrical potential across the membrane. Channels whose permeability varies with the electrical potential across the membrane are said to be *electrically gated* or *voltage gated.* A change in the conformation or configuration of the membrane protein is responsible for changes in the permeability of the channel (Fig. 2–11).

Ions (atoms or radicals having a positive or negative charge) cannot diffuse freely through the lipid bilayer of the plasma membrane. Thus, a channel that is permeable to a given ion must be present for that ion to diffuse through cell membranes. **Most channels are permeable only to a single specific ion or a small number of specific ions. This characteristic is important from a clinical standpoint, as some drugs are relatively specific for a given type of channel. With the use of these agents, the movement of a specific ion across cell membranes can be regulated. For example, the inward movement of calcium into cells of the heart can be regulated with such drugs, and this is beneficial in certain types of cardiac arrhythmias (abnormalities in the electrical activity of the heart).**

The rate and direction of passage of a charged ion through a channel depends on two factors that may act synergistically. That is, both may have the same affect on the rate and direction of movement. Or they may act antagonistically, each having opposite effects on rate and direction of movement. One factor is the concentration gradient between the two sides of the membrane for the particular ion. Because of diffusion, ions have net movement through permeable channels from areas of higher concentration to areas of lower concentration. The second factor is any electrical gradient generated by concentration differences among other charged ions on the two sides of the membrane. In all animal cells, the concentrations of charged ions on the two sides of the cell membrane are normally such that the inside of the cell is negative to the outside (Fig. 2–11). The net negative charge on the inside of the cell inhibits the inward diffusion of negatively charged ions (anions), while it promotes the inward diffusion of positively charged ions (cations). The term *electrochemical gradient* is used to refer to the combined effects of the concentration gradient and electrical gradient on the diffusion rate of an individual ion.

Facilitated diffusion is the same as simple or free diffusion in that it operates passively down the concentration or electrochemical gradient. However, facilitated diffusion requires a *carrier system* in the membrane to assist the crossing. The carrier system is a transmembrane protein that binds the diffusing molecule or molecules on one side of the membrane and then transfers them to the other side, where the transported molecules are released (Fig. 2–12). The movement or transport across the membrane probably entails a change in the shape of the protein, but it does not require any direct use of ATP for energy as in active transport.

Sugars, especially glucose, depend on facilitated diffusion to enter cells by joining with carrier proteins upon reaching the lipid bilayer of the membrane. The glucose carrier complex transports glucose down the glucose concentration gradient to the inside of the cell membrane. Here the carrier releases the glucose to enter the cell. The carrier remains in the membrane and reconfigures itself so that it is available for more transport. Other substances besides glucose, such as amino acids, also depend on facilitated diffusion to cross cell membranes.

Closed Channel

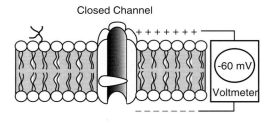

Open Channel

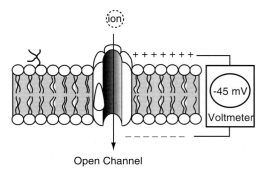

Figure 2-11. Electric-gated channel opens and closes with changes in the electrical potential across the cell membrane.

Outside

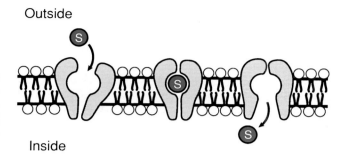

Figure 2-12. Facilitated diffusion of solute (*small circles*) across a cell membrane by the action of a carrier protein. (Reprinted with permission from Johnson, L. R. *Essential Medical Physiology*. 2nd ed. Philadelphia: Lippincott-Raven, 1998.)

Inside

The rate at which facilitated diffusion occurs also depends on the number of carrier proteins available in the membrane. In the case of glucose, the speed of entry into many cells, such as skeletal muscle, is greatly increased by the hormone insulin, which the pancreas secretes. Insulin facilities the entry of glucose into skeletal muscle, in part by increasing the number of carrier proteins in the cell membrane of these cells.

Osmosis

Osmosis is movement of water across membranes. Like many solutes, water does not diffuse freely through the lipid bilayer of cell membranes but rather must diffuse through water channels formed by transmembrane proteins. These proteins are aquaporins. If the intracellular fluid within a cell has a higher concentration

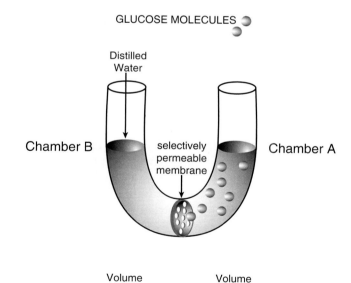

Figure 2-13. Osmosis and osmotic pressure. A membrane impermeable to solute particles prevents their diffusion from chamber A into chamber B. Distilled water from chamber B migrates into chamber A until the difference in the height of the water columns equals the osmotic pressure of the solution in chamber A.

of undiffusable solutes than the interstitial fluid bathing the cell, water will move into the cell from the interstitial fluid until the concentrations are the same on both sides of the membrane. As the water moves in, the volume in the cell increases. The driving force moving water from the solution on the side of the lower solute concentration to the side with the higher solute concentration is **osmotic pressure.**

The osmotic pressure of an aqueous solution can be measured with the use of a **U**-tube in which the two sides are separated by a semipermeable membrane, which is permeable only to water (Fig. 2–13). The solution is placed in one side of the **U**-tube, and distilled water is placed in the other. The force of osmosis moves water through the membrane from the side containing distilled water to the side containing the solution. This movement continues until the hydrostatic pressure generated by the increased height of the fluid column on the solution side is equal to the osmotic force (Fig. 2–13). The units of osmotic pressure may be given in centimeters of water (height of water column), or converted to millimeters of mercury (mm Hg) (height of a column of mercury creating an equivalent amount of hydrostatic pressure).

Osmotic pressure is an important mechanism in maintaining cellular volume by determining whether water will enter or leave cells. If the concentration of solutions on each side of a membrane is the same, as seen with cells in blood, the bathing fluid is said to be **isotonic** (isosmotic) in relation to the cells. This means that the osmotic pressure is the same on both sides of the membrane. **A 0.9% solution of sodium chloride is considered to be isotonic with mammalian red blood cells and for this reason is called a** *normal or physiologic saline solution.* **Normal saline can be used to moisten exposed tissues, such as open wounds, without damaging the cells.**

If the bathing fluid has a lower osmotic pressure than the cells, it is said to be **hypotonic,** and water tends to cross the membrane and enter the cells. In the case of red blood cells in hypotonic plasma, the water entering the cells can swell and finally burst them, a condition called hemolysis.

Red blood cells in a **hypertonic** plasma (more concentrated than the cell cytoplasm) lose water to the plasma and become wrinkled. The wrinkling of red cells is called crenation. In relation to mammalian cells, a solution less concentrated than 0.9% sodium chloride is said to be hypotonic; one more concentrated than 0.9% sodium chloride is said to be hypertonic; and of course a 0.9% sodium chloride solution is isotonic.

The osmotic pressure of a solution is determined by the number of solute particles: the more solute particles in a volume of fluid, the greater the osmotic pressure. The number of particles is determined by the **molar concentration** of the solution and by the number of ions formed if the solute is an electrolyte. For example, glucose is not an electrolyte, having one particle per molecule, but sodium chloride is an electrolyte, giving two particles (Na^+ and Cl^-) per molecule when placed in solution. A 1-molar solution of sodium chloride has twice the osmotic pressure of a 1-molar solution of glucose, because the sodium chloride solution has twice the number of particles in solution.

These concepts of osmosis and osmotic pressure become important when intravenous fluids are administered to animals for problems such as dehydration, anorexia, milk fever, and diarrhea. Furthermore, they are important principles in normal functions of animals, such as the flow of blood and lymph, the excretion of wastes in the urine by the kidneys, and the digestion and absorption of food, as is discussed in subsequent chapters.

Active Transport

Some molecules and ions can move across cell membranes (either in or out of cells) against concentration or electrical gradients. The term *against* as used here means that the particles are moving in the direction opposite to that of diffusion. This movement across the cell membrane consumes energy produced by the cell and is called **active transport.**

The best-recognized example of a primary active transport system is the **sodium–potassium (Na–K) pump.** This pump is actually a membrane protein that is also an enzyme. The protein reversibly binds three Na^+ and two K^+ ions simultaneously. The enzymatic activity of this protein permits it to hydrolyze ATP to gain energy. By a poorly understood mechanism, the gain of energy causes the protein to change its shape so that the Na^+ and K^+ are moved to the other side of the membrane. There the ions are released, and the protein returns to its original shape. These movements are summarized in Fig. 2–14. The Na–K pump, or **Na–K–AT-Pase,** is a component of the membrane of all cells, and it is always arranged in the membrane so that Na^+ moves out of the cell and K^+ moves into the cell. The continuous operation of this transport system is a major factor in keeping the intracellular concentration of Na^+ relatively low in all cells, while the intracellular concentration of K^+ is relatively high in all cells.

Secondary active transport also requires a membrane protein carrier and cellular energy, but the carrier proteins are not ATPases (enzymes that can use ATP directly). The uptake of glucose from the lumen of the intestine and the lumen of renal tubules by epithelial cells is an example of secondary active transport. In both types of epithelial cells, a membrane protein that acts as a carrier is found in the portion of cell membrane facing the lumen. This protein is capable of binding Na^+ and glucose simultaneously when both are in the lumen. After both

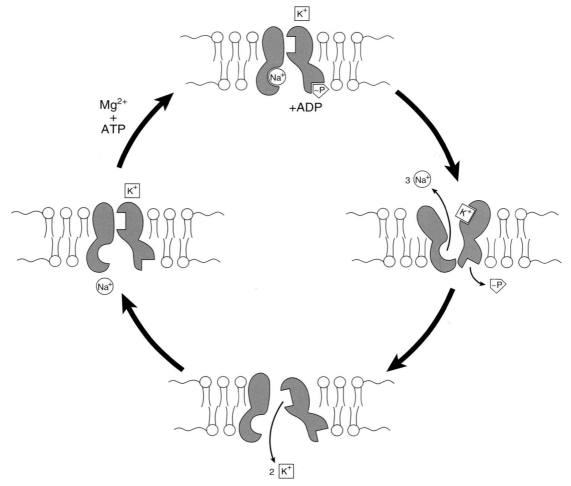

Figure 2-14. The possible operation of the Na^+–K^+ pump, (Na^+–K^+)-ATPase. (Reprinted with permission from Johnson, LR. *Essential Medical Physiology*. 2nd ed. Philadelphia: Lippincott-Raven, 1998.)

Na^+ and glucose are bound, the protein changes its shape so that both are moved to the opposite side of the membrane. There they are released into the interior of the cell. This transport can move glucose against its concentration gradient because of the potential energy of the concentration gradient for Na^+. Recall that the low intracellular Na^+ concentration in all cells is maintained by the continuous operation of the Na–K–ATPase. Thus, ATP is used directly in maintenance of the low intracellular concentration of Na^+, and this energy is used indirectly or secondarily to transport glucose.

An important characteristic of primary and secondary active transport systems is their degree of *specificity*. In most cases, a given transport protein transports only specific ions or molecules. For example, the Na–K pump transports only Na^+ and K^+. Other electrolytes are not transported by this system.

Membrane Potentials and Excitable Cells

Resting Membrane Potential

There is a relatively small difference in the amounts of charged ions locally on the opposite sides of the outer cell membrane of all animal cells. In most conditions (i.e., resting conditions), the outside of the cell membrane has a small excess of positive ions (cations), and the inside of the cell membrane has a small excess of negative ions (anions). The excess negative and positive charges tend to attract each other, so they line up on each side of the membrane, creating an *electrical potential* across the membrane (Fig. 2–11). The measurable voltage difference is the *membrane potential*. The size of the membrane potential varies among types of cells from -10 mV (millivolts) to -100 mV. In many nerve and muscle cells, it is about -85 mV. This means that the inside of the membrane is 85 mV more negative than the outside.

The concentrations of various cations and anions throughout the intracellular and extracellular fluids are maintained relatively constant in normal, healthy animals. As a result, two features of the membrane primarily determine the magnitude of the membrane potential. These are the transport mechanisms available to move cations and anions across the membrane and permeability of the membrane to the different ions.

Recall that all cell membranes contain the Na–K pump or Na–K–ATPase system (Fig. 2–14). The net effect of the Na–K–ATPase system is constant movement of Na^+ out of the cell and K^+ into the cell. The system actually moves in three Na^+ ions for every two K^+ ions that move out. This difference contributes to the net negative charge found on the inside of the membrane.

In resting conditions, cell membranes are relatively impermeable to Na^+ (and proteins, which tend to be anionic) but are quite permeable to K^+. Even though some Na^+ tends to leak back into the cell down the concentration gradient, the relatively low membrane permeability to Na^+ and the continuous operation of the Na–K pump maintain the intracellular concentration of Na^+ (10 mEq/L) less than that in the extracellular fluid (140 mEq/L).

In contrast, the intracellular potassium concentration (140 mEq/L) is much greater than its extracellular concentration (5 mEq/L). Because the cell membrane is quite permeable to K^+, it can freely diffuse out of the cell down the concentration gradient. This exit of a positively charged cation is a major contributor to the relative excess of negatively charged ions on the inside of the membrane. **The importance of this exit of K^+ is illustrated by the effects of changes in the concentration of extracellular K^+ on the electrical activity of the heart. Abnormal increases in extracellular K^+ concentration, such as may occur with kidney disease, are often associated with abnormal electrical activity of the heart (cardiac arrhythmias), and these can threaten life.**

In the typical cell in resting conditions, sodium and potassium are the major determinants of the membrane potential. However, in some cell types and in certain conditions, the membrane permeability to other ions, hence passage of these ions across the membrane, may be a significant contributor to the membrane potential. For example, if the membrane permeability to Cl^- increased, Cl^- would diffuse into the cell down the concentration gradient, and the inside of the cell would become more negative.

Excitable Cells and Action Potentials

Nerve and muscle cells are **excitable cells.** In response to the proper stimulus, their cell membrane potential can undergo a rapid but short-lived reversal in electrical potential, so that the inside is positive to the outside. This event is known as an **action potential** (Fig. 2–15). The reversal of the resting membrane potential is described as **depolarization** of the membrane, because during this period the membrane potential is closer to zero. Stimuli that elicit action potentials can be physical, chemical, or electrical. When a stimulus is strong enough to cause an action potential, it is a **threshold stimulus.**

The changes in membrane potential during an action potential are due to rapid changes in membrane permeability to different ions and movement of those ions across the membrane. The rapid changes in permeability are due to the opening and/or closing of membrane channels (i.e., channels formed by transmembrane proteins). The channel itself may respond to physical, chemical, or electrical stimuli, and the response of the channel is the link between threshold stimuli and action potentials. A threshold stimulus is one that causes enough change in channel status to bring on a rapid reversal of the membrane potential.

When an action potential occurs at a single site on an excitable cell, the membrane potential of adjacent areas along the membrane of the same cell also changes. The change in potential in the adjacent area is due to the movement of charge (ions) between the two areas (Fig. 2–16). If the membrane in the adjacent area has membrane channels sensitive to changes in voltage (voltage-gated channels) and if the change in membrane potential in the adjacent area reaches a threshold voltage, another action potential in the adjacent area is elicited. This can occur again and again, so that a series of action potentials moves along the surface of a cell (Fig. 2–16). This movement of action potentials is **propagation** of the action potential. This type of propagation is typical of all excitable cells (muscle and nerve cells).

Disrupting the activity of membrane channels can prevent action potentials and their propagation. For example, propagation of action potentials in peripheral nerves depends on the rapid opening of Na$^+$ channels. Local anesthetics, such as lidocaine, block these sodium channels and prevent action potential propagation when applied along a peripheral nerve.

Membrane Receptors and Intracellular Signaling

The cell membrane protects the cell from the extracellular environment by restricting ex-

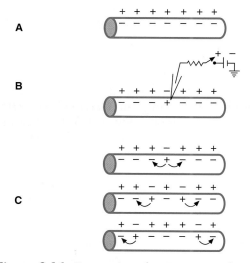

Figure 2-16. Propagation of action potentials. *A)* Resting membrane potential. *B)* Initial threshold stimulus. *C)* Propagation. (Reprinted with permission from Johnson, L.R. *Essential Medical Physiology.* 2nd ed. Philadelphia, New York: Lippincott-Raven, 1998.)

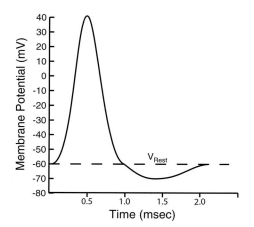

Figure 2-15. Nerve action potential.

change between the intracellular and extracellular fluid spaces. However, cells must also be able to detect the presence of certain chemical substances in the extracellular fluid and alter appropriate intracellular functions when these chemicals are present. These abilities are essential for communication between individual nerve cells, between nerve and muscle cells, and between cells of endocrine glands and the cells affected by the hormones secreted by endocrine glands. The recognition of the specific chemical in the extracellular fluid and the response to its presence are based on the interaction between the chemical and a membrane protein. **Ligand** is the general term applied to any chemical that is capable of interacting with, or binding to, a membrane protein, or membrane receptor. Important characteristics of the ligand–receptor relationship are reversibility, specificity, affinity, and saturation.

The binding of a ligand to a membrane receptor is usually **reversible,** for it is due to relatively weak chemical attractions. The weakness of this binding is also a reason for some of the other characteristics of the ligand–receptor relationship. Membrane receptors can bind to only a limited number of particular ligands or chemicals; that is, receptors demonstrate **specificity** for certain ligands. However, even though a receptor may be capable of binding any of a number of ligands, the **affinity,** or strength of binding, between the receptor and ligand may not be the same for both chemicals. Ligands that form a strong bond with a receptor are described as having a high affinity for the receptor.

The number of membrane receptors on any given cell or cell population is finite. Thus, it is possible to provide enough ligand that all receptor molecules have ligand bound to them. A receptor is described as occupied when it has a ligand bound to it. **Saturation** of receptors occurs when all are occupied with ligand.

These concepts and characteristics of ligands and receptors are the basis for a variety of pharmaceutical agents. For example, the β-blocker drugs are ligands that bind to β-adrenergic receptors but do not produce any biologic response. However, because the β-blocker occupies the receptor, the binding of any other ligand is prevented. Thus, β-blockers are used when it is desirable to reduce the biologic activity of β-adrenergic receptor stimulation. The binding of the β-blocker to the β-receptor prevents normal endogenous agents (epinephrine and norepinephrine) from binding to the receptor and bringing about a biologic response.

The binding of a ligand to a membrane receptor is but the first step in the process by which a chemical in the extracellular fluid can alter the function of a cell without entering the cell. The second step depends on the particular type of membrane receptor. In some cases, the membrane receptor is also a membrane channel. The binding of a ligand to these types of receptors is associated with a change in the permeability of the channel; hence, these channels are described as being **ligand gated.** Other membrane receptors are also enzymes that are activated by the binding of a ligand. These enzymes have active sites facing the interior of the cell, so intracellular functions are changed as a result of the ligand–receptor interaction.

Yet another way that the function of a cell can be changed after a ligand binds membrane receptors involves another specific group of membrane proteins known as **G proteins.** G proteins are within the cell membrane and closely associated with certain receptor proteins. The G protein acts as an intermediate in the chain of events between ligand binding and cellular response. As a result of the ligand–receptor binding, the associated G protein acts to activate or inhibit an enzyme or membrane channel. The potential actions of G proteins are summarized in Fig. 2–17.

Adenyl cyclase is a cell membrane enzyme whose activity is regulated by ligand–receptor interactions. In some cases, the enzyme also acts as the cell membrane receptor, but in other cases, the enzyme is linked to a receptor via a G protein. Adenyl cyclase catalyzes the intracellular formation of **cyclic adenosine monophosphate** (**cAMP**), which in turn can activate intracellular **kinases.** These activated kinases can activate other intracellular proteins to change cellular function. In this general scheme, cAMP is said to be a **second messenger** in that it transfers a chemical signal from the membrane to the interior of the cell. cAMP is the second messenger for many of the peptide hormones that bind to membrane recep-

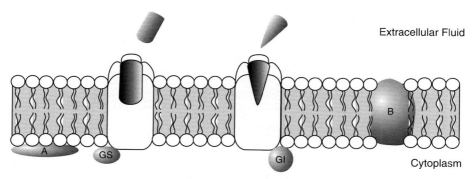

Figure 2-17. The G-proteins associated with membrane receptors can be stimulatory (GS) or inhibitory (GI). The G-proteins will act on associated membrane enzymes (A) or channels (B) after the appropriate ligand binds to the membrane receptor that is exposed to the extracellular fluid.

tors. Examples include parathyroid hormone, glucagon, and luteinizing hormone.

Membrane proteins may also act as receptor sites for attachment of disease-causing agents, such as viruses. After binding to an appropriate membrane receptor, the cell endocytoses the virus receptor complex. This provides a means by which the virus can infect the susceptible cell.

Cytoplasm and Cytoplasmic Organelles

Cytoplasm

Cytoplasm is the material filling the inside of the cell and containing the intracellular organelles and nucleus. *Organelles* are intracellular structures organized for a particular function within the cell. These include the Golgi apparatus, endoplasmic reticulum (smooth and rough), mitochondria, centrioles, free ribosomes, lysosomes, peroxisomes, and a variety of crystals, granules, and droplets (formerly called inclusions, collectively). The relatively liquid component of cytoplasm is *cytosol;* the organelles are arranged within the cytosol by a complex system of intracellular filaments and microtubules called the **cytoskeleton.**

Dissolved or suspended within the fluid cytosol are a variety of proteins, sugars, and salts. Many of the proteins are enzymes that function in the metabolic activities of the cell. Within some cells are proteins that function as cytosolic receptors binding ligands that have gained

access to the cytosol after passing through the cell membrane.

The Golgi Apparatus

The **Golgi apparatus** varies in size and location in cells of different tissues but generally appears as a stack of flattened membranous sacs (lamellae) near the nucleus (Fig. 2–18). It functions as the site of the final stages of synthesis and packaging of secretory products of the cell. Within the Golgi, secretory products are enclosed within a membrane vesicle for temporary storage in the cell or for transport to the plasma membrane, where exocytosis releases the products into the extracellular fluid as a form of secretion. Mucopolysaccharides may form in the Golgi apparatus, and glycoproteins are terminally synthesized there as combinations of carbohydrates and proteins that have been transported to the Golgi apparatus by the smooth and rough endoplasmic reticulum.

The Endoplasmic Reticulum and Ribosomes

The **endoplasmic reticulum** is a membranous network found throughout the cytoplasm of the cell (Fig. 2–18). It was first described in the endoplasm (the cytoplasm deepest in the cell), giving rise to the name endoplasmic reticulum. Although still called the endoplasmic reticulum, it has been observed in all parts of the cytoplasm and may be continuous with the outer

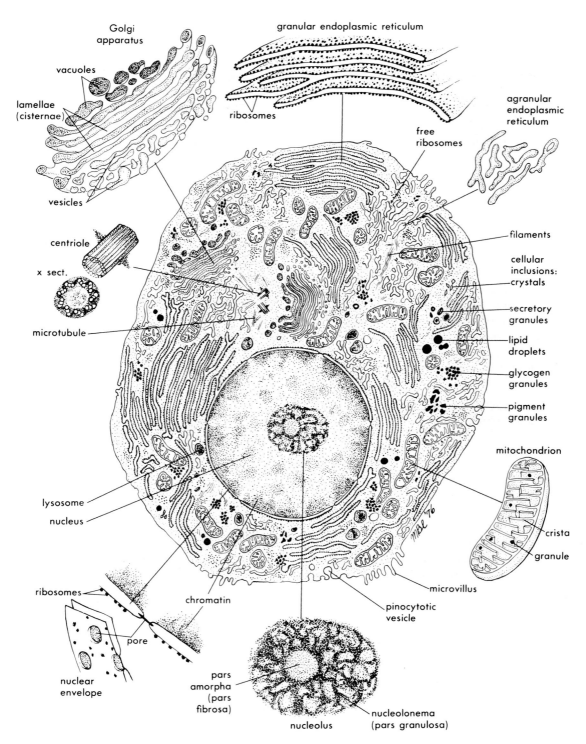

Figure 2-18. General organization of a typical cell. (Reprinted with permission from Crouch, J.E. *Functional Human Anatomy.* 4th ed. Philadelphia: Lea & Febiger, 1985.)

nuclear membrane. The endoplasmic reticulum is in the form of tubules and sheets, with occasional enlarged sacs or vesicles called **cisternae.**

In some sites, the endoplasmic reticulum is associated with ribosomes, which appear like beads along the membrane. Granular or **rough endoplasmic reticulum** (Fig.2–18) is endoplasmic reticulum associated with ribosomes; agranular or **smooth endoplasmic reticulum** (Fig. 2–18) has no ribosomes associated with it.

Mitochondria

Mitochondria are ovoid organelles about 10 μm long. The double membrane of the mitochondrion, with the cristae projecting into the interior, provides a large surface area for attachment of enzymes (Fig. 2–18). Studies of fragmented mitochondria indicate that all of the enzymes associated with oxidation of nutrients to carbon dioxide, ATP, and water are found in the mitochondria. Thus, all of the enzymes and coenzymes involved in the **tricarboxylic acid cycle** (also called the Krebs cycle, or citric acid cycle) are largely local to the mitochondria.

Oxidation during the tricarboxylic acid cycle releases carbon dioxide and hydrogen atom pairs (H_2). The H_2 furnishes its electrons to the mitochondrial electron transport system to drive a series of reduction reactions, culminating in the formation of water and storage of the energy in the form of ATP. The ATP is formed by the oxidative phosphorylation of ADP (**adenosine diphosphate**), which adds one inorganic phosphate molecule to ADP, creating a higher-energy compound. The energy incorporated into ATP becomes available for any cellular activity that requires energy, such as protein synthesis, muscle contraction, and active transport. Energy is released during the reconversion of ATP to ADP and an inorganic phosphate. Most of the cellular processes requiring energy take place outside of the mitochondria.

Since the mitochondria produce the energy for the cell, it follows that the more mitochondria in a cell, the more active the cell can be. Mitochondrial ATP production depends on oxygen, so highly active cells also need a ready supply of oxygen. The enzymes of the glycolytic pathway, using glucose as a substrate, can produce ATP without oxygen in the cytoplasm. However, this pathway is less efficient than mitochondrial production; it produces less ATP per molecule of substrate.

Mitochondria contain their own DNA and RNA for reproducing themselves. They also carry on partial synthesis of proteins and lipids and have their own ribosomes. Mitochondrial reproduction can be stimulated by increased demands for cell energy and is not dependent on cellular division.

Lysosomes

Lysosomes are membrane-bound vesicles of digestive (hydrolytic) enzymes. They are larger than ribosomes but smaller than mitochondria, ranging in diameter from 0.25 to 0.75 μm. Lysosomes apparently originate from the endoplasmic reticulum and the Golgi apparatus.

Lysosomes contain a variety of enzymes that degrade all types of biologic molecules. Normally, the membrane of the lysosome prevents lysosomal enzymes from acting on molecules within the cytoplasm. However, in certain conditions, the enzymes are released into the cytosol, which may then lyse (destroy) the cell itself.

Cytoplasmic vesicles formed by the phagocytosis of extracellular material may fuse with lysosomes, thereby permitting the enzymatic digestion of the contents of the vesicle while protecting the cell itself from lysis. White blood cells, which act as scavenger cells by phagocytizing bacteria, dead tissue, and damaged cell debris, contain many lysosomes. Lysosomes also engulf and degrade intracellular organelles. This is a means by which individual cells can remove and recover components of damaged parts of themselves. The only mammalian cells that are known not to contain lysosomes are the red blood cells.

When cells contain inactive lysosomes, disease can follow. An example is Pompe's disease, in which the lysosomes cannot digest glycogen. Also, changes caused by sunburn occur when the ultraviolet light of the sun ruptures lysosomes in the skin cells.

Other Structures

Peroxisomes are smaller than lysosomes and are most numerous in cells of the liver and kidney. Peroxisomes contain enzymes responsible for degrading lipids, alcohols, and a variety of potentially toxic substances. Hydrogen peroxide is produced within the peroxisome as a result of this enzymatic action. Other enzymes within the peroxisome rapidly degrade the potentially toxic hydrogen peroxide to protect the cell.

Microtubules, intermediate filaments, and microfilaments are rodlike organelles that make up the **cytoskeleton,** which primarily functions to determine the shape of the cell and assist with cell movement. Microtubules are scattered throughout the cytoplasm in most cells and are the largest and most rigid of the three cytoskeletal components (Fig. 2–19). Microtubules are spindle fibers in cell division, motile elements in cilia, assisters of transport of molecules within some cells, such as in the processes of neurons (nerve cells). Intermediate filaments are primarily found in association with specialized cell-to-cell junctions, such as desmosomes (Fig. 2–9). Microfilaments are thinner than microtubules, but they make up most of the cytoskeleton. Microfilaments are composed of actin, a protein involved in cell movement and muscle contraction.

The centriole is a short cylinder about 0.2 μm wide and 0.4 μm long. Centrioles, composed of nine triplets of microtubules, usually occur at the bases of cilia, where they are called basal bodies. A pair of centrioles, the centrosome, also occurs in all cells near the nucleus and organizes the microtubules, which form the mitotic spindle during cell division.

Nucleus

Structure of the Nucleus

The **nucleus** contains the genetic material of the cell encoded in molecules of DNA. With light microscopy, DNA and its associated proteins are seen as a more diffusely staining **chromatin** in the nondividing cell and as **chromosomes** in the dividing cell. The nuclei of somatic cells contain the information necessary for determining the form and structure of new cells, and the nuclei of sex cells contain the information necessary to determine the characteristics of a new individual. The **nucleoli** consist largely of clustered DNA, which codes for ribosomal RNA; the nucleoli are seen as densely staining spherical bodies in the nucleus (Fig. 2–18).

The nuclear envelope (Fig. 2–18), which surrounds the cell nucleus, is composed of two distinct membranes separated by about 20 nm. The outer membrane is continuous with the endoplasmic reticulum. Pores (small gaps or interruptions) in the nuclear envelope permit ex-

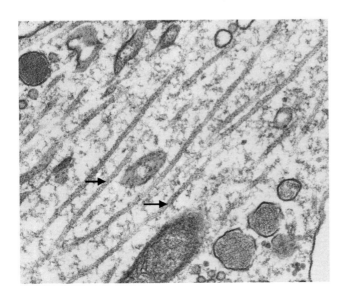

Figure 2-19. Microtubules in axons of neurosecretory neurons. (Reprinted with permission from Dellman, HD and Eurell, J. *Textbook of Veterinary Histology.* 5th ed. Baltimore: Lippincott Williams & Wilkins, 1998.)

change between the protoplasm of the nucleus (nucleoplasm) and the cytoplasm outside the nucleus, including the movement of RNA synthesized in the nucleus out into the cytoplasm.

The functional activity and the continued life of the cell depend on the presence and functional integrity of a nucleus. A cell from which the nucleus has been removed (enucleated) gradually ceases activity, atrophies, and finally dies. However, if the nucleus is replaced with a nucleus from a cell from the same species prior to irreversible atrophy, function of the cell can be restored. The only cells in higher animals that do not have nuclei are mature red blood cells. This lack of nucleus is associated with their short lifespan, only 120 days.

The primary functions of the nucleus are (1) to regulate protein synthesis in the cell, thereby regulating the biochemical activities of the cell, and (2) to ensure the passage of genetic material (the chromosomes and their component genes) to subsequent generations of cells and/or organisms.

DNA and DNA Replication

The genetic material necessary to direct cellular functions is primarily composed of chains of DNA. The chains of DNA are formed by joining small units (**nucleotides**), each containing a phosphate, a sugar (deoxyribose), and either a purine or pyrimidine base. The purine bases in DNA are adenine and guanine, and the pyrimidine bases are thymine and cytosine (Fig. 2–20).

Watson and Crick determined the structure of DNA to be a **double helix,** something like a spiral staircase or twisted metal ladder. The outside rails consist of two long chains of sugar–phosphate molecules, and the rungs are made up of paired bases that hold the two parts of the double helix together. Adenine is always paired with thymine, and guanine is always paired with cytosine. The two strands are joined by hydrogen bonds between the bases (Fig. 2–21). The two strands of the DNA double helix are not identical but are complementary. In other words, whenever adenine appears on one strand, thymine is in the same position on the opposite strand, and whenever guanine

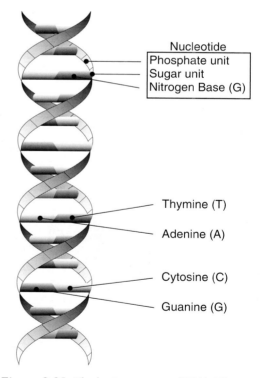

Figure 2-21. The basic structure of DNA. There are four nucleotides. The symbols in the upper right show how the nucleotides pair in DNA. (Adapted with permission from Cohen, B.J. and Wood, D.L. Memmler's *The Human Body in Health and Disease.* 9th ed. Philadelphia: Lippincott Williams & Wilkins, 2000.)

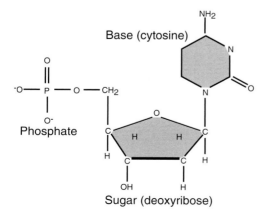

Figure 2-20. General structure of a nucleotide (subunits of DNA and RNA).

is on one strand, cytosine is in the same position on the other strand.

To pass on the genetic information to the next generation of cells or animals, the DNA double helix must be replicated. Replication of DNA begins with unwinding of the helix and splitting of the chain at the point of junction of complementary bases. Each separated strand serves as a *template,* or model, for the formation of its complementary strand, which produces two double DNA helices, replicas of the original. Each new double helix consists of one strand of the original double helix and one newly synthesized strand (Fig. 2–22). Errors in the duplication of DNA strands during replication give rise to *genetic mutations.* Errors may occur spontaneously, or their frequency may be increased through the effects of numerous external factors, or *mutagens* (e.g., ionizing radiation, exposure to certain chemicals).

The genetic information in DNA is coded by the specific sequence of purine and pyrimidine bases in a DNA molecule. This sequential arrangement of bases and its control of hered-ity, both on the cellular and the species level, have been called the *genetic code,* or the language of life. The interpretation of this code results in the synthesis of specific proteins. The only cellular constituent whose synthesis is specifically directed by the genetic code is protein. Such proteins include those that are secreted as cellular products, those that are found in the cell membrane, and those that function within the cytosol or within cellular organelles.

The DNA code is said to be a *triplet code,* for each group of three nucleotides in the DNA chain ultimately calls for a specific amino acid in the process of protein synthesis. There are approximately 20 amino acids in the cell. With four bases that may be included in a triplet, there are more than enough potential triplet codes to represent the 20 amino acids. Other triplet codes in the DNA serve as signals to demarcate the segment of the DNA chain that represents a particular protein and to regulate the initial and terminal steps in protein synthesis.

A *gene* is a segment of DNA that contains the triplet codes for all amino acids in one or more

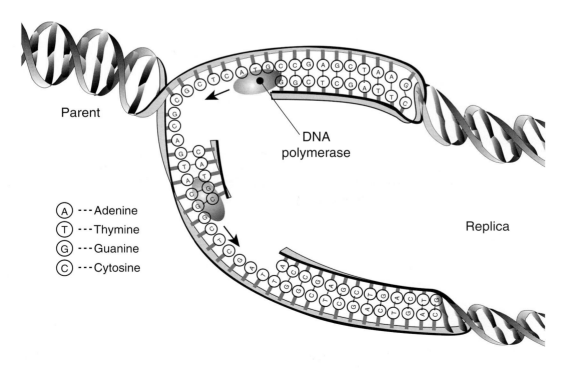

Figure 2-22. Semiconservative replication of DNA. (Adapted with permission from Bell, G.H., et al. *Textbook of Physiology and Biochemistry.* 8th ed. Baltimore: Williams & Wilkins, 1979.)

proteins and the signal sequences necessary to regulate the processing of the DNA segment. However, interspersed within a gene are also sequences of nucleotides that are not regulators of the process and do not contain necessary triplet codes. These noncoding, nonregulatory segments are **introns.** The DNA coding segments in a gene are **exons.** A single gene may have multiple exons and introns throughout its length.

RNA: Transcription and Translation

The processes by which the genetic code is interpreted and proteins are synthesized require the participation of three forms of RNA (ribonucleic acid). The three forms of RNA are **messenger RNA** (mRNA), **transfer RNA** (tRNA), and **ribosomal RNA** (rRNA). Like DNA, all three forms of RNA consist of nucleotide units that contain a sugar (ribose), a phosphate, and a purine or pyrimidine base. The two purines that are found in DNA, adenine and guanine, are also found in RNA, as is the pyrimidine cytosine. However, RNA does not contain the pyrimidine thymine that is found in DNA. Instead, RNA contains the pyrimidine uracil. Whereas the structure of DNA was two strands or chains of nucleotides joined together in a double helix, RNA exists only as a single strand.

The first step in the interpretation of the genetic code, **transcription,** results in the formation of a mRNA. This process is similar to DNA replication except that DNA now serves as a template for the synthesis of a mRNA instead of a new complementary strand of DNA. A specific nuclear enzyme, **RNA polymerase II,** and other nuclear proteins collectively known as **general transcription factors** bind together at a specific site on the DNA to initiate the transcription of a specific gene. The site on the DNA at which binding occurs and transcription begins is known as a **promoter.** A special segment of DNA adjacent to the promoter region contains a start sequence of nucleotides to signal RNA polymerase II to begin the synthesis of mRNA. Other regulatory proteins that act as **enhancer** or **repressor** transcription factors can also influence the rate of transcription of a specific gene. These regulatory transcription factors may bind to sites on DNA that are distant from the promoter region but because of the folding and curling of the DNA strand, they can interact with the proteins bound at the promoter region.

Using the DNA as a template, RNA polymerase II synthesizes a single complementary strand of nucleotides. As with DNA, each group of three nucleotides in the newly synthesized mRNA is the code for a specific amino acid. Each group of three nucleotides in the mRNA is a **codon.** When the end of the segment of DNA that represents a particular protein is reached, a stop sequence in the DNA terminates the mRNA synthesis, and the mRNA strand detaches from the RNA polymerase. Figure 2–23 summarizes the steps of transcription.

Recall that the segment of DNA that represents a gene and serves as the template for mRNA contains both exons and introns (i.e., both coding and noncoding regions). Thus, the newly synthesized mRNA must be processed to remove the segments that correspond to the introns in the DNA. This processing is done before the mRNA exits the nucleus and enters the cytoplasm, where protein synthesis will take place. The segments of mRNA that correspond to the noncoding introns are excised, and the segments that correspond to the coding exons are spliced together by a complex consisting of RNA and a protein called a **spliceosome.** During the splicing, the spliceosome sometimes omits segments of the initial mRNA that correspond to some of the coding exons. This omission results in **alternately spliced** mRNAs and ultimately the synthesis of different proteins from the transcription of a single gene.

Within the cytoplasm, the processed mRNA binds to a **ribosome.** This binding occurs at a specific end of the mRNA under the direction of a start codon at that site. The start codon also signals the binding of an initial tRNA with a specific amino acid attached. There is at least one specific tRNA for each of the approximately 20 amino acids in the cell. After the first tRNA is bound, a second tRNA with its attached amino acid arrives and binds to the next codon in line. Ribosomal enzymes then detach the amino acid from the first tRNA and link the two amino acids to begin the formation of a peptide chain. The first tRNA can be detached from the ribosome and transfer another amino acid. The ribosome now directs the binding of a third tRNA with its appropriate amino acid and the subsequent linkage of the third amino acid to the second. Figure 2–24 summarizes these initial steps in protein synthesis.

This basic process of tRNA binding and amino acid linking continues as the ribosome moves along the mRNA strand. The result is a specific sequence of amino acids that are appropriate for the codons contained in the mRNA strand. A stop codon at the end of the mRNA signals the ribosome to detach the newly synthesized amino acid chain from the mRNA. The mRNA remains intact and may be reused multiple times. The decoding of the mRNA and the synthesis of the appropriate amino acid chain constitute *translation.*

Biotechnology

Genetic engineering and **biotechnology** are general terms used to describe the myriad of techniques used to alter the genetic code in organisms. Because the same principles of genetic information storage and transfer apply in all living organisms (from viruses through the hierarchy of plants, invertebrates, vertebrates, and humans), these techniques and procedures are widely applied. **Because of the commonality of chemicals involved (DNA and RNA), it is also possible to move genetic material from one species to another. For example, mammalian DNA has been placed into the genome of *Escherichia coli*, which have then produced mammalian proteins.** *Recombinant DNA* is the general term describing DNA that contains novel segments inserted by biotechnological techniques. An animal or plant that contains DNA from another organism is said to be *transgenic.*

The discovery of a group of enzymes known as **restriction nucleases** was a key factor in the development of recombinant DNA techniques. These enzymes cut DNA into shorter segments by splitting the linkages between nucleotides. The enzymes do not act at random sites through the DNA strand; instead, each individual nuclease acts at a specific site termed its restriction

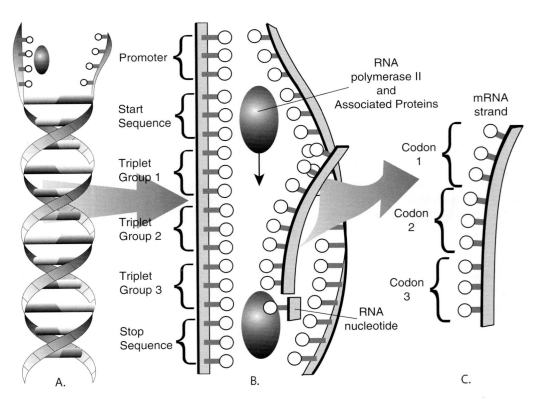

Figure 2-23. Transcription. A) Separation of a DNA double helix. B) RNA polymerase II uses triplet groups as code to synthesize mRNA. C) Codons in completed mRNA correspond to triplet groups in DNA. A minimal number of triplets and codons are shown for clarity.

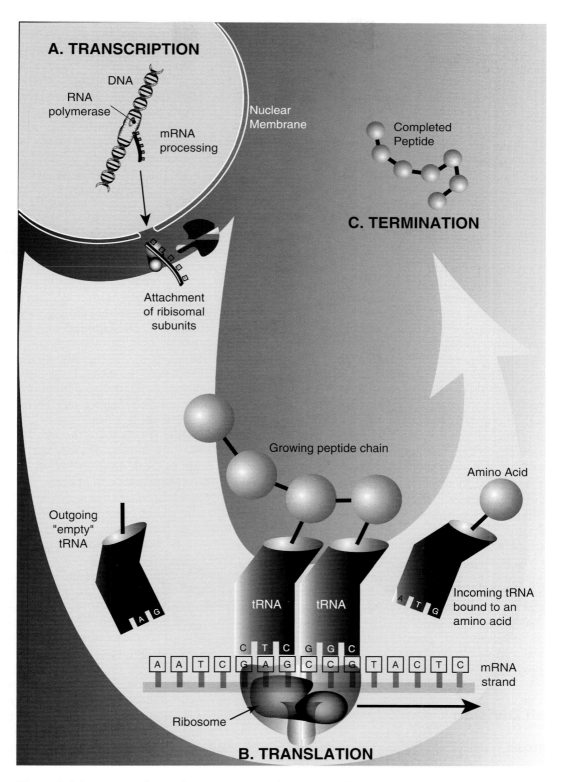

Figure 2-24. Protein synthesis. A) Transcription results in processed mRNA which exits nucleus. B) Translation of the mRNA produces a peptide chain. C) The completed peptide is released.

site. If DNA from two different organisms are treated with the same nuclease, the nuclease will fragment the DNA at similar restriction sites in both. This yields segments of DNA with similar characteristics at their ends, but the sequences within the segments may be quite different. Because the ends of the segments from the two organisms are similar, **DNA ligase** (an enzyme that reestablishes the nucleotide linkages) can be used to join the different DNA segments. The final result is a DNA strand that contains DNA from two different organisms.

To produce a transgenic organism, recombinant DNA must be inserted into the genome of an organism. In domestic animals, this has been accomplished by microinjection of recombinant DNA into a **pronucleus** of single-cell embryos. The pronucleus is a nucleuslike structure in the embryo that contains genetic material from one parent. One-cell embryos have two pronuclei that ultimately fuse so that the genetic material from the two parents can be joined in the new individual. Recombinant DNA has also been transferred into embryos by infecting early-stage embryos with **retroviruses** containing recombinant DNA in their genome. Retroviruses are a specific group of viruses that insert their own genetic material into the genome of organisms they infect. As they insert their own genetic material, they also insert the recombinant DNA.

Clones are genetically identical individuals produced by asexual means. Cloning has been accomplished by splitting an early-stage multicell embryo into single cells, which continue their development into identical individuals. This technique has been successfully used in domestic animals. Clones have also been produced by **nuclear transfer.** In this technique, nuclei obtained from cells of adult animals are transferred into oocytes with their original nucleus removed. The oocytes with the transferred nucleus can be placed in the uterus of an appropriate female for gestation.

Cell Division

Mitosis

Each day millions of cells in the body of any normal animal die and are degraded or sloughed from epithelial surfaces. These cells must be replaced if normal life is to continue, and the replacement cells must be replicas of the original cells. **Mitosis,** the division of somatic cells to produce two daughter cells, includes the duplication of genetic material for each daughter cell. Even though the process of cell division is normally a continuous process, it has been divided into periods, or phases, for ease of communication about the process. The active phases are primarily based on nuclear changes visible by light microscopy. They are prophase, metaphase, anaphase, and telophase (Fig. 2–25).

Interphase. The period between active cell divisions is interphase. It may vary from a matter of hours in actively proliferating tissue to an almost permanent condition in cells that no longer divide, such as mature cardiac muscle cells. The replication of DNA during interphase prepares the cell to begin mitosis.

Prophase. Prophase, the first of the active phases, is characterized by condensation of chromatin into twisted filamentous threads (**chromatids**). (The term mitosis comes from the Greek word *mitos,* meaning thread.) Also during prophase, the nuclear envelope and the nucleolus begin to break down and disappear, and the two centrioles move to opposite poles of the cell. Microtubules become organized and arranged in a fan shape, radiating outward from the centrioles to the equator of the cell. This arrangement is the **mitotic spindle.**

Metaphase. Metaphase is the period when the nuclear envelope and nucleolus totally disappear. The chromatids move and line up across the cell's equator in the middle of the spindle, and the spindle microtubules attach to the centromere region of the chromatids.

Anaphase. Anaphase is the stage in which each centromere divides, separating the two chromatids, now properly called **chromosomes** again. The cell now contains twice as many chromosomes as it had originally. Half of the chromosomes begin to migrate toward one centriole at a pole of the spindle, and the other half migrates to the other centriole.

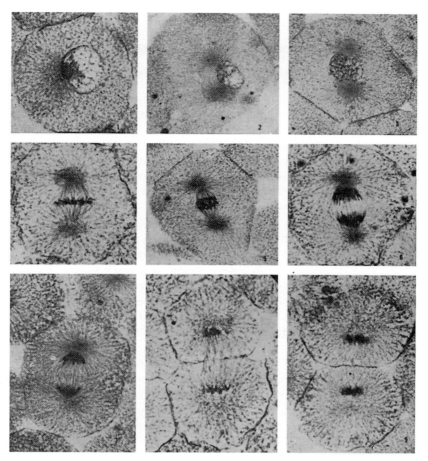

Figure 2-25. States of mitosis in cells of the whitefish blastula: *1)* Interphase, with cell center adjacent to nucleus. *2)* Early prophase, showing development of astral centers. *3)* Late prophase, with astral centers at opposite ends of the cell. *4)* Metaphase. *5)* Early anaphase. *6)* Late anaphase. *7)* Early telophase. *8)* Mid telophase, showing cleavage furrow. *9)* Telophase interphase following separation of daughter cells. (Courtesy of Phillip G. Coleman, Michigan State University.)

Telophase. Telophase begins when half of the chromosomes have been drawn by the microtubules to each pole of the cell. A nuclear envelope forms around each set of daughter chromosomes, and a nucleolus appears in each new nucleus. The spindle tubules disappear, and the chromosomes begin to unwind into filaments. Ultimately the chromosomes lose their visible identity and become the chromatin of the interphase period.

The cell itself next divides into two daughter cells. The division of the cytoplasm is called *cytokinesis.* It starts with invagination of the plasma membrane around the equator of the cell and ends by pinching off the two halves, with a nucleus in each half, creating the daughter cells. Each centriole is also replicated, and each daughter cell is now a replica of the parent cell. Mitosis is complete.

Meiosis

Meiosis (reduction division) differs from mitosis in a number of ways. It occurs during *gametogenesis,* the formation of ova in the female (*oogenesis*) and spermatozoa in the male (*spermatogenesis*). These processes are discussed in detail in Chapters 25 and 27. Since fertilization doubles the number of chromosomes in the fertilized ovum, equal numbers being contributed by the male and female, there must be a mechanism to reduce the somatic, or *diploid,* number of chromosomes in each gamete prior to fertilization.

Meiosis not only reduces the diploid number of chromosomes by half to the *haploid* number, it also increases the genetic variability of the offspring by *crossing over.* Homologous chromosomes in the primary sex (germ) cells pair up during prophase of meiosis. Homologous chromosomes are similar chromosomes that were contributed by the two parents of the individual. These paired homologous chromosomes may then *cross over* and exchange similar areas, resulting in two chromosomes that are different from either parent chromosome.

Regulation of Cell Growth and Replication

Most cell types in the body can grow beyond normal size (hypertrophy). However, not all cell types in the mature animal have the same ability to replicate and produce two new daughter cells. Some cell types, for example the epithelium lining the small intestine and certain blood cells, are continuously replicating to replace cells that are lost from the body or die. Other cell types, for example cardiac and skeletal muscle cells, do not normally replicate and produce new daughter cells. What determines the ability of cells to replicate and divide is not fully understood. However, a variety of chemical signals stimulate cell growth and in some cases, cell division. Chemical signals with these capabilities are said to be *growth factors.* Typically, growth factors stimulate only certain populations of cells. For example, colony-stimulating growth factors stimulate bone marrow cells to produce blood cells, while insulin-like growth factors stimulate cartilage proliferation at growth plates in bone to promote an increase in body size.

Unregulated cell growth and replication are a factor in the development of cancer. A mass of cells undergoing uncontrolled growth is a *tumor.* A tumor is said to be *benign* if it is local and does not invade other tissues. *Malignant* tumors are capable of invading surrounding tissues and spreading to other sites throughout the body (*metastasis*).

Sometimes normal cells must undergo spontaneous, or programmed, death and be removed without an inflammatory response so that normal function of a tissue or organ can proceed. For example a corpus luteum formed in an ovary during an estrus cycle must be removed before another cycle can begin. The term *apoptosis* is applied to spontaneous or programmed death of normal cells. In some cases the development of tumors may also include a decrease in the rate of normal apoptosis.

Chapter 3

EMBRYOLOGY

Development of Germ Layers
Neurulation
Differentiation of Other Tissues

*E**mbryology* is the study of the early prenatal development of an animal. It begins with the fertilization of the egg (*ovum*) by a *spermatozoon* to form a *zygote.* The ovum and spermatozoon each contribute half of the nuclear chromosomes to the newly formed zygote. The cells of the zygote undergo division, migration, and differentiation to become successively a morula, a blastula, a gastrula, and then an embryo. Strictly speaking, the *period of the embryo* ends when the various organs and organ systems are formed. The embryo then becomes a fetus that more or less resembles an adult of the same species. The *period of the fetus* primarily entails increase in size and functional differentiation of organs. In cattle, the embryo becomes a fetus approximately at the end of the second month of gestation. The fetus becomes a *neonate* (newborn animal) at *parturition* (birth).

Development of Germ Layers

The one-celled zygote undergoes the first mitotic divisions, known as *cleavage,* shortly after fertilization. Cleavage increases the number of cells (called *blastomeres*) without increasing the volume of the developing embryo, so that after each cell division, the daughter cells have smaller cytoplasmic mass. However, the nuclei of the daughter cells are normal in size and contain a full complement

47

of chromosomes. The cluster of small cells resulting from cleavage has a lobulated appearance resembling a berry; hence, the name **morula** (Latin, *small mulberry*) is given to this stage (Fig. 3–1).

When the morula reaches the uterus, a cavity, the **blastocele,** forms within it, transforming the morula into a hollow ball called a **blastula.** The blastula comprises a layer of cells, the **trophoblast,** surrounding the blastocele, into which a collection of cells, the **inner cell mass,** protrudes. The inner cell mass eventually forms the body of the embryo. The trophoblast will develop into the extraembryonic tissues, including the placenta.

The portion of the inner cell mass closest to the trophoblast is the **epiblast,** and the portion adjacent to the blastocele is the **hypoblast.** As the inner cell mass develops, a cavity forms dorsal to the epiblast; this is the **amniotic cavity.** Simultaneously, proliferating hypoblast cells migrate to line the blastocele. This lining becomes the **endoderm,** the germ line destined to become the lining of the gastrointestinal and respiratory systems, the epithelial parts of glands associated with the digestive system, and parts of the reproductive system.

Sometime before the end of the second week of development, the epiblast begins to thicken with proliferating cells on the longitudinal axis of the embryo. This thickening is the **primitive streak,** and here the epiblast cells migrate into the interior of the embryo, taking up residence between the outer layer of cells (now called **ectoderm**) and the endoderm. This migration of cells is **gastrulation** (Fig. 3–2); with it the embryo establishes the three primary cell lines that will give rise to all of the tissues in the adult body.

The ectoderm on the dorsal surface of the embryo will become skin and nervous tissue. The cells between ectoderm and endoderm become **mesoderm,** the germ line that gives rise to muscle, the skeleton, urinary and cardiovascular systems, and parts of the reproductive system.

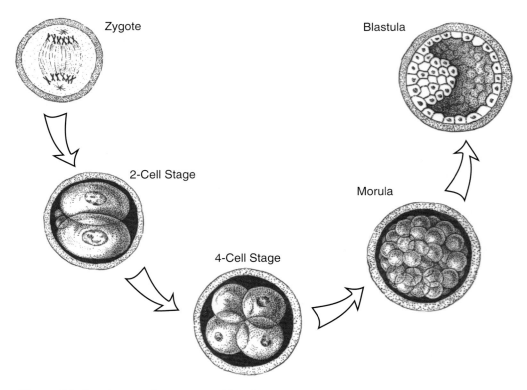

Figure 3-1. Development from zygote to blastula.

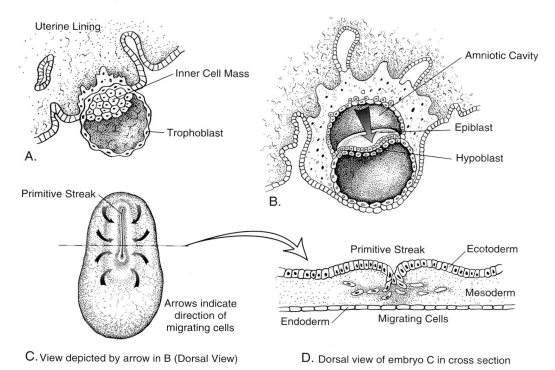

Figure 3-2. Gastrulation. *A)* and *B)* Around the time of implantation, when the embryo embeds in the wall of the uterus, the inner cell mass becomes a disc of two distinct layers, epiblast and hypoblast. *C)* Embryo viewed from above, as indicated by the arrow in B. Cells of the epiblast begin to proliferate and migrate toward the longitudinal primitive streak on the dorsal midline. *D)* Cross-section through the region of the primitive streak. Migrating cells move to the interior of the embryo, where they become mesoderm.

Neurulation

Around the second week of development, the mesoderm on the dorsal midline of the developing embryo condenses into a longitudinal rod, the **notochord.** The notochord in vertebrates is essential to inducing the formation of the overlying nervous system and the differentiation of adjacent mesoderm into definitive vertebrae.

Ectoderm overlying the notochord is induced by it to thicken, forming the **neural plate.** From this point, these cells, destined to become the nervous system, constitute the **neurectoderm.** The lateral edges of the neural plate thicken and grow dorsad, turning the neural plate into a **neural groove.** The dorsal growth of the edges of the neural groove continues until they meet and fuse, forming the **neural tube** (Fig. 3–3). The formation of the

neural tube proceeds from cranial to caudal, so that the brain develops before the caudal portions of the spinal cord. The lumen of the neural tube persists in the adult as the ventricular system of the brain and the central canal of the spinal cord.

Differentiation of Other Tissues

Mesodermal cells on each side of the notochord condense into a series of blocklike paired masses. These are the segmentally arranged **somites,** which in turn develop into vertebrae and muscles. Mesoderm lateral to the somites is called **nephrogenic (intermediate) mesoderm.** It will give rise to urogenital organs (Fig. 3–4).

The most lateral mesoderm, the **lateral plate mesoderm,** splits into two layers, forming a cavity, the **celom.** The celom will eventually

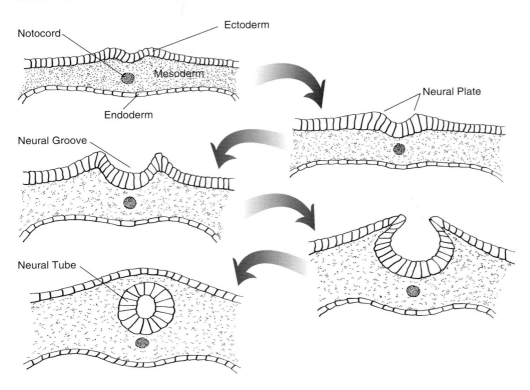

Figure 3-3. Neurulation. Shown in cross-section, the ectoderm overlying the notochord is induced to thicken, forming the neural plate. Differential growth of cells of the neural plate produces a depression, the neural groove. The edges of the neural groove approach one another and fuse, creating the neural tube, the precursor to the spinal cord and brain.

become the thoracic, abdominal, and pelvic cavities.

The outer layer of the lateral plate mesoderm and the adjacent ectoderm make up the **so-matopleure,** which forms part of the body wall and enters into the formation of the fetal membranes. The inner layer of the lateral plate mesoderm and the endoderm form the **splanchno-pleure,** which forms the wall of the gut (Fig. 3–5).

Differentiation of the relatively indifferent cells of each of the three germ layers to form specialized tissue cells is called **histogenesis.** Much is known about when and where various tissues and organs develop, and developmental biologists are beginning to unravel the molecular and genetic events that underlie development. For instance, cell surface molecules that instruct cells to migrate and aggregate have been identified, as have others that cause cells to change the expression of their genes. Once a

cell has altered the expression of its genome so as to assume a more specialized role, it is said to be **committed.** Each of the three germ lines is committed to form certain kinds of tissues (Table 3–1). **Differentiation** occurs as these cells assume the appearance and functions characteristic of the cell type to which they are committed.

Early embryonic cells are capable of differentiating into multiple tissue types, a characteristic called **pluripotency.** These early pluripotent cells are often called **embryonic stem cells.** Unlike most differentiated tissues, they are capable of long-term survival in culture (outside the body). Embryonic stem cells are profoundly interesting to biomedical researchers, as it appears that cultured stem cells can be induced to differentiate into a wide variety of tissue types. This technique offers promise of a novel way of treating diseases involving loss of normal tissue. A few of the many possibilities include use of

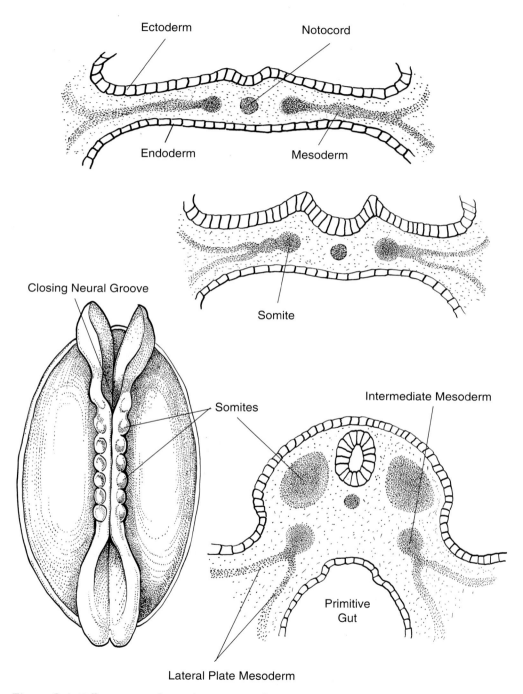

Figure 3-4. Differentiation of mesoderm. Somites form most medially. These will give rise to the muscles and bones associated with the vertebral column. Lateral to the somites is the intermediate mesoderm, which will differentiate into tissues of the urogenital system. Most laterally, the lateral plate mesoderm will become parts of the gastrointestinal wall and body wall.

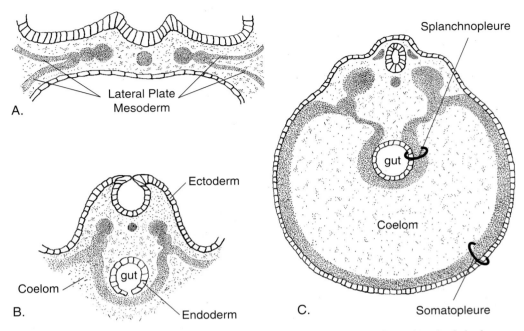

Figure 3-5. A) Lateral plate mesoderm splits early in development, creating the coelom (early body cavity). B) The external layer associates with overlying ectoderm, while the internal layer associates with endoderm of the developing gut. C) Ectoderm plus the external layer of lateral plate mesoderm constitutes the somatopleure; it will become the body wall. The internal mesoderm and endoderm are called splanchnopleure, which becomes the wall of the gastrointestinal tract.

stem cells to create (1) hematopoietic cells to regenerate normal blood precursors for treatment of blood and immune disorders, (2) cartilage and bone to replace damaged skeletal components, and (3) neuronal precursors to replace the neurons lost in Parkinson's disease or Alzheimer's disease. Research with human embryonic stem cells is fraught with contentious ethical considerations, since these cells are generally acquired from aborted embryos and fe-

Table 3-1. The Germ Layer Origin of Tissues

Ectoderm	Mesoderm	Endoderm
Epidermis, including cutaneous glands, hair, nails (claws, hoofs), lens	Muscle (all types)	Epithelia of:
	Cartilage	Pharynx, including root of tongue, auditory tube, tonsils
	Bone	
Epithelia of sense organs, nasal cavity, paranasal sinuses, oral cavity	Blood, bone marrow	Larynx, trachea, lungs
	Endothelium	Thyroid, parathyroids, thymus
Dental enamel	Mesothelium (lining of serous cavities)	Digestive tube and glands
Nervous tissue		Urinary bladder
Adenohypophysis	Epithelium of kidney and ureter	Vagina, vestibule
Chromaffin cells of adrenal gland	Epithelium of gonads, genital ducts	Urethra and associated glands
	Adrenal cortex	
	Synovium	

tuses. Research using animal embryos tends to be less ethically problematic, but it will naturally lead to intense debate as techniques developed in animal models are extrapolated for use in human medicine.

The study of embryology is a basic interest to individuals working in the animal industry, since abnormalities of embryonic and fetal development can produce malformations or death of the fetus or neonate. Development of the embryo and fetus is covered in greater detail in standard textbooks on embryology. This subject, especially when treated as a descriptive discipline, is also called *developmental anatomy.*

Chapter 4

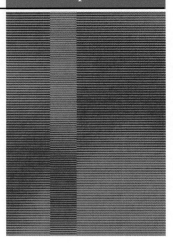

The Skeletal System

The study of the bones that make up the skeleton, or framework of the body, is ***osteology.*** The skeleton gives a basis for the external structure and appearance of most vertebrate animals as we know them (Figs. 4–1 and 4–2). All mammals share a basic body plan with striking similarities in skeletal structure. Differences reflect adaptations to specific lifestyles.

The skeleton of a living animal is made up of bones that are themselves living structures. They have blood vessels, lymphatic vessels, and nerves; they are subject to disease; they can undergo repair; and they adjust to changes in stress. The functions of bones include providing protection, giving rigidity and form to the body, acting as levers, storing minerals, and forming the cellular elements of blood.

Functions of Bones

Protection of vital organs is one of the important functions of bones. The central nervous system is protected by the skull and vertebral column; the heart and lungs, by the rib cage; and internal parts of the urogenital system, by the pelvis.

In the vertebrates, locomotion, defense, offense, grasping, and other activities of this type depend largely upon the action of muscles that attach to levers. Almost without exception, these levers are made of bone and are integral parts of the skeleton.

The entire skeleton serves as a dynamic storage area for minerals, particularly calcium and

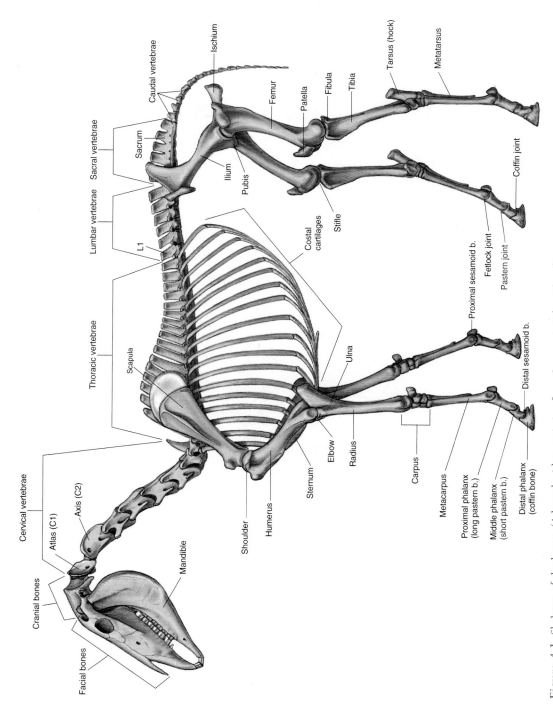

Figure 4-1. Skeleton of the horse. (Adapted with permission from *Spurgeon's Color Atlas of Large Animal Medicine*. Baltimore: Lippincott Williams & Wilkins, 1999, p 5.)

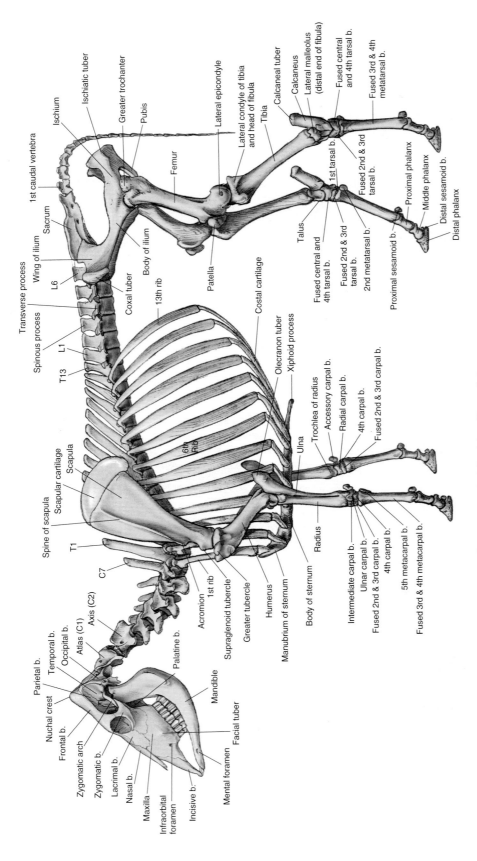

Figure 4-2. Skeleton of the ox. (Adapted with permission from *Spurgeon's Color Atlas of Large Animal Medicine.* Lippincott Williams & Wilkins, 1999, p 35.)

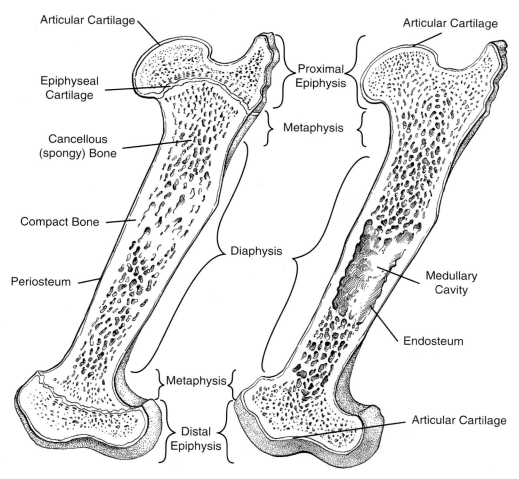

Figure 4-3. Longitudinal section of the equine femur. *Left)* Immature (growth plates open). *Right)* Mature (growth plates fused).

phosphorus. These minerals are deposited and withdrawn as needed in the ongoing homeokinetic process. Blood formation is not strictly a function of bone itself but of the marrow within the cavity of long bones and the spongy substance of all young bones.

Terminology

Certain terms (Fig. 4–3) routinely used in reference to bones, particularly long bones, include the following:

Compact (dense or *cortical) bone* is the hard layer that covers most bones and forms almost the entire shaft of long bones.

Cancellous (spongy) bone is composed of spicules arranged to form a porous network. The spaces are usually filled with marrow.

The *medullary cavity (marrow cavity)* is the space surrounded by the cortex of a long bone. In young animals it is filled with *red marrow,* which gradually is replaced by fatty *yellow marrow* as the animal ages.

Epiphysis refers to either end of a long bone. The end closest to the body is the proximal epiphysis, and the end farthest from the body is the distal epiphysis.

The *diaphysis* is the cylindrical shaft of a long bone between the two epiphyses.

The *metaphysis* of a mature bone is the flared area adjacent to the epiphysis. It is generally the widest part of a long bone.

Epiphyseal cartilage or *disk* (*physis*) is a layer of hyaline cartilage that separates the diaphysis and epiphysis within the metaphysis of an immature bone. This is the only area in which a bone can lengthen.

Articular cartilage is a thin layer of hyaline cartilage that covers the articular surface of a bone.

Periosteum is a fibrous membrane that covers the surface of a bone except where articular cartilage is. *Osteoblasts* (bone-producing cells) of the periosteum are responsible for increases in the diameter of bones, and activity of periosteal cells is important in the healing of fractures.

Endosteum is a fibrous membrane that lines the marrow cavity and *osteonal canals* (*osteons*) of a bone. Erosion of existing bone by os-teoclasts (bone-destroying cells) in the endosteum determines the size of the marrow cavity and the thickness of the diaphyseal cortex. Both periosteum and endosteum contain osteoblasts and osteoclasts (see Chapter 5).

Many of the projections from and depressions in bones have general names that depend to some extent on their size and function. Both projections and depressions may be articular or nonarticular. If they are articular, they form an integral part of a joint and are covered with articular cartilage. Nonarticular projections and depressions are outside of joints. Many of them provide areas for attachment of muscle tendons or of ligaments. Table 4–1 lists some common bony features.

Table 4-1. Bony Features

		Example
Articular Projections		
Head	Spherical articular projection	Head of femur
Condyle	Approximately cylindrical articular mass	Medial & lateral femoral condyles
Trochlea	Pulleylike articular mass	Trochlea of distal humerus
Facet	Relatively flat articular surface	Articular facets between carpal bones
Nonarticular Projections		
Process	General term for bony projection	Spinous process or transverse process of vertebra
Tuberosity (Tuber)	Relatively large nonarticular projection	Deltoid tuberosity of humerus and tuber sacrale of pelvis
Tubercle (tuberculum)	Smaller projection	Greater and lesser tubercles of humerus
Spine	Pointed projection or ridge	Nasal spine of palatine bone and spine of scapula
Crest	Sharp ridge	Median sacral crest
Neck	Cylindrical part of bone to which a head is attached	Femoral neck
Line (linea)	Small ridge or mark on bone	Gluteal lines of ilium
Articular Depressions		
Fovea	Small depression (may be articular or not)	Fovea capitis on head of femur
Glenoid Cavity	Shallow articular concavity	Glenoid cavity of scapula
Notch	Indentation (may be articular or not)	Semilunar notch of ulna and alar notch of atlas
Nonarticular Depressions		
Fossa	Large nonarticular depression	Supraspinous fossa of scapula
Foramen	Circumscribed hole in bone	Foramen magnum at base of skull
Canal	Tunnel through one or more bones	Vertebral canal through length of vertebral column

Classification of Bones According to Gross Appearance

Any bone may be classified in one of the following groups: long, short, flat, sesamoid, pneumatic, or irregular.

Long bones are greater in one dimension than any other. Each consists of a relatively cylindrical shaft (the diaphysis) and two extremities, the epiphyses, with a metaphysis between each epiphysis and the diaphysis. Long bones function chiefly as levers and aid in support, locomotion, and prehension. The best examples of long bones are in the extremities. In the thoracic limb the long bones include the humerus, radius, ulna, metacarpals, and phalanges. In the pelvic limb, the long bones are the femur, tibia, fibula, metatarsals, and phalanges.

Short bones are cuboid, or approximately equal in all dimensions. There is no single marrow cavity, but the interior is composed of spongy bone filled with marrow spaces. The exterior is formed by a thin layer of compact bone. Short bones absorb concussion, and they are found in complex joints such as the **carpus** (the knee of the thoracic limb) and **tarsus** (**hock**), where a variety of movements as well as absorption of shock occur.

Flat bones are relatively thin and expanded in two dimensions. They consist of two plates of compact bone, the **lamina externa** and **lamina interna,** separated by spongy material called **diploë.**

Flat bones function chiefly for protection of vital organs such as the brain (skull), the heart and lungs (scapulae and ribs), and the pelvic viscera (pelvis), but many provide large areas for attachment of muscles. The scapulae and pelvic bones have large areas for muscle attachment.

Sesamoid bones are so called because of their fancied resemblance to a sesame seed, although many sesamoid bones of domestic animals have distinctly unseedlike shapes. Sesamoid bones occur along the course of tendons to reduce friction, increase leverage, or change the direction of pull. The **patella** (kneecap) is the largest sesamoid bone in the body.

Pneumatic bones contain air spaces or sinuses that communicate with the exterior. The frontal bones and maxillary bones of the skull are examples of this type of bone.

Irregular bones are unpaired bones on the median plane; they include the vertebrae and some of the unpaired bones of the skull. These bones do not fit well into any other classification. They feature prominent processes and offer protection, support, and muscular attachment.

Axial Skeleton

The **axial skeleton** includes bones on or attached to the midline (axis) of the body and comprises the skull, vertebral column, sternum, and ribs. Table 4–2 lists the bones of the axial skeleton by regions.

Table 4-2. Bones of the Axial Skeleton

Skull				
Cranial Part	**Facial Part**	**Vertebrae**	**Ribs**	**Sternum**
Ethmoid	Incisive	Cervical	True (joined to sternum by cartilages)	Sternebrae
Frontal	Lacrimal	Thoracic		Manubrium
Interparietal	Mandible	Lumbar	False (not directly connected to sternum)	Xiphoid process
Occipital	Maxilla	Sacral		
Parietal	Palatine	Caudal	Floating (fixed only at vertebrae; last 1 or 2 pairs)	
Pterygoid	Nasal			
Sphenoid	Turbinates (conchae)			
Temporal	Zygomatic			
Vomer	Hyoid apparatus			

Skull

The part of the skeleton that shapes the head is the **skull.** It protects the brain, supports many of the sense organs, and forms passages for entry to the digestive and respiratory systems. The skull consists of a cranial part (braincase), which surrounds the brain, and the remainder, which is the facial part (Figs. 4–4 and 4–5). The term *cranium* is sometimes used to denote the entire skull but more commonly refers only to the braincase, not the facial bones. Most of the observable species differences, as far as the head is concerned, depend on variations in the facial part of the skull.

The caudal and dorsal walls of the cranium are formed by the **occipital, parietal, interparietal,** and **frontal bones.** In domestic animals that possess them, the horns have at their core bony projections that arise from the frontal bones. These projections are the **cornual processes.**

Laterally and ventrally the walls are formed by the **temporal bones,** which contain the middle and inner ears, and the **sphenoid bone,** which supports the brain and pituitary gland. Rostrally, the unpaired **ethmoid bone** presents numerous openings for passage of the olfactory nerves associated with the sense of smell.

The facial portion of the skull can be divided into orbital, nasal, and oral regions.

The **orbit,** which means circle, designates the bony socket that protects the eye. The orbit is surrounded by portions of the **frontal, lacrimal,** and **zygomatic bones.** Frontal, zygomatic, and temporal bones all participate in the formation of the prominent **zygomatic arch** that borders the ventral and caudal parts of the orbit.

The air passages through the nasal part of the skull are bounded dorsally by the **nasal bones,** laterally by the **maxillae** and **incisive bones,** and ventrally by the **palatine processes** of the maxillae, incisive, and **palatine bones.** Right and left nasal passages are separated longitudinally by the **vomer bone** and a cartilaginous septum. Scroll-like **conchae** (**turbinate bones**) arise from the lateral walls of the nasal cavity and project into the nasal passages. The conchae are covered with highly vascular mucous membrane that helps warm and humidify the inspired air; conchae in the caudal parts of the nasal cavity feature the **olfactory epithelium,** which contains the nerve cells specialized to detect odors.

The maxilla and zygomatic bone of the horse feature a sharp ridge, the **facial crest,** that is readily seen and felt on the lateral aspect of the horse's head, ventral and rostral to the eye.

Communicating with the nasal cavity are diverticula, known as **sinuses,** within some of the bones. The bones that may contain these sinuses include the frontal, maxillary, nasal, sphenoid, and palatine bones. Because it features a diverticulum that extends into the cornual process, the frontal sinus in cattle may be exposed by dehorning mature animals.

The oral (mouth) portion of the skull is roofed by the maxillae and incisive bones and by the palatine bone. The maxillae and incisive bones contain the teeth of the upper dental arcade (although the incisive bones lack teeth in ruminants).

Ventrolaterally, the **mandible** completes the oral portion. The mandible pivots on a fossa of the temporal bone just in front of the opening of the ear. The mandible contains all of the lower teeth and gives attachment to some of the muscles associated with chewing and swallowing.

The **hyoid apparatus** is a bony framework (Fig. 4–6) that gives support to the pharynx (throat) and provides attachment to some pharyngeal, laryngeal, and lingual muscles. It is between the right and left portions of the mandible and is attached to the **styloid process** of each temporal bone.

Vertebral Column

The **vertebral column** is composed of median unpaired irregular bones called **vertebrae.** The following letters are typically used to designate the respective regions:

C   Cervical vertebrae, neck region
T   Thoracic, chest
L   Lumbar, loin
S   Sacral, pelvis, fused vertebrae
LS Fused lumbar and sacral (birds)
Cd Caudal (coccygeal), tail

A **vertebral formula** for a given species consists of the letter symbol for each region fol-

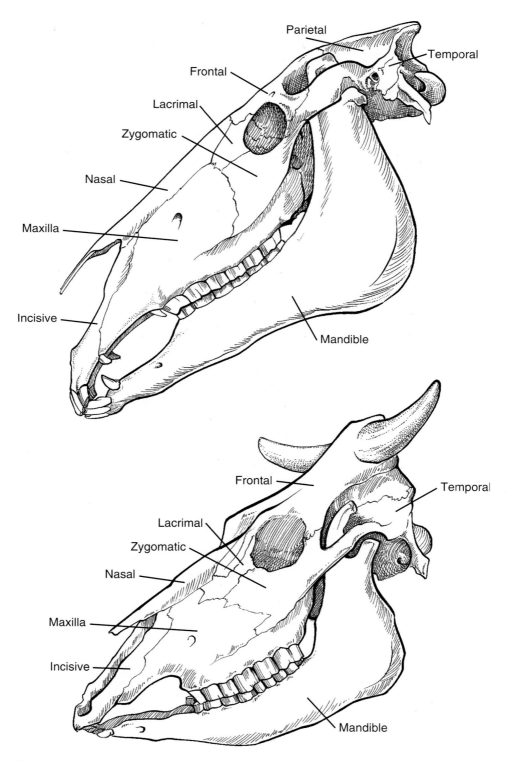

Figure 4-4. Equine (*left*) and bovine (*right*) skulls, lateral view.

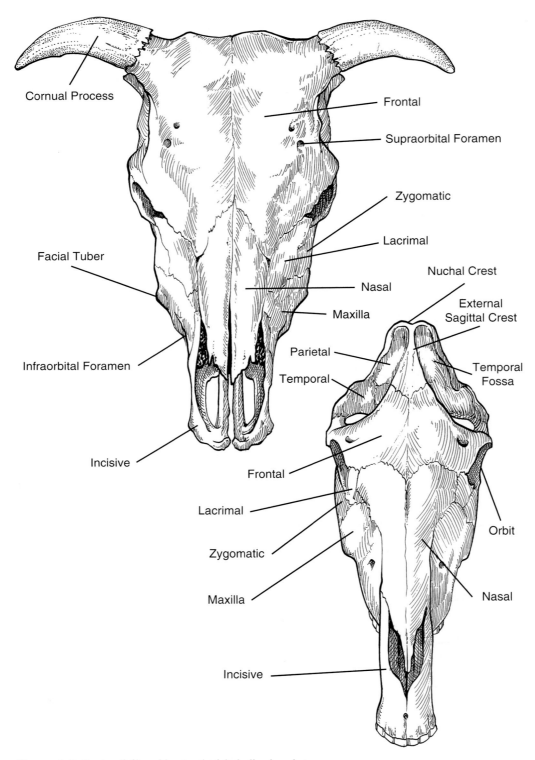

Figure 4-5. Equine (*left*) and bovine (*right*) skulls, dorsal view.

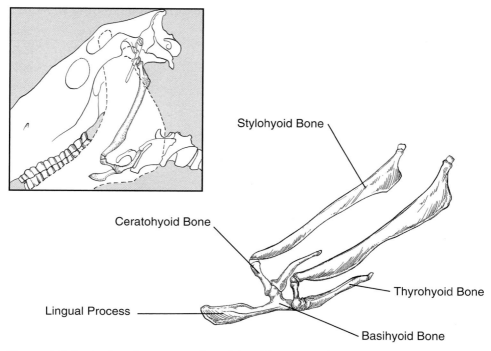

Figure 4-6. Equine hyoid apparatus. The stylohyoid bones articulate with the styloid processes of the skull, and the thyrohyoid bones articulate with the larynx. The prominent lingual process extends into the base of the tongue and affords an attachment site for some lingual muscles.

lowed by the number of vertebrae in that region in the given species. Vertebral formulas of common domestic animals and humans are shown in Table 4–3. The parts of a typical vertebra include the body, the arch, and the processes (Fig. 4–7).

The **body** is a cylindrical mass forming the ventral aspect of the vertebra and the vertebral foramen.

Dorsally, the **arch** completes the **vertebral foramen,** which contains the spinal cord. When vertebrae are placed in series, the adjacent arches form the **vertebral canal,** through which the spinal cord runs longitudinally.

Cranial and caudal **articular processes** form joints with adjacent vertebrae and ribs in the thoracic region.

The **spinous process** projects dorsad to form the spine of the vertebra. In the horse, the very tall spinous processes of the first few thoracic vertebrae form a dorsal prominence called the **withers.**

Transverse processes project laterad from the arch.

The **intervertebral foramina** are formed by the alignment of notches on adjacent vertebrae. Spinal nerves exit the vertebral canal via the intervertebral foramina on their way to innervating peripheral structures.

The **cervical vertebrae** have well-developed articular processes to accommodate the large range of motion of the neck. The other processes are less well developed in cervical vertebrae than in other regions. All domestic mammals have seven cervical vertebrae.

The **atlas** is the first cervical vertebra. The spinous process is absent. The atlas articulates with the occipital condyles of the skull cranially and with the axis caudally.

The **axis** is the second cervical vertebra. Its spinous process forms a longitudinal sail on its dorsum. The body of the axis features a cranial projection called the **dens** (for its resemblance

Table 4-3. Vertebral Formulas of Common Domestic Animals and Humans

Species	Cervical	Thoracic	Lumbar	Sacral	Caudal
Horse	7	18	6	5	15–20
Ox	7	13	6	5	18–20
Sheep	7	13	6–7	4	16–18
Goat	7	13	7	4	12
Hog	7	14–15	6–7	4	20–23
Dog	7	13	7	3	20–23
Chicken	14	7	14 (lumbosacral)		6
Human	7	12	5	5	4

to a tooth), which articulates with the body of the axis in a pivot joint.

The remaining cervical vertebrae are similar to one another, with small spinous processes and rather large transverse and articular processes. With the exception of the last cervical vertebra (C7), each cervical transverse process contains a *transverse foramen.*

Thoracic vertebrae are characterized by well-developed spinous processes and articular facets for the ribs. *Costal fovea* on the bodies of adjacent thoracic vertebrae form cavities for articulation with the heads of the ribs. Each transverse process also features a fovea for articulation with the tubercle of the rib of the same number as the vertebra.

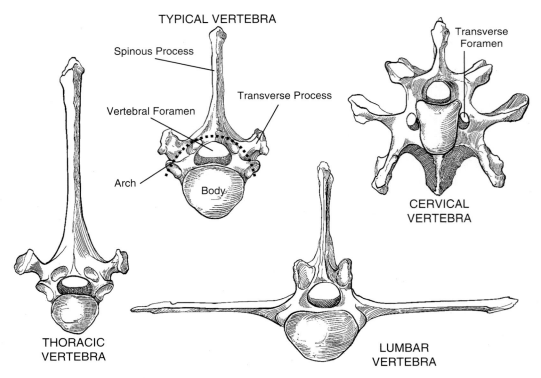

Figure 4-7. Typical vertebrae.

Lumbar vertebrae have large, flat transverse processes that project laterad. The spinous processes are similar to those of the last few thoracic vertebrae. The articular processes are more robust than those of the thoracic vertebrae, but not as large as the articular processes in the cervical region. The body and caudal articular processes of the last lumbar vertebra articulate with the sacrum.

The *sacral vertebrae* are fused to form a single wedge-shaped bone, the *sacrum,* which articulates with the last lumbar vertebra cranially, with the first caudal vertebra caudally, and with the wings of the ilia craniolaterally. The intervertebral foramina of the sacrum are represented by dorsal and ventral rows of *sacral foramina* on dorsal and ventral sides of the sacrum. These foramina, as with other intervertebral foramina, give passage to spinal nerves.

Caudal (coccygeal) vertebrae form the bony basis for the tail. Depending on the length of the tail, the number varies considerably from species to species and even within the same species. Size of the vertebrae decreases rapidly in a caudal direction, until the last few caudal vertebrae are merely small rods of bone.

Sternum and Ribs

The *sternum* forms the floor of the bony thorax and gives attachment to the *costal cartilages* of the ribs as well as providing a bony origin for the pectoral muscles. The cranial extremity of the sternum is the *manubrium;* the middle portion is the *body;* and the caudal extremity is the *xiphoid process.* The cranial extremity of the manubrium in the horse is the keellike *cariniform cartilage.* The sternum consists of individual bones called *sternebrae* that tend to fuse as age advances. The number of sternebrae varies with species as follows: pig and sheep, six each; ox and goat, seven; and horse and dog, eight.

The *ribs* form the lateral walls of the bony thorax. Usually the number of pairs of ribs is the same as the number of thoracic vertebrae. Rarely an extra rib or pair of ribs lies either cranial or caudal to the thoracic vertebrae. A typical rib consists of a *shaft,* a sternal extremity ventrally, and a vertebral extremity dorsally.

Except for the last one or two pairs of ribs, the sternal extremity is connected to the sternum by the costal hyaline cartilage; ribs so attached are called *sternal (true) ribs.* The vertebral extremity consists of a spherical *head* connected to the rib by a constricted *neck* and a *tubercle* that articulates with the transverse process of a thoracic vertebra. The head articulates with the bodies of two adjacent vertebrae at the costal fovea.

The number of sternal ribs corresponds to the number of sternebrae in the animal. The ribs caudal to the sternal ribs are called *asternal (false) ribs* because they are not directly connected to the sternum. The costal cartilages at the ventral extremity of most of the asternal ribs overlap and thus indirectly connect the asternal and sternal ribs. Sometimes the last pair or two of ribs have no connection with other ribs at the ventral end. Such ribs are called *floating ribs.* The spaces between adjacent ribs are the *intercostal spaces,* numbered to correspond to the number of the rib cranial to the space.

Appendicular Skeleton

The *appendicular skeleton* is made up of the bones of the limbs. The bones of the thoracic limb are compared to those of the pelvic limb by region in Table 4–4.

Pectoral Limbs

The *scapula* (shoulder blade) in all animals is a relatively flat triangular bone (Fig. 4–8). The distal portion is the ventral angle, and it forms the only true joint between the scapula and another bone in most domestic animals. Birds and higher primates have a *clavicle* (collarbone), which forms a joint with the scapula, but in most quadrupeds, the clavicle is represented only by the *clavicular tendon,* a connective tissue band within the brachiocephalicus muscle. The fused clavicles are called the *furcula,* or *wishbone,* in birds. Birds have a *coracoid* as a separate bone in addition to the scapula and clavicle. The coracoid in humans and domestic mammals has been reduced to the *coracoid*

Table 4-4. Comparison of Bones of Thoracic and Pelvic Limbs

Thoracic Limb		Pelvic Limb	
Part of Limb	*Bones*	*Part of Limb*	*Bones*
Thoracic (shoulder) girdle	Scapula, clavicle, coracoid	Pelvic girdle	Sacrum Pelvis: ilium, ischium, pubis
Brachium (arm)	Humerus	Thigh	Femur
Antebrachium (forearm)	Radius, ulna	Crus (true leg)	Tibia, fibula
Carpus (knee)	Carpal bones	Tarsus (hock)	Tarsal bones
Metacarpus (cannon and splint bones)	Metacarpal bones	Metatarsus (cannon and splint bones)	Metatarsal bones
Phalanges (digit)	Proximal, middle, and distal phalanges Proximal and distal sesamoid bones	Phalanges (digit)	Proximal, middle, and distal phalanges Proximal and distal sesamoid bones

process (a bony prominence), which protrudes mediad from the scapula near the ventral angle in most species.

The lateral face of the scapula has a ridge called the **spine** extending from the ventral angle to the dorsal border. In some species the distal end of the spine is flattened to form the **acromion process.** The spine divides the lateral face into the **supraspinous fossa,** which is cranial to the spine, and the **infraspinous fossa,** which is caudal and ventral to the spine. The costal (medial or deep) face of the scapula gives attachment to many of the muscles that connect the limb to the body.

The **humerus** (arm bone) is a long bone that varies only in minor details from one animal to another. It has a shaft and two extremities. The proximal end joins the ventral angle of the scapula to form the **scapulohumeral (shoulder) joint.** The proximal end of the humerus also features a number of irregular tuberosities and tubercles, providing sites of attachment to muscles of the shoulder region. The palpable prominence produced by this end of the humerus is called the **point of the shoulder.** The distal end of the humerus forms the elbow joint with the proximal ends of the radius and ulna.

The **radius** and **ulna** are the bones of the **antebrachium** (forearm). In mammals, the radius is the larger of the two, although in birds it is smaller than the ulna. The radius enters into the elbow joint proximally and the carpus distally.

The radius can be felt directly beneath the skin on the medial side of the forearm.

The **ulna** varies in its degree of development from species to species. The prominent **olecranon process (point of the elbow)** is found in all mammals proximal and caudal to the elbow joint. This process forms a lever for attachment of the muscles that extend the elbow. In the horse, the proximal portion of the shaft of the ulna is well developed but fused to the radius. The ox, sheep, goat, and pig each have a complete ulna, but with little or no movement between the ulna and radius. The cat and dog have considerably more movement between these complete bones, but not nearly as much as primates, who can pronate and supinate their hands.

The **carpus** in all animals is a complex region that includes two rows of small bones. This region corresponds to the human wrist, and is frequently, although erroneously, called the knee by horsemen. Carpal bones in the proximal row are called (from medial to lateral) **radial, intermediate,** and **ulnar,** while those in the distal row are numbered 1 to 4 from medial to lateral. In addition, an **accessory carpal bone** projects caudad from the lateral side of the carpus. The numbering of the carpal bones of the distal row is based on an ancestral four, but among common domestic farm animals only the pig consistently has four carpal bones in this distal row. The first carpal bone of the horse, when present, is small

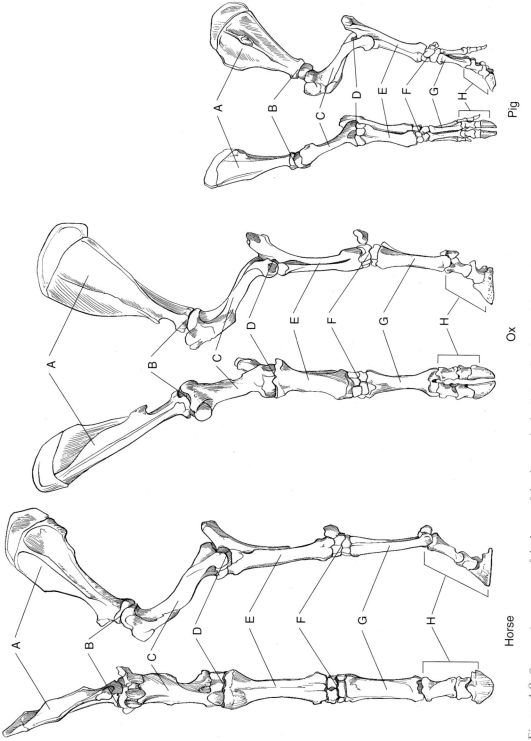

Figure 4-8. Comparative anatomy of the bones of the thoracic limb. *A*) Scapula, *B*) Scapulohumeral (shoulder joint), *C*) Humerus, *D*) Elbow joint, *E*) Antebrachium (radius & ulna), *F*) Carpus, *G*) Metacarpus, *H*) Digit (Phalanges).

Horse

Ox

Pig

and non–weight bearing. The first carpal is not present in ruminants, and the second and third carpal bones are fused in these species.

The **metacarpus** is immediately distal to the carpus. In the horse it includes one large **metacarpal (cannon) bone,** the base for the third digit (corresponding to the middle finger), and two small metacarpal (**splint**) bones. The second metacarpal bone is on the medial side, and the fourth is on the lateral side. Trauma to these small bones with consequent excess bone formation results in **splints.** Splints in horses sometimes produce lameness but often constitute only a **blemish,** a disfigurement not associated with unsoundness (Figure 4–9).

The cannon bone of the ox and sheep is a fusion of the third and fourth metacarpal bones. A vertical groove on the dorsum of the cannon bone indicates the embryonic line of fusion.

The pig has four metacarpal bones. The first

is absent; the second and fifth are reduced; and the third and fourth bear most of the weight.

The **digits** number one to five, depending on the species. The horse, having only one digit, literally walks on the tip of the middle finger, or third digit. The digits, like the metacarpal bones, are numbered from one to five from medial to lateral. Each complete digit is made up of three **phalanges (proximal phalanx, middle phalanx,** and **distal phalanx**). In the horse the proximal phalanx is also called the **long pastern bone;** the middle phalanx, the **short pastern bone;** and distal phalanx, the **coffin bone.** Each digit also includes two **proximal sesamoid bones** at the palmar aspect of the joint between the 3rd metacarpal bone and proximal phalanx and a **distal sesamoid (navicular) bone** at the junction of the middle and distal phalanges.

Horsemen refer to the joint between the cannon bone and the proximal phalanx (the metacarpophalangeal joint) as the **fetlock.** The portion of the digit between the fetlock and the hoof is the **pastern.**

The ox, sheep, and goat have two principal digits, the third and fourth, while the second and fifth digits are represented only by the small **dewclaws** at the back of the pastern. In the pig the dewclaws are more fully developed as digits (Figure 4–8).

Pelvic Limbs

The **pelvis** consists of a circle of bones by which the pelvic limbs articulate with the vertebral column (Fig. 4–10). Each **hemipelvis** (half a pelvis) comprises three bones, which are fused to form the **os coxae,** or **pelvic bone** (Figure 4–11). The two **ossa coxarum** are firmly attached to one another at the **pelvic symphysis** ventrally and are joined to the sacrum of the axial skeleton by two strong **sacroiliac joints.** The three bones entering into the formation of each ox coxae are the **ilium,** the **ischium,** and the **pubis.** All three of these participate in the formation of the acetabulum of the hip joint.

The **ilium** is the largest and most dorsal of the pelvic bones. It is irregularly triangular, with the apex at the acetabulum and the base projecting craniodorsad. The medial angle, the

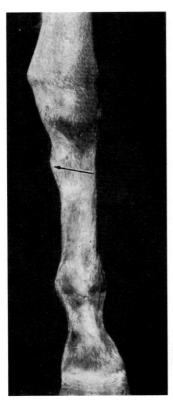

Figure 4-9. Medial splint. (Reprinted with permission from Stashak, T.S.: *Adams' Lameness in Horses.* 5th ed. Baltimore, Lippincott Williams & Wilkins, 2002.)

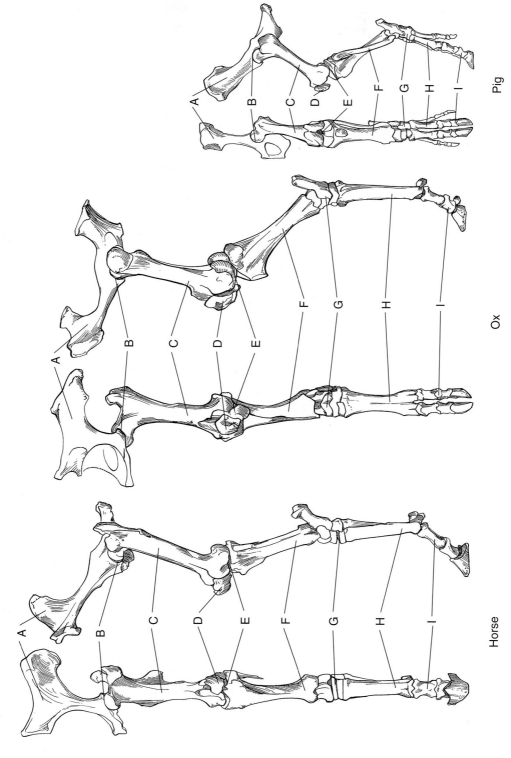

Figure 4-10. Comparative anatomy of the bones of the pelvic limb. *A)* Pelvis, *B)* Coxofemoral (Hip) joint, *C)* Femur, *D)* Patella, *E)* Stifle (Knee) joint, *F)* Crus (Tibia & Fibula), *G)* Tarsus (Hock), *H)* Metatarsus, *I)* Digit (Phalanges).

Horse

Ox

Pig

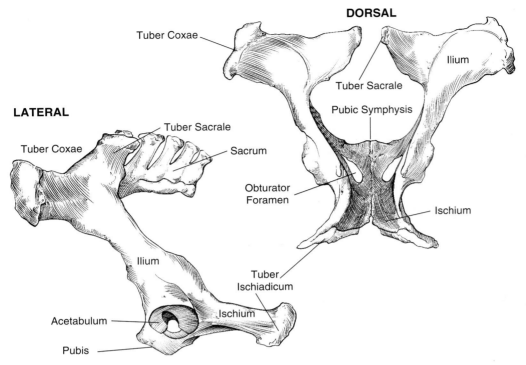

Figure 4-11. The pelvis of the ox . Cranial (*left*) and lateral (*right*) views.

tuber sacrale, is close to the sacroiliac joint near the midline. The lateral angle, the *tuber coxae,* is known as the *point of the hip* (often called the *hook bone* by cattlemen). A fracture of the tuber coxae in the horse results in obvious asymmetry in the two points of the hips, as viewed from behind. Horsemen call this condition a *knock-down hip.*

The broad, flat portion between the tuber coxae and tuber sacrale is the *wing* of the ilium, and the dorsal margin is the *iliac crest.* The body of the ilium projects ventrad and caudad between the wing and acetabulum and helps form the lateral wall of the pelvic cavity.

The *ischium* projects backward and ventrad from the acetabulum, forming much of the floor of the pelvic cavity. The ischium has a large roughened caudal prominence, the *tuber ischiadicum,* commonly called the *pin bone* in cattle.

The *pubis,* the smallest of the three pelvic bones, forms the cranial part of the floor of the pelvic cavity. The pubis also enters into the formation of the acetabulum and meets the pubis

of the opposite side at the symphysis. The pubis and ischium form the boundaries of the *obturator foramen.*

The *femur* (thigh bone) extends from the *coxofemoral* (*hip*) *joint* to the *stifle* (the joint corresponding to the human knee) (Fig. 4–9). The proximal end of the femur has a nearly spherical *head* that articulates with the acetabulum of the os coxae to form the hip joint. There are also several roughened prominences, the *trochanters,* for the attachment of heavy thigh and hip muscles. The shaft of the femur is nearly circular on cross-section and has considerable length. The distal end has two condyles for articulation with the tibia and a trochlea for articulation with the *patella,* a sesamoid bone embedded in the tendon of insertion of the large quadriceps muscle.

The *tibia* and *fibula* are the bones of the true leg (*crus*), the portion of the pelvic limb between stifle and hock. The tibia, the larger of the two, is palpable beneath the skin medially. The fibula, which is much smaller, is on the lateral side of the leg.

The tibia has an expanded proximal end that participates in the stifle joint. Its shaft is triangular in cross-section. The distal end of the tibia has two concave depressions that form the hinge joint of the hock with the **talus** (***tibiotarsal bone***).

In the dog, pig, and humans, the fibula is a long, thin bone extending from the proximal end of the tibia to the lateral aspect of the hock. The horse has both the proximal end and a portion of the shaft, whereas only a vestige of the proximal end of the fibula is present in domestic ruminants. All domestic species have the distal extremity of the fibula, forming the prominent ***lateral malleolus*** of the hock. The lateral malleolus is fused to the tibia in the horse but is a separate small bone articulating with distal tibia in ruminants.

The ***tarsus*** (***hock***) is composed of small bones much like the carpus in the thoracic limb; it corresponds to the human ankle. The proximal row of tarsal bones consists of two large bones. The ***talus*** dorsally has two spool-like ridges for articulation with the tibia. The ***calcaneus*** projects proximad and caudad to form the point of the hock. The calcaneus, which corresponds to the human heel, acts as a lever for the muscles extending the hock.

In the horse, the central row of tarsal bones is reduced to a single ***central tarsal bone.*** The bones of the distal row are numbered 1 to 4 from medial to lateral, with tarsal bones 1 and 2 fused into a single bone. In cattle, tarsal bones 2 and 3 are fused, as are the central and 4th.

The metatarsus and digits of the pelvic limb are similar to the metacarpus and digits of the thoracic limb.

Chapter 5

Microscopic Anatomy and Growth and Development of Bone

Microscopic Anatomy and Formation of Bone

About a third of the weight of bone consists of an organic framework of fibrous tissue and cells. This organic matter mainly consists of collagen and polysaccharides called **glycosaminoglycans** (**GAGs**), which contain chondroitin sulfate. They give resilience and toughness to bones. The remaining two-thirds of the weight of bone consists of inorganic calcium and phosphorus salts in the organic framework. About 80% of these salts are calcium phosphate, and the remainder is primarily calcium carbonate and magnesium phosphate. The calcium phosphate is primarily found in **hydroxyapatite** crystals formed with calcium hydroxide. These salts give hardness and rigidity to bones and make them resist the passage of x-rays. If the inorganic salts are removed by soaking a bone in dilute acid, the resulting decalcified bone will retain its original form but will be flexible enough to be tied in a knot. On the other hand, if the organic matter is removed by charring in a furnace so that only the inorganic salts remain, the bone will retain its form but be brittle and break unless handled with extreme care.

Mature bone consists of **osteocytes** (bone cells) surrounded by an intercellular matrix composed of calcified **osteoid** material. The osteocytes are in small cavities in the bone called **lacunae** (meaning little lakes) (Fig. 5–1). A system of tiny canals called canaliculi connects the lacunae within the substance of the bone. Even

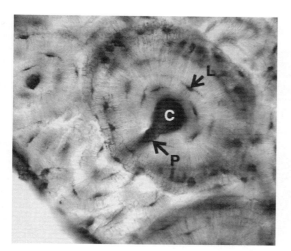

Figure 5-1. Unstained ground bone. Osteocytes in lacunae (L) and fine canaliculi extend from each lacuna. The central (C) and perforating (P) canals contain blood vessels, nerves, and lymphatics. (Reprinted with permission from Dellmann, H.D. and Eurell, J. *Textbook of Veterinary Histology*. 5th ed. Baltimore: Lippincott Williams & Wilkins, 1998.)

though bone is highly vascular, with capillaries close together, the canaliculi transmit tissue fluid that is essential for maintaining the life of the osteocytes.

Both the lacunae and canaliculi are formed because cytoplasmic processes connect the *osteoblasts* (bone-forming cells) at the time the osteoid material is laid down. Thus the cells and their processes act as a mold until the osteoid tissue is set and mineralized. The cytoplasm is then partially withdrawn, leaving the cells, now known as osteocytes, in the lacunae, which are connected by canaliculi containing cytoplasmic extensions.

Cancellous bone, or spongy bone, consists of a network of fingerlike bony spicules, or *trabeculae.* This type of bone is found in the extremities of long bones, where resistance to compression without excessive weight is needed. Flat bones between two layers of compact bone, as in the skull, are also cancellous. The spicules of bone are arranged so as to resist stresses and strains imposed on the bone by weight or pull of muscles.

Compact bone, found in the shafts of long bones, consists primarily of many laminated tubes known as *osteonal* systems (formally termed haversian systems). Each osteon consists of one central canal containing vessels and nerves surrounded by circular plates of bone (*osteonal lamellae*) forming the laminated cylinder (Fig. 5–2). These plates are laid down in a centripetal fashion (from the periphery toward the center). After the bone is formed, the osteoblasts that became embedded in the bone substance are called osteocytes. In general these osteons are added on the periphery of the shaft of a bone as the bone increases in diameter. Blood vessels extend from the periosteum to central canals through *perforating canals* (also known as *Volkmann's canals*), which often travel at right angles to the central canals (Fig. 5–2).

Osteoblasts usually come from mesenchymal cells, the parent cells of all connective tissues. The osteoblasts divide readily, but only a portion of the new cells actually secretes osteoid substance and forms bone; the rest is held in reserve as the osteogenic layer of the *periosteum* and *endosteum* within the marrow cavity and central canals. These reserve cells divide and form more osteoblasts whenever more bone is needed, as in repair of fractures, response to stress, or growth. Because the intercellular matrix is unyielding, bone can be added only on the surface, and the osteocytes (mature osteoblasts) probably have lost the ability to divide.

As the shaft of a long bone enlarges in diameter as a result of the activity of the osteogenic layer of the periosteum, bone along the inner surface is normally resorbed to increase the size of the marrow cavity (Fig. 5–3). Resorption of bone may also occur under abnormal conditions, such as during a period of calcium deficiency. Whenever bone is resorbed (under normal or abnormal conditions), large multinucleated cells called *osteoclasts* (bone-destroying cells) usually are found (Fig. 5–4). These cells, derived from macrophages, take an active part in bone destruction by releasing organic acids and enzymes.

Ossification

Ossification is the formation of true bone by deposition of calcium salts in a matrix of osteoid tissue. *Calcification* refers to the deposi-

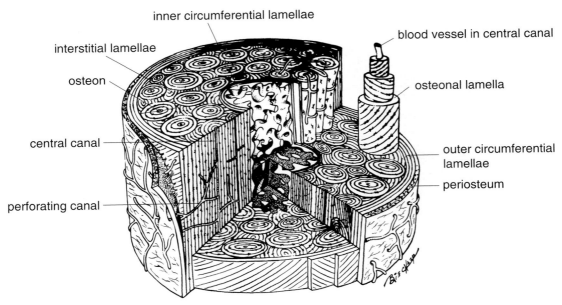

inner circumferential lamellae

interstitial lamellae

osteon

central canal

perforating canal

blood vessel in central canal

osteonal lamella

outer circumferential lamellae

periosteum

Figure 5-2. The structural unit of compact bone is the osteon. An osteon is telescoped to show the concentric layers of bone that surround a central canal. Interstitial lamellae of bone fill the space between osteons, and the inner and outer surfaces are formed by inner and outer circumferential lamellae. (Reprinted with permission from Dellmann, H.D. and Eurell, J. *Textbook of Veterinary Histology.* 5th ed. Baltimore: Lippincott Williams & Wilkins, 1998.)

tion of calcium salts in any tissue. Calcification of tissue other than osteoid is usually associated with some pathologic process.

Regardless of the location, the sequence of actual bone formation consists of osteoblasts laying down osteoid tissue that is subsequently calcified under the influence of the enzyme alkaline phosphatase. A local area of bone formation is called a *center of ossification* (Fig. 5–5). The environment in which bone forms determines whether the type of ossification is endochondral or intramembranous.

Endochondral (Intracartilaginous) Ossification

During fetal development, most of the skeleton first develops as a cartilage pattern or model, and then the cartilage of this model is gradually replaced by bone. This process is called endochondral ossification. The center of ossification that develops in the midshaft region of a long

bone is the *primary ossification center* (Fig. 5–5). Secondary ossification centers then develop near the ends of long bones. These ossification centers grow and expand, but a region of cartilage, the *physis,* still separates the centers during growth and development. *Chondrocytes* within this region continue to proliferate and produce cartilage to provide this separation and thus allow for continued growth in the length of the long bone.

The midshaft region of a long bone that contains the primary ossification center is the *diaphysis;* each end that contains a secondary ossification center is an *epiphysis* (Fig. 5–5). As animals grow and mature, the region of cartilage that separates the bony diaphysis and epiphyses continues to narrow. *Epiphyseal plate,* another term used to describe this region of cartilage in growing animals, emphasizes how narrow it may become.

When the cartilage in the epiphyseal plates is completely replaced by bone, increases in length, hence growth in stature of the animal, is impossible. This is epiphyseal closure. An epi-

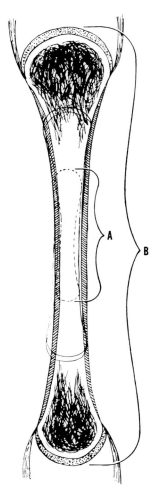

Figure 5-3. Remodeling that occurs as a long bone increases in size. Both resorption and deposition of bone take place. *A)* Size and shape of young bone. *B)* Size and shape of mature bone. (After Grant, J. C. *A Method of Anatomy.* Baltimore: Williams & Wilkins, 1971.)

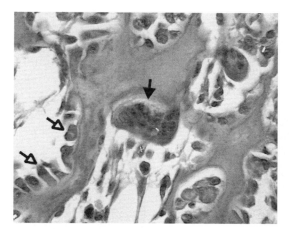

Figure 5-4. Osteoclast (*solid arrow*) resorbs bone. Osteoblasts (*open arrows*) form bone. (Reprinted with permission from Dellmann, H.D. and Eurell, J. *Textbook of Veterinary Histology.* 5th ed. Baltimore: Lippincott Williams & Wilkins, 1998.)

physeal line can often be seen on bones where this closure has occurred. The region of a long bone where the diaphysis and an epiphysis meet is a *metaphysis* (Fig. 5–5).

Several hormones affect the rate of growth of long bones, but *growth hormone* and sex hormones (*androgens* and *estrogens*) are key regulators. In general, growth hormone promotes elongation of long bones, while the sex hormones promote growth and epiphyseal closure. Growth hormone itself has little direct effect on chondrocytes within epiphyseal plates. It stimulates other cells within the area

of the plates and in the liver to produce peptides, *insulinlike growth factors* (IGFs), which in turn stimulate the chondrocytes to proliferate and increase their rate of cartilage production. This provides more cartilage in which bone can form to increase the length of the long bone. **The critical role of IGFs has been confirmed in some human dwarfs and African pygmies who have normal blood levels of growth hormone but who fail to grow because of low levels of IGFs.**

Androgens, such as the sex hormone testosterone, and estrogens have a variety of complex effects on the rates of bone growth. The well-recognized growth spurt associated with puberty is thought to be due to stimulatory effects of androgens and estrogens that increase in circulation at this time. Androgens appear to have a greater stimulatory effect than estrogens, and this difference is responsible in part for differences in body size between males and females. The stimulatory effects of androgens on growth are in part due to their ability to increase the secretion of growth hormone. While sex hormones are capable of stimulating the rate of growth, they also bring about epiphyseal closure, which ultimately limits body size. The mechanisms responsible for this effect are not completely understood, but differences in

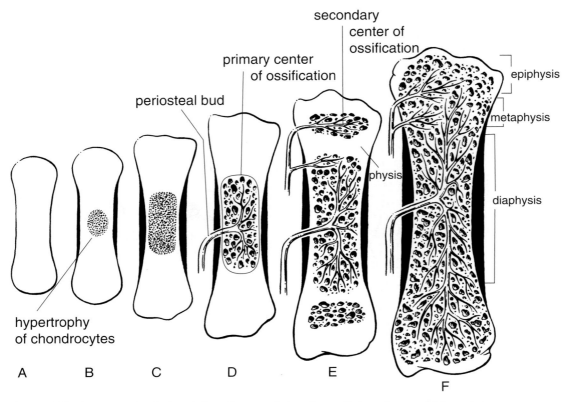

Figure 5-5. The stages of endochondral ossification of a long bone. *A)* A cartilage model forms initially. *B)* The chondrocytes in the center of the model hypertrophy. *C)* Blood vessels from the periosteum (periosteal bud) invade the cartilage model, bringing bone-forming cells to initiate the primary center of ossification. *D)* The physis and secondary centers of ossification are established. *E)* The growth plate closes in the mature bone and a confluent marrow cavity from the epiphysis to the diaphysis is formed. (Adapted with permission from Dellmann, H.D. and Eurell, J. *Textbook of Veterinary Histology.* 5th ed. Baltimore: Lippincott Williams & Wilkins, 1998.)

the magnitude of their stimulatory effect on ossification versus their stimulatory effect on cartilage production may be responsible.

Intramembranous Ossification

Many of the flat bones, such as bones of the skull, are preformed in a fibrous membrane, or matrix, which is infiltrated with osteoid tissue. The osteoid tissue calcifies to form true bone. The layers of periosteum on either side of the bone then form additional bone. Like long bones of the limbs, large flat bones in mature animals consist of compact bone surrounding a cancellous bone core.

Physiology of Bone

Bone Mechanics and Remodeling

Elasticity is the characteristic of a substance that enables it to change shape when subjected to stress but return to its original shape when the stress is removed. Mature bone is relatively inelastic. A rod of bone can be elongated only about 0.5% of its length before breaking. However, even this much deformity is not perfectly elastic; the deformity is permanent, and the bone will not return completely to its original length if stretched near its breaking point. This characteristic of deforming under stress without returning to the original shape is exaggerated in bone diseases such as rickets.

In addition to tension (stretching), bone may be subjected to stresses of compression, shearing, bending, and torsion (twisting). A bone will support considerably more weight in a static situation (supporting weight without moving) than under a dynamic load. A dynamic load results from impact between the bone and another object. For example, the leg bones of a horse bear a static load when the horse is standing quietly but bear a dynamic load when the horse is running, jumping, or kicking. Compression, bending, and shearing of the leg bones are all stresses produced by this type of activity. When a horse or other animal pivots with one or more feet bearing weight, torsion or twisting is added to the other stresses. This is seen particularly well in the action of cutting horses. Muscles and tendons that run parallel to a bone tend to act like guy wires and reduce stresses, particularly bending and shearing stresses.

Bone, even in a fresh carcass, appears hard, dense, inelastic, and almost lifeless. Actually bone is quite a dynamic tissue, and all bone is constantly being formed and resorbed. The continuous turnover of bone in mature animals is termed **remodeling.** Through remodeling, bone can shrink (atrophy), increase in size (hypertrophy), repair breaks, and rearrange its internal structure to best resist stresses and strains. In both normal and pathologic conditions, bone can reshape itself according to good engineering principles to sustain a maximum of stress with a minimum of bone tissue. **Atrophy of bone occurs when pressure is constant and excessive or when there is little or no stress, as in weightlessness in space or when a limb is immobilized and not bearing weight. Proliferation of bone may occur in response to concussion or intermittent pressure. Thus, pressure can cause either atrophy or proliferation, depending on the degree and duration of stress and the maturity of the bone. Excessive pressure on growing bone slows or stops growth, while in mature bone it may stimulate either excessive growth or rearrangement of structure.**

Calcium of Bone

In 100 cc of bone there is 10 g of calcium, as compared with 6 mg per 100 cc for most tissues and about 10 mg per 100 mL for blood. Thus, bone serves as a reservoir of minerals, especially calcium, that is constantly being either replenished or depleted. Through the action of osteoclasts and osteocytes, calcium can be taken from this reservoir when serum calcium levels are low. The reservoir can be replenished by the action of osteoblasts and osteocytes.

The activity of the cells within bone is subject to regulation by the hormones **parathyroid hormone (PTH)** and **calcitonin.** The sources of these hormones and the regulation of their secretion are discussed in Chapter 12. The overall effect of PTH is to increase serum calcium by increasing the net release of calcium salts from bone. This effect is due in part to increased osteoclast activity and inhibition of osteoblast activity. PTH also affects osteocytes in mature bone, and these cells also play a role in the rapid release of calcium salts in response to PTH. However, the mechanism by which osteocytes promote a rapid release of calcium is poorly understood. The primary effect of calcitonin is to reduce osteoclast activity, which tends to lower serum calcium. Thus, the normal regulation of serum calcium concentrations involves a balancing of the effects of PTH and calcitonin on the cells of bone.

Fractures and Fracture Healing

A fracture of bone is simply a break in the continuity of a bone. Among the many types of fractures described are the following (Fig. 5–6):

A **simple fracture** is one in which the skin over the fracture site is unbroken.

An **open fracture** is one in which a wound from the exterior contacts the bone at the point of the fracture. This may be caused by a broken end of bone perforating the skin or by a penetrating object, such as a bullet, causing the fracture.

A **greenstick fracture** is one in which one side of the bone is broken or splintered and the

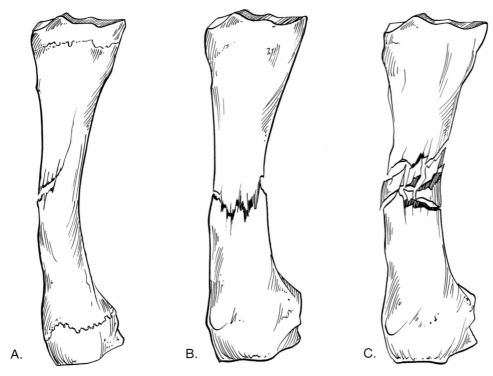

Figure 5-6. Types of fractures. *A)* Greenstick. *B)* Complete. *C)* Comminuted. (After Kahn, F. *Man in Structure and Function.* New York: Alfred A. Knopf, 1943.)

other side only bent. This type of fracture usually is found only in young animals.

A *complete fracture* is one in which the bone is broken entirely across.

A *physeal fracture* (formally known as epiphyseal fracture) is one that occurs at the junction of an epiphysis and the diaphysis of a bone. This type of fracture is limited to young animals.

A *comminuted fracture* is one in which the bone was splintered or crushed, producing small fragments.

If the broken ends of a fractured bone are brought into apposition (touch) and are immobilized (prevented from moving), the normal process of healing will take place (Fig. 5–7). When the fracture occurs, some blood vessels are ruptured, releasing blood around the broken ends of the bone. This forms a clot that is invaded by connective tissue cells forming *granulation tissue* (term for mass of tissue consisting largely of fibroblasts and capillaries). The osteoblasts from the surface of the bone,

from the periosteum, and from the endosteum lining the marrow cavities and haversian canals divide rapidly and produce a massive amount of osteoid tissue called a *callus.* The osteoid tissue fills the gap between the broken ends of the bone, fills the marrow cavity for a distance, and completely encircles the broken ends of the bone, forming an effective splint that usually prevents movement between the segments. The callus becomes mineralized, changing into true bone. Remodeling of the callus to form a typical bone shaft with a marrow cavity completes the healing process. Misalignment of the fractured bone is corrected to some extent by the action of osteocytes and osteoclasts, which also remove excessive internal and external callus. As soon as the bone is put to use, functional orientation of the callus begins, with a tendency to straighten imperfections in the alignment of the bone. The callus will increase in size on the concave side, where stress is greatest, and tend to erode on the convex side, thus tending to correct any deformity.

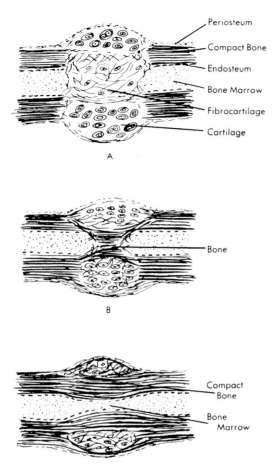

Periosteum
Compact Bone
Endosteum
Bone Marrow
Fibrocartilage
Cartilage

A

Bone

B

Compact Bone
Bone Marrow

C

Figure 5-7. Some stages in healing of a fracture of a long bone. *A)* Early soft callus replaces blood clot. *B)* Intermediate callus. *C)* Nearly healed hard callus.

The amount of spontaneous correction that is possible in fractures depends on a number of factors, including age of the animal, blood supply to the bone, degree of correction necessary, presence or absence of infection, and amount of damage to surrounding tissues. Excessive separation of fragments, which may be caused by too much traction or incomplete immobilization of a fracture, may result in nonunion, with fibrous tissue filling the gap between fragments.

Quickest fracture healing occurs in young animals, particularly if the fracture site has a good blood supply and is completely immobilized with the ends of the fragments in apposition. In man, a fracture may heal completely within a month in an infant, but a similar fracture in a person past middle age may require 6 months or longer to heal.

If bone healing is delayed or a major defect has resulted from a severe fracture or surgical removal of bone, grafting or transplanting bone into the damaged area may stimulate healing. Bone for grafts may be obtained from the same animal that is receiving the graft (*autogenous graft*) or from another animal of the same species (*allograft*). Autogenous grafts are typically cancellous bone obtained from a site such as the proximal end of the humerus. Allografts of cortical bone may be used relatively intact or as bone chips to fill deficient areas. Autogenous grafts have an advantage in that the portion of the bone in contact with tissue fluid may survive and the osteoblasts become active. At the same time, osteoclasts remove the dead portions of the graft, which are replaced by healthy bone if the graft is functional and subjected to the proper amount of stress. Osteoblasts in allografts die, because the animal body tends to reject any foreign protein.

Other Pathologic Conditions

Other pathologic conditions of bones may be caused by infections, tumors, endocrine disturbances, or nutritional imbalances. Tuberculosis of bone and *osteomyelitis* (inflammation of the bone and bone marrow) are two infections sometimes seen in bone. In man, osteomyelitis usually is caused by staphylococci or streptococci that gain access to the bone by way of the blood stream and develop into a general infection or by way of a wound, in which case the infection may remain local.

Benign (slow growing, noninvasive, and not likely to cause death) bone tumors are named according to the cells of bone from which they originate. A tumor of bone tissue itself is called an *osteoma. Chondromas* may develop from the epiphyseal cartilage or from unabsorbed islands of cartilage that preceded the developing bone. Tumors develop and grow as a result of intrinsic changes in the cells of origin, but bony growths may also occur on the surface of a bone simply in response to prolonged irritation. Such growths are called *exostoses.*

Malignant tumors grow rapidly, metastasize (spread to other locations), and are often fatal if not treated. *Osteogenic sarcomas* are malignant tumors of bone that most commonly develop near the ends of long bones. *Sarcoma* is a general term for malignant tumors originating from tissues of mesodermal origin, such as connective tissue.

Osteodystrophy is a general term for any abnormality in bone development. Many osteodystrophies are due to some abnormality in the normal regulation of calcium and phosphorus. The abnormality could be produced as a result of an inappropriate diet or some disease state disrupting calcium and phosphorus regulation.

Rickets in young, growing animals and *osteomalacia* in adults are conditions of inadequate mineralization of osteoid. Without appropriate mineralization, bones are relatively weak and flexible. Both rickets and osteomalacia usually are due to a lack of vitamin D, which is required for normal absorption of calcium from the gastrointestinal tract. However, they may also be caused by an imbalance or lack of calcium and/or phosphorus in the diet. Rickets chiefly affects the growing areas in bone, while osteomalacia, sometimes called adult rickets, affects the entire bone, since there are no rapidly growing areas in adult bone.

Achondroplasia is a hereditary condition in which the metaphyses fuse early in life but the bones continue to increase in diameter. An animal affected with it is called an achondroplastic dwarf. The dachshund is a breed of dogs selectively bred for this condition. Dwarfism in cattle closely resembles achondroplasia.

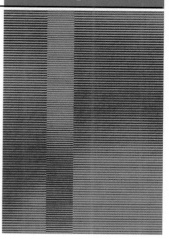

JOINTS

*S*yndesmology *(arthrology)* is the study of the *articulations* (unions) between bones, which are commonly called *joints.* Joints can be classified by a variety of schemes, usually anatomy or degree of movement. The tissue that unites the bones of a joint is generally fibrous tissue or cartilage. The structure and arrangement of these tissues is specialized for the joint's specific task.

Classification of Joints

Based on their structure and the material that unites them, joints may be classified as fibrous, cartilaginous, or synovial. These classifications can be combined as follows:

Fibrous Joints

Fibrous joints have no joint cavity. The bones are united by fibrous tissue (Fig. 6–1).

    Syndesmosis refers to a joint united by fibrous tissue that permits only slight movement. The normal union of the shafts of the splint bones and cannon bone of the horse is an example of syndesmosis.

    Suture is the junction between bones of the skull, which is fibrous tissue early in life but may ossify after maturity.

    Gomphosis is the specialized articulation of teeth in their alveoli (sockets) in the mandible and maxilla. The collagenous tissues and fibro-

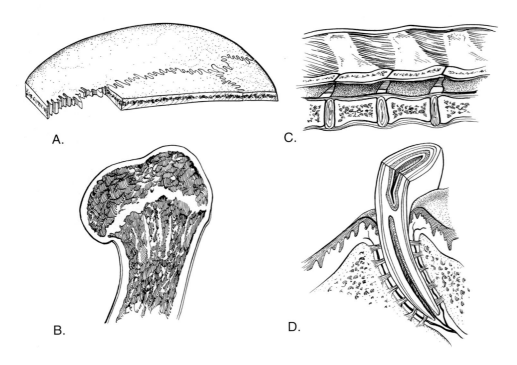

Figure 6-1. Types of fibrous joints. *A)* Suture. *B)* Synchondrosis (growth plate). *C)* Symphysis (an intervertebral disk). *D)* Gomphosis.

blasts that join the tooth to the socket constitute the *periodontium.*

Cartilaginous Joints

The bones of a *cartilaginous joint* are united by cartilage, with no intervening joint cavity.

Synchondrosis is an immovable joint in which the uniting medium is hyaline cartilage. The union of the diaphysis and epiphysis of an immature bone is an example of synchondrosis. (Fig. 6–1)

Symphyses (fibrocartilaginous joints) are united by flattened discs of fibrocartilage as found between adjacent pubic bones and between the bodies of adjacent vertebrae and sternebrae.

The fibrous or cartilaginous tissues separating adjacent bones in syndesmoses, synchondroses, and symphyses can be replaced by bone, as a result of either aging or degenerative processes. When this occurs, the joint is sometimes called a *synostosis.*

Synovial Joints

Most *synovial* (formerly called diarthrodial) *joints* have similar general structure, which includes articular surfaces, articular cartilages, articular cavity, joint capsule, and ligaments (Fig. 6–2).

The *articular surfaces* are specialized layers of compact bone on the surfaces that articulate with other bones.

The *articular cartilage* is a layer of hyaline cartilage covering the articular surface.

The *articular cavity* is a space between the adjacent bones of the joint surrounded by the joint capsule. Because the space is normally very small, having within it only a very small amount of lubricating fluid, it is called a potential space. Inflammation can expand the space with accumulation of fluid, a condition called *joint effusion.*

The *joint capsule* consists of two layers. The deeper layer is the *synovial membrane,* a delicate layer of specialized connective tissue extending from the edges of the articular carti-

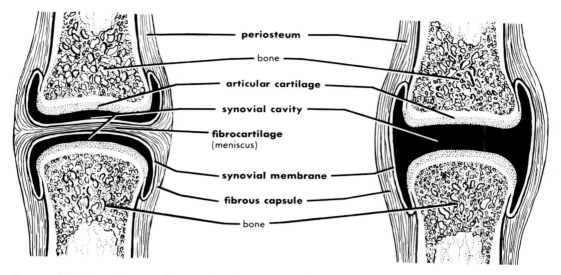

Figure 6-2. Synovial joints. (Reprinted with permission from Crouch, J.E. *Functional Human Anatomy.* 4th ed. Philadelphia: Lea & Febiger, 1985.)

lages of the adjacent bones but not covering the articular cartilage. This membrane secretes the **synovial fluid (synovia),** which lubricates the normal joint. The synovial membrane's surface area may be increased by folds (**plicae synoviales**), which may contain fat pads and which project into the joint cavity. Villi (**villi synoviales**), fingerlike projections, may also project into the joint cavity.

The superficial layer of the joint capsule is the **fibrous membrane,** a heavier fibrous sleeve adjacent to the synovial membrane. This fibrous layer may be thickened in certain areas to form the extracapsular (or periarticular) ligaments that connect adjacent bones and help stabilize the joint.

Ligaments, in relation to the musculoskeletal system, are connective tissue bands that extend from bone to bone. (Folds of serous membrane as seen in the thoracic, abdominal, and pelvic cavities are also called ligaments and are described with the appropriate organs in other chapters.) **Tendons** are connective tissue bands that connect muscle to bone and are described in Chapter 7.

Intracapsular (intra-articular) ligaments are found within joints and are surrounded by the synovial membrane. The cruciate ligaments of the stifle are intracapsular ligaments.

Extracapsular (periarticular) ligaments are external to the joint capsule; they include collateral, dorsal, palmar, plantar, and annular ligaments. **Collateral ligaments** lie on the medial and lateral aspects of a joint. **Dorsal** and **palmar (or plantar) ligaments** lie in front of and behind the joint. **Annular ligaments** surround the joint, and their fibers generally circle the joint to strengthen and protect the capsule.

Menisci (fibrocartilage discs) are interposed between surfaces of some joints, where they contribute to the congruency of the articular cartilages and probably play a role in complex joint movements. Menisci are truly intracapsular in that they are not covered by synovial membrane. Prominent menisci are found in the stifle and the temporomandibular joint.

Other Synovial Structures

Synovial membrane is also associated with two other structures, discussed more completely in Chapter 7. A **bursa** is a small, fluid-filled sac lined with synovial membrane. Bursae act as cushions and are generally found where tendons cross over a bony prominence.

Tendons may also be protected from bony prominences by a **synovial sheath,** a synovial membrane–lined tube that wraps around the tendon's circumference. Synovial sheaths are particularly noteworthy in the distal limbs, where long tendons pass over joints. Inflammation of a synovial sheath and its tendon, or *tenosynovitis,* may follow trauma or penetrating injury and can result in a very obvious and painful distension of the sheath. Tendons and synovial sheaths are discussed more completely in Chapter 7.

Movements of Joints

Synovial joints may exhibit one or more of the following movements: gliding or sliding, flexion, extension, hyperextension, rotation, adduction, abduction, and circumduction (Fig. 6–3).

Gliding or *sliding* movement occurs between two more or less flat surfaces in plane joints.

Flexion is movement in the sagittal plane that tends to decrease the angle between segments making up a joint. The carpus must be

flexed when a horse's front foot is picked up for trimming.

Extension is the reverse of flexion and is movement in the sagittal plane that tends to increase the angle between segments forming the joint.

Hyperextension is movement in which the angle between segments is increased beyond 180°, or a straight line. The fetlock of the horse is hyperextended while in the normal standing position. Other joints do not normally hyperextend unless fatigued or stressed or when poor conformation provides inadequate support to the joint. Hyperextension of the equine carpus, for example, may occur late in a race, when the galloping horse is fatigued, and can result in injury to the joint. A horse whose carpi are hyperextended because of poor confirmation is said to be *calf-kneed* and is prone to go lame with hard work.

Rotation consists of a twisting movement of a segment around its own axis. Shaking the head "no" is a good example of rotation, in this

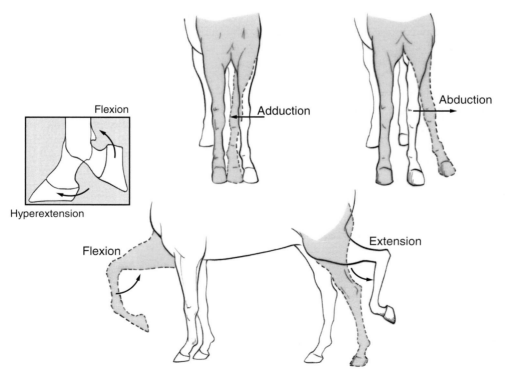

Figure 6-3. Joint movements of the thoracic limb. The fetlock joint is hyperextended in the normal standing position.

case between the atlas and axis of the vertebral column.

Adduction is movement of an extremity toward the median plane. *Abduction* is movement of an extremity away from the median plane.

Circumduction combines the other types of movement except rotation; it may be defined as a movement in which an extremity describes a cone, with the distal end of the extremity describing a circle. A horse that paddles (an undesirable outward swinging of the feet while in motion) is exhibiting circumduction.

Pronation tends to rotate an extremity so that the dorsum is up. *Supination* is a movement that tends to rotate an extremity so that the palmar or plantar aspect of the limb is up. Pronation and supination are rarely seen to any extent in domestic animals.

Types of Synovial Joints

Synovial joints are classified according to the type of joint surface and movements. *Simple joints* involve only two articulating bones, while *composite joints* include more than two bones within the same joint capsule. The types of synovial joints commonly found in domestic animals include ginglymus, plane, trochoid, and spheroid. Additional types of joints, described particularly in the dog, are condyloid, ellipsoid, and saddle.

Ginglymus (*hinge*) *joints* move only in their sagittal plane. The movements in this type of joint are flexion, extension, and in some joints, hyperextension. The fetlock is a good example of a ginglymus joint.

Plane joints have only a slight gliding movement between relatively flat apposed surfaces. These surfaces are called *facets*. The joints between adjacent carpal bones are examples of plane joints.

A *trochoid* (*pivot*) *joint* is one in which rotary movement occurs around one axis. The atlantoaxial joint is the only good example of a trochoid joint in domestic animals.

Spheroid (*ball and socket*) *joints* permit movement in nearly any direction. A spherical head on one bone fits into a cup-shaped depression in the other segment of the joint. Flex-

ion, extension, adduction, abduction, rotation, and circumduction are all possible in spheroid joints. The *coxofemoral* (*hip*) *joint* is the best example of a spheroid joint.

In the *condylar joint,* convex articular condyles articulate with somewhat concave articular surfaces. The *temporomandibular* and *femorotibial* (*stifle*) *joints* are examples. They resemble ginglymus joints but permit more movement.

The *ellipsoid joint* has an articular surface that is expanded more in one direction than another, forming an ellipse. The joint between the distal end of the radius and proximal row of carpal bones is ellipsoid. In domestic animals this has been called a ginglymus joint.

The *saddle joint* has surfaces that resemble an English saddle. It permits all types of movement except rotation. The carpometacarpal joint of the human thumb is the best example, but the interphalangeal joints of the dog are sometimes classified as saddle joints.

Joints of the Axial Skeleton

The joints of the skull are chiefly of the suture type, with adjacent bones united by fibrous tissue. In old age these typically ossify, becoming synostoses. The *fontanel* (soft spot) in a baby's head is an example of fibrous tissue connecting adjacent bones. In addition to the sutures associated with the braincase, the skull also features the symphysis of the mandible, the synchondrosis at the junction of the sphenoid bone and occipital bone at the base of the skull, and the temporomandibular joint.

The *temporomandibular joint* between the mandible and the temporal bone of the skull consists of an articular surface on the skull and one on the mandible, with a plate of cartilage (articular disk or meniscus) between. The temporomandibular joint acts as a ginglymus joint when the mouth opens and closes and as a plane joint when the jaw moves from side to side and forward and back, as in grinding food. The temporomandibular joint may be described as a condylar joint.

The *atlanto-occipital joint* between the occipital bone of the skull and first cervical vertebra (the atlas) is strictly a ginglymus joint. Two condyles on the occipital bone fit into corresponding depressions in the atlas. The only movements possible are flexion and extension in the sagittal plane, as in nodding the head "yes."

Rotation of the head occurs almost entirely between the atlas and axis, at the *atlantoaxial joint.* The *dens,* a toothlike projection from the cranial extremity of the axis, projects into the vertebral foramen of the atlas, where it is held by a group of strong ligaments that permit considerable rotary movement. The atlantoaxial joint is the best example of a pivot joint, in which one segment rotates around the long axis of another.

The symphyseal (fibrocartilaginous) joints between adjacent vertebrae throughout the rest of the vertebral column exhibit relatively little motion. The bodies of adjacent vertebrae are united by a heavy disk of fibrocartilage, the *intervertebral disk* (**IVD**), that is flexible enough to permit some bending in any direction, even twisting. This fibrocartilage has a soft center, the *nucleus pulposus,* which may abnormally protrude through the surrounding *annulus fibrosus* into the vertebral canal. The resulting condition, a ruptured intervertebral disk, may cause significant injury to the overlying spinal cord.

The articular processes of adjacent vertebrae have flat surfaces that are apposed to form plane joints with limited gliding movements. These surfaces are larger and the movements more extensive near the head, decrease in the thoracic region, and are again more extensive in the lumbar region. The joints between sacral vertebrae fuse completely, and the sacrum becomes a single bone with the segments joined by synostoses.

The ribs are attached to the vertebral column by two separate joints. One is between the head of the rib and the costal fovea formed by the bodies of two adjacent thoracic vertebrae; the other is between the tubercle of the rib and a facet on the transverse process of the vertebra of the same number as the rib. The first joint is the pivot type, and the second is the plane type. The heads of the paired ribs on each side of an intervertebral space are joined by an *intercapital ligament,* which forms a reinforcing band across the dorsal side of the intervertebral disk. The presence of the intercapital ligament helps explains why disk protrusions are rare in the thoracic region of the vertebral column.

Joints of the Appendicular Skeleton

The Thoracic Limb

The scapula, or shoulder blade, has no true bony connection with the thorax. It is held in place by a number of muscles and ligaments. This type of joint is sometimes called a *synsarcosis.*

The *shoulder* (*scapulohumeral*) *joint* is spheroid. Movements in all directions, including rotation, are possible. However, in domestic animals the arrangement of shoulder muscles practically limits movement to a hinge type of action in the sagittal plane. Thus, extension and flexion are the chief movements. The head of the humerus is a large sphere much more extensive than the comparable cavity of the scapula. The joint capsule is extensive, with poorly developed ligaments. The tendons of the muscles crossing the shoulder joint on all sides act effectively as ligaments, with the added advantage of being able to contract or relax, thus giving greater mobility to the joint.

The *elbow* is a true ginglymus joint formed by the humeral condyle meeting the proximal ends of the radius and ulna. The proximal end of the radius is slightly concave and expanded to give an extensive surface for support. Combined with semilunar notch to the ulna, the radius forms a half-circle embracing the humeral condyle. In the horse and ox movement in the elbows is limited to flexion and extension. In humans and to a lesser degree in carnivores, the joint between the radius and ulna permits supination and pronation.

The *carpus* (Fig. 6–4) is a complex joint that permits flexion and extension not only between the radius and proximal row of carpal bones (*radiocarpal joint*) but also to a lesser degree between the proximal and distal rows of carpal bones (*midcarpal joint*). The entire joint is capable of absorbing considerable shock because of the many small arthrodial joints formed by adjacent carpal bones connected by short ligaments. The joint between the distal row of

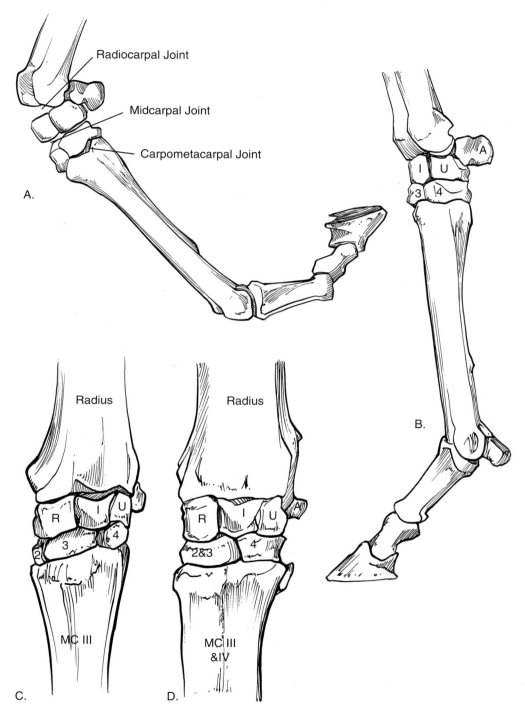

Figure 6-4. Carpus and distal joints of limb. *A)* Equine thoracic limb in flexion. Most of the carpal flexion derives from flexion at radiocarpal and intercarpal joints; the carpometacarpal joint has little movement. *B)* Lateral view of equine thoracic limb in weight-bearing position. *C)* Dorsal view of the equine carpus. *D)* Dorsal view of the bovine carpus.

carpal bones and the metacarpus (*car-pometacarpal joint*) is almost entirely a plane joint, which allows only limited gliding movements and makes almost no contribution to the degree to which the entire carpus can flex.

The fibrous layer of the joint capsule of the carpus is extensive, being a long sleeve extending from the radius to the metacarpus and enclosing the carpal bones. The synovial membrane, however, forms three separate sacs: a *radiocarpal sac,* a *midcarpal sac,* and a *car-pometacarpal sac.*

In the horse there is normally little movement between the large metacarpal III and the smaller metacarpals II and IV (splint bones). Excessive movement or trauma results in inflammation, hence a splint. Acutely, the splint is a painful swelling where the shafts of the large and small metacarpal bones meet. Later this swelling may ossify and form a bony prominence that may not cause any lameness at all (see Fig. 4–9).

In the ox and sheep, the third and fourth metacarpal bones are fused to form the single cannon bone, which articulates proximally with the distal carpal bones and distally with the proximal phalanges. In the dog and pig, the proximal end of adjacent metacarpal bones abut one another in a series of plane joints (*intermetacarpal joints*).

The *metacarpophalangeal (fetlock) joint* of the horse is formed by the distal end of the metacarpus; the proximal end of the first phalanx, or long pastern bone; and the two proximal sesamoid bones. It is a ginglymus joint that in the normal standing position is hyperextended.

The *proximal interphalangeal (pastern) joint* is a ginglymus joint between the first and second phalanges (the long and the short pastern bones). Although it is a ginglymus joint, it is rather limited in motion. Degenerative changes in this joint are called a **high ringbone.**

The *distal interphalangeal joint (coffin joint)* is formed by the second and third phalanges and the distal sesamoid (navicular) bone. The coffin joint is largely encased within the hoof and is essentially a ginglymus joint. Horsemen refer to degenerative joint disease in this joint as a **low ringbone.** A similar pattern of articulations is followed for each digit in animals possessing more than one digit per foot (e.g., ruminants and pigs).

The Pelvic Limb

The **sacroiliac joint** is the only bony connection between the axial and appendicular skeletons. In the young animal, this joint exhibits features of both synchondroses and synovial joints, although its mobility is progressively diminished in the adult. The articular surface of the sacrum is held in tight apposition to the wing of the ilium by a number of short, strong ligaments. Movement in this joint is normally severely limited, but it may become more extensive just prior to parturition, when the ligaments stretch under the influence of the hormone **relaxin** (see Chapter 28). Ligaments in this area include dorsal and ventral **sacroiliac** and **sacrotuberous ligaments.** The latter is a strong, wide band in the ox, sheep, and horse that extends from the sacrum to the tuber ischiadicum and helps form the lateral wall of the pelvis.

The sacroiliac joint can be partially separated (a *sacroiliac subluxation*) by a fall or other trauma. Such an injury produces pain and muscle spasm and often becomes a source of chronic soreness. Sometimes visible asymmetry in the two tubera sacrales develops, with the subluxated side displaced upward. Horsemen refer to this sign as *hunter's bump* (Fig. 6–5).

The **coxofemoral (hip) joint** is the best example of a spheroid (ball and socket) joint. The head of the femur is about two-thirds of a sphere that fits into the less extensive acetabulum of the os coxae. The margin of the acetabulum is reinforced and deepened by a marginal cartilage.

The joint capsule of the hip joint is extensive, but not so extensive as that of the shoulder. The **ligament of the femoral head (round ligament)** connects the head of the femur with a nonarticular area within the acetabulum. The hip joint of the horse is reinforced by an **accessory ligament** that extends from the prepubic tendon to the head of the femur. It is presumed to prevent significant abduction of the pelvic limb. Movements in nearly all directions are possible in the hip joint, but as in the shoulder joint, extension

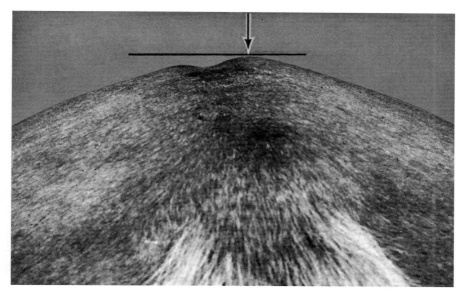

Figure 6-5. Hunter's bump, an asymmetry of the tubera sacrales produced by subluxation of the sacroiliac joint. The higher tuber sacrale is the affected side. (Reprinted with permission from Stashak, T. S. *Adams' Lameness in Horses.* 5th ed. Baltimore: Lippincott Williams & Wilkins, 2002.)

and flexion are the movements chiefly employed in normal locomotion.

The **stifle joint** corresponds to the human knee (Fig. 6–6). It comprises the condyles of the distal femur, separated from the proximal tibia by two intra-articular **menisci.** Each meniscus is a half-moon–shaped disk that conforms to the surface of the proximal tibia and is concave on the upper surface to fit the respective condyle of the femur. These menisci help keep the joint congruent and absorb shock. The stifle is held in apposition by a **medial** and a **lateral collateral ligament** and by two intra-articular **cruciate ligaments** that form an X as they cross from the tibia to the femur in the middle of the joint.

Also associated with the stifle is the **patella** (**kneecap**), a sesamoid bone embedded in the tendon of insertion of the large cranial muscles of the thigh. This muscle group (see Chapter 7) is a powerful extensor of the stifle, acting through its connection to the cranial aspect of the proximal tibia via one (pig) or three (horses and ruminants) strong **patellar ligaments.** In the horse, the **medial patellar ligament** is attached to the medial aspect of the patellar via a large, hook-shaped fibrocartilage. The combined carti-

lage and tendon create a stout loop that can be locked over the medial ridge of the femoral trochlea at will (Fig. 6–6). In this position, the stifle is held in extension without muscular effort; this anatomic arrangement therefore contributes to the ability of the horse to stand while sleeping.

The **tarsus** (**hock**) **joint,** like the carpus, is a composite joint (Fig. 6–7). The ginglymus portion is formed between the distal end of the tibia and the talus. This portion of the joint is held together by strong medial and lateral collateral ligaments of the hock.

The calcaneus projects proximad and caudad to form a lever for attachment of the **common calcaneal tendon (Achilles tendon)**, hence the extensor muscles of the hock. The calcaneus is firmly attached to the other tarsal bones by many short, strong ligaments. The ligaments are less extensive over the craniomedial aspect of the hock. In this location, the joint capsule is immediately beneath the skin, and distension of this joint results in an obvious soft bulge that horsemen call a **bog spavin.** In the horse, movement between adjacent tarsal bones is limited to a small degree of gliding. However, in the ox, sheep, and pig, the proximal intertarsal joint

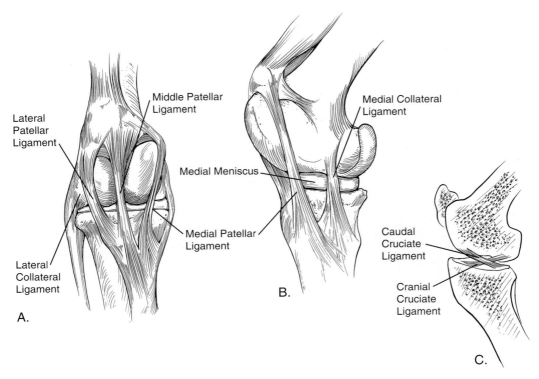

Figure 6-6. Equine stifle. *A)* Cranial view of right stifle. Note the medial patellar ligament's relationship to the medial ridge of the femoral trochlea and the presence of the medial and lateral menisci within the femorotibial articulation. *B)* Medial view of right stifle. In this position the patella is locked over the trochlea and no muscular effort is required to keep the joint extended. *C)* A sagittal section of the stifle showing the cruciate ligaments, whose intra-articular location provides cranial-to-caudal stability to the joint.

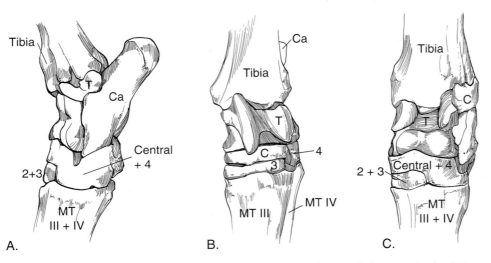

Figure 6-7. Hock. *A)* Lateral view of left bovine hock. *B)* Cranial view of left equine hock. *C)* Cranial view of left bovine hock.

has some hinge movement. Distal to the hock the joints are similar to those of the forelimb.

Pathology of Joints and Related Structures

Since synovial joints depend on free movement for effective functioning, anything that interferes with their mobility can produce gait abnormalities. Disorders affecting joints are commonly due to injuries, infections, or inflammations.

Injuries to joints include dislocations, fractures, sprains, cuts, and puncture wounds. A **dislocation,** also known as a **luxation,** is a condition in which articular surfaces undergo a significant loss of congruency (less severe dislocations are **subluxations**). Dislocation of a joint nearly always includes stretching or tearing of ligaments, and if the dislocation is severe enough, the joint capsule also may tear. The usual treatment for dislocation consists of replacing the joint in its normal position (**reducing** the luxation), surgical repair of severely disrupted elements if necessary, and external support and/or fixation. Reduction may be difficult unless the animal is fully anesthetized so that all muscles are relaxed. Early treatment is important to prevent the joint cavity from filling with connective tissue. Because of the excessive stretching or tearing of ligaments, recovery from a dislocation may be less satisfactory and take longer than recovery from a properly treated fracture.

Occasionally a reasonably functional joint, called a **false joint,** may develop at the site of a chronic luxation. In a false joint, the fibrous connective tissue that develops in response to the inflammation and abnormal stresses at the luxation may provide enough stability to permit considerable movement, even though no joint capsule or cartilage develops as in true joints. False joints may also form at a fracture site if the ends of the fracture are not immobilized.

Fractures, or breaks of bones, may affect one or more of the segments making up a joint. Fractures within or close to a joint are often difficult to reduce adequately, since even minor discontinuities in the articular surface can lead to severe arthritic changes. Immobilization following reduction is also often difficult because of the short length of at least one of the segments.

A **sprain** is a condition in which the ligaments are stretched but the joint does not remain subluxated following removal of the displacing force. The term *strain* is sometimes used in place of sprain, although **strain** is used more frequently to denote excessive stretching of a muscle or tendon. Although a considerable amount of swelling may follow a sprain, the affected joint usually recovers spontaneously if rested adequately.

Cuts such as those from barbed wire may extend into a joint cavity, causing loss of synovial fluid. A condition of this nature may be serious and difficult to treat. The danger is not from the loss of synovial fluid but from infection of the joint cavity. Synovial fluid is a good medium for bacterial growth, and the many recesses of most joint cavities make drainage and treatment of an infected joint difficult. There is danger of permanent damage to the articular cartilage from infection.

Puncture wounds to joints may result from penetration by a sharp object such as a nail, wire, or wood sliver. Such wounds are especially dangerous, since the wound is often not obvious, it usually drains poorly, and the environment into which the bacteria are introduced is frequently anaerobic (not exposed to air). In such conditions, a puncture wound can precipitate a particularly severe infection.

Infection may also reach the joint by way of blood or lymph. **Erysipelas** of swine and umbilical infections arising from a variety of bacteria in foals frequently result in joint infections. Certain viral illnesses, for example caprine arthritis–encephalitis (**CAE**) virus of goats, can cause nonseptic arthritis of multiple joints.

Arthritis, or more correctly, **osteoarthritis,** is inflammation of the components of a joint, causing swelling and pain; it usually accompanies each of the conditions previously mentioned. In addition, injury from kicks, blows, and falls may result in inflammation of a joint without any infection. Chronic inflammation is likely to produce bony and cartilaginous changes that can permanently affect the joint's function. **Degenerative joint disease** (**DJD**) is the medical expression often

Table 6-1. Pathologic Disorders of Joints and Related Structures

Name of Condition	Pathology
Bicipital bursitis	Inflammation of bursa between tendon of *m. biceps brachii* and humerus
Bog spavin	Distension of joint capsule of hock; swelling on the craniomedial aspect of hock
Bone spavin (jack spavin)	DJD of distal intertarsal and tarsometatarsal joints
Bowed tendon (tenosynovitis)	Inflammation, usually due to stretching, of digital flexor tendons and their synovial sheaths caudal to cannon bone; usually thoracic limbs affected
Bursitis	Inflammation of any bursa
Capped elbow	Inflammation of bursa over olecranon process (point of elbow)
Capped hock	Inflammation of bursa over calcaneus (point of hock)
Carpitis (popped knee)	Inflammation of carpal joint capsule and/or ligaments
Curb	Thickening of long plantar ligament on caudal aspect of hock
Dislocation (luxation)	Components of joint displaced
Fistulous withers	Inflammation or infection with draining tract from bursa over spinous processes
Herniated (slipped) intervertebral disk	Prolapse of nucleus pulposus of IVD, usually into the vertebral canal; can cause spinal cord damage
Hunter's bump	Subluxation of sacroiliac joint
Laminitis (founder)	Inflammation of laminae between hoof wall and distal phalanx
Navicular disease	Inflammation of navicular bursa and bone, often with involvement of associated tendons
Osselets	Periostitis of proximal phalanx and/or distal metacarpus III, with capsulitis of fetlock joint
Osteoarthritis	Inflammation of any joint. Because term includes the boney elements of joint, it is more descriptive than arthritis.
Poll evil	Inflammation or infection of bursa over atlas (C1)
Quittor	Infection of collateral cartilages of distal phalanx
Ring bone	Osteophyte formation of interphalangeal joints
Side bone	Ossification of collateral cartilages of distal phalanx
Splints	Inflammation and exostosis involving joint between cannon bone and a splint bone (usually medial)
Sprain	Stretching of ligaments of any joint
Stifling (upward fixation of the patella)	Inadvertent locking of patella over medial ridge of femoral trochlea; holds patella and hock in extension
Strain	Excessive stretching of muscle and/or tendon
Subluxation	Partial dislocation of any joint
Synovitis	Inflammation of any synovial membrane
Thorough-pin	Synovitis of deep digital flexor tendon sheath proximal to hock
Trochanteric bursitis	Inflammation of bursa between greater trochanter of femur and tendon of middle gluteal muscle
Wind puffs (wind gall)	Synovitis of fetlock joint or tenosynovitis of digital flexor tendons in region of fetlock

used to describe the multiple changes in a chronically inflamed joint; it includes loss of articular cartilage, erosion of underlying bone, and the development of bone spurs (*osteophytes* or *exostoses*) around the margins of the joint. The obvious enlargements associated with high and low ringbone in horses are due to the osteophytes associated with the osteoarthritic pastern and coffin joints, respectively. These and other disorders affecting joints or related structures (mostly in horses) are listed in Table 6–1.

Osteoarthritis is commonly treated with nonsteroidal antiinflammatory drugs (e.g., aspirin, phenylbutazone), which reduce the pain associated with inflammation but do not reverse DJD. Recently, much anecdotal and some clinical evidence has supported the use of chondroprotective agents. These drugs, many of which are used as food additives, may inhibit formation of destructive enzymes and prostaglandins in the diseased joints and increase production of the molecular constituents of synovial fluid and cartilage.

Chapter 7

ANATOMY OF THE MUSCULAR SYSTEM

A note on nomenclature is appropriate before a survey of the muscles of domestic animals. Traditionally, muscles are given Latin names, and as these are foreign words, they are italicized. The Latin names are usually highly descriptive of the function and/or appearance of the muscle, and the student is encouraged to use a medical dictionary to explore their meaning. In Latin, as in many Romance languages, the noun is written first, followed by adjectives that describe it. Hence, the *musculus triceps brachii* (literally, the three-headed muscle of the arm) begins with the noun, *musculus,* usually abbreviated as *m.,* plural *mm.* In English, nouns are generally preceded by their descriptors, so the abbreviation for muscle is placed at the end of the string of adjectives, for example, *deep digital flexor m.* In Latin, the same muscle is *m. flexor digitalis profundus.* This text uses English or Latin, whichever is in wider use.

Types of Muscle Tissue

The three types of muscle are skeletal, smooth, and cardiac. The bulk of the muscle in the body is **skeletal muscle,** and it is responsible for producing the voluntary movements of the limbs, trunk, and head. It is also the muscle tissue we are most familiar with as the meat of our domestic animals. The muscle cells (fibers) of skeletal muscle tissue are grouped into distinct organs of variable size called **muscles.** These muscles are usually attached to the bones of the skeleton (hence the term skeletal muscle) and are under voluntary control of the animal. Under the microscope, skeletal muscle fibers exhibit a characteristic striped pattern arising from the orderly arrangement of the contractile proteins within the cells (see Fig. 1–11). As a consequence, skeletal muscle is also called **striated muscle.**

Smooth (**involuntary** or **unstriated**) **muscle** is composed of muscle cells that have no striations visible with a microscope. Smooth muscle is found in systems of the body with automatic function. Thus, smooth muscle is a major component of the wall of organs of the digestive and urogenital systems and most blood vessels. Contraction of smooth muscle is an intrinsic property of the fibers themselves, which means that contraction does not generally require stimulation by a nerve; however, the contractility of smooth muscle is regulated and coordinated by the autonomic nervous system.

Cardiac muscle is characterized by fibers with visible striations, so it is considered a type of striated muscle. However, cardiac muscle, like smooth muscle, contracts intrinsically and is not under voluntary control. Cardiac muscle is restricted to the heart, where it constitutes most of the thickness of the wall. Its rhythmic contraction is responsible for the circulation of blood.

Functions of the Muscular System

The varied functions of the muscular system are all based on **contraction** (shortening) of muscle fibers. Layers of smooth muscle in the walls of the stomach and intestines contract to mix and propel food along the gastrointestinal tract; smooth muscle layers in the walls of blood vessels control the distribution of blood, which is propelled by the contraction of the cardiac muscle of the heart. In the eye, smooth muscle fibers adjust the diameter of the pupil and thickness of the lens for optimal vision, while in the skin, contraction of smooth muscles causes the hair to stand up. Skeletal muscles permit locomotion by contracting to change the relative positions of bones during movement and by maintaining joint angles against the pull of

gravity during support. The skeletal muscles of respiration move air into and out of the lungs by contracting to change the volume of the thoracic cavity. In addition, heat production through shivering is the result of brief repetitive contractions of skeletal muscle throughout the body.

The remainder of this chapter describes the locations, attachments, and actions of the major skeletal muscles. Figures 7–1 to 7–3 illustrate many of these muscles of the horse and ox.

Skeletal Muscle Organization

Muscle fibers are arranged in bundles surrounded by fibrous connective tissue. The connective tissue between individual muscle fibers is called **endomysium.** The sheath surrounding bundles of muscle fibers is called **perimysium,** and the connective tissue around an entire muscle is known as **epimysium.**

Muscle fibers may be arranged in parallel sheets, as in the abdominal muscles, or bands, as in the sartorius muscle on the medial side of the thigh; the muscle fibers in these **strap muscles** are parallel to one another. Other arrangements of muscle fibers include **fusiform** muscles and various **pennate,** or **penniform** (featherlike), arrangements (Fig. 7–4). In the penniform arrangements, a tendon represents the quill, and the muscle fibers attaching to the tendon at an angle represent the vane of the feather. If the fibers come from only one side, the arrangement is called **unipennate;** from two sides, **bipennate;** and from three or more sides, **multipennate.**

The parallel arrangement of muscle fibers in strap muscles provides the greatest potential for overall muscle shortening but is a relatively weak arrangement, while the pennate arrangement increases the power of a muscle but at the expense of distance over which it can contract.

Muscle Attachments

If a muscle appears to arise directly from the bone, it is said to have a **fleshy attachment.** In reality, the muscle fibers attach to very short tendons, which in turn attach to the periosteum

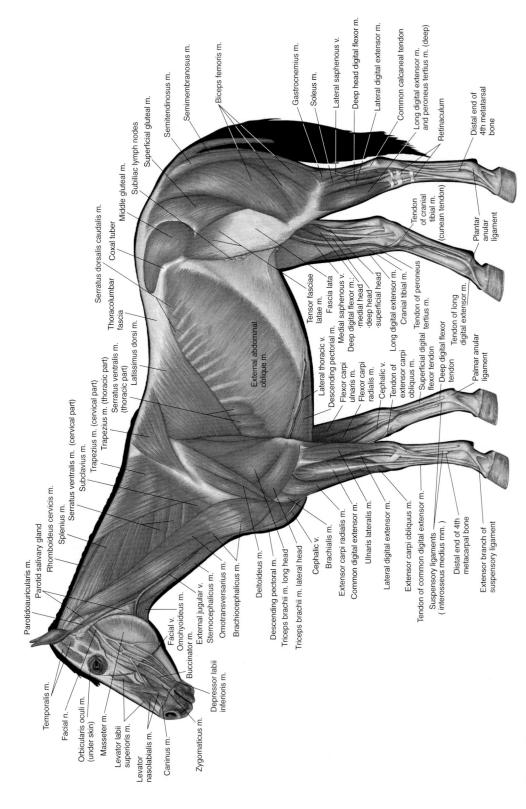

Figure 7-1. Superficial muscles of the horse. (Reprinted with permission from McCracken et al. *Spurgeon's Color Atlas of Large Animal Anatomy*. Baltimore: Lippincott Williams & Wilkins, 1999.)

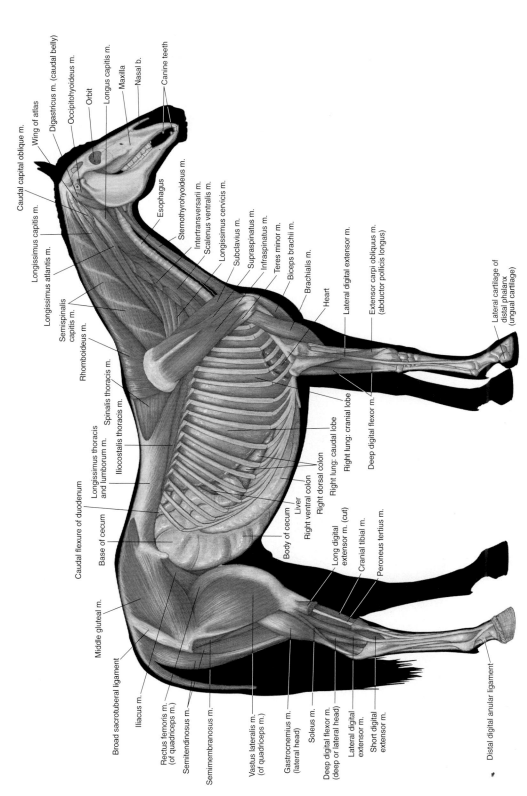

Figure 7-2. Deeper muscles of the horse. (Reprinted with permission from McCracken et al. *Spurgeon's Color Atlas of Large Animal Anatomy*. Baltimore: Lippincott Williams & Wilkins, 1999.)

The labels in the figure are:

Caudal capital oblique m.
Wing of atlas
Digastricus m. (caudal belly)
Occipitohyoideus m.
Orbit
Longus capitis m.
Maxilla
Nasal b.
Canine teeth
Longissimus capitis m.
Longissimus atlantis m.
Semispinalis capitis m.
Rhomboideus m.
Spinalis thoracis m.
Iliocostalis thoracis m.
Longissimus thoracis and lumborum m.
Esophagus
Sternothyrohyoideus m.
Intertransversarii m.
Scalenus ventralis m.
Longissimus cervicis m.
Subclavius m.
Supraspinatus m.
Infraspinatus m.
Teres minor m.
Biceps brachii m.
Brachialis m.
Heart
Lateral digital extensor m.
Extensor carpi obliquus m. (abductor pollicis longus)
Lateral cartilage of distal phalanx (ungual cartilage)
Caudal flexure of duodenum
Base of cecum
Body of cecum
Liver
Right ventral colon
Right dorsal colon
Right lung: caudal lobe
Right lung: cranial lobe
Deep digital flexor m.
Long digital extensor m. (cut)
Cranial tibial m.
Peroneus tertius m.
Middle gluteal m.
Broad sacrotuberal ligament
Iliacus m.
Rectus femoris m. (of quadriceps m.)
Semitendinosus m.
Semimembranosus m.
Vastus lateralis m. (of quadriceps m.)
Gastrocnemius m. (lateral head)
Soleus m.
Deep digital flexor m. (deep or lateral head)
Lateral digital extensor m.
Short digital extensor m.
Distal digital anular ligament

97

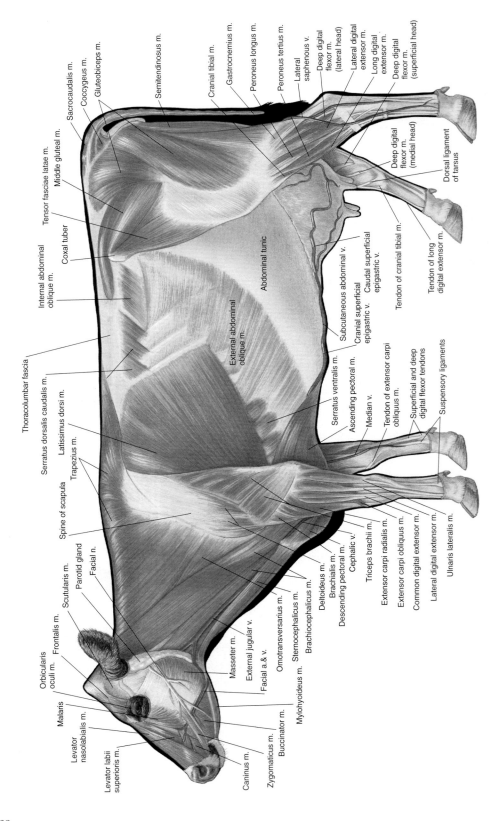

Figure 7-3. Superficial muscles of the cow. (Reprinted with permission from McCracken et al. *Spurgeon's Color Atlas of Large Animal Anatomy.* Baltimore: Lippincott Williams & Wilkins, 1999.)

Orbicularis oculi m.

Frontalis m.

Malaris

Levator nasolabialis m.

Levator labii superioris m.

Caninus m.

Zygomaticus m.

Buccinator m.

Scutularis m.

Parotid gland

Facial n.

Masseter m.

External jugular v.

Facial a. & v.

Omotransversarius m.

Sternocephalicus m.

Brachiocephalicus m.

Mylohyoideus m.

Deltoideus m.

Brachialis m.

Descending pectoral m.

Cephalic v.

Triceps brachii m.

Extensor carpi radialis m.

Extensor carpi obliquus m.

Common digital extensor m.

Lateral digital extensor m.

Ulnaris lateralis m.

Serratus ventralis m.

Ascending pectoral m.

Median v.

Tendon of extensor carpi obliquus m.

Superficial and deep digital flexor tendons

Suspensory ligaments

Subcutaneous abdominal v.

Cranial superficial epigastric v.

Caudal superficial epigastric v.

Abdominal tunic

External abdominal oblique m.

Tendon of cranial tibial m.

Tendon of long digital extensor m.

Dorsal ligament of tarsus

Deep digital flexor m. (medial head)

Deep digital flexor m. (superficial head)

Long digital extensor m.

Lateral digital extensor m.

Deep digital flexor m. (lateral head)

Lateral saphenous v.

Peroneus tertius m.

Peroneus longus m.

Gastrocnemius m.

Cranial tibial m.

Semitendinosus m.

Gluteobiceps m.

Coccygeus m.

Sacrocaudalis m.

Middle gluteal m.

Tensor fasciae latae m.

Coxal tuber

Internal abdominal oblique m.

Thoracolumbar fascia

Serratus dorsalis caudalis m.

Latissimus dorsi m.

Trapezius m.

Spine of scapula

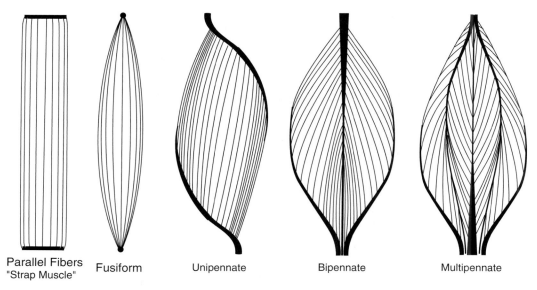

Figure 7-4. Arrangements of muscle fibers: Parallel (a strap muscle), fusiform, unipennate, bipennate, multipennate.

of the bone or may even penetrate the surface of the bone for a short distance. The muscles attaching to the scapula have fleshy attachments.

Tendons, fibrous bands of collagen connecting muscles to bone, are composed of dense, regular connective tissue in parallel bundles. Most tendons are cords or bands that attach spindle-shaped or pennate muscles to bones. Other tendons are flat sheets known as ***aponeuroses,*** usually associated with flat muscles. The heavy fibrous sheets that cover the muscles of the loin are good examples of aponeuroses.

Most muscles have attachments to two bones. The less mobile attachment is called the ***origin,*** and the more movable attachment is called the ***insertion.*** For example, the m. *biceps brachii* extends from the scapula to the radius. The scapula usually moves less than the radius during contraction of the biceps, so the origin of the biceps is its attachment to the scapula, and the insertion is its attachment to the radius. In the extremities, the origin usually is proximal and the insertion distal. Since the only thing a muscle can actively do is contract, it nearly always tends to bring its origin and insertion closer together, causing one or both of the bones to move.

Some muscles have distinctive divisions, called ***heads,*** that have separate origins. The triceps is an example of a muscle with multiple heads, in this case three.

Functional Grouping of Muscles

If a muscle is on the side of the limb toward which a joint bends (decreasing the angle between the segments), it is a ***flexor*** of that joint. A muscle on the opposite side is an extensor. The m. *biceps brachii,* on the cranial side of the limb, flexes the elbow. The m. *triceps brachii,* on the caudal aspect of the limb, takes origin from the scapula and humerus and inserts on the ulna. Thus the triceps is an ***extensor*** of the elbow (Fig. 7–5).

Muscles that tend to pull a limb toward the median plane are ***adductors,*** and those that tend to move the limb away from the median plane are ***abductors.*** Muscles that pass over more than one joint often have different classifications depending on the joint on which they are acting. The m. *gastrocnemius* (the large muscle in the gaskin or calf of the leg) is a flexor of the stifle and an extensor of the hock.

Muscles that surround an opening, whether they are striated or smooth, are ***sphincters.*** The smooth muscle surrounding the opening between the stomach and the intestine forms the

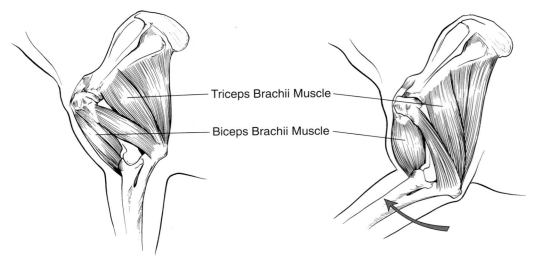

Figure 7-5. Functional grouping of muscles. The *m. biceps brachii* is a flexor of the elbow, and the *m. triceps brachii* is an extensor. In this case, the *m. biceps brachii* is an agonist for elbow flexion, while the *m. triceps brachii* acts as an antagonist. Any muscles that assist elbow flexion indirectly by stabilizing other joints are considered synergists of that movement.

pyloric sphincter, which controls passage of food from the stomach. The *m. orbicularis oculi* is composed of striated muscle fibers in the eyelids, and its contraction closes the eyelids.

Cutaneous muscles occur in the superficial fascia (a layer of connective tissue) between the skin and the deep fascia covering the skeletal muscles. These cutaneous muscles attach to the skin and are responsible for movement of the skin. When a fly rests on a horse, the cutaneous muscles enable the horse to shake the skin to dislodge the fly.

The muscles involved in a specific action, such as extension of the elbow, may also be classified according to the part each plays in the action. The **agonists (prime movers)** are the muscles directly responsible for producing the desired action. The **antagonists** are muscles that oppose the desired action; they have an action directly opposite that of the agonists. **Synergists** are muscles that oppose any undesired action of the agonists. For example, in extension of the elbow, a movement produced by the *m. triceps brachii* (the agonist for extension of the elbow), the *m. biceps brachii* and *m. brachialis* are antagonists because they produce the opposite action, flexion of the elbow. Since the long head of the triceps can flex the shoul-

der joint as well as extend the elbow, any muscle that opposes flexion of the shoulder joint is a synergist of elbow flexion. The *m. supraspinatus* and *m. brachiocephalicus* are synergists for this particular action.

Whether a given muscle is classified as an agonist, an antagonist, or a synergist depends entirely on the specific action. If flexion (instead of extension) of the elbow is the desired action, the *m. biceps brachii* and *m. brachialis* become agonists, while the *m. triceps brachii* and anconeus m. become antagonists.

Synovial Structures

Synovial structures of the body include **joint capsules, bursae,** and **synovial (tendon) sheaths.** The inner layer of each consists of a connective tissue membrane that produces synovial fluid to reduce friction. Synovial joints were described in detail in Chapter 6.

A **bursa** is a synovial sac between two structures that tend to rub against each other (Fig. 7–6). Clinically important bursae include (1) the **bicipital bursa**, between the biceps brachii tendon and the proximal end of the humerus; (2) the **atlantal bursa**, between the ligamentum nuchae and atlas; (3) the **supraspinous bursa,** between the ligamentum nuchae and the spinous process of the second thoracic vertebra; (4) **superficial bursae,** between the skin and olecranon process of the ulna at the point of the elbow and between the skin and superficial digital flexor tendon at the point of the hock; and (5) the **navicular bursa,** between the deep digital flexor tendon and the navicular (distal sesamoid) bone. Normally a bursa contains only enough fluid to reduce friction between adjacent parts.

Inflammation of a bursa, often associated with excessive fluid, is called *bursitis.* Enlargement of bursae can be due to trauma, as is usually the case with *capped hock, capped elbow* (*shoe boil*) and *carpal hygroma.* Inflammation followed by formation of a draining tract, which is fairly common, underlies the equine conditions *poll evil* (at the atlantal bursa) and *fistulous withers* (at the supraspinous bursa).

A bursa gives adequate protection to structures that move only a short distance in relation to each other. However, tendons that must travel a long distance (sometimes as much as several inches) over a bone or other structure require protection and friction-free movement for their entire length. This is afforded by a **synovial sheath** (Fig. 7–6).

A synovial sheath resembles an elongated bursa placed between the tendon and underlying tissue, with the edges of the bursa (sheath) reflected around the tendon until they meet. This results in an inner layer of synovial membrane surrounding the tendon and a superficial layer of the synovial membrane outside the tendon, forming a closed sac that contains synovial fluid to reduce friction between the tendon and adjacent structures. The double fold of membrane formed where the edges of the synovial sheath meet is the **mesotendon.**

Inflammation of a synovial sheath and its tendon is called *tenosynovitis.* Low-grade trauma (for instance, as associated with rigorous schooling of young horses) can result in a mild, painless tenosynovitis of the digital flexor tendon sheath (*windpuffs*) or the deep digital flexor tendon sheath proximal to the hock (*thoroughpin*).

Muscles of the Thoracic Limb

Muscles Acting on the Shoulder Girdle

The scapula can make complex movements in man, but in the domestic animals the chief movement is a pendulous swing forward and

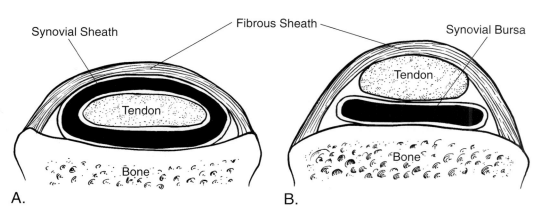

Figure 7-6. Synovial structures. *A)* A synovial sheath surrounds a tendon over a greater distance and facilitates its frictionless movement. *B)* A bursa lies interposed between a tendon or ligament and a bony prominence.

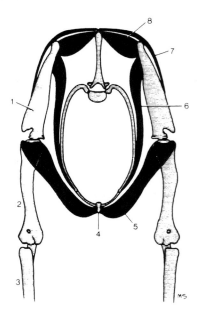

Figure 7-7. Muscular suspension of the thorax between the thoracic limbs. *1)* Scapula. *2)* Humerus. *3)* Radius and ulna. *4)* Sternum. *5) M. pectoralis profundus. 6) M. serratus ventralis. 7) M. trapezius. 8) M. rhomboideus.* The attachment of limbs to the trunk is achieved through a synsarcosis, rather than by a bony joint.

backward of the distal end of the bone (Figs. 7–7 and 7–8). The muscles that hold the scapula in place contribute to this swinging movement. Superficial muscles include the **m. trapezius** and the **m. omotransversarius**. The **m. rhomboideus** and the **m. serratus ventralis** are deep (Fig. 7–7).

The **m. trapezius** is a triangular flat muscle that takes origin along the dorsal midline from the head to the lumbar vertebrae. The *m. trapezius* inserts chiefly on the spine of the scapula. The portion taking origin cranial to the scapula helps swing the scapula forward; the one attaching behind draws it back. The entire *m. trapezius* also aids in holding the scapula against the body.

The **m. rhomboideus** is a heavier muscle just deep to the trapezius. The *m. rhomboideus* also takes origin from the dorsal midline both cranial and caudal to the scapula. The *m. rhomboideus* inserts on the deep (medial) face of the dorsal end of the scapula.

The **m. serratus ventralis** is the largest and most important muscle attaching the thoracic limb to the trunk. It is a large, fan-shaped mus-

cle. The origin of the *m. serratus ventralis* is the widest part and extends from the transverse processes of the cervical vertebrae and ribs along a curved line just above the sternum as far back as the tenth costal cartilage. The insertion is on the medial side of the dorsal portion of the scapula. The *m. serratus ventralis* on each side together form a sling that supports the trunk between the thoracic limbs. The cervical portion, on contraction, tends to rotate the distal part of the scapula backward, while the thoracic portion rotates it forward.

The **m. omotransversarius** is a separate muscle of the shoulder region in most domestic species. It takes origin from the transverse processes of the more cranial cervical vertebrae and inserts on the distal part of the spine of the scapula (clavicular tendon in the horse). With these attachments, the omotransversarius usually pulls the distal end of the scapula forward, although with the limb in weight-bearing position, it instead assists lateral flexion of the neck.

Muscles Acting on the Shoulder Joint

The shoulder, being a ball-and-socket joint, can make all types of movement. In the quadruped its chief actions are extension and flexion.

Extensors of the Shoulder. The **m. brachiocephalicus,** as the name implies, extends from the head to the arm. The origin is from the occipital bone of the skull and transverse processes of the cervical vertebrae. It inserts on the lateral side of the proximal part of the humerus proximal to the deltoid tuberosity. The *m. brachiocephalicus* is the heavy muscle covering the cranial aspect of the point of the shoulder. It raises and advances the shoulder. The *m. brachiocephalicus* is also the principal extensor of the shoulder and acts as a lateral flexor of the neck when the limb is weight bearing.

The *m. brachiocephalicus* is subdivided into the **m. cleidobrachialis,** extending from the clavicular tendon (representing the vestigial clavicle) to the humerus, and the **m. cleidocephalicus,** extending from the clavicular tendon to the head and neck. In species other than the horse, the *m. cleidocephalicus* is often further

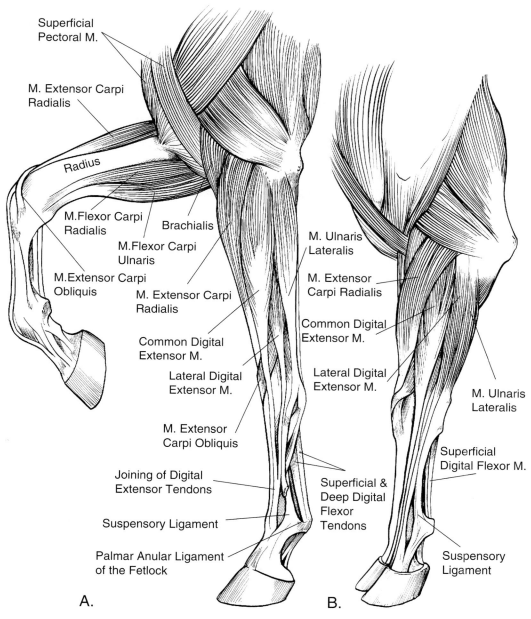

Superficial Pectoral M.

M. Extensor Carpi Radialis

Radius

M.Flexor Carpi Radialis

M.Flexor Carpi Ulnaris

Brachialis

M.Extensor Carpi Obliquis

M. Extensor Carpi Radialis

Common Digital Extensor M.

Lateral Digital Extensor M.

M. Extensor Carpi Obliquis

Joining of Digital Extensor Tendons

Suspensory Ligament

Palmar Anular Ligament of the Fetlock

A.

M. Ulnaris Lateralis

M. Extensor Carpi Radialis

Common Digital Extensor M.

Lateral Digital Extensor M.

M. Ulnaris Lateralis

Superficial Digital Flexor M.

Superficial & Deep Digital Flexor Tendons

Suspensory Ligament

B.

Figure 7-8. Muscles of the thoracic limb. *A)* Equine. *B)* Bovine.

subdivided into a mastoid part attaching to the mastoid process of the temporal bone and either an occipital part (in ruminants and pigs) or a cervical part (in carnivores). The *m. cleido-brachialis* is comparable to the anterior deltoid muscle of humans.

The ***m. supraspinatus*** originates from the supraspinous fossa of the scapula cranial to the spine. It inserts on the greater tubercle (both greater and lesser in the horse) of the humerus. The *m. supraspinatus* may assist in extending the shoulder but acts chiefly as a ligament of the shoulder joint. This is one of the muscles that atrophies (shrinks) in ***sweeny*** in horses, in which its motor innervation, the suprascapular nerve, is damaged.

Flexors of the Shoulder. The *m. teres major* originates from the dorsal part of the caudal border of the scapula and inserts on the teres major tuberosity on the medial side of the shaft of the humerus. It is a strong flexor of the shoulder joint.

The *m. latissimus dorsi* is a wide, triangular muscle that originates from the spinous processes of the thoracic and lumbar vertebrae by means of a wide aponeurosis, the **thoracolumbar fascia.** It inserts with the *m. teres major* on the medial side of the humerus and is a strong flexor of the shoulder. Also, it pulls the thoracic limb caudad or if the limb is fixed, advances the trunk.

The *m. infraspinatus* originates from the infraspinous fossa just caudal and ventral to the spine of the scapula. It inserts into the caudal part of the greater tubercle of the humerus. The *m. infraspinatus* also acts as a strong collateral ligament of the shoulder joint and may abduct, flex, and outwardly rotate the shoulder. This muscle also atrophies in cases of sweeny.

The *m. teres minor* lies just distal to the infraspinatus muscle and has the same action as the *m. infraspinatus*. The *m. teres minor* originates from the distal caudal border of the scapula and inserts on the teres minor tuberosity of the humerus just distal to the greater tubercle of the humerus.

Adductors of the Shoulder. The *pectoral muscles* form the substance of the brisket. They originate from the sternum and insert mainly on the proximal part of the humerus. Commonly they are divided into the **superficial pectoral muscle (m. pectoralis superficialis)** and the **deep pectoral muscle (m. pectoralis profundus)**. These pectoral muscles are strong adductors of the forelimb, and the deep pectoral muscle also advances the trunk when the limb is fixed on the ground (weight bearing).

The *m. coracobrachialis* is a small muscle extending from the coracoid process on the medial side of the scapula to the medial side of the shaft of the humerus.

The *m. subscapularis* holds the shoulder in close apposition. It originates from the subscapular fossa on the medial side of the scapula below the attachments of the *m. rhomboideus* and *m. serratus ventralis*. It inserts on the lesser tuberosity of the humerus and adducts the shoulder joint.

Abductors of the Shoulder. The *m. deltoideus* extends from the spine of the scapula to the deltoid tuberosity of the humerus. It is an abductor and flexor of the shoulder joint.

Muscles Acting on the Elbow

Since the elbow is a hinge joint, the muscles acting on it are either flexors or extensors. In quadrupeds, the extensors are stronger than the flexors because they support the weight of the body by maintaining the limbs in extension (Fig. 7–8).

Extensors of the Elbow. The *m. triceps brachii* has three heads. The **long head** originates from the caudal border of the scapula, while the **medial** and **lateral heads** originate from the respective sides of the humeral diaphysis. Carnivores have an **accessory head** that also originates from the humerus between the medial and lateral heads (although this arrangement gives the carnivore four heads on this muscle, it is still called a triceps). All heads insert on the olecranon process of the ulna. The triceps is the strongest extensor of the elbow. The long head may also act to flex the shoulder.

The *m. anconeus,* deep to the *m. triceps brachii,* is a rather small muscle that covers the caudal aspect of the joint capsule of the elbow. It also originates on the humerus, inserts on the olecranon process, and extends the elbow.

The *m. tensor fasciae antibrachii* originates via a thin aponeurosis that is blended with the long head of the triceps muscle and the *m. latissimus dorsi*. The flattened muscle belly lies on the caudomedial aspect of the arm and inserts via a second aponeurosis on the olecranon and antebrachial fascia. The muscle's name reflects its action on the antebrachial fascia (it tenses it), but through these fascial connections the *m. tensor fasciae antibrachii* also assists the triceps in extension of the elbow.

Flexors of the Elbow. The *m. biceps brachii* originates on the supraglenoid tubercle just dorsal and cranial to the articular surface of the scapula. It inserts on (1) the radial tuberosity on the cranial aspect of the proximal radius, (2) the medial collateral ligament of the elbow, and (3) the antebrachial fascia. The tendinous blending with the antebrachial fascia forms a palpable cordlike structure on the flexor surface of the elbow called the **lacertus fibrosus.** The biceps assists in holding the shoulder joint in apposition and may extend it to some extent. However, the chief action of the *m. biceps brachii* is flexion of the elbow.

The *m. brachialis* is strictly a flexor of the elbow, since it originates on the humerus and inserts on the cranial aspect of the radius (and sometimes the ulna).

The *m. pronator teres* is primarily a flexor of the elbow, although it may tend to pronate the antebrachium of the dog and cat. It originates on the medial epicondyle of the humerus and inserts on the medial side of the radius. In the horse, this muscle is usually absent, occasionally reduced to a fibrous band.

Extensor muscles of the carpus and digit (discussed in the next section), which originate on the lateral epicondyle of the humerus, may assist in flexion of the elbow as a secondary function.

Muscles Acting on the Carpus

The carpus, like the elbow, acts essentially as a hinge joint. However, the extensors of the carpus lie on the craniolateral aspect of the limb, and the flexors are found on the caudomedial side.

Extensors of the Carpus. The *m. extensor carpi radialis* is the largest extensor of the carpus. It extends from the lateral epicondyle of the humerus to the proximal end of the metacarpal region. It inserts on the metacarpal tuberosity on the dorsal surface of the proximal end of the metacarpus. This is the most prominent muscle on the front of the forearm and is the most cranial muscle of the group. As the name implies, the *m. extensor carpi radialis* acts primarily as an extensor of the carpus.

The *m. extensor carpi obliquus* is flat, trian-

gular extensor of the carpus lying deep to the digital extensor muscles of the antebrachium. It arises from the craniolateral aspect of the distal half of the radius (and ulna in species with a complete ulna). Its oblique tendon crosses mediad on the cranial aspect of the carpus, superficial to the tendon of the *m. extensor carpi radialis,* to insert on the most medial metacarpal bone, which is the second in the horse and the third in the cow and sheep. In humans, this muscle is one of the well-developed abductors and extensors of the thumb (the pollex) and so in this species is called the *m. abductor pollicis longus.* This name is only infrequently used in veterinary anatomy, since most domestic species lack a well-developed first digit.

The *m. extensor carpi ulnaris* (*m. ulnaris lateralis*) is the most caudal of the extensor muscles. It also takes origin from the lateral epicondyle of the humerus but passes downward over the lateral side of the carpus to insert on the most lateral metacarpal bone. In most domestic animals this muscle produces weak flexion of the carpus, although by origin and nerve supply it belongs with the extensor group. It also produces some outward rotation of the forearm. In addition, the extensor muscles of the digits whose tendons pass over the dorsal surface of the carpus may act secondarily as extensors of the carpus.

Flexors of the Carpus. On the medial side of the forearm, the *m. flexor carpi radialis* is just caudal to the radius, which is palpable directly beneath the skin. It takes origin from the medial epicondyle of the humerus and inserts on the palmar aspect of the proximal end of the metacarpus (medial side).

On the lateral side, the *m. flexor carpi ulnaris* exerts considerable leverage as a flexor of the carpus by inserting on the accessory carpal bone, which projects in a palmar direction from the lateral aspect of the carpus.

These muscles are, of course, primarily flexors of the carpus, but they may act slightly in extension of the elbow. Recall, too, that in spite of its common name, the *m. extensor carpi ulnaris* is a flexor of the carpus in domestic animals (for this reason, many veterinary anatomists recommend the alternate name, *m. ulnaris lateralis*).

Muscles Acting on the Digits

Extensors of the Digit. The *common digital extensor muscle (m. extensor digitorum communis)* is the longest extensor muscle in the thoracic limb. It originates from the lateral epicondyle of the humerus close to the *m. extensor carpi radialis.* Its tendinous insertion is on the extensor process of the distal phalanx and on the proximal ends of the middle and proximal phalanges. The tendon is single in the horse, double in the cow, sheep, and goat, and split into four separate tendons in the pig and carnivores, in which it inserts on the second through the fifth digits. This muscle is an extensor of all joints of the digit, including the fetlock. It may also assist in extending the carpus and even in flexing the elbow.

The common digital extensor m. of two-toed animals has several distinct heads. One of these gives rise to its own tendon that inserts on the third digit (the medial toe). In these species, this head of the common digital extensor m. is sometimes identified as a separate muscle, the medial digital extensor muscle.

The *lateral digital extensor m. (m. extensor digitorum lateralis)* is found in all species. Its origin is just caudal to the common digital extensor m., and the insertion varies according to the number of digits present. In the carnivores, it inserts on the fifth digit; in two-toed animals, on the fourth digit; and in the horse, on the proximal phalanx of the third (and only) digit.

Flexors of the Digit. In all animals the principal digital flexors are the superficial and the deep digital flexor muscles. The *deep digital flexor m. (m. flexor digitorum profundus)* lies the closest to the metacarpal bones. It originates from the humerus, radius, and ulna. Its long, stout tendon extends distad through the carpal canal, then along the palmar side of the metacarpus to insert on the palmar surface of the distal phalanges. As with the common digital extensor tendon, the number of insertions depends on the number of digits, with the main tendon dividing into individual slips, one per digit, just proximal to the fetlock. The deep digital flexor is the only muscle that flexes the distal interphalangeal joint. Secondarily, it also flexes the more proximal joints of the digit and the carpus. The deep digital flexor m. also is important in supporting the fetlock.

The *superficial digital flexor m. (m. flexor digitorum superficialis)* is similar to the deep digital flexor m., but it inserts primarily on the proximal part of the middle phalanx of each digit. In the horse, the superficial digital flexor tendon inserts on the palmar aspects of the proximal end of the middle phalanx and the distal end of the proximal phalanx. Tendons of both the superficial and deep digital flexor mm. can be palpated palmar to the cannon bone. The expression **bowed tendons** describes a traumatic condition of horses involving tendonitis of one or both of these tendons in the cannon region (Fig. 7–9).

Interosseous muscles lie between the metacarpal bones of carnivores and humans. In the larger animals most of the muscle tissue has been replaced with connective tissue, and these

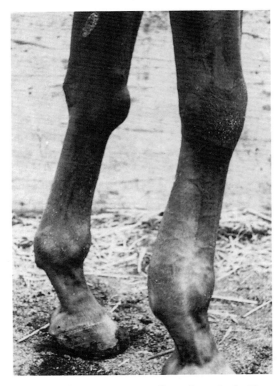

Figure 7-9. Tenosynovitis (bowed tendon). Note swelling on the palmar aspect above the fetlock in the area of the flexor tendons.

structures are known as the **suspensory ligaments.**

Muscles of the Pelvic Limb

The hip is a ball-and-socket joint and as such can move in nearly any direction (Fig. 7–10). However, the chief movements are extension and flexion of the femur. Adduction and abduction are also fairly common movements, and some rotation is possible.

Muscles Acting on the Hip Joint

Extensors of the Hip. The chief extensors of the hip are the so-called **hamstring muscles,** which pass caudal to the hip from the tuber ischiadicum to the proximal end of the tibia, fibula, or calcaneus of the tarsus. They include the **m. biceps femoris** (the most lateral of the caudal muscles of the thigh), the **m. semitendinosus** (the middle muscle of the caudal group), and the **m. semimembranosus** (the medial muscle of this group). The divisions between these muscles can be seen as vertical grooves in animals that are not very fat. In the horse, the m. biceps femoris and m. semitendinosus extend dorsad over the rump to attach to the sacral and caudal (coccygeal) vertebral spines. In many other animals the hamstring muscles originate only from the tuber ischiadicum. In ruminants, the m. biceps femoris is blended with the superficial gluteal muscle and is therefore called the **m. gluteobiceps.** It is a powerful extensor of the hip, stifle, and hock.

The **middle gluteal muscle (m. gluteus medius)** is another strong extensor of the hip. It originates from the wing of the ilium and inserts on the greater trochanter of the femur, a lever projecting above the hip.

Flexors of the Hip. Flexors of the hip are cranial to the femur. The most important are the **m. iliacus** and **m. psoas major,** which insert on the lesser trochanter on the medial side of the femur. Together they are called the **iliopsoas muscle.** The m. iliacus originates from the ventral surface of the wing of the ilium. The m. psoas major originates from the ventral surfaces of the lumbar transverse processes.

The **m. sartorius** is a thin, straplike muscle that extends from the tuber coxae to the tibia, diagonally crossing the medial surface of the thigh. The **m. rectus femoris** (one head of the m. quadriceps femoris) and the **m. tensor fasciae latae** also flex the hip and are also described as extensors of the stifle.

Abductors of the Hip. Abductors of the hip extend laterally over the hip joint so as to move the limb away from the median plane. The **deep gluteal muscle (m. gluteus profundus)** extends from the spine of the ischium laterad over the hip joint to insert on the greater trochanter.

The **superficial gluteal muscle (m. gluteus superficialis)** extends from the sacral vertebral spines to the third trochanter just distal to the greater trochanter. The **m. tensor fasciae latae** extends from the tuber coxae to the lateral femoral fascia, which attaches to the patella. In addition to abducting the hip joint, this muscle flexes the hip joint and extends the stifle.

Adductors and Rotators of the Hip. Adductors of the hip pull the limb toward the median plane. They are all on the medial aspect of the thigh, extending from the pelvis to either the femur or the tibia. The **m. gracilis** is the most medial muscle extending from the symphysis of the pelvis to the tibia.

The **m. pectineus,** a small spindle-shaped muscle deep to the m. gracilis, is both an adductor and flexor of the hip.

The **m. adductor** is the largest muscle on the medial side of the thigh. It extends from the ventral aspect of the pelvis to the medial side of the femur and tibia. It is a strong adductor but may also help to extend the hip.

The **m. quadratus femoris** is an adductor of the thigh. Several other small muscles in this deep layer of hip musculature extending from the area of the obturator foramen are outward rotators of the thigh. They include the **internal** and **external obturator muscles (mm. obturatorius internus et externus),** and the **mm. gemelli.**

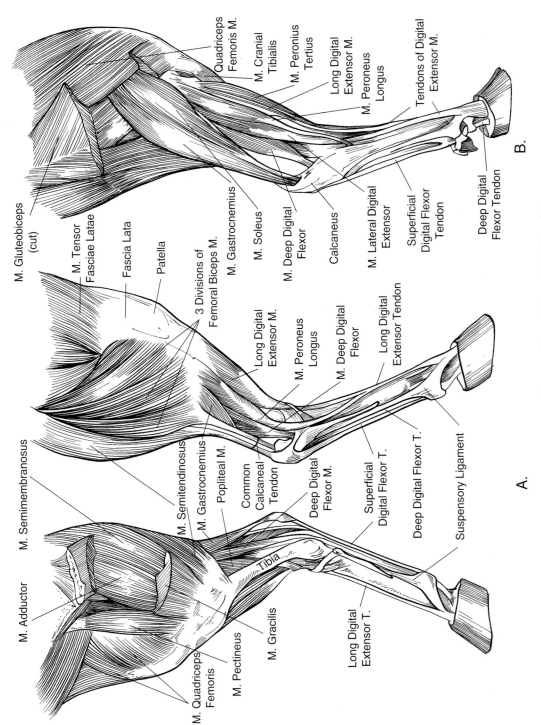

M. Adductor

M. Semimembranosus

M. Gluteobiceps (cut)

M. Tensor Fasciae Latae

Fascia Lata

Patella

3 Divisions of Femoral Biceps M.

M. Gastrocnemius

Quadriceps Femoris M.

M. Cranial Tibialis

M. Peronius Tertius

Long Digital Extensor M.

M. Peroneus Longus

Tendons of Digital Extensor M.

Long Digital Extensor M.

M. Peroneus Longus

M. Deep Digital Flexor

Long Digital Extensor Tendon

M. Soleus

M. Deep Digital Flexor

Calcaneus

M. Lateral Digital Extensor

Superficial Digital Flexor Tendon

Deep Digital Flexor Tendon

B.

M. Semitendinosus

M. Gastrocnemius

Popliteal M.

Common Calcaneal Tendon

Deep Digital Flexor M.

Superficial Digital Flexor T.

Deep Digital Flexor T.

Suspensory Ligament

Tibia

M. Quadriceps Femoris

M. Pectineus

M. Gracilis

Long Digital Extensor T.

A.

Figure 7-10. Muscles of the pelvic limb. *A)* Equine. *B)* Bovine: Lateral view. Left) medial view. Right) lateral view.

Muscles Acting on the Stifle

The stifle is essentially a hinge joint, so the muscles acting on it are either extensors or flexors.

Extensors of the Stifle. One large muscle, the **m. quadriceps femoris,** is the primary extensor of the stifle. This muscle has four heads; their distinct origins and clearly distinguishable muscle bellies make it common practice to name them as separate muscles. The longest head, the **m. rectus femoris,** originates from the ilium just above the acetabulum. The other three heads, **m. vastus medialis, m. vastus intermedius,** and **m. vastus lateralis,** originate from the respective areas of the shaft of the femur. All four heads insert on the patella. The patella, being fastened to the front of the tibia by the patellar ligaments, extends the stifle when it is pulled proximad by the *m. quadriceps femoris.* Because of its origin on the ilium, the *m. rectus femoris* also flexes the hip.

Flexors of the Stifle. The chief flexors of the stifle are the hamstring muscles, which also extend the hip (*m. biceps femoris, m. semitendinosus, m semimembranosus;* discussed earlier). In addition, the extensor muscles of the hock that originate on the caudal surface of the distal end of the femur may also flex the stifle. These muscles include the *m. gastrocnemius* and the superficial digital flexor m. (discussed later). The **m. popliteus** is a relatively small muscle caudal to the stifle. Its chief action is flexion of the stifle, although it may slightly rotate the leg (tibia and fibula) mediad.

Muscles Acting on the Hock

The principal actions of the hock are extension and flexion.

Extensors of the Hock. Extensors of the hock primarily attach to the calcaneus (point of the hock) by way of the **common calcanean tendon.** The **m. gastrocnemius** and **superficial digital flexor m.** originate from the caudal aspect of the distal femur, and their tendons make up the bulk of the common calcanean tendon. They are joined in part by portions of the *m. biceps femoris, m. gracilis, and m. semitendinosus,* which also assist in extending the hock and hip and flexing the stifle. The deep digital flexor m. also extends the hock.

Flexors of the Hock. Flexors of the hock include the **m. tibialis cranialis** and the **peroneal muscles,** whose tendons pass over the dorsal surface of the hock to insert on the tarsus and metatarsus. The *m. peroneus tertius* is the only named peroneal muscle in the horse. Additionally, the *m. peroneus longus* is found on the ox, sheep, goat, pig, and dog. The *m. peroneus brevis* is also found in carnivores. The digital extensors also flex the hock, because their tendons pass over the flexor surface of the hock.

Muscles Acting on the Digit

Digital extensors of the thoracic limb also tend to extend the carpus, while digital extensors of the pelvic limb tend to flex the hock. Likewise, digital flexors of the thoracic limb produce flexion of the carpus, while digital flexors of the pelvic limb produce extension the hock. Muscles acting on the digits of the pelvic limb are similar in arrangement to those of the thoracic limb.

Extensors of the Digit. The *long digital extensor muscle* (*m. extensor digitorum longus*) originates from the distal end of the femur and passes distad to insert on the distal phalanx of each digit. As with the common extensor in the thoracic limb, the tendon has one part in the horse, two parts in the ox, goat, and sheep, and four parts in the pig and carnivores.

The *lateral digital extensor muscle* (*m. extensor digitorum lateralis*) lies between the extensor and flexor groups of muscles of the crus. In the horse, its tendon joins that of the long digital extensor m. about the middle of the cannon. In ruminants, it inserts via a separate tendon on the proximal middle phalanx of the fourth digit. In pigs, it resembles the ruminant condition, with the addition of a small deep part of the muscle that features a separate tendon inserting on the fifth digit.

Flexors of the Digit. The *superficial* and *deep digital flexor mm.* are arranged in the pelvic limb similarly to the thoracic limb. However, the tendon of the superficial digital flexor muscle also attaches to the calcaneus.

Muscles of the Head

Muscles of Mastication

Muscles of mastication are those that have attachments to the mandible and whose contractions produce the jaw movements associated with chewing (Fig. 7–11). As a general rule, considerably more muscle mass (and therefore strength) is devoted to the elevation (closure) of the mandible than to depression (opening). Most of the muscles of mastication are innervated by the trigeminal nerve (see Chapter 9).

The **m. temporalis** is a strong muscle arising from the sagittal crest and the expansive temporal fossa of the lateral cranium and inserting on the coronoid process of the mandible. Its action is to elevate the mandible, bringing the upper and lower teeth together.

The **m. masseter** is especially well developed in herbivorous species. This powerful masticatory muscle arises from the maxillary region of the face and the zygomatic arch. It inserts on the caudal mandible, and its primary actions are to elevate the mandible and to draw it laterad. The broad expanse of the horse's cheek is formed by the masseter muscle.

Medial to the mandible are two **pterygoid muscles (mm. pterygoideus)**. These arise from the ventral parts of the skull (the pterygoid and palatine bones) and insert on the mandible. These muscles assist in closing the mandible and play an important role in the side-to-side grinding movements typical of herbivore mastication.

Opening of the jaw is largely assisted by gravity, but forceful depression of the mandible is primarily the function of the **m. digastricus.**

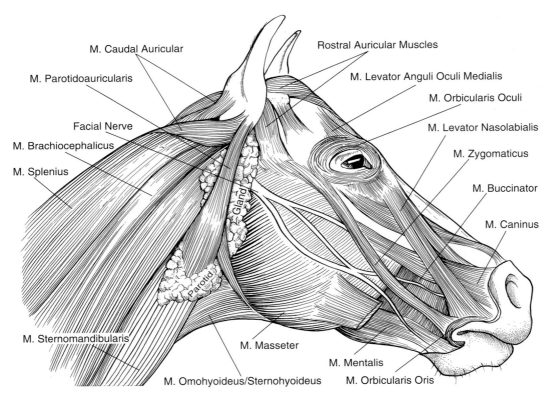

Figure 7-11. Muscles of the equine head.

This muscle arises from the region caudal to the temporomandibular joint and inserts on the angle of the mandible. As the name implies, the muscle has two bellies, indistinctly divided near the muscle's center.

Muscles of Facial Expression

The muscles that move the skin and appendages of the face and head are the **muscles of facial expression** or **mimetic muscles.** These are generally thin cutaneous muscles innervated by the facial nerve (see Chapter 9).

The **auricular muscles** are roughly divided into a rostral and a caudal group. The contraction of auricular muscles produces the range of ear movements characteristic of domestic animals.

The **m. orbicularis oculi** is a sphincterlike muscle that surrounds the **palpebral fissure** (the opening of the eyelids). Contraction of the m. orbicularis oculi produces a forceful closure of the fissure.

A large number of muscles produce movements of the lips and cheeks; these are important in prehension of food and assist with mastication by keeping food in the mouth and positioned between the teeth. A sphincterlike muscle, the **m. orbicularis oris,** surrounds the lips; its contraction purses the lips. The **m. buccinator** forms the wall of the cheek. Other mimetic muscles lift and depress the lips, change the shape of the nostrils, and produce other facial movements.

Other Muscles of the Head

A number of striated muscles lie within the orbit associated with the globe of the eye. These **extraocular eye muscles** (so called as they are attached to the outside of the eyeball) move the globe of the eye in the many directions of which it is capable. The extraocular eye muscles are described in Chapter 11 with the anatomy of the visual apparatus.

A large number of muscles associated with the pharynx and soft palate are important in **deglutition** (swallowing) and **phonation** (**vocalization**). Their various functions are to lift or depress the palate and to constrict or dilate the pharynx. This same region contains many muscles that originate or insert on the hyoid apparatus. These act to move the hyoid apparatus relative to the tongue and larynx or when the hyoid apparatus is fixed in place, to move these latter structures relative to it. The individual muscles in this complex group are beyond the scope of this book.

The tongue of domestic animals is an organ capable of extraordinary movements; it is used in the prehension and mastication of food, drinking of water and suckling of milk, and as a grooming tool. The **intrinsic muscles** of the tongue are arranged in fascicles that run longitudinally, transversely and vertically, allowing the tongue to change shape in multiple planes. **Extrinsic muscles** of the tongue, those that arise from outside the tongue, include the **m. genioglossus,** which arises from the rostral part of the mandible (the **genu**) and inserts in the base of the tongue so that its contraction draws the entire tongue rostrad. The **m. hyoglossus** arises from the hyoid apparatus and inserts in the base of the tongue; it draws the tongue caudad. The **m. mylohyoideus** lies transversely between the rami of the mandible. It is not, therefore, strictly a muscle of the tongue, but its contraction lifts the floor of the mouth, hence the tongue.

Muscles of the Trunk and Neck

Extensors of the Vertebral Column

The group of muscles dorsal to the transverse processes of the vertebrae on either side of the spinous processes are the **epaxial muscles.** These make up the loin muscles and continue forward to the head. Collectively, they are referred to as the **m. erector spinae.** In domestic animals, the largest of these muscles is known as the **m. longissimus.** It is composed of innumerable small bundles of muscle fibers that extend from vertebral transverse processes to spinous processes, from transverse processes to transverse processes, or between spinous processes. As these attachments may extend from one vertebra to the next or overlap one or more vertebrae, there are many possibilities for naming individual muscles and a variety of individual muscle actions. As a general description, however, these muscles are responsible for extension and when acting unilaterally, lateral flexion of the spinal column. They may also cause slight rotation (twisting) of the spinal column, as seen when a bucking horse throws the front feet to one side and hind feet to the opposite side.

Other epaxial muscle groups include the medial *transversospinalis system,* whose fibers span one or more vertebrae from transverse to spinous processes, and the *iliocostalis system.* The latter is the most lateral group of the epaxial muscles (Fig. 7–12).

The same general arrangement of muscles is continued into the neck, where much greater

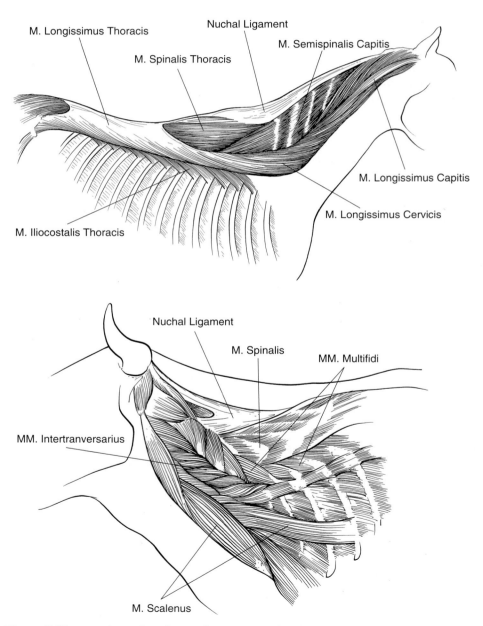

Figure 7-12. Epaxial muscles. A) Superficial muscles of the horse. B) Deeper muscles of the ox.

flexibility is evidenced. The dorsal neck muscles, which extend (raise) the head and neck, are well developed to support the head. The large extensor muscles of the head originate from the vertebrae in the region of the withers and insert on the occipital bone of the skull. The most superficial of these muscles (other than the *m. trapezius*, which does not originate from the vertebrae) is the *m. splenius*, and deep to it is the *m. complexus* (Figs. 7–1 to 7–3). Other muscles that actively extend the head and neck include the *m. rhomboideus*, continuations of the *m. longissimus*, and the *rectus capitis* and *obliquus capitis* groups. Deeper muscles that extend from one vertebra to the next also aid in movements of the neck. In addition to these muscles, a heavy elastic band, the *ligamentum nuchae*, reaches from the withers to the skull. The ligamentum nuchae gives considerable aid to the muscles that extend the head and neck.

Flexors of the Vertebral Column

Muscles ventral to the transverse processes of the vertebrae are the *hypaxial muscles*. They tend to flex the trunk, neck, and head. These include the *m. sternocephalicus*, which extends from the sternum to the mandible in the horse and to the mandible and mastoid process of the skull in ruminants. In addition, the *m. sternothyroideus, m. sternohyoideus, m. longus colli*, and *m. longus capitis* are flexors.

Abdominal Muscles

The muscles that form the bulk of the abdominal wall support the organs of digestion and many of the reproductive organs, particularly the gravid (pregnant) uterus. The abdominal muscles may act to flex the vertebral column. If contracting on one side only, they flex it laterally or even twist the vertebral column. These muscles are important in emptying the contents of the digestive tract (defecation), urinary tract (urination, also called micturition), and female reproductive tract at birthing (parturition). The abdominal muscles are used in regurgitation and vomiting and serve as strong muscles for

forced expiration of air from the lungs, as seen during coughing or sneezing.

The abdominal muscles are arranged in layers much like plywood, with the muscle fibers running in different directions. Most of these muscles have broad aponeurotic insertions that meet at the midventral line known as the *linea alba* (white line).

The *external abdominal oblique m. (m. obliquus externus abdominis)* is the most superficial. The fibers of this muscle lie obliquely ventrad and caudad. Its origin is from the last few ribs and thoracolumbar (lumbodorsal) fascia over the back and loins. The insertion is by means of a broad flat tendon (aponeurosis) that meets the insertion of the muscle from the opposite side at the linea alba. Caudally, the muscle is continued by an aponeurosis, sometimes called the *inguinal ligament*, at the junction of abdominal wall to pelvic limb. This ligament forms the superficial wall of the *inguinal canal* for the passage of the spermatic cord of the male. It contains a slit, the *superficial inguinal ring*, through which the spermatic cord passes from the inguinal canal into the scrotum.

The *internal abdominal oblique m. (m. obliquus internus abdominis)* is immediately deep to the external abdominal oblique muscle. Its fibers pass obliquely ventrad and craniad, and the muscle also inserts on the linea alba by means of an aponeurosis. In some animals, this muscle forms the deep wall of the inguinal canal and also the *deep inguinal ring*. The most caudal group of fibers from the internal abdominal oblique muscle passes through the inguinal canal with the spermatic cord and attaches to the outer covering of the testicle. This muscle is the *cremaster m.*, which pulls the testicle toward the inguinal canal. In some animals, such as rodents and elephants, the testicle is retracted into the abdominal cavity except during breeding seasons.

The *m. transversus abdominis* is the deepest of the abdominal muscles. It originates from the deepest layer of thoracolumbar fascia, and the fibers are directed perpendicular to the long axis of the body to insert on the linea alba.

The *m. rectus abdominis* forms the muscular floor of the abdomen. It originates from the cartilages of the ribs and the sternum. The fibers run directly caudad in a horizontal plane to attach to the pubis by means of a strong **prepubic tendon.** The *m. rectus abdominis* characteristically is divided by a series of **tendinous intersections.**

Muscles of Respiration

The muscles of respiration are either expiratory, forcing air out of the lungs by decreasing the size of the thorax, or inspiratory, causing air to enter the lungs by increasing the size of the thorax.

The **diaphragm** is the chief muscle of inspiration. It is a dome-shaped sheet of muscle separating the thoracic and abdominal cavities. It projects into the thorax. Contraction of the fibers of the diaphragm tends to flatten the diaphragm and force the abdominal viscera caudad, further into the abdomen. This in effect increases the volume of the thorax and lowers intrathoracic pressure, drawing air into the lungs.

The **external intercostal mm.** (**mm. intercostales externi**) extend from each rib to the next rib behind. The fibers are directed ventrad and caudad similarly to the external abdominal oblique muscle. When these muscles contract, they tend to rotate the ribs upward and forward, increasing the size of the thorax. The **internal intercostal mm.** (**mm. intercostales interni**), which lie deep to the external intercostal muscles, run from each rib to the next one in front, and the fibers are directed ventrad and craniad. Although not all studies are in agreement, most anatomists describe their action as reducing the volume of the thorax and therefore aiding in forced expiration. Some authorities believe that both the external and internal intercostal muscles may function in both inspiration and expiration.

As mentioned previously, the abdominal muscles may act as muscles of expiration by forcing the abdominal viscera against the diaphragm, decreasing the size of the thorax.

Microscopic Anatomy and Physiology of Muscle

The basis for movement in living cells is contractile proteins, which can convert chemical energy into the mechanical energy of tension and motion. Muscle cells are highly specialized for contraction, and their primary constituents are contractile proteins. However, proteins with contractile properties have also been extracted from many other types of cells. For example, such proteins are responsible for the migration of some white blood cells from capillaries into peripheral tissues, for the movements of mitochondria, and for the movement of the cilia on some epithelial cells.

Skeletal Muscle

Structure

The skeletal muscle fiber (also called voluntary striated muscle fiber) is actually a long, multinucleated cell with visible striations. Immediately beneath the outer cell membrane (sarcolemma) are numerous nuclei, reflecting the end-to-end fusion of shorter primitive muscle cells during development. The interior of the fiber is packed with elongated protein strands (**myofibrils**), and filling the clefts and spaces between these strands is an extensive network of smooth **endoplasmic reticulum (sarcoplasmic reticulum)** and associated tubular invaginations of sarcolemma (**transverse,** or **T, tubules**) (Fig. 8–1).

Although skeletal muscle fibers look virtu-

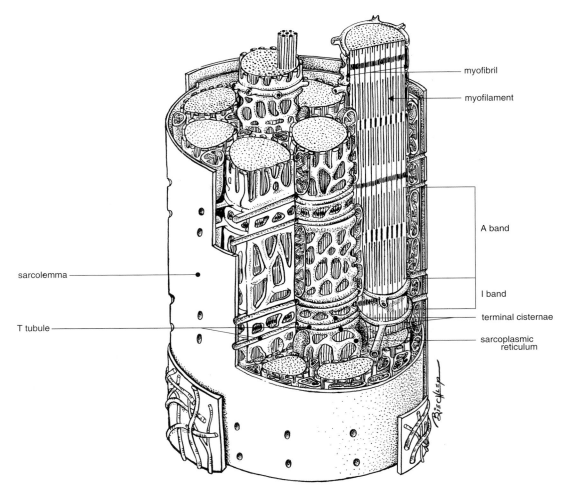

myofibril

myofilament

A band

I band

terminal cisternae

sarcoplasmic reticulum

sarcolemma

T tubule

Figure 8-1. The myofibrils of a skeletal muscle cell are surrounded by sarcoplasmic reticulum. T tubules extend into the sarcoplasm from the sarcolemma to surround the myofibrils. (Reprinted with permission from Delmann D., and Eurell J. *Textbook of Veterinary Histology.* 5th ed. Baltimore: Lippincott Williams & Wilkins, 1998.)

ally identical on routine histologic stains (see Fig. 1–11), their biochemical differences can be appreciated with histochemical techniques. Staining for the activity of myosin adenosine triphosphatase (ATPase), the enzyme that splits adenosine triphosphate (ATP) to yield energy for muscle contraction, reveals that some muscle fibers stain darkly (**type II fibers**), others lightly (**type I fibers**) (see Fig. 2–6). These histochemical results correlate with the physiologic properties of the muscle fibers themselves: type I fibers contract slowly (**slow twitch**) but can contract for long periods. Type II fibers contract fast (**fast twitch**) but are more suscep-

tible to fatigue. Speed of contraction is therefore a property of the activity of myosin ATPase and the rate of ATP hydrolysis; endurance is related to the intracellular content and activity of mitochondria and the ability to generate ATP for contraction by oxidative or aerobic metabolism.

The specific types of muscle fibers that make it up determine the functional characteristics of a whole muscle. Muscles that require sustained contraction, such as the antigravity muscles, typically contain more slow-twitch endurance fibers than do the muscles that contract briefly but quickly and with great force. It is even possible to show a difference among breeds of horses with regard to the muscle fiber composition of the same muscle; the middle gluteal muscle of the sprinting quarter horse is usually characterized by more of the large, fast-twitch but low-endurance type II fibers than is the same muscle of the slower but long-winded Arabian.

On casual examination with a light microscope, the cross-striations of skeletal muscle appear to be disks throughout the entire fiber. However, the electron microscope shows the striations only in the myofibrils and not in the sarcoplasm (cytoplasm of muscle cell). The alternate light and dark bands of all myofibrils appear at the corresponding places in the fiber (Fig. 8–2). The fact that corresponding bands of adjacent myofibrils are in register makes it appears that these bands extend across the whole fiber (Figs. 8–1 and 8–2). The apparent bands of myofibrils are due to relative density and partial overlapping of **thick** and **thin filaments.** Letters are used to designate the different bands.

The light zones, or bands, called **I bands,** consist of thin filaments only. The darker regions, called **A bands,** are composed of overlapping thick and thin filaments (Fig. 8–2). Thus, alternating A and I bands produce the banding pattern on the myofibril.

A dense line, the **Z line,** bisects each I band (in fact, one end of each thin filament is attached to the Z line; the opposite end of each thin filament is free). The segment of myofibril between adjacent Z lines is the **sarcomere,** the fundamental unit of contraction in striated muscle (Fig. 8–2).

Each striated muscle fiber contains hundreds or thousands of myofibrils, and each myofibril contains approximately 1500 thick and 3000 thin **myofilaments.** Each thick filament is composed of hundreds of molecules of **myosin,** a golf club–shaped protein molecule with a molecular weight of 332,000 (by comparison, hydrogen has a molecular weight of 2). A thin filament is composed principally of chains of molecules of **actin,** a globular protein of molecular weight 70,000. The structure of these filaments and details of their actions in contraction are described in more detail in a later section.

The sarcoplasmic reticulum is agranular (contains no ribosomes) and functions in excitation–contraction coupling (discussed later in this chapter). A Golgi apparatus, large numbers of mitochondria, and glycogen inclusions also are found in muscle fibers.

The transverse tubules (or T systems) are continuous with the plasma membrane and extend into the interior of the muscle fiber at right angles in the myofibrils and sarcoplasmic reticulum. The T system propagates action potentials from the sarcolemma into the interior of the muscle fiber (Fig. 8–1) to initiate contraction of the entire fiber.

Skeletal muscle fibers range in diameter from 10 to 100 μm. In general, the large fibers appear to be longer and tend to be found in large rather than small muscles. Animals on full feed are reported to have larger fibers than animals on restricted feed. It is generally accepted that males have larger muscle fibers than females. Length of skeletal muscle fibers varies widely with the length of the muscle and arrangement of muscle fibers (parallel or pennate). Some fibers in parallel muscles probably extend the entire length of the muscle.

It is generally believed that skeletal muscle fibers are such specialized cells that little if any multiplication of fibers or formation of new fibers occurs after birth. All increases in size of muscles at any stage in life following birth are due to hypertrophy (increase in size) of individual muscle fibers, with the synthesis of more myofibrils and an increased vascular supply. It is well known that exercise can increase muscular development, as is seen in weight lifters. This, of course, is accomplished by increase in size of existing individual muscle fibers. **If the nerve supply to a muscle is destroyed, the muscle fibers decrease to practically nothing, a condition called *denervation* or *neurogenic atrophy*. This was seen in sweeny of draft horses, when the suprascapular nerve was crushed by a collar, resulting in shrinking of the supraspinatus and infraspinatus muscles of the shoulder.**

Excitation, Contraction, and Relaxation

Skeletal muscle contraction is triggered by the generation of an action potential on the sarcolemma. This action potential is initiated by

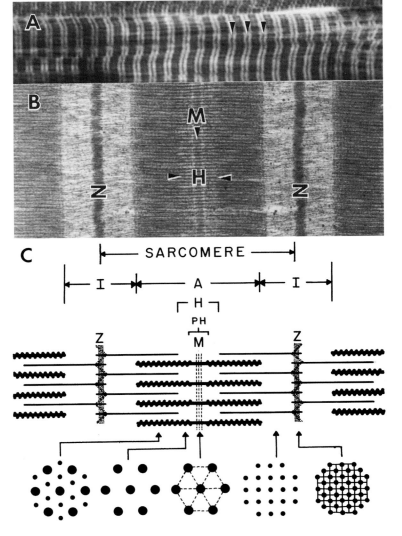

Figure 8-2. Light micrograph (*A*) and electron micrograph (*B*) of longitudinal skeletal muscle and schematic representation (*C*) of a sarcomere. (Reprinted with permission from Dellmann D. and Eurell J. *Textbook of Veterinary Histology.* 5th ed. Baltimore: Lippincott Williams & Wilkins, 1998.)

the firing of a motor neuron whose axon branch terminates at the **neuromuscular junction** near the midpoint of the muscle fiber. The neuromuscular junction (Fig. 8–3) is a type of excitatory synapse.

The action potential of the nerve is not propagated directly onto the adjacent muscle cell. Instead, depolarization of the motor nerve ending releases a chemical neurotransmitter, **acetylcholine** (ACh). When ACh diffuses across the synaptic cleft of the neuromuscular junction, it binds to specific cell membrane receptors (nicotinic ACh receptors) on the postjunctional membrane of the muscle fiber (Fig. 8–3). The binding of ACh to its receptors brings

about the opening of ligand-gated membrane channels, which allow sodium ions to enter the muscle cell. The entrance of sodium (a positively charged cation) shifts the membrane electrical potential in a positive direction (**depolarization**). The effect of ACh persists only momentarily, since another enzyme, **acetylcholinesterase,** quickly degrades ACh.

ACh is synthesized in the cytoplasm of the presynaptic nerve endings and stored in membrane-bound synaptic vesicles in the end of the nerve fiber (Fig. 8–3). Each action potential reaching the end of the nerve stimulates the release of a set number of vesicles and thus a set amount of ACh. Continuous

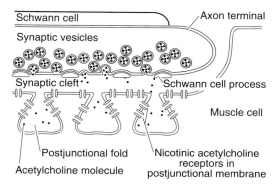

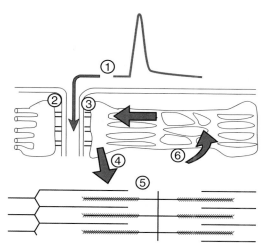

Figure 8-3. Structural features of a neuromuscular junction. The terminal end of the axon contains synaptic vesicles with the neurotransmitter ACh. Nicotinic ACh receptors are on the cell membrane of the skeletal muscle cell. (Reprinted with permission from Rhoades R.A. and Tanner G.A. *Medical Physiology.* Boston: Little, Brown, 1995.)

Figure 8-4. The cyclic movements of calcium during excitation–contraction coupling in skeletal muscle. Action potential enters the T tubule (*1*). The T tubule conducts the action potential into the body of the cell (*2*). The action potential on the T tubule (*3*) stimulates the release of calcium from the sarcoplasmic reticulum (*4*). Muscle contraction occurs (*5*). Calcium is transported back into the sarcoplasmic reticulum and muscle relaxation results (*6*). (Reprinted with permission from Rhoades R.A. and Tanner G.A. *Medical Physiology.* Boston: Little, Brown, 1995.)

synthesis maintains a constant supply of vesicles so that ACh is not depleted even with intense exercise.

End-Plate and Action Potentials. The local depolarization of the sarcolemma at the neuromuscular junction is called an **end-plate potential.** This change in potential produces a local flow of current that depolarizes adjacent areas on the sarcolemma. Normally, the depolarization of the adjacent sarcolemma is enough to reach the threshold potential of electrically gated channels in these areas of the cell membrane. When this occurs, these channels open to allow the inward diffusion of sodium, and another action potential results. Local flow of current occurs again, and other action potentials are generated in other areas adjacent to the site of the first action potential. The process is repeated, and the overall effect is the propagation of action potentials over the entire sarcolemma of the muscle fiber. This process is similar to that for propagation of action potentials along the axon of a nerve cell (see Fig. 2–16).

Since the T tubules are inward continuations of the sarcolemma, the action potential (or impulse) travels along these tubules throughout the muscle fiber (Fig. 8–4). In certain sites where the T tubules pass immediately adjacent to the sarcoplasmic reticulum, there is a struc-

tural link between a protein in the sarcolemma of the T tubule (**dihydropyridine receptor**) and a membrane protein channel in the sarcoplasmic reticulum. When an action potential occurs on the sarcolemma in the area of the dihydropyridine receptor, the channel in the sarcoplasmic reticulum becomes **permeable to Ca^{2+}**. The permeable change is possible because of the link between the two membrane proteins.

Before stimulation, the Ca^{2+} concentration within the sarcoplasmic reticulum is much greater (more than 100-fold) than within the sarcoplasm. When the Ca^{2+} channels in the sarcoplasmic reticulum open, Ca^{2+} diffuses into the surrounding sarcoplasm of the muscle fiber and into the myofibrils. The increase in Ca^{2+} in the myofibrils leads to the interaction of thick and thin filaments, and movement (sliding) of the thin filaments past the thick filaments toward the center of the sarcomere. This sliding movement shortens the sarcomeres, which shortens the myofibrils, which shortens the entire muscle fiber. Figure 8–4 summarizes the movements of Ca^{2+} during **excitation–contraction coupling** in skeletal muscle.

Hyperkalemic periodic paralysis (HyPP) is an inherited disease of horses caused by a genetic mutation of a transmembrane protein. The electrically gated sodium channel (described earlier as participating in the generation of action potentials on the cell membranes of skeletal muscle) is defective in affected animals, and as a result, the permeability of the channel to sodium may be increased inappropriately. This permits the entrance of sodium, membrane depolarization, and involuntary muscular contractions. Hyperkalemia is an increase in serum potassium concentration, and this is one stimulus that can increase the permeability of the abnormal channels, hence the name of the condition. Clinical signs include muscle spasms, tremors, sweating, and weakness. This condition is also known as Impressive syndrome, because it is primarily seen in quarter horses and other descendants of the quarter horse sire Impressive.

Myosin and Actin Filaments. Each thick filament in a sarcomere is a bundle of myosin molecules. Each molecule has two parts: (1) a filamentlike part that lies parallel to similar parts of other myosin molecules, making up the length of the thick filament; and (2) a part that projects outward like an arm from the end of the filament (Fig. 8–5). An enlargement at the end of the arm is termed the **myosin head.** The arm attaching the myosin head to the filament is flexible, like a hinge, where it joins the filament segment and also where it joins the head. Myosin heads protrude from all around the thick filament. They extend away from the center in both directions, toward the surrounding thin filaments (Fig. 8–5).

Each thin filament is made up of three proteins: actin, **tropomyosin,** and **troponin.** Actin molecules are the most prominent and are arranged in two long strands wound around each other in a spiral. Tropomyosin molecules are also joined in a strand that spirals around strands of actin. The third protein, troponin, is found attached to tropomyosin at specific sites

along the strand. Together they are called the **troponin–tropomyosin complex** (Fig. 8–5).

The stands of tropomyosin lie over sites on the actin strand where myosin heads can bind. Calcium ions released from the sarcoplasmic reticulum bind to the troponin part of the troponin–tropomyosin complex and induce a molecular change in the tropomyosin strand. This change uncovers myosin binding sites on the actin strands so that the myosin head can attach.

Binding of the myosin head to actin leads to the release of adenosine diphosphate (ADP) and phosphate, which were bound to the myosin head. The myosin head also rotates from its resting position toward the center of the sarcomere; this movement pulls the actin chain to which it is bound past the thick filament (Fig. 8–5).

The myosin head remains at its final angle and bound to the actin of the thin filament until an intact ATP molecule binds to another site on the myosin head. (This site on the myosin head is ATPase, which also promotes the hydrolysis of ATP prior to movement of the head.) With the binding of a new ATP, the myosin head detaches from the actin chain and resumes its resting angle, ready to repeat the process of attaching to actin, moving from resting to final angle and pulling the attached thin filament farther toward the center of the sarcomere, and detachment with the binding of still another ATP molecule.

The cycle of events that produces the shortening of each sarcomere, the **sliding filament model of muscle contraction,** is summarized in Figure 8–5. The resultant contraction shortens the sarcomere and shortens the I bands. The A band always remains the same length. During shortening, the thin filaments slide over the thick filaments as they are drawn from both ends, pulling the Z lines closer together (Fig. 8–2). The filaments themselves do not shorten.

Relaxation. Muscle contraction will continue as long as there is an excess of Ca^{2+} in the sarcoplasm, but when the effect of the action potentials on the sarcolemma ends, the Ca^{2+} is sequestered back into the sarcoplasmic reticulum (Fig. 8–4). Ion pumps in the membrane of the sarcoplasmic reticulum use the energy of ATP to pump the Ca^{2+} from the sarcoplasmic fluid back into storage, so that it can be ready for the next depolarization. (Without ATP the muscle

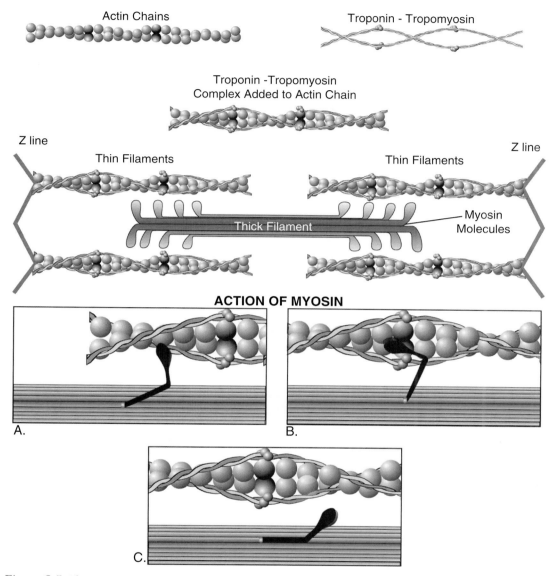

Figure 8-5. The primary components ant the organization of thin and thick filaments are shown in the top-half of the figure. Boxes A, B, and C illustrate the sequential action of myosin as it binds to actin and then rotates to move the thin filament past the thick filament (from right to left in the figure).

cannot relax.) Only a small amount of Ca^{2+} is left out in the sarcoplasm of the relaxed resting muscle, not enough to act on the troponin–tropomyosin complex. Therefore, during relaxation the thin and thick filaments are dissociated, allowing the elasticity of the muscle to return it to its resting length, which pulls the Z lines and thin filaments back to their original positions.

Replenishment of ATP. A great amount of ATP is needed because the energy for contraction is derived from hydrolyzed (dephosphorylated) ATP. Also, the muscle fiber uses ATP to sequester Ca^{2+} back into the sarcoplasmic reticulum. It is also needed for complete recovery of the membrane after depolarization—the Na–K–ATPase system.

The concentration of ATP in resting skeletal

muscle is relatively small, supplying only enough energy to maintain contraction for a brief period. Since muscles continue to contract after the initial supply of ATP has been used up, the resulting ADP is phosphorylated again from another source, **creatine phosphate** (CP).

There is normally about five times as much CP as ATP stored in the sarcoplasm of skeletal muscle. When the ATP is used for contraction and relaxation, transphosphorylation occurs from CP to the resulting ADP, forming ATP again. This replenishment reaction occurs almost as fast as ATP is used. Therefore, the ATP level changes little until the concentration of CP gets low. CP acts as the immediate energy source for the resynthesis of ATP. This is a convenient means of transferring energy for muscle contraction.

The concentration of CP is also limited. Thus, if muscle contraction continues for longer than a few seconds, the CP and new ATP eventually have to be reconstituted by the citric acid cycle (Krebs cycle) in the mitochondria of the muscle fibers. If muscle activity outstrips the ability of the mitochondria to produce ATP aerobically, anaerobic metabolism of carbohydrate fuel begins and lactic acid accumulates in the muscle cell. Glucose (the major carbohydrate fuel) is obtained from the blood supply to the muscle and from the **glycogen** stored in the muscle fibers. Glycogen is broken down by **glycogenolysis.** Glycogenolysis and **glycolysis** are complex processes involving a number of reactions, enzymes, and intermediate compounds.

Oxygen from the blood must also be supplied to the mitochondria in muscles for the citric acid cycle to operate and result in oxidative phosphorylation of ADP to ATP. While lactic acid was mostly being produced anaerobically during muscle contraction, an **oxygen debt** was building up. This oxygen debt must be repaid during relaxation before optimal muscle activity can resume.

The chain of reactions involved in supplying energy for muscle contraction and recovery is shown in Table 8–1.

Strength of Contraction

Whenever a single muscle fiber receives a nervous impulse and action potentials are generated on the muscle fiber, the action potentials will be propagated over the entire fiber and cause the whole fiber to contract. This is the **all-or-none law** of muscle contraction.

The all-or-none law applies to a single muscle fiber or a **single motor unit** (a motor neuron and all of the muscle fibers it supplies); it does not apply to an entire muscle, such as the *m. biceps brachii.* The all-or-none law also does not state that a muscle fiber will always contract with the same speed or the same force but only that for the conditions at the time of stimulation the muscle fiber will contract to its maximum. The force of contraction does depend on the state of the fiber at the time; that is, whether it is fatigued, stretched to its optimal length, and so on.

The sliding filament mechanism is possible because of overlap of the thin and thick filaments. This overlap permits the binding between actin and myosin. Experimental studies have demonstrated that the amount of overlap of the filaments before contraction begins, affects the contraction strength of individual muscle fibers. When muscle fibers are stretched before being stimulated, contraction strength increases up to an optimal amount of stretch. Any further stretching produces a decrease in

---

Table 8-1. Chain of Reactions That Supply Energy for Muscle Contraction and Recovery

ATP →	ADP + phosphoric acid + energy (for immediate use in contraction)
CP →	Creatine + phosphoric acid + energy (for resynthesis of ATP from ADP)
Glucose (glycogen or blood) →	Lactic acid + energy (for resynthesis of CP from creatine and phosphoric acid)
Lactic acid + oxygen →	Water + carbon dioxide + energy (for resynthesis of ATP and CP)

ATP, adenosine triphosphate; ADP, adenosine diphosphate; CP, creatine phosphate.

contraction strength. This same relationship is true for the other striated muscle, cardiac muscle, and is an important factor in the regulation of cardiac contraction strength.

Summation. Each gross muscle, which is composed of multiple motor units and many individual muscle fibers, is capable of contracting with varying degrees of strength. This is the result of summing the contractions in two ways. *Motor unit summation* (recruitment) occurs when more motor units are stimulated to contract simultaneously in the gross muscle. Therefore, more muscle fibers and bundles are contracting and producing greater strength in the whole muscle. *Temporal summation* occurs when the frequency of stimulation to one or more motor units is increased. That is, the frequency of stimulation is such that the first contraction is not over by the time the second contraction begins. The two become additive, which increases the contraction strength (Fig. 8–6). Ordinarily, in normal muscle function, both types of summation occur at the same time.

Tetany (Tetanus). When the frequency of stimulation becomes so rapid that further increases in frequency will not increase the strength of contraction, the greatest force that the muscle can develop has been reached. This is called *tetany, tetanus,* or tetanization. All of these terms are defined as a continuous tonic spasm of muscle or a steady state of contraction (Fig. 8–7). **The disease caused by the toxin from *Clostridium tetani*, which produces spasm of the masseter muscles (lockjaw) followed by a spasm of other muscles, is also specifically referred to as tetanus. The *Clostridium* toxin produces skeletal muscle tetany by inhibiting the release of inhibitory neuromediators within the central nervous system. These inhibitors normally act within the spinal cord to regulate the activity of motor neurons to skeletal muscle. Without these inhibitors, any motor activity can result in spastic or tetanic contractions of the skeletal muscle. Loud noises or sudden movements can cause affected animals to tense their muscles and may induce generalized spasms.**

Fatigue. *Fatigue* is a decrease in work capacity caused by work itself. Fatigue may occur at the level of the individual muscle fiber, or it may be a generalized state affecting the animal as a whole. On a whole-animal basis, resistance to fatigue entails some poorly defined factors such as motivation. The factors contributing to fatigue of an individual muscle fiber have been best studied in muscle cells in isolated in vitro preparations outside of the body. These stud-

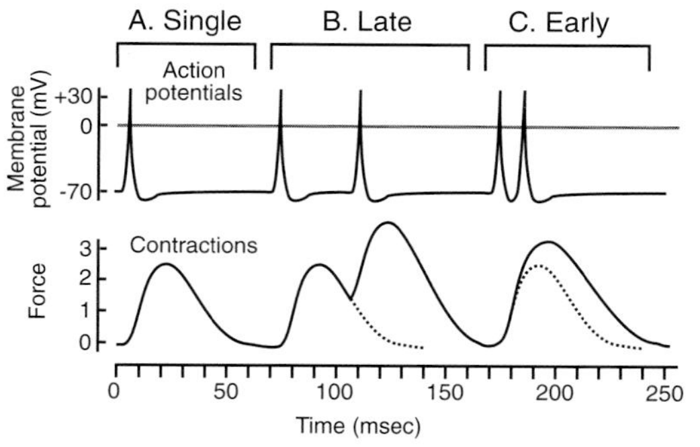

Figure 8-6. Temporal summation of muscle twitches. The first contraction (*A*) is due to a single action potential. The second contraction (*B*) illustrates summation because a second action potential arrives before the muscle can relax completely. The third contraction (*C*) illustrates summation when a second action potential arrives before the muscle can begin to relax. (Reprinted with permission from Rhoades R.A. and Tanner G.A. *Medical Physiology.* Boston: Little, Brown, 1995.)

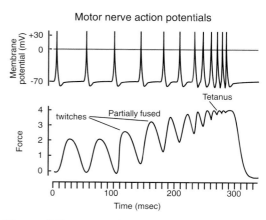

Figure 8-7. Tetany. The interval between action potentials steadily decreases until no relaxation can occur between action potentials. (Reprinted with permission from Rhoades R.A. and Tanner G.A. *Medical Physiology.* Boston: Little, Brown, 1995.)

ies indicate that fatigue is a function of the muscle cell itself and is not due to failure or fatigue of the neurons that innervate skeletal muscles.

At the individual cell level, one contributor to fatigue is a decrease in the availability of ATP, as its use increases with increased muscle contractions. However, even with strenuous prolonged exercise ATP is never totally depleted, because the intracellular generation of ATP is also increased during exercise. Increases in intracellular concentrations of various metabolites generated as a result of contraction also contribute to fatigue. Among these are the phosphate from the splitting of ATP to ADP and organic acids such as **lactic acid.** Lactic acid can diffuse out of the cell and reduce the pH of the interstitial fluids within a muscle. Accumulations of lactic acid within muscles contribute to pain and soreness of muscles following strenuous exercise.

The rate at which ATP is generated within an exercising muscle depends on the availability of substrates for the different metabolic pathways that produce ATP. If a muscle primarily uses the glycolytic pathway, glucose must be readily available. Glucose may be stored within the muscle cell as glycogen or delivered via the circulation. If a muscle uses the oxidative pathway to produce ATP, oxygen must be available in addition to fatty acids or other similar substrates. The oxygen of course must arrive via the circulation. Adequate blood flow during exercise to deliver oxygen, fatty acids, and/or glucose to skeletal muscle is a key factor in resisting fatigue.

Drugs That Affect Skeletal Muscle Function

Almost as soon as ACh initiates the impulse for muscle contraction, the enzyme acetylcholinesterase inactivates the ACh. This enzyme, which degrades ACh, is found within the area of the neuromuscular junction. Agents that are capable of inhibiting the action of the acetylcholinesterase enzyme are referred to as **anticholinesterases.** The effect of anticholinesterases at the neuromuscular junction is to prolong the availability and effects of the ACh.

These actions may be desirable in some disease states, and neostigmine and physostigmine are commonly used anticholinesterase drugs. However, too much anticholinesterase activity can produce a toxicity characterized by muscular spasms and asphyxiation due to spasms of skeletal muscles necessary for respiration. The signs of anticholinesterase toxicity also include constriction of the pupil of the eye, intestinal cramps, vomiting, and diarrhea. These signs are due to the increased availability of ACh at neural synapses within the parasympathetic division of the autonomic nervous system. Parasympathetic nerves are discussed in more detail in Chapter 10.

Anticholinesterase activity is the basis for some effective insecticides and the so-called nerve gases that have been studied extensively by the armed forces since World War II. Most of these compounds are alkyl phosphates, and the insecticides are also known as *organic phosphates* or *organophosphates.* The insecticides include such products as malathion, parathion, and diazinon. Products for both external application and oral administration are included in the organophosphate insecticides. If improperly used, any of the organophosphates is extremely dangerous, not only to domestic animals but also to the person using it. Therefore, it is imperative that this class of insecticides be used under proper supervision and that instructions for use are followed exactly.

Another group of drugs affecting the neuromuscular junction are the curariform drugs. These drugs act like **curare,** the deadly poison that South American Indians use on their arrowheads. These agents bind to ACh receptors on the postjunctional membrane, so that ACh cannot bind to the receptors and produce an end-plate potential. Curare is not destroyed by acetylcholinesterase. Death can result from asphyxiation because of paralysis of muscles needed for respiration. The paralysis induced by curariform drugs depends on the concentration of the drug, and such agents are used therapeutically to produce varying amounts of paralysis, such as for muscle relaxation during certain types of surgery.

Botulinum toxin, which is produced by the bacterium *Clostridium botulinum,* also acts at the neuromuscular junction. It prevents the release of ACh from the nerve ending by preventing synaptic vesicles containing ACh from binding to the cell membrane for exocytosis. Flaccid paralysis results because action potentials cannot be produced on the sarcolemma to bring about muscle contraction. The term *limberneck* has been applied to the characteristic flaccid paralysis of the neck in poultry intoxicated with botulinum toxin.

Types of Muscle Contraction

The primary function of muscle is to contract, that is, develop tension and shorten. However, contraction is often described as four types: concentric (shortening), eccentric (lengthening), isometric (same length but increased tension), and isotonic (same tension but length changes).

Concentric contraction is the usual form, in which the muscle moves a bone or segment by shortening. An example is flexion of the elbow by contraction of the *m. biceps brachii.*

Isometric contraction occurs naturally whenever a limb or portion of the body is held stationary against equal resistance, such as gravity. To hold the head up in a fixed position, the dorsal neck muscles must contract isometrically.

Eccentric contraction occurs in the extensor muscles of the neck when an animal lowers its head gradually. Antagonistic muscles may also undergo eccentric contraction when unsuccessfully opposing the actions of a prime mover.

Isotonic contraction occurs when the length of the muscle changes but the tension remains the same, primarily when a muscle lifts a given weight. The weight is constant; therefore tension does not change.

Rigor and Rigor Mortis. If most of the ATP in a muscle is depleted, the myosin heads cannot separate from the actin in the thin filaments and the calcium can no longer be sequestered back into the sarcoplasmic reticulum by the calcium pump. Therefore, relaxation cannot occur, because the actin and myosin filaments are bound in a continuous contracted state. This is termed *rigor,* and it is sustained until more ATP is made available. *Rigor mortis* is rigor that occurs a few hours after death, when ATP is no longer available. The muscles of the whole animal progressively become stiff and rigid; without ATP to sequester the calcium and separate the cross-bridges, the filaments remain locked together. The rigidity continues until cell autolysis and protein degradation break down the muscle.

Tone. The term *muscle tone* refers to the slight tension exhibited by all muscles at rest. It is due to the continuous transmission of impulses at very low frequency from the spinal cord to the muscles. Tone keeps muscles in a partially contracted state and prevents them from becoming flaccid (flabby), as occurs in paralysis.

When an animal becomes anxious, fearful, or excited, the muscle tone intensifies. Therefore, the muscles become taut (tension increases), and the animal can respond faster to any stimulus. This is often seen in the skittish, nervous, or jumpy animal. During sleep, muscle tone is low to allow for optimal relaxation.

Smooth Muscle

Smooth muscle is sometimes called *involuntary muscle* because it is found in structures that are not voluntarily or consciously regulated (e.g., gastrointestinal tract, blood vessels, reproductive tract). About 99% of the smooth muscle of the animal body is of the *visceral type,* which is also called *single-unit* or *unitary smooth muscle.* Cells of this type of smooth muscle are joined with gap junctions to provide mechanical and electrical connections between cells. The electrical connections permit the propagation of action potentials directly from cell to cell. The spreading of action potentials and the contraction that is elicited allow a group of muscle cells to act together as a single unit. This type of activity is appropriate for generalized activities of an entire organ, such as the contraction of the stomach.

About 1% of the smooth muscle of the animal body is *multiunit smooth muscle* (e.g., iris and ciliary body of the eye and pilomotor fibers that erect the hair in the skin). In this type of smooth muscle, the contraction of each individual smooth muscle cell is more dependent on its autonomic innervation. Gap junctions are not prevalent between these cells.

Structure

The smooth muscle cell is a fusiform (spindle shaped) contractile unit with a central nucleus. Size of smooth muscle fibers varies considerably. Most cells are 50 to 250 μm long and 5 to 10 μm in greatest diameter. The major portion of the cell consists of sarcoplasm. No cross-striations, myofibrils, or sarcolemma is easily visible with the light microscope (see Fig. 1–11). Filaments are present as actin and myosin molecules, but there are no orderly arrangements to form striations. Interactions between actin and myosin filaments (i.e., sliding filaments) are believed to be the basis for smooth muscle contractions, but the characteristic shortening of sarcomeres is not seen because there is no distinct organization of the filaments. A sarcoplasmic reticulum, which accumulates calcium, is present, but it is not as extensive or as highly organized as in skeletal muscle.

Like skeletal muscle, smooth muscle cells can hypertrophy to increase the size of organs. However, unlike skeletal muscle, smooth muscle cells can also divide mitotically to increase the number of cells. For example, the increase in size of the uterine wall during pregnancy to several times its nonpregnant volume is due in considerable measure to an increase in the amount of smooth muscle in the wall. Some of the increase is due to an increase in size of individual muscle fibers, but there is also an increase in the number of cells. This hypertrophy and hyperplasia in the uterus are under the influence of reproductive hormones. Late in pregnancy there is also a change in the structure of the cell membranes of uterine smooth muscle cells. An increase in gap junctions between cells in late pregnancy sets the stage for the mechanical and electrical coupling between smooth muscle cells that will be necessary for normal parturition. In general, the structure and function of smooth muscle are more subject to modification by external factors, such as hormones, than are those of skeletal muscle.

Stress–Relaxation

Smooth muscle exhibits a special property called **stress–relaxation,** or **plasticity.** This is the ability to adjust to stretching without increasing the final tension or the pressure exerted on the contents within a hollow viscus surrounded by smooth muscle. As the muscle stretches, the tension increases at first, but then in a few seconds or a few minutes the smooth muscle relaxes again to its original tension, even though it is still elongated.

This stress–relaxation occurs in the stomach when it is filling with food, in the intestines as the processed food moves along, in the blood vessels when the blood volume increases, in the urinary bladder as it increases its volume of urine, and in the uterus as pregnancy develops.

Plasticity allows expansion of stretch within physiologic limits without an increase in pressure and without pain; the smooth muscle does not lose its contractile ability. The reverse occurs upon emptying of a visceral organ when the stretched muscle shortens back to its original length: all tension is lost at first but returns shortly. Plasticity is believed to be due to changes in the arrangement or binding of the myosin and actin filaments upon stretching or shortening.

Contraction and Relaxation

All skeletal muscle contraction depends on ACh release at a neuromuscular junction and the generation and propagation of action potentials on the cell membrane. This is not the case for smooth muscle. The stimuli that bring about smooth muscle contraction and relaxation are quite variable. Thus, smooth muscle is a much more functionally diverse tissue than skeletal muscle.

The contraction and relaxation of most smooth muscle are much slower events than the rapid muscle twitch that is characteristic of skeletal muscle. This permits the maintenance of a relatively constant pressure with the use of little cell energy. This is characteristic of smooth muscle in organs that require a constant state of tone or some degree of contraction for normal function (e.g., smooth muscle in the walls of blood vessels).

Role and Sources of Calcium

As in skeletal muscle, contraction and relaxation of smooth muscle are linked to the Ca^{2+} concentration in the cytosol of smooth muscle cells. However, how this concentration is regulated and the role of Ca^{2+} in the contraction process is quite different in the two types of muscle. Some calcium is stored in the sarcoplasmic reticulum of smooth muscle cells, but many types of smooth muscle cells also contain a significant number of **calcium channels** in the outer cell membrane. These calcium channels may be either **voltage-gated or ligand-gated,** and the smooth muscle within a given organ may have both types of channels or primarily only one type of channel. When these channels open in response to the appropriate stimulus (changes in membrane potential or presence of specific ligands), calcium can diffuse into the cell to initiate contraction. Receptors that are specific for many different ligands (e.g., hormones and neurotransmitters) are found on the smooth muscle of different organs. This is important functionally, because a given hormone produces contraction only of organs with receptors for that specific hormone. Calcium entering from the outside via the channels may stimulate the release of further calcium from the sarcoplasmic reticulum, which further strengthens the contractions.

An understanding of the role of calcium channels in the outer cell membrane of smooth muscle cells lead to the development of a group of drugs termed calcium channel blockers. These agents are capable of binding to and inactivating these calcium channels, and this tends to reduce the strength of contractions. Smooth muscle cells in the walls of many arterial blood vessels have these types of channels, and this type of drug has been proved effective to lower blood pressure in both humans and animals.

When the cytosolic Ca^{2+} concentration increases within smooth muscles, the calcium ions bind to a regulatory protein (**calmodulin**), and these bindings results in contraction. Unlike skeletal muscle, whose regulatory proteins are associated with the actin filaments, the calmodulin in smooth muscle is associated with the heads of myosin molecules in myosin filaments. The binding of calcium to calmodulin activates a **kinase,** also associated with myosin, and this kinase **phosphorylates** other sites on myosin. This phosphorylation ultimately results in contraction, so **myosin phosphorylation** is a key regulatory step. This is in contrast to skeletal muscle, whose myosin does not require phosphorylation. For relaxation, the phosphorylation of myosin is reversed by other intracellular enzymes that are always present and active. This reversal and relaxation can occur when the cytosolic calcium concentration is reduced. Calcium is removed from the cytosol by the transport back into the sarcoplasmic reticulum or out of the cell. Most of this transport is done by an active transport system (Ca^{2+}–ATPase) on the membrane of the endoplasmic reticulum and the outer cell membrane.

Unlike skeletal muscle, some smooth muscle responds to certain stimuli by relaxation or a reduction in contraction strength. For example, stimulation of β_2-adrenergic receptors on airway smooth muscle in the lungs produces relaxation and an increase in airway diameter. In general this type of relaxation is due to either a reduction in the number or availability of calcium channels in the cell membrane or a reduction in the phosphorylation of myosin within the myofilaments of smooth muscle cells.

Action Potentials and Slow Waves

Not all smooth muscle cells have action potentials on their cell membranes during contraction and relaxation. Cells with predominantly ligand-gated calcium channels in their cell membranes may undergo a contraction–relaxation cycle without action potentials. The cell membrane may depolarize slightly because of the entry of calcium, but no action potential is seen. Smooth muscle cells that do have action potentials during contraction have both sodium and calcium electrically gated channels in their cell membrane.

Action potentials in skeletal muscle occur after the binding of ACh to its cell membrane receptors. In smooth muscle, action potentials can be elicited by a variety of stimuli. Some smooth muscle is similar to skeletal muscle in that action potentials occur only after the binding of ligands to cell membrane receptors, but action potentials may also occur in smooth muscle in response to **mechanical stretch** or during **slow-wave electrical activity.** The smooth muscle that responds to stretch is believed to have membrane channels that are subject to mechanical stimulation.

The visceral or single-unit smooth muscle in some organs (the gastrointestinal tract being the classic example) exhibit a unique type of membrane electrical activity termed slow waves. These are waves, or periods, of spontaneous fluctuations in the resting membrane potential that spread throughout a body of smooth muscle and typically occur at some regular rhythm (Fig. 8–8). Slow waves alone do not cause contractions, but action potentials may occur at the peak of these waves, and the action potentials are associated with contractions (Fig. 8–8). Because action potentials and contractions are seen only at the peak of the slow waves, the rate at which slow waves develop determines the rate at which smooth muscle contractions can occur. The precise origin of the slow waves is uncertain, but a variety of stimuli, such as hormones, neurotransmitters, and the local chemical environment, can determine whether action potentials occur at the peak of the slow waves. The relationship between slow-wave activity and action potentials is important in the regulation of gastrointestinal motility and is discussed in more detail in Chapter 21.

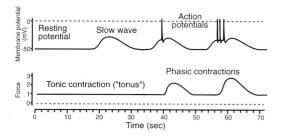

Figure 8-8. Slow-wave electrical activity in smooth muscle with action potentials and phasic contractions corresponding to peak of slow waves. (Reprinted with permission from Rhoades R.A. and Tanner G.A. *Medical Physiology.* Boston: Little, Brown, 1995.)

Action potentials spread across groups of single-unit smooth muscle fibers because of gap junctions between the fibers (where the plasma membranes of adjacent cells touch). Thus, single-unit smooth muscle cells can be linked electrically while remaining independent chemically (no secretion of transmitter substance from cell to cell is required).

Autonomic Innervation

In visceral or single-unit smooth muscle, the fibers of the **autonomic nervous system** travel between the smooth muscle cells in a branching network of terminal fibrils. These fibrils have varicosities (beadlike enlargements) at intervals along their axons. When action potentials depolarize them, the transmitter substance is released and diffuses to the smooth muscle cell membranes of several cells, where stimulation occurs. In multiunit smooth muscle, a branch of an autonomic nerve innervates each muscle fiber. This provides more direct neural control of each muscle cell, but the junction between neuron and muscle is less highly structured than the neuromuscular junction of skeletal muscle. For both types of smooth muscle, the innervation is usually dual; that is, both divisions of the autonomic nervous system innervate smooth muscle. Important exceptions are blood vessels (arteries, arterioles, and veins), which have predominantly sympathetic innervation, and in the skin, where the pilomotor fibers and sweat glands receive only sympathetic innervation.

Acetylcholine is released from the ***parasympathetic postganglionic*** nerve fibers and ***norepinephrine,*** from the ***sympathetic postganglionic*** fibers. The response of smooth muscle (contraction or relaxation) to these neuromediators depends on the type of autonomic receptor (Tables 10–1 and 10–2) on the smooth muscle and the intracellular events initiated by the binding of the neuromediators to their receptors. For example, stimulation of β_2-adrenergic receptors causes smooth muscle relaxation, while stimulation of α_1-adrenergic receptors causes smooth muscle contraction. Some smooth muscle can also be stimulated to contract by stimulation of muscarinic receptors by ACh. Individual smooth muscle cells may have multiple types of receptors in their cell membranes and respond to both autonomic neurotransmitters. In this case, the overall response of the smooth muscle also depends on the relative levels of the different neurotransmitters.

Cardiac Muscle

Cardiac muscle (sometimes known as involuntary striated muscle) has many anatomic characteristics that are similar to those of striated skeletal muscle fibers, although the striations are fainter than in skeletal muscle. Both types of muscle consist largely of sarcoplasm, myofibrils, a sarcoplasmic reticulum, transverse tubules, nuclei, and a sarcolemma. The most striking difference is the tendency for cardiac muscle fibers to branch and join, forming a network. The heart is made up of cells that are separate entities; however, unique structures, found where cardiac muscle meet end to end, are the **intercalated disks.** These disks can be seen with the light microscope (Fig. 1–6) and are interposed between muscle cells. The disks represent apposed cell membranes and gap junctions. The gap junctions provide a mechanical attachment between cells and permit electrical transmission from one cardiac muscle cell to the next. Action potentials can readily spread from cell to cell, causing cardiac muscle to act electrically and mechanically as a functional **syncytium,** as if it were a single cell mass.

Blood vessels and lymphatic vessels are both plentiful in cardiac muscle. A generous blood supply is essential, because most ATP production depends on aerobic metabolism. In humans disruption of the blood supply to cardiac muscle quickly results in myocardial ischemia and the symptoms of a heart attack. Cardiac muscle may also undergo necrosis (cell death) if the loss of blood supply is prolonged or extremely severe.

Excitation and Contraction

Individual cardiac muscle cells do not require nerve stimulation to contract, but action potentials must occur on the cell membrane. Action potentials first occur spontaneously within specialized myocardial **pacemaker cells** within the heart, and these are propagated throughout the heart by a specialized conduction system and from cell to cell via the gap junctions (at intercalated disks). The **impulse generation and conduction system** is described in detail in Chapter 18. Autonomic nerves innervate the pacemaker cells, and these serve to modify the rate of spontaneous action potentials, which in turn determines contraction rate of the entire heart.

The cardiac action potential is much slower than that of skeletal muscle. It lasts for hundreds of milliseconds (1 msec = 1/1000 second), as opposed to 5 to 10 msec in skeletal muscle. Also, the contraction time in cardiac muscle lasts as long as the action potential does. Instead of a sharp spike potential, the cardiac action potential has a long plateau, which extends the time of both the action potential and the muscle contraction.

As is true for the other two types of muscle, an increase in intracellular Ca^{2+} must occur to bring about cardiac cell contraction. In cardiac cells the Ca^{2+} enters the cell via electrically gated cell membrane channels and is also released from an extensive sarcoplasmic reticulum network. Thus, cardiac muscle has some similarities to both smooth and skeletal muscle. The Ca^{2+} binds to regulatory proteins on the actin filaments, and contraction occurs in a manner similar to that in skeletal muscle.

Cardiac Hypertrophy

Hypertrophy (increase in cell size) occurs in cardiac muscle when the heart has excessive work to do, but like skeletal muscle, mature cardiac muscle cells do not readily regenerate or undergo hyperplasia. **Living at high altitude may cause hypertrophy of the heart in both man and animals, partly because of increased vascular resistance and blood pressure in the lungs.** *Brisket disease* **(high mountain disease) of cattle occurs when hypertrophy of the heart cannot adequately compensate for the increased vascular resistance. A common clinical sign is edema of the brisket. Cardiac hypertrophy also occurs in people and animals who undergo strenuous athletic training.**

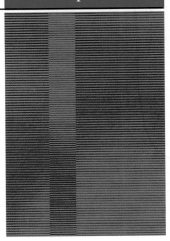

Chapter 9

Anatomy of the Nervous System

The nervous system consists of the **brain,** the **spinal cord,** and the **peripheral nerves,** which connect the various parts of the body to either the brain or spinal cord. A variety of cell types are found within the nervous system, but the primary functional cell is the **neuron.** A major function of the other cell types appears to be to support the activity of the neurons.

The basic functions of the nervous system can be summarized thus:

1. Initiate and/or regulate movement of body parts by initiating and/or regulating the contraction of skeletal, cardiac, and smooth muscles
2. Regulate secretions from glands
3. Gather information about the external environment and about the status of the internal environment of the body, using senses (sight, hearing, touch, balance, taste) and mechanisms to detect pain, temperature, pressure, and certain chemicals, such as carbon dioxide, hydrogen, and oxygen
4. Maintain an appropriate state of consciousness
5. Stimulate thirst, hunger, fear, rage, and sexual behaviors appropriate for survival

All functions of the nervous system require the rapid transmission of information from one site within the body to another. This transmission is possible in part because neurons have the property of **excitability.** This property (see Chapter 2) permits neurons to develop **action** *potentials* and rapidly propagate them along their individual cellular processes (axons). When an action potential reaches the end of an axon, the information encoded in the action potential is transmitted to another neuron or some other type of cell. This transmission is accomplished at specialized junctions known as *synapses.*

For descriptive purposes the entire nervous system (Fig. 9–1) can be divided into two parts: the *central nervous system (CNS)*, which includes the brain and spinal cord, and the *peripheral nervous system (PNS)*, which consists of cranial nerves and spinal nerves going to somatic (body) structures. A further distinction is often made: the *autonomic nervous system (ANS)*, which integrates activity of visceral structures (smooth muscle, cardiac muscle, and glands). The ANS has elements in both the central and peripheral nervous systems, and it features both sensory and motor components.

In the PNS, *sensory (afferent) nerves* gather information about the external and internal environments and relay this information to the CNS. The information is obtained by specialized organs or cells that react to specific environmental energies and initiate action potentials in associated sensory neurons. The specialized organs or cells that detect specific stimuli are *sensory receptors.* Sensory systems are discussed more completely in Chapter 11.

The CNS interprets information arriving via the PNS, integrates that information, and initiates appropriate movement of body parts, glandular secretion, or behavior in response. Communication between the CNS and muscles and glands is accomplished via *motor (efferent) nerves* of the PNS.

Microscopic Neuroanatomy

The individual nerve cell is called a *neuron* (Fig. 9–2). Neurons possess the usual features of cells, but in keeping with their function of communication over long distances, they also exhibit a number of specializations. Each neuronal cell body gives rise to one or more *nerve processes,* cytoplasmic extensions of the cell. The nerve processes are called *dendrites* if they transmit electrical signals toward the cell bod-

ies; they are called *axons* if they conduct electrical signals away from the cell bodies. The axon (each neuron gives rise to only one, which may branch) arises from a conical mound of cytoplasm, the *axon hillock,* and its terminus branches into an arborization called the *telodendrion.* The telodendrion makes contact with other neurons or effector organs. In mammals, *effector organs* stimulated either directly or indirectly by the telodendrion include muscles and glands.

The junction between the axon of one neuron with another neuron or target cell is the *synapse.* The neuron belonging to the axon is the *presynaptic neuron,* and the one receiving information from the axon is the *postsynaptic neuron.* A synapse may be between the axon of one neuron and the cell body, dendrites, and/or axon of the postsynaptic neuron. Typically, each neuron synapses with many other neurons through the extensive branching of its terminal ends and of its axon; branches of the main axon are *axon collaterals.*

Neurons may be classified morphologically according to their number of nerve processes (Fig. 9–3). *Unipolar neurons* have one process; *bipolar neurons* have one dendrite and one axon; and *multipolar neurons* have a number of dendrites in addition to their single axon. The nervous systems of adult mammals do not have true unipolar neurons, but many sensory neurons have their single dendrite and axon fused so as to give the appearance of a single process. This configuration is *pseudounipolar.*

Nervous tissue consists not only of neurons but also of supportive cells. In the CNS, these supportive cells are the *neuroglia,* comprising a variety of *glial cells,* while most of the supporting tissue of the PNS is ordinary white fibrous connective tissue.

Nerve fibers may be *myelinated* or *unmyelinated.* Myelinated fibers are surrounded by a white sheath of fatty material. This *myelin sheath* actually consists of many layers of cell membrane of a specialized glial cell, wrapped around axons so that in cross-section the myelin sheath resembles a slice of jelly roll. In the PNS, the myelinating cell is the *Schwann cell (neurolemmocyte)*, whereas in the CNS, the *oligodendrocyte* fulfills this function. Unmyelinated nerve fibers are not exposed directly to the ex-

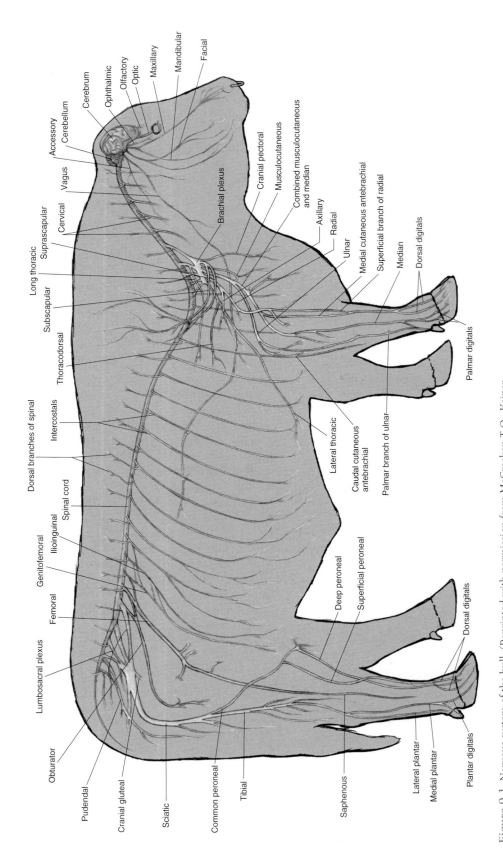

Figure 9-1. Nervous system of the bull. (Reprinted with permission from McCracken T.O., Kainer R.A. and Spurgeon T.L. *Spurgeon's Color Atlas of Large Animal Anatomy.* Baltimore: Lippincott Williams & Wilkins, 1999.)

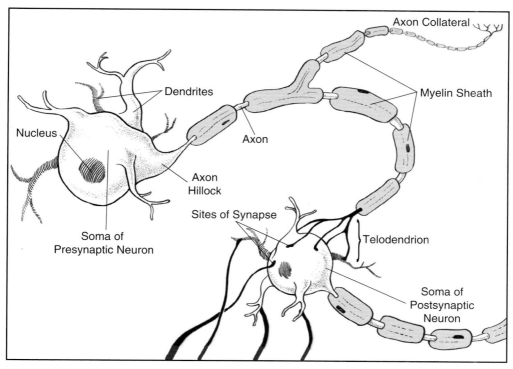

Figure 9-2. Cellular anatomy of a multipolar neuron.

tracellular fluid; rather, they are invaginated into the cell membrane of an adjacent Schwann cell. In this way all nerve fibers, myelinated or not, are covered by at least one layer of glial cell membrane. Several unmyelinated fibers may be invaginated into separate areas of the same Schwann cell (Fig. 9–4).

Groups of nerve cell bodies within the CNS are generally called **nuclei**, while groups of nerve cell bodies in the PNS are called **ganglia**. Do not confuse a nucleus of the CNS with the nucleus of an individual cell. Bundles of nerve processes within the CNS are frequently called **tracts**, or **fasciculi**, while bundles of processes in the PNS are called **nerves**. In general terms, aggregates of neuronal cell bodies form the **gray matter** of the CNS, whereas regions characterized primarily by tracts are **white matter.**

Embryology

The nervous system is the first organ system to begin to form in the embryo (see Chapter 3). Shortly after gastrulation, ectodermal cells on the dorsum just cranial to the primitive streak begin to proliferate and differentiate into a **neural plate.** The neural plate proliferates faster along its lateral margins than on the midline, creating the **neural groove,** the edges of which (the **neural folds**) ultimately meet dorsally to form the **neural tube** (Fig. 9–5). The entire CNS is formed from the cells of the neural tube. The lumen of the neural tube persists in the adult as the central canal of the spinal cord and as the ventricles of the brain (discussed later).

Closure of the neural tube is not simultaneous throughout the embryo. Fusion develops first at the level that will eventually become the medulla oblongata (the most caudal part of the brainstem) and proceeds craniad and caudad from there. The openings at the cranial and caudal end of the closing tube are called the **rostral** and **caudal neuropores,** respectively (see Fig. 3–4).

The rostral neuropore closes early in development; failure to do so disrupts development of the brain, leading to profound underdevelopment of the head. In its most severe form

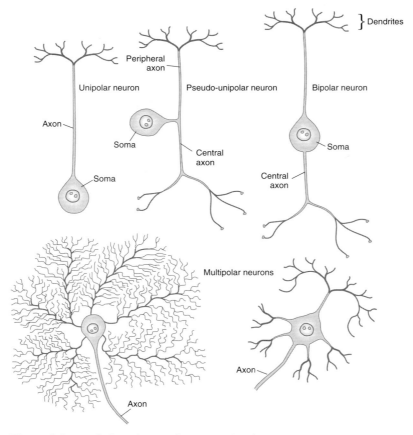

Figure 9-3. Morphological types of neurons. Classification is based on number of processes extending from the cell body. Unipolar neurons are not found in adult vertebrate nervous systems. Pseudounipolar and bipolar neurons are characteristic of sensory systems. Most neurons in the nervous system are multipolar and can assume a variety of shapes. (Reprinted with permission from Kingsley R.E. *Concise Text of Neuroscience.* Baltimore: Williams & Wilkins, 1996.)

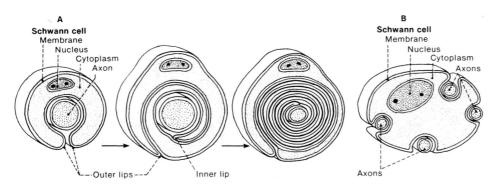

Figure 9-4. *A)* Cross-section of the development of a myelinated axon. In the peripheral nervous system, the myelinating glial cell is a Schwann cell; in the CNS the oligodendrocyte lays down myelin wraps. *B)* Some Schwann cells in the peripheral nerves envelop multiple axons without forming the wrappings of myelin. Axons thus embedded are considered nonmyelinated. (Reprinted with permission from DeMyer W. *Neuroanatomy.* Baltimore: Williams & Wilkins, 1988.)

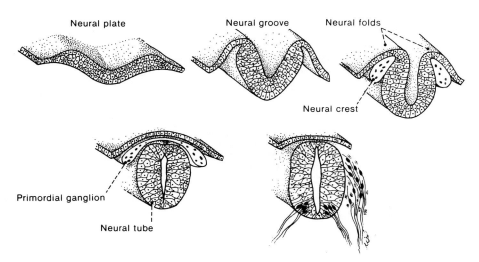

Figure 9-5. Formation of the neural tube. The thickened ectoderm of the neural plate develops into a groove that subsequently fuses on the dorsal side to form a closed tube. Neural crest cells adjacent to the neural folds differentiate into many tissues, including the neurons of the ganglia. (Reprinted with permission from DeMyer W. *Neuroanatomy*. Baltimore: Williams & Wilkins, 1988.)

(short of embryonic death), *anencephaly* **(a complete absence of the brain, often with concurrent absence of meninges and skull) results. The caudal neuropore closes later. Failure of closure in the caudal part of the neural tube results in a variety of spinal cord abnormalities called** *myelodysplasias.* **These are sometimes also associated with vertebral anomalies, such as** *spina bifida.*

As the edges of the deepening neural groove approach one another at the dorsal midline, a longitudinal column of cells differentiates at the union between the ectoderm and the neuroectoderm on each side of the groove. These cells, the **neural crest,** end up lateral to the neural tube on each side of it and eventually form sensory and autonomic ganglion cells, Schwann cells, and other related tissues. In addition, the neural crest gives rise to a variety of other cell types, including parts of the meninges and many of the bones and muscles of the head.

Development of the spinal cord continues by an increase in the thickness of the wall of the neural tube. As cells divide and differentiate, three concentric layers of the neural tube emerge: an inner ventricular zone, a middle intermediate zone, and a superficial marginal zone (Fig. 9–6).

The thin **ventricular zone** of cells (also called **ependymal zone**) surrounds the lumen of the neural tube and is the site of mitosis of neuronal and glial precursors in the developing nervous system. It will ultimately form the ependyma of the central canal of the spinal cord and of the ventricles of the brain.

As cells are born in the germinal layer, they migrate outward to form the **intermediate zone** (also called **mantle zone**). The intermediate zone comprises neurons and neuroglia and becomes the gray matter near the center of the cord. The dorsal parts of the intermediate zone develop into the **dorsal horns.** It is here that sensory processing takes place. The ventral intermediate zone becomes the **ventral horns,** the location of the motor neurons whose axons will extend out into the periphery to innervate muscles and glands.

The **marginal zone,** which is most superficial, consists of nerve processes that make up the white matter of the spinal cord. The white color comes from the fatty myelin sheaths. The spinal cord white matter is divided into **dorsal, lateral,** and **ventral funiculi,** which are delimited by the dorsal and ventral horns of gray matter.

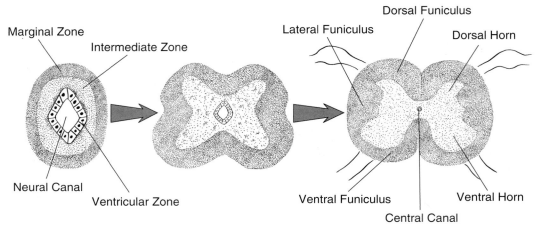

Figure 9-6. Cross-sectional view of the development of the spinal cord.

Development of the brain (Fig. 9–7) begins before the neural tube is fully closed caudally. It grows rapidly throughout embryonic and fetal life and into the neonatal period. The first gross subdivisions of the brain create the three-vesicle stage. These subdivisions, which consist of three dilations of the presumptive brain, are the *prosencephalon,* or forebrain; *mesencephalon,* or midbrain; and *rhombencephalon,* or hindbrain. The prosencephalon develops lateral extensions, the **optic vesicles,** the precursors of the optic nerves and retinas.

In the five-vesicle stage of development, the prosencephalon further subdivides to form the *telencephalon* (future cerebrum) and the **diencephalon,** and the rhombencephalon divides into the **metencephalon** (future pons and cerebellum) and the **myelencephalon** (future medulla oblongata). The mesencephalon does not subdivide.

Central Nervous System

Brain

The gross subdivisions of the adult brain include the *cerebrum, cerebellum,* and **brainstem** (Figs. 9–8 and 9–9). The cerebrum devel-

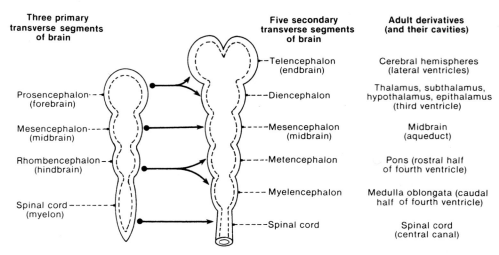

Figure 9-7. Dorsal view of the neural tube. The early brain divides into three vesicles that further differentiate into five vesicles. These give rise to the main regions of the adult brain. (Reprinted with permission from DeMyer W. *Neuroanatomy.* Baltimore: Williams & Wilkins, 1988.)

ops from the embryonic telencephalon. The components of the brainstem are defined in a number of ways; for our purposes, we include the *diencephalon, midbrain, pons,* and *medulla oblongata* as parts of the brainstem.

Telencephalon. The telencephalon, or *cerebrum,* comprises the two *cerebral hemispheres,* including the *cerebral cortex,* the *basal nuclei,* and other subcortical nuclei, and the *rhinencephalon.* The telencephalon encloses the cavities of the lateral ventricles and the rostral portion of the third ventricle.

The surface area of the cerebrum in domestic mammals is increased by numerous foldings to form convex ridges, called **gyri** (singular **gyrus**), which are separated by furrows called *fissures* or *sulci.* A particularly prominent fissure, the *longitudinal fissure,* lies on the median plane and separates the cerebrum into its right and left hemispheres. Unlike the spinal cord, in the cerebrum the neurons (and conse-

quently the gray matter) are on the exterior. This layer of cerebral gray matter is called *cerebral cortex.* In humans and some animals, the cortical areas have been extensively mapped to localize specific sensory and motor functions. Anatomic regions defined by consistent features and general function are referred to as *lobes.* The cerebral cortex is the site at which voluntary movements are initiated, sensations are brought to consciousness, and higher functions, such as reasoning and planning, take place.

Deep to the cerebral cortex are aggregates of subcortical gray matter called the *basal nuclei* (an older term, basal ganglia, is discouraged, as the word *ganglion* usually refers to an accumulation of cell bodies outside the CNS). The basal nuclei are important in initiation and maintenance of normal motor activity. In humans, *Huntington's chorea* and *Parkinson's disease* are movement disorders caused by degeneration of parts of the basal nuclei.

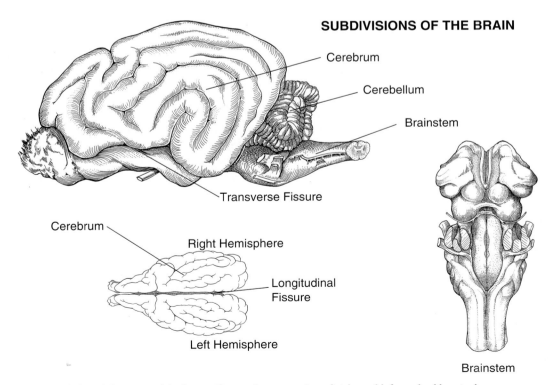

Figure 9-8. Subdivisions of the brain. The cerebrum consists of right and left cerebral hemispheres. (Reprinted with permission from Miller M.E., Christensen G.C., and Evans H.E. *Anatomy of the Dog.* 3rd ed. Philadelphia: W.B. Saunders, 1993.)

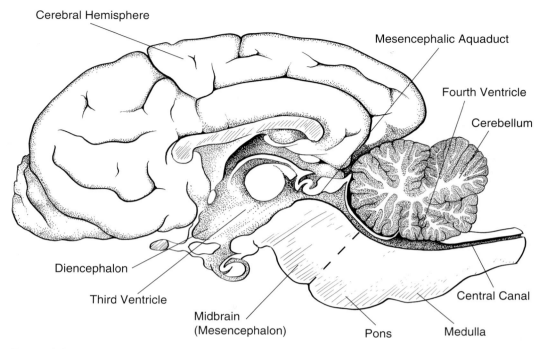

Figure 9-9. Midsagittal section of the brain. The lateral ventricles, one in each cerebral hemisphere, are not seen on this view, as they lie lateral to the midline.

The ***rhinencephalon*** is, from the evolutionary standpoint, one of the oldest parts of the cerebrum. It comprises a series of ventral and deep cortical structures associated primarily with the sense of smell (olfaction) and is therefore sometimes called the olfactory brain. The rhinencephalon has prominent connections to the parts of the brain that control autonomic functions, emotional behaviors, and memory, a fact that accounts for the striking ability of odors to affect these functions.

Diencephalon. The ***diencephalon*** is a derivative of the prosencephalon. The thalamus, epithalamus, hypothalamus, and the third ventricle are included in the diencephalon.

The ***thalamus*** is an important relay center for nerve fibers connecting the cerebral hemispheres to the brainstem and spinal cord. The ***epithalamus,*** dorsal to the thalamus, includes a number of structures, notably the ***pineal gland,*** which is an endocrine organ in mammals. Its primary secretion, ***melatonin,*** appears to be important in circadian (daily) rhythms and sleep induction. In addition, activity of the pineal gland is likely to be important in species with markedly seasonal reproductive cycles.

The ***hypothalamus,*** ventral to the thalamus, surrounds the ventral part of the third ventricle and comprises many nuclei that function in autonomic activities and behavior. Attached to the ventral part of the hypothalamus is the ***hypophysis,*** or ***pituitary gland,*** one of the most important endocrine glands. The neuronal connections between the hypothalamus and the hypophysis constitute a critical point of integration of the two primary communication systems of the body, the nervous and endocrine systems.

Mesencephalon. The ***mesencephalon,*** or ***midbrain,*** lies between the diencephalon rostrally and the pons caudally. The two cerebral peduncles and four colliculi are the most prominent features of the midbrain.

The ***cerebral peduncles,*** also called ***crura cerebri,*** are large bundles of nerve fibers connecting the spinal cord and brainstem to the cerebral hemispheres. These peduncles consist of both sensory and motor fiber tracts.

The *colliculi* (*corpora quadrigemina*) are four small bumps (*colliculus* is Latin for little hill) on the dorsal side of the midbrain. They consist of right and left *rostral colliculi* and right and left *caudal colliculi.* The rostral colliculi coordinate certain visual reflexes, and the caudal colliculi are relay nuclei for audition (hearing).

Metencephalon. The *metencephalon* includes the *cerebellum* dorsally and the *pons* ventrally. The cerebellum features two *lateral hemispheres* and a median ridge called the *vermis* because of its resemblance to a worm. The surface of the cerebellum consists of many laminae called *folia.* In the cerebellum, like the cerebrum, the white matter is central, and the gray matter is peripheral in the *cerebellar cortex.* The cerebellum is critical to the accurate timing and execution of movements; it acts to smooth and coordinate muscle activity.

The pons is ventral to the cerebellum, and its surface possesses visible *transverse fibers* that form a bridge from one hemisphere of the cerebellum to the other. Many other fiber tracts and cranial nerve nuclei make up the remainder of the pons.

Myelencephalon. The *myelencephalon* becomes the *medulla oblongata* in the adult. It is the cranial continuation of the spinal cord, from which it is arbitrarily distinguished at the foramen magnum. The medulla oblongata (often simply called the medulla) contains a number of important autonomic centers and nuclei for cranial nerves.

Ventricular System. The *ventricles* of the brain are the remnants of the lumen of the embryonic neural tube (Fig. 9–10). Right and left *lateral ventricles* lie within the respective cerebral hemispheres. They communicate with the midline *third ventricle* by way of the *interventricular foramina.* Most of the third ventricle is surrounded by the diencephalon. The third ventricle connects with the *fourth ventricle* by way of the *mesencephalic aqueduct* (cerebral aqueduct) passing through the midbrain.

The fourth ventricle, between the cerebellum above and pons and medulla below, communicates with the *subarachnoid space* surrounding the CNS through two *lateral apertures.* Each ventricle features a *choroid plexus,* a tuft of blood capillaries that protrudes into the lumen of the ventricle. The plexus of capillaries is cov-

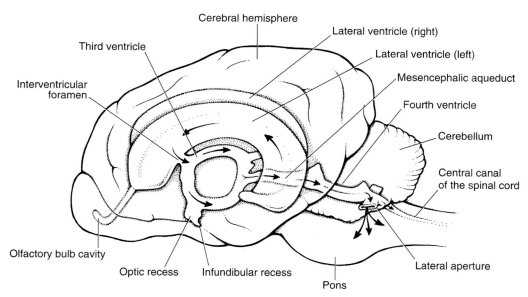

Figure 9-10. Ventricular system of the brain. *Arrows* indicate the direction of flow of CSF, which is produced in the ventricles and flows via the lateral apertures into the subarachnoid space surrounding the brain and spinal cord. (Reprinted with permission from Smith B.J. *Canine Anatomy.* Philadelphia: Lippincott Williams & Wilkins, 1999.)

ered by a layer of ependymal cells that are continuous with the lining membrane of the ventricles.

Cerebrospinal fluid (CSF), filling the ventricular system and surrounding the CNS, is formed primarily by the choroid plexuses, with a smaller contribution made by the ependyma lining the ventricles. CSF is a modified transudate, formed primarily through active secretion by the ependymal cells, especially those of the choroid plexuses.

The circulation of cerebrospinal fluid begins in the two lateral ventricles (where the majority is produced), flows through the interventricular foramina into the third ventricle, then by way of the cerebral aqueduct into the fourth ventricle, and finally through the lateral apertures into the subarachnoid space, where it surrounds both the brain and spinal cord. CSF is reabsorbed back into the venous blood via special modifications of the meninges called *arachnoid granulations.* These tiny structures protrude into the blood-filled dural sinuses (discussed later) and act as one-way valves for the return of CSF from the subarachnoid space to the venous blood. Reabsorption of CSF is passive, driven by the pressure gradient across the arachnoid granulations (i.e., the higher pressure of CSF within the subarachnoid space drives the CSF into the low pressure sinus).

Any obstruction in cerebrospinal circulation can injure the brain, since the choroid plexuses produce CSF independent of the pressure within the ventricular system. Buildup of CSF will expand the affected ventricular spaces at the expense of nervous tissue, which can be markedly compressed as a result. If this occurs during development (as often happens when the mesencephalic aqueduct is inadequately formed), the head can become markedly enlarged and the cerebral tissue extremely attenuated. This is the condition called *hydrocephalus* (literally, water head). In an older individual whose cranial bones are fully formed and fused at the sutures, buildup of CSF does not visibly enlarge the head; the elevated pressure inside the cranial vault, however, can profoundly affect the brain within.

Meninges

The coverings of the brain and spinal cord are the *meninges* (singular *meninx*). They include, from deep to superficial, the *pia mater,* the *arachnoid,* and the *dura mater* (Fig. 9–11).

The *pia mater,* the deepest of the meninges, is a delicate membrane that invests the brain and spinal cord, following the grooves and depressions closely. The pia mater forms a sheath around the blood vessels and follows them into the substance of the CNS.

The middle meninx arises embryologically from the same layer as the pia mater but separates from it during development so that a space forms between them. Remnants of their former connection in the adult take the form of many filaments of connective tissue that extend between them. Because of the weblike appearance of these filaments, this middle layer is called the *arachnoid* (arachnoidea, arachnoid mater), and the connecting filaments are the *arachnoid trabeculae.* Together, the pia mater and arachnoid constitute the *leptomeninges* (from the Latin word *lepto,* delicate), reflecting their fine, delicate nature. The space between the two layers, bridged by arachnoid trabeculae, is the *subarachnoid space.* It is filled with CSF. It is from this space that CSF is collected when a spinal tap is performed.

The *dura mater* is the tough fibrous outer covering of the CNS. Within the cranial vault the dura mater is intimately attached to the inside of the cranial bones and so fulfills the role of periosteum. It also forms the *falx cerebri,* a median sickle-shaped fold that lies in the longitudinal fissure and partially separates the cerebral hemispheres. Another fold of dura mater, the *tentorium cerebelli,* runs transversely between the cerebellum and the cerebrum. In some locations within the skull, the dura mater splits into two layers divided by channels filled with blood. These *dural sinuses* receive blood from the veins of the brain and empty into the jugular veins. They are also the site of reabsorption of CSF back into the circulation.

The pia mater and the arachnoid of the spinal meninges are much as they are within the cranial vault. The dura mater of the spinal meninges, however, is separated from the pe-

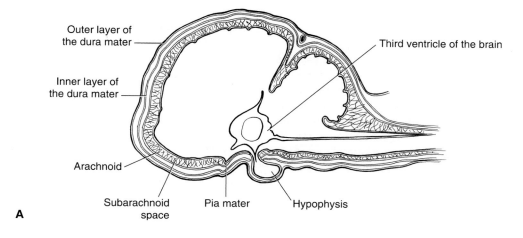

A

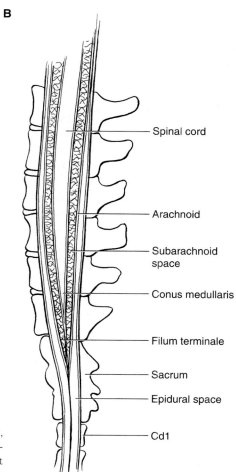

B

Figure 9-11. Meninges. *A)* Cranial meninges. *B)* Spinal meninges, depicted at the caudal end of the spinal cord. (Reprinted with permission from Smith B.J. *Canine Anatomy.* Philadelphia: Lippincott Williams & Wilkins, 1999.)

riosteum of the vertebral canal by a fat-filled space, the **epidural space.**

It is into the epidural space that physicians and veterinarians introduce local anesthetics to produce anesthesia in the caudal parts of the body. This procedure, *epidural anesthesia,* is often done for obstetric procedures. One common application is the injection of anesthetic between the first and second caudal vertebrae of the ox as an aid to repairing and reducing uterine, vaginal, or rectal prolapses.

Spinal Cord

The spinal cord (Figs. 9–12 and 9–13) is the caudal continuation of the medulla oblongata. Unlike that of the cerebrum, the spinal cord's gray matter is found at the center of the cord, forming a butterfly shape on cross-section. Myelinated fiber tracts, the white matter, surround this core of gray matter. A **spinal cord segment** is defined by the presence of a pair of spinal nerves. Spinal nerves are formed by the conjoining of **dorsal** and **ventral roots.**

Sensory neurons of neural crest origin are present in aggregates, called **dorsal root ganglia,** lateral to the spinal cord. The neurons within these ganglia are pseudounipolar, and they give rise to axons that enter the dorsal horn of the spinal cord and other fibers that join with motor fibers from the ventral horn neurons to become a **spinal nerve** extending into the periphery. The processes that extend from the spinal nerve to the spinal cord, which are sensory, are collectively called the **dorsal root.**

The **ventral root** of the spinal nerve consists largely of motor fibers that arise from the nerve cells in the ventral horn of the spinal cord. The dorsal and ventral roots unite to form the spinal nerve close to the intervertebral foramen between adjacent vertebrae. The dorsal root ganglion is usually very close to this conjoining of dorsal and ventral roots; it frequently can be found just within the intervertebral foramen. In this location it is susceptible to compression when an intervertebral disk protrudes; to a large degree, it is this compression that causes the intense, electric pain associated with disk disease.

Tracts of the Spinal Cord. A *tract* is a bundle of functionally related axons in the CNS. Tracts that carry **sensory** information are **ascending** tracts, whereas those carrying **motor** commands are **descending** tracts. The white matter of the spinal cord in which the tracts are found can be roughly divided into three columns on each half of the cord: a **dorsal funiculus** (often called the **dorsal column**), a **lateral funiculus,** and a **ventral funiculus.**

Sensory Tracts. The **dorsal funiculi** contain afferent tracts that primarily carry information

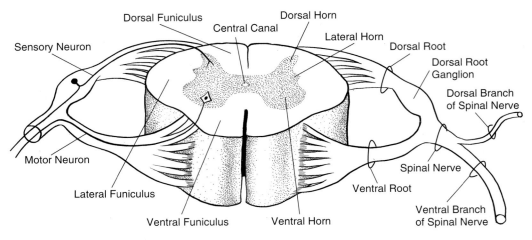

Figure 9-12. Cross-sectional anatomy of the spinal cord and spinal nerves.

about body position from joints, tendons, and muscles. This type of sense is called **proprioception**. Injury to this pathway produces uncoordinated, inaccurate movements, as the cortex lacks some of the information it needs to make ongoing adjustments in the planning and execution of voluntary movements. Such incoordination is **sensory ataxia**.

Proprioceptive information also ascends the spinal cord in several **spinocerebellar tracts,** located superficially on the lateral funiculus. As the name suggests, these tracts are headed for the cerebellum, where the proprioceptive information is used to shape voluntary movements so that they are accurate and smooth.

Information about pain is carried by a large number of described pathways, but these are often grouped under the name **spinothalamic tract** or **anterolateral system.** This large group of fibers is found in a wide band through the lateral and ventral funiculi. Some of these tracts terminate in the brainstem, where they mediate reflexes associated with painful stimuli. Others make connections that alert the entire cortex and initiate aversive behaviors. Still others are relayed directly to the parts of the cortex that create conscious awareness of the painful stimulus.

Like pain, touch information is carried in a variety of ascending tracts. Some of these are found in the dorsal columns and others in the spinothalamic system.

Motor Tracts. Motor systems are often functionally grouped into two main categories: a ventromedial motor system, largely local to the ventral funiculus, and a dorsolateral motor system, found in the dorsal part of the lateral funiculus.

The **ventromedial motor system** primarily is responsible for activity in the axial and proximal limb muscles, especially extensors and antigravity muscles. Activity in the tracts of this system assists with the supportive phase of gait, when limbs are in weight-bearing position with joints extended. A particularly noteworthy tract of the ventromedial motor system is the **lateral vestibulospinal tract,** which originates in the region of the pons and medulla.

The **dorsolateral motor system** is in many ways complementary to the ventromedial system. Dorsolateral tracts tend to control the muscles of the distal limb, especially the flexors. Activity here is important in the flexion or swing phase of gait, when limbs are lifted from the ground and advanced while flexed. In quadrupeds, the most prominent tract in the dorsolateral motor system is the **rubrospinal tract,** which arises from the midbrain. In primates and most especially humans, the **corticospinal tracts** arising from the motor cortex of the cerebrum are especially well developed.

Peripheral Nervous System

The PNS includes the nerves and ganglia outside the CNS. Its purpose is to convey sensory information to the brain and spinal cord and to produce movement of muscle and secretion from glands via its motor nerves.

Spinal Nerves

With the exception of cervical and caudal nerves, a pair of spinal nerves (one right and one left) emerges caudal to the vertebra of the same serial number and name (Fig. 9–13). For example, the first pair of thoracic nerves emerges through the intervertebral foramina between the first and second thoracic vertebrae; the last pair of thoracic nerves emerges through the intervertebral foramina between the last thoracic and first lumbar vertebrae, and the second pair of lumbar nerves emerges through the foramina between the second and third lumbar vertebrae. Thus there are the same number of pairs of thoracic, lumbar, and sacral nerves as there are similar vertebrae.

The first pair of cervical nerves emerges through the lateral vertebral foramina of the atlas, and the second pair between the atlas (C1) and axis (C2). Therefore, there are eight pairs of cervical nerves although only seven cervical vertebrae.

Usually there are fewer pairs of caudal nerves than caudal vertebrae. Five or six pairs are typically seen in domestic ungulates.

Dorsal and ventral roots arise from the spinal cord and fuse, generally close to the intervertebral foramen. At this point, the conjoined sensory fibers of the dorsal root and motor fibers of

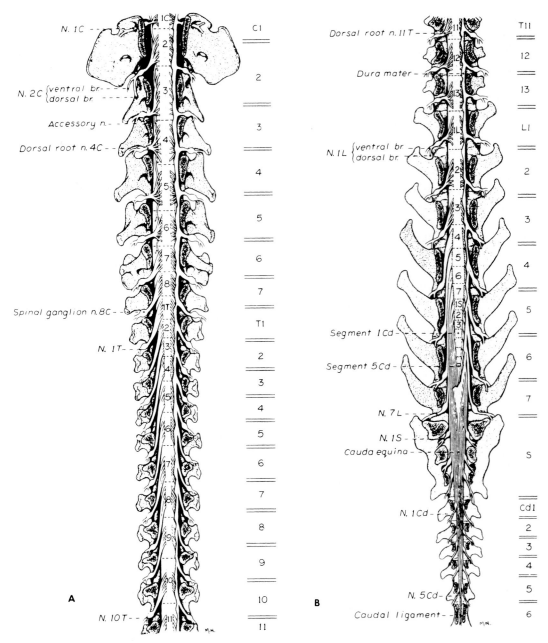

Figure 9-13. Spinal cord of the dog. View is from dorsal side, with the vertebral arches removed to expose the cord within the vertebral canal. Note the relation of the spinal nerves to the vertebral bodies. The spinal cord is shorter than the vertebral column, so that the more caudal spinal cord segments lie within vertebrae whose name and number are more cranial (e.g., spinal cord segment L6 lies within vertebra L4). The nerve roots are progressively longer in these more caudal parts of the vertebral column as they extend from the cord to the foramen of exit. (Reprinted with permission from Fletcher T.F. and Kitchell R.L. Anatomical studies on the spinal cord segments of the dog. A.J.V.R. 1966;27:1762.)

the ventral root become the **spinal nerve,** characterized as a **mixed nerve,** since it has both sensory and motor elements.

Almost as soon as the spinal nerve emerges through the intervertebral foramen, it divides into a **dorsal branch** and a **ventral branch.** Both of these branches are mixed nerves, because each contains both sensory and motor fibers.

In general, the dorsal branches of spinal nerves innervate structures (muscles and skin) that are dorsal to the transverse processes of the vertebrae. The ventral branches supply structures ventral to the transverse processes and most of the thoracic and pelvic limbs.

The spinal nerves tend to innervate the re-gion of the body in the area adjacent to where they emerge from the vertebral column. The limbs, however, are supplied with sensory and motor fibers within tangled arrangements of spinal nerves known as **plexuses.** The regions of the spinal cord supplying the plexuses are visibly greater in diameter because they have more sensory and motor neurons supplying the mass of the limbs. These enlargements are called **intumescences.**

Brachial Plexus. Each thoracic limb is supplied by a **brachial plexus,** a network of nerves derived from the last three cervical and first one or two thoracic nerves (Figs. 9–1 and 9–14). The spinal cord enlargement associated with

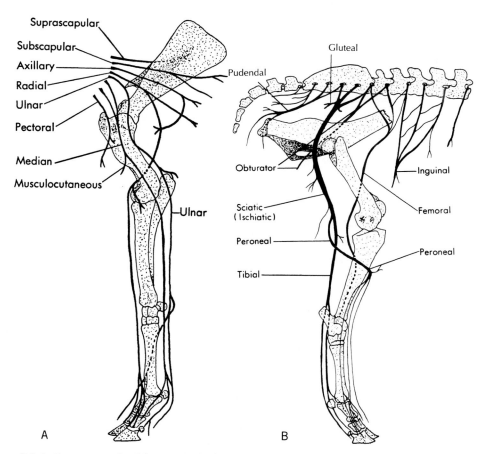

Figure 9-14. *A)* Nerve supply of thoracic limb of the ox. These nerves arise from the brachial plexus. *B)* Nerve supply of pelvic limb of the ox. These nerves arise from the lumbosacral plexus. (After McLeod W.M. Bovine Anatomy. 2nd ed. Minneapolis: Burgess Publishing, 1958.)

the brachial plexus lies primarily in the caudal cervical vertebrae and is consequently described as the **cervical intumescence**.

The brachial plexus gives rise to specific named nerves that innervate the muscles of the thoracic limb and supply sensation to the same general regions of the skin. Table 9–1 lists the nerves arising from the brachial plexus and the region and muscles supplied by each.

Lumbosacral Plexus. The right and left **lumbosacral plexuses** supply nerves to the respective pelvic limbs (Figs. 9–1 and 9–14). The lumbosacral plexuses are made up of the ventral branches of the last few lumbar and first two or three sacral nerves. The nerves derived from the lumbosacral plexus are described in Table 9–2.

Cranial Nerves

Classically, 12 pairs of **cranial nerves** arising from the brain are described (Fig. 9–15). They are designated by Roman numerals, numbered from most rostral (I) to most caudal (XII). With the exception of cranial nerves I (olfactory) and

Table 9-1. Nerves of Brachial Plexus

Nerve	Muscles Innervated	Cutaneous Distribution
Suprascapular	*Supraspinatus & infraspinatus*	No sensory fibers
Pectorals	Superficial, deep pectoral	No sensory fibers
Subscapular	*Subscapularis*	No sensory fibers
Musculocutaneous	*Biceps brachii* *Coracobrachialis* *Brachialis*	Medial aspect of antebrachium, carpus; craniomedial aspect of metacarpus
Axillary	*Teres minor et major* Deltoid	Shoulder region
Radial	*Triceps brachii* *Anconeus* *Extensor carpi radialis* Common and lateral digital extensors *Ulnaris lateralis* *Extensor carpi obliquus* *Supinator*	Craniolateral aspect of antebrachium
Ulnar	*Flexor carpi ulnaris* Deep digital flexor Intrinsic mm of digit (when present)	Caudal aspect of antibrachium, craniolateral aspect of Metacarpus, pastern/foot
Median	*Flexor carpi radialis* Superficial and deep digital flexor *Pronator teres* (when present)	Caudal metacarpus, pastern/foot
Thoracodorsal	*Latissimus dorsi*	No sensory fibers
Lateral thoracic	*Cutaneous trunci*	No sensory fibers

Table 9-2. Nerves of Lumbosacral Plexus

Nerve	Muscles Innervated	Cutaneous Distribution
Cranial gluteal	Middle and deep gluteal, *tensor fasciae latae*	No sensory fibers
Caudal gluteal	Superficial gluteal	No sensory fibers
	Parts of middle gluteal, *semitendinosus, biceps femoris* in horse	
Femoral	*Sartorius*	Medial aspect of thigh
	Quadriceps femoris	
	Iliopsoas	
Obturator	*Adductor*	No sensory fibers
	Gracilis	
	Pectineus	
	Obturator externus	
Sciatic	*Semitendinosus et semimembranosus*	Sensory fibers arise from distal branches (peroneal & tibial nn.)
	Biceps femoris	
	Obturator internus	
	Gemelli	
	Quadratus femoris	
Peroneal	*Tibialis cranialis*	Dorsal metatarsus and pastern/foot
	Extensor digitorum longus et lateralis	
	Peroneus	
Tibial	*Gastrocnemius*	Caudal crus, plantar metatarsus, pastern/foot
	Flexor digitorum superficialis et profundus	
	Tibialis caudalis	
	Popliteus	

II (optic), the cranial nerves arise from the midbrain, pons, and medulla oblongata and in general resemble ordinary spinal nerves. They do not, however, have discernible dorsal and ventral roots, and some are strictly motor or sensory (as apposed to spinal nerves, which are all mixed nerves).

Cranial nerve II, the optic nerve, only superficially resembles an actual nerve of the PNS. Its fibers are a tract of the CNS, invested with meninges and with myelin provided by oligodendrocytes. Features of the 12 cranial nerves are outlined in Table 9–3.

Autonomic Nervous System

The ANS is the part of the nervous system that regulates activity in viscera and other structures not normally under voluntary control (Fig. 9–16). The common representation of the ANS as a motor subdivision of the peripheral nervous system ignores the facts that (1) sensory fibers from viscera make up a large proportion of the fibers in autonomic nerves and (2) some CNS tracts and nuclei integrate and control visceral activity. Nonetheless, for purposes of this introduction, we consider only the peripheral

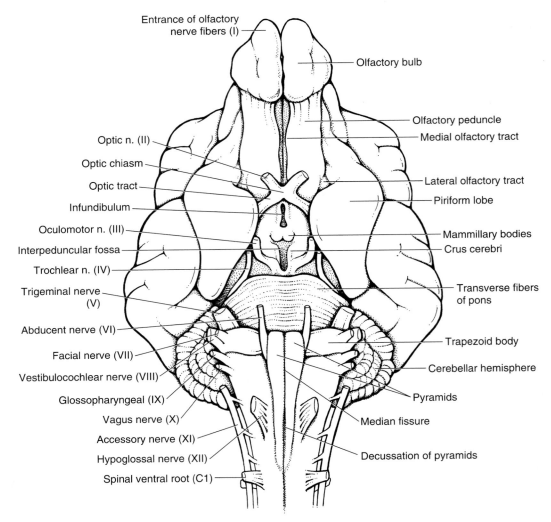

Figure 9-15. Ventral view of the canine brain. (Reprinted with permission from Smith B.J. *Canine Anatomy*. Philadelphia: Lippincott Williams & Wilkins, 1999.)

motor components of the ANS. These are the nerves that influence activity in smooth muscle, cardiac muscle, and glands.

In motor nerves to voluntary muscle, the cell bodies of neurons directly innervating the target are found in the ventral horn of the spinal cord, and the telodendria of these neurons make direct contact with the target. Motor nerves of the ANS, in contrast, consist of a series of *two* neurons. The first has its cell body in the CNS, and its axon extends into the periphery, where it synapses on the cell body of a second neuron. It is the axon of the second neuron that contacts the visceral target. Because of this two-neuron

arrangement, autonomic nerves are characterized by *autonomic ganglia,* peripheral collections of the cell bodies of the second neurons. Using the autonomic ganglion as a point of reference, the first neuron is called *preganglionic,* and the second, *postganglionic.*

The motor output of the ANS is concerned with *homeokinesis,* the dynamic process of regulating the internal environment to meet the needs of the organism. As a consequence, the ANS is functionally and anatomically divided into two parts. The *sympathetic division* of the ANS prepares the organism to meet a stress by producing a combination of physiologic

Table 9-3. Synopsis of Cranial Nerves

Number	Name	Type	Arises From	Function and Distribution
I	Olfactory	Sensory	Olfactory bulb	Olfaction (smell); nasal mucosa
II	Optic	Sensory	Diencephalon	Vision; retina
III	Oculomotor	Motor	Midbrain	Motor to extraocular eye muscles; parasympathetic innervation to iris sphincter and ciliary muscles
IV	Trochlear	Motor	Midbrain	Dorsal oblique muscle of eye
V	Trigeminal	Mixed	Pons	
	Ophthalmic division	Sensory		Sensory to eye and dorsal parts of head
	Maxillary division	Sensory		Sensory to maxillary region, nasal cavity, palates, upper teeth
	Mandibular division	Mixed		Sensory to tongue, lower teeth and jaw; Motor to muscles of mastication
VI	Abducens	Motor	Medulla	Lateral rectus and retractor bulbi muscles of eye
VII	Facial	Mixed	Medulla	Sensory (taste) to rostral two-thirds of tongue; parasympathetic to salivary and lacrimal glands; motor to muscles of facial expression
VIII	Vestibulocochlear	Sensory	Medulla	Hearing (cochlear division) and sense of acceleration (vestibular division)
IX	Glossopharyngeal	Mixed	Medulla	Sensory (taste) to caudal third of tongue; parasympathetic to salivary glands; motor to pharyngeal muscles
X	Vagus	Mixed	Medulla	Sensory to pharyngeal, laryngeal mucosa, most viscera; parasympathetic to cervical, thoracic and most abdominal viscera; motor to pharyngeal, laryngeal muscles
XI	Accessory	Motor	Medulla & Cervical Spinal Cord	Motor to cervical, shoulder muscles (e.g., *trapezius*)
XII	Hypoglossal	Motor	Medulla	Muscles of tongue

changes often called the fight-or-flight response. The ***parasympathetic division*** of the ANS is in many respects the opposite of the sympathetic division. Parasympathetic activity leads to digestion and storage of fuel molecules and acts to bring the organism to a state of rest. This is sometimes called the rest-and-digest response. The physiologic effects of the two divisions are covered more completely in Chapter 10.

Sympathetic Nervous System

Sympathetic nerve fibers arise from thoracic and lumbar segments of the spinal cord, and so the sympathetic division is sometimes called the ***thoracolumbar division***. Preganglionic sympathetic neurons have their cell bodies in a small ***lateral horn*** of the spinal cord gray matter, between dorsal and ventral horns. The myelinated axons of these fibers leave via the ventral root,

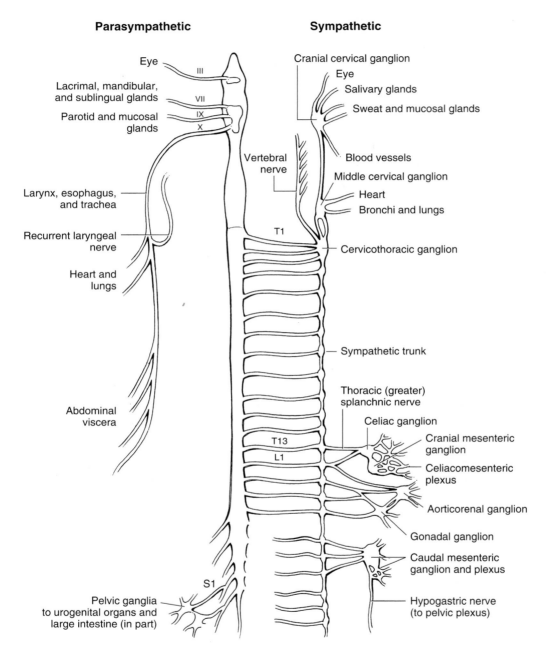

Figure 9-16. The autonomic nervous system. *Left)* The parasympathetic outflow with cranial nerves III, VII, IX, and X and sacral spinal cord segments carrying parasympathetic fibers. *Right)* The sympathetic division. Thoracic and cranial lumbar segments make contributions to the sympathetic trunk. These projections are bilateral and are shown on one side only in this drawing for purposes of clarity.

enter the spinal nerve, and then leave it just outside the intervertebral foramen to join a longitudinal chain of autonomic ganglia. One string of these ganglia lies on each side of the vertebral column. Each receives preganglionic fibers from the spinal nerves only in thoracic and lumbar regions, although the chains themselves extend from the cranial cervical region to the most caudal parts of the vertebral column. The ganglia, together with the nerve fibers that link them longitudinally, are called the *sympathetic trunk.* The ganglia themselves are most correctly called the *ganglia of the sympathetic trunk,* although they are also called *paravertebral ganglia.* Cell bodies of many of the postganglionic sympathetic neurons are found here. From the sympathetic trunk ganglia, the unmyelinated axons of postganglionic neurons reach their targets either following spinal nerves or via unique autonomic nerves.

In some cases, preganglionic axons pass through the trunk without synapsing and instead synapse on other sympathetic ganglia outside the sympathetic trunk. This second group, collectively known as *prevertebral ganglia,* tends to be associated with the large, unpaired arterial branches of the abdominal aorta, after which they are usually named.

No sympathetic preganglionic cell bodies lie cranial to the thoracic spinal cord, so sympathetic innervation to head structures (e.g., the pupil, sweat glands, salivary glands) arrives at its targets by traveling craniad in right and left bundles of fibers in the ventral neck. These are the cranial continuation of the sympathetic trunks in the thorax. These preganglionic sympathetic fibers are bound in a connective tissue sheath with fibers of each vagus nerve (cranial nerve X); the combined fibers are the *vagosympathetic trunk,* readily identified dorsolateral to and parallel with the trachea (windpipe). Sympathetic fibers in the vagosympathetic trunk synapse in the *cranial cervical ganglion,* found deep to the tympanic bulla of the skull, and from this ganglion the postganglionic fibers spread to the structures of the head.

No sympathetic preganglionic cell bodies exist caudal to the midlumbar region, so sympathetic innervation to pelvic organs (rectum and urogenital organs) arrives via the right and left *hypogastric nerves,* a continuation of the cau-

dal parts of the sympathetic trunk. The fibers of the hypogastric nerve become admixed with parasympathetic fibers in a diffuse network of autonomic nerves on the lateral surface of the rectum called the *pelvic plexus.*

The sympathetic innervation to the *adrenal gland* (see Chapter 11) is unique in that preganglionic sympathetic fibers synapse directly on the chromaffin cells of the adrenal medulla without an intervening ganglion. Sympathetic stimulation causes this tissue to release *catecholamines* (epinephrine and norepinephrine) into the blood stream, producing a widespread, pronounced, and prolonged fight-or-flight response. This is another physiologically important site at which the rapid communication system of the body (the nervous system) is integrated with the slow, more lingering communication system of the body (the endocrine system).

Parasympathetic Nervous System

The parasympathetic division of the autonomic nervous system arises from cranial nerves and sacral segments of the spinal cord; for this reason, it is sometimes called the *craniosacral division.* Fibers of the cranial portion are distributed via four cranial nerves: the oculomotor, facial, glossopharyngeal, and vagus nerves. The first three of these supply parasympathetic fibers to smooth muscle and glands of the head. The vagus nerve supplies parasympathetic fibers to the viscera of the thorax and neck and to nearly all of the abdominal viscera. The distal part of the digestive tract (including transverse colon and caudal to it) and the pelvic viscera are innervated by parasympathetic fibers from the sacral portion of the parasympathetic nervous system. These pelvic fibers intermix with sympathetic nerves to form the pelvic plexus.

Enteric Nervous System

Neuroanatomists recognize another subdivision of the nervous system, the *enteric nervous sytem.* This is the network of motor and sensory neurons embedded in the walls of the gastrointestinal tract and its accessory glands (e.g., pancreas, liver). Activity in the enteric nervous system is influenced by the parasympathetic and sympathetic divisions of the ANS, but the system is functional without input from outside the viscera. Two dense networks of neurons are found in the walls of these organs. One, the **submucosal (Meissner's) plexus,** is just deep to the inner lining of the gut. The other, the **myenteric (Auerbach's) plexus,** is found within the muscular layer.

Normally the motor output of the ANS controls the overall activity of the viscera, but in large part the intrinsic neurons of the enteric nervous system control local events. Sensory neurons monitor local stretch, chemical composition of the gut's contents, and gastrointestinal hormones. Activity in these sensory neurons stimulates local reflex movements, mediated by the motor neurons of the enteric nervous system. In this way, motility of the gut, dilation of local blood vessels, and secretions can be adjusted to meet the immediate local demands of digestion.

Chapter 10

PHYSIOLOGY OF THE NERVOUS SYSTEM

Physiology of the Nerve Impulse

Nerves rapidly transmit information from one body site to another via nerve impulses (i.e., action potentials propagated along the axons of neurons within the nerves). The genesis of a resting membrane potential and the development of action potentials and their propagation are described in detail in Chapter 2 and are only briefly reviewed here.

The resting membrane potential of neurons depends mainly on **nongated potassium channels** in the cell membrane and the **electrogenic Na–K–ATPase,** or **Na–K, pump.** The continuous exit of potassium from the cell down its concentration gradient and the continuous activity of the pump maintain a difference in charge across the membrane so that the interior is negative relative to the exterior (i.e., resting membrane potential).

The axonal cell membranes of neurons contain **voltage-gated sodium channels.** These channels are closed at normal resting membrane potentials but rapidly open when the membrane potential is brought to threshold voltage. This results in the inward movement of sodium (down its concentration gradient) and a large, rapid membrane **depolarization** (Fig. 10–1). At the peak of the action potential (maximal depolarization), the sodium channels close and some additional **voltage-gated potassium channels** are open. The closing of the sodium channels and the

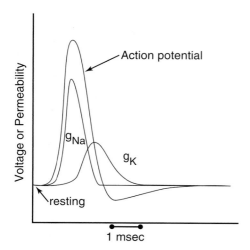

Figure 10-1. Change in sodium and potassium permeability during neuron action potential. The lines labeled *Na* and *K* show the respective changes in membrane permeabilities, and the changes are drawn to illustrate their time course relative to the action potential.

exit of additional potassium **repolarizes** the membrane. The exit of additional potassium produces a small **afterhyperpolarization** until resting conditions can be reestablished (Fig. 10–1).

When an action potential occurs on the axon of a neuron, the membrane potential of adjacent areas is altered by local movement of charge. Normally this causes the sodium channels in the adjacent area to reach their threshold voltage, and another action potential is elicited. By this means action potentials can be propagated along axons (Fig. 2–16). Propagation normally occurs in only one direction, in part because the sodium channels where the action potential just occurred are **refractory** to another stimulus. This refractory period is a characteristic of normal sodium channels, and the channels rapidly pass through this period, so that they are no longer refractory when another normal impulse arrives.

Conduction Velocity and Myelination

As described in Chapter 9, the axons of neurons may be either unmyelinated or myelinated. Unmyelinated axons have voltage-gated sodium channels throughout their cell membrane, and thus the propagation of action potentials along unmyelinated axons is as described earlier. The myelin sheath that surrounds myelinated axons contains the lipid **sphingomyelin**, which is a good insulator against ionic flows. Each Schwann cell covers about a 1-mm distance along the axon, and the junction between two Schwann cells is called the **node of Ranvier.** No myelin is present at these nodes, and voltage-gated sodium channels are especially prevalent in the axonal cell membrane at the node. Therefore, the circuits of current must flow from node to node, and action potentials occur only at the nodes. Since this is analogous to jumping from one node to the next, it is given the name **saltatory conduction** (from Latin *saltare,* to jump) (Fig. 10–2). This type of conduction contributes to the increased rate of impulse conduction in myelinated axons.

Conduction velocities of axons also depend on their diameter. Large-diameter axons propagate action potentials at higher velocities than do small-diameter axons, because large axons have less internal resistance to the flow of current. Large myelinated fibers, 20 μm in diameter, approach conduction velocities of 250 mph (130 m/second). At this rate an impulse could travel 6 feet in about 15 msec. The smallest unmyelinated fibers of the body, about 0.5 μm in diameter, conduct at only about 20 inches per second (0.5 m/sec).

Synaptic Transmission

Synapses are specialized junctions where information is exchanged between neurons or between a neuron and the cell or cells that it in-

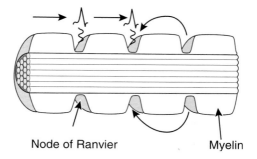

Figure 10-2. Propagation of the action potential in a myelinated axon. Action potentials occur at each node of Ranvier.

nervates. Two general types of synapses, *electrical* and *chemical,* are found between neurons in the nervous system, with chemical synapses being more prevalent. Electrical synapses are essentially gap junctions between the cell membranes of adjacent neurons that permit ionic exchange.

Information exchange at chemical synapses entails the release of a chemical *neurotransmitter* from the presynaptic neuron. When an action potential arrives at the terminal end of the presynaptic neuron, the change in membrane potential is believed to be responsible for opening voltage-gated calcium channels. The calcium concentration within the cytosol is lower than the calcium concentration in the extracellular fluid, so calcium can diffuse through the open channels into the cell down its concentration gradient. The increase in intracellular calcium within the terminal end of the presynaptic neuron is associated with exocytosis of neurotransmitters stored in secretory vesicles within the presynaptic neuron. Typically, an individual neuron contains vesicles with only one primary neurotransmitter, but a wide variety of substances have been found to function as neurotransmitters. These are discussed later in this chapter.

The cell membranes of presynaptic and postsynaptic neurons (or other target cells) are not in immediate contact. A small but distinct separation exists, and the space between is the *synaptic cleft.* Neurotransmitters released by the presynaptic neuron must diffuse across the synaptic cleft to have their effect on postsynaptic neurons, or target cells. However, this diffusion occurs almost instantaneously because of the very small size of the cleft (average 20 nm, or about a millionth of an inch). The events of synaptic transmission are summarized in Figure 10–3.

Neurotransmitters typically bind to cell membrane receptors on postsynaptic neurons or target organs. At synapses between neurons, the binding changes the postsynaptic membrane's permeability to ions (either directly or indirectly via second messengers), and this in turn produces a change in the membrane potential of the postsynaptic neuron. Synapses and the neurotransmitters that depolarize the postsynaptic neuron are *excitatory synapses* and *excitatory*

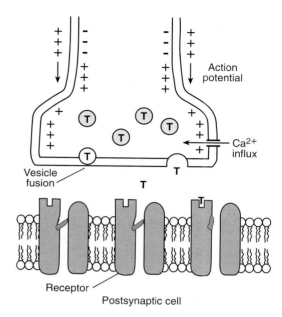

Figure 10-3. Summary of events involved in synaptic transmission. *1)* Action potential arrives and stimulates release of neurotransmitter (shown as T) by exocytosis. *2)* Neurotransmitter diffuses to site of its receptor and binds. *3)* Binding produces change in postsynaptic cell (e.g., opening of membrane channel). (Reprinted with permission from Rhoades R.A. and Tanner G.A. *Medical Physiology.* Boston: Little, Brown, 1995.)

neurotransmitters, while synapses and neurotransmitters that *hyperpolarize* the postsynaptic neuron are *inhibitory.* The change in postsynaptic membrane potential produced by excitatory neurotransmitters is an *excitatory postsynaptic potential* (**EPSP**), while an inhibitory neurotransmitter produces an *inhibitory postsynaptic potentials* (**IPSP**). Typically, excitatory neurotransmitters cause membrane depolarization by increasing the membrane's permeability to sodium, while inhibitory neurotransmitters increase the membrane's permeability to either potassium or chlorine. Hyperpolarization of the cell membrane can be brought about by either an increased rate of potassium exit from a cell or an increased rate of chlorine entry into the cell down their respective concentration gradients.

The amount of excitatory neurotransmitter released by a single action potential in a single presynaptic neuron is constant. However, it is also typically insufficient to depolarize the post-synaptic neuron to a threshold voltage at which an action potential can be elicited. Therefore, to reach threshold voltage in a postsynaptic neuron, the change in voltage produced by multiple EPSPs must be **summated.** Summation of EPSPs is classified as either *temporal* or *spatial.* Temporal summation occurs when a single presynaptic neuron releases neurotransmitter repeatedly before the effect of each single release is lost. When effective summation occurs, the additive effects of the multiple releases are enough to produce an action potential in the postsynaptic neuron. Spatial summation occurs when simultaneous or nearly simultaneous neurotransmitter release occurs at more than one synapse on the postsynaptic neuron. Spatial summation is possible because neuron cell bodies typically have multiple junctions with many presynaptic neurons.

After a neurotransmitter has been released and had its desired effect on the postsynaptic neuron, it must be removed to prevent continuous stimulation of the postsynaptic neuron. The specific mechanisms by which neurotransmitters are removed from neural synapses vary among neurotransmitters. However, in general these can be any one or a combination of the following: (1) enzymes in the area of the synapse degrade the neurotransmitter; (2) cell membrane transport systems absorb the neurotransmitter; or (3) the neu-

rotransmitter diffuses away from the area of the synapse.

Typically, as described earlier, a single neuron and its dendrites contain multiple synaptic junctions and receive synaptic input from multiple presynaptic neurons, so a single neuron may receive impulses from several sources. This pattern or organization is described as *convergence* (Fig. 10–4). *Divergence* is the opposite: each axon branches, so that synaptic connections are made with many neurons (Fig. 10–4). These organizational patterns permit information to be widely distributed throughout a neural network (divergence) or permit multiple sources of information to be brought to focus on a single neuron for a focused response (convergence). These are very simple illustrations of how the organization of neuronal networks can contribute to the processing and integration of information. For example, a single neuron can be simultaneously stimulated by excitatory and inhibitory neurotransmitters from different presynaptic neurons (a converging network). The property of spatial summation permits the neuron receiving these converging inputs to integrate the different stimuli and respond appropriately.

Neurotransmitters

Most neurotransmitters can be classified as amino acids, monamines (modified amino acids), or polypeptides. While more than 20 com-

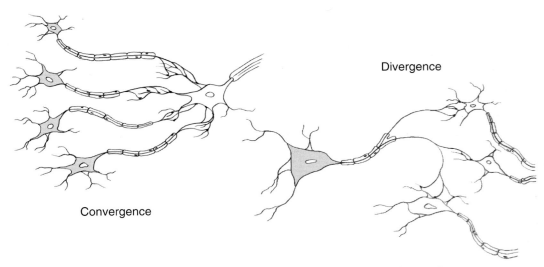

Divergence

Convergence

Figure 10-4. Simple patterns to illustrate convergence and divergence in neural networks.

pounds have been proved to function as neurotransmitters (and the list will surely grow), some are especially prevalent throughout the nervous system and should receive individual consideration.

Acetylcholine (derived from the amino acid choline) is the neurotransmitter released at the neuromuscular junction on skeletal muscle (see Chapter 8) by some peripheral neurons of the autonomic nervous system (ANS) (discussed later) and found at many synapses throughout the central nervous system (CNS). Neurons releasing acetylcholine are classified as **cholinergic,** and this term is also applied to synapses for which acetylcholine is the neurotransmitter. Two general classes of acetylcholine (also termed cholinergic) receptors, **nicotinic** and **muscarinic,** are found at cholinergic synapses. The enzyme *acetylcholinesterase* is responsible for rapidly degrading acetylcholine and thus terminating its action at cholinergic synapses.

Norepinephrine is the neurotransmitter used by most peripheral neurons in the sympathetic division of the ANS (discussed later) and at synapses at several sites in the CNS. Presynaptic neurons and synapses using norepinephrine are termed **adrenergic,** and this term is also applied to cell membrane receptors that bind norepinephrine. The term *adrenergic* has been applied to these receptors because **epinephrine,** or **adrenaline,** also binds to these receptors. (Adrenaline is the British term for epinephrine, which is released from the adrenal gland.) Adrenergic receptors may be classified as α_1, α_2, β_1, or β_2 according to their relative binding affinities for various adrenergic agonists. Epinephrine and norepinephrine are both classified as **catecholamines** because of their chemical structure and because they are derived from the amino acid tyrosine. *Dopamine* is another catecholamine that functions as a neurotransmitter within the central and peripheral nervous systems, and specific dopamine receptors also exist.

γ-Aminobutyric acid (GABA) is the most prevalent inhibitory amino acid neurotransmitter in the CNS. Binding of GABA to its receptor produces neuronal hyperpolarization (inhibition). **Several agents that act as sedatives, tranquilizers, and general muscle relaxants have part of their effect via promoting GABA's effects on the CNS. These include alcohol, barbiturates, and the benzodiazepines (e.g., diazepam and chlordiazepoxide). Some of these agents bind directly to GABA receptors; others seem to facilitate the action of endogenous GABA. The GABA receptors may also be the principle target for some general anesthetics.**

Glutamate is the predominant excitatory neurotransmitter in the CNS, and several subtypes of glutamate receptors have been identified. One subtype of glutamate receptor, the NMDA receptor (named for the agonist N-methyl-D-aspartate), are found in high concentrations in areas within the brain that are involved with memory and learning. Stimulation of NMDA receptors is believed to bring about long-term potentiation of transmission in neural pathways in these areas.

Neural Control of Skeletal Muscle

As described in Chapter 7, each contraction of skeletal muscle requires stimulation of the muscle by a somatic motor neuron. Somatic motor neurons have their cell bodies within the CNS, and their axons extend from the CNS to contact skeletal muscle cells at neuromuscular junctions. Each time an action potential passes down the axon of a single motor neuron, all skeletal muscle cells that are innervated by that motor neuron are stimulated to contract. A single motor neuron can stimulate more than one skeletal muscle cells, since its axon branches, but a single skeletal muscle cell receives input from only one motor neuron. Thus, all contractions of any single skeletal muscle cell must be initiated by action potentials arriving via the same motor neuron. **A clinical classification applied to the motor neuron that extends from the CNS to skeletal muscle fibers is *lower motor neuron (LMN).* (More specifically, this is the somatic LMN, but *somatic* is often omitted in common usage.) Any contraction of skeletal muscle depends on an intact and properly functioning LMN, and the classic sign of a dysfunctional LMN is *flaccid paralysis* (a total lack of movement and muscle tone of the affected muscle).**

Typically, a single neuron receives inputs

from multiple other neurons because of convergence in neural networks. Therefore, a single LMN is subject to regulation by multiple inputs from other neurons within the CNS. **Upper motor neuron (UMN)** is the general term applied to a neuron within the CNS that acts to regulate the activity of a LMN. UMNs are responsible for initiating voluntary movement and maintaining relatively stable body posture and position relative to gravity, so that voluntary movements are normal. If the LMNs to a muscle are intact but some of the UMNs that normally regulate those LMNs are dysfunctional, both reflex and voluntary activity of the muscle are possible, but the character of both reflexes and voluntary activity may be abnormal.

Reflexes Involving Skeletal Muscle Contraction

A **reflex** action is an automatic, or unconscious, response to an appropriate stimulus. In the case of reflexes involving skeletal muscle, the response is skeletal muscle contraction. The simplest reflex requires two neurons. The first is an afferent neuron, which detects the appropriate stimulus and transmits that information via action potentials to the CNS. Within the CNS the afferent neuron synapses with and stimulates action potentials in an efferent neuron. The efferent neuron exits the CNS and stimulates skeletal muscle contraction. The entire neural circuit from stimulus detection to response is a **reflex arc,** and in the simplest case, in which only one synapse is involved, the reflex arc is a **monosynaptic reflex** (Fig. 10–5). Very few reflexes are monosynaptic; usually one or more interneurons are interposed between the afferent and efferent neurons.

Reflexes can be classified according to the segments or parts of the CNS that are required to complete the reflex arc or circuit. Among the simplest of reflex arcs are those that can be completed within segments of the spinal cord (**spinal reflexes**). A typical spinal reflex is the **patellar tendon reflex,** or knee jerk reflex (Fig. 10–5). The knee jerk is elicited by tapping the patellar ligament (tendon), which causes the knee or stifle to extend. The sudden stretching

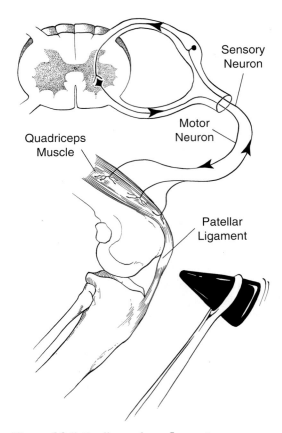

Figure 10-5. Patellar tendon reflex arc is a monosynaptic spinal reflex.

of the muscle simulates muscle spindles (see Chapter 11) related to the quadriceps muscle. Action potentials are transmitted along axons of primary afferent neurons and into the spinal cord by way of the dorsal root. A synapse occurs between the afferent neuron and appropriate motor neurons in the ventral gray horn of the spinal cord. Action potentials then are transmitted via the efferents to the muscle fibers of the **m. quadriceps femoris** of the thigh (in this case the muscle in which the stimulus originated), causing it to contract. This type of **stretch reflex** is also known as a **postural reflex** because it aids in maintaining a standing position. Sudden flexing of the stifle stretches the quadriceps muscle, which initiates the reflex that causes the stifle to support the weight of the animal. The same reflex occurs in humans when the area just below the knee is struck.

The fact that the patellar tendon reflex arc

can be completed within a limited region of the spinal cord does not mean that other segments of the CNS cannot affect the characteristics of the reflex response. Through the actions of either inhibitory or excitatory UMNs that affect the activity of the LMNs participating in the reflex arc, the strength or character of the reflex response can be changed. As described earlier, the patellar tendon reflex is an example of a postural reflex that functions to maintain a normal posture and body position. By affecting the character of the reflex, UMNs can also assist in the maintenance of posture and body position. More information about the regulation of UMNs is given later in this chapter.

Reflex center is a general term used to describe the area within the CNS where afferent information is integrated to produce the efferent activity or reflex response. In the case of simple spinal reflexes, the reflex center is within the spinal cord (i.e., the synapses are between the afferent and efferent neurons). Reflexes can be quite complex and may require integration by reflex centers within the brain or brainstem. **For example, vomiting is a reflex that can be stimulated by a variety of diverse stimuli and that requires a series of highly coordinated contractions of skeletal muscles in the diaphragm, esophagus, and pharynx. These actions are coordinated by a reflex center in the brainstem. This center receives afferent information from quite diverse areas (such as the stomach lining and the vestibular apparatus) and stimulates efferent neurons to all participating skeletal muscles. This center can be stimulated pharmacologically by the administration of any of a variety of *emetic* drugs.**

In the dog, *spinal reflexes* that are used in various types of clinical examinations include the *withdrawal reflex,* in which the limb is withdrawn when the footpad or toe is pinched; patellar tendon reflex, in which extension of the stifle results from tapping the patellar ligament; and *extensor postural thrust reflex,* in which the limb extends when the foot is pushed toward the body, as would occur in normal body support.

Attitudinal and postural reactions include the *tonic neck reflexes,* in which passively extending the neck (raising the head) increases the tone of extensor muscles of the forelimbs

and decreases the tone of extensor muscles of the hind limbs. This may be a partial explanation for the value of raising a horse's head to prevent kicking. Conversely, when a horse that gets its head down is much more likely to kick or buck. The *extensor postural thrust* enables the limbs to support the weight of the body without conscious thought on the part of the animal.

Reflexes associated with the cranial nerves include the *corneal reflex,* in which the eyelids close in response to stimulation of the cornea of the eye, and the *palpebral reflex,* in which gentle palpation or tapping of the eyelids causes closure. General anesthesia depresses reflex responses, and these last two reflexes are often used to evaluate the depth of anesthesia.

Voluntary Movement and Its Regulation

Animals cannot be asked about their intentions or thoughts while moving about. Therefore, much of what is known or assumed about voluntary movement in animals is based on information from humans; that is, humans are the experimental animals. Much of the information from humans is based on studies of individuals with naturally occurring diseases or acquired neural deficits due to trauma. Studies on animals with similar lesions or deficits suggest that the underlying mechanisms are the same in humans and animals.

A classic diagram in textbooks on human physiology defines an area of the cerebral cortex, the *motor cortex,* and shows areas within it that control various groups of skeletal muscles (Fig. 10–6). While this does not mean that neurons from this area make direct synaptic connections with skeletal muscle cells, a functional association between these areas and specific skeletal muscles can be demonstrated by eliciting contractions of specific muscles by stimulation of discrete areas within the motor cortex. However, the precise linkage between the desire for and initiation of a specific voluntary movement (e.g., reaching for, grasping, and lifting a cup of coffee) and how the necessary muscles are appropriately stimulated to bring about that movement are not completely understood.

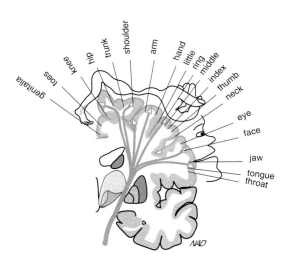

Figure 10-6. Cross-section of an area of motor cortex showing the areas that control the various parts of the body. The human features are drawn to show the relative amount of representation within the cortex. In humans a large area is devoted to control of the digits. In farm animals such as the horse, the area devoted to control of the digits is small. The size of the area depends on the need for fine motor control. (Reprinted with permission from Johnson L.R. *Essential Medical Physiology*. 2nd ed. Philadelphia: Lippincott-Raven, 1998.)

What is understood about normal voluntary movement, and is more relevant to animals, is that it requires a great deal of afferent information before and during the movement, and this information is used for the coordination of voluntary movements. This afferent information is primarily derived from *proprioceptors* (specialized sensory receptors designed to provide information about body position discussed in Chapter 11) in muscles, tendons, and joints throughout the body. This information is vital for coordinated movements. For example, to reach for a cup of coffee and grasp it, the position of arms, hands, and fingers must be known first. When the cup is lifted, continuous adjustments must be made in muscle contraction so that the movement is smooth regardless of the weight of the cup or the amount of coffee in it. Much of the afferent information on body position is received and used by the brain without any conscious awareness.

The *cerebellum* receives much of the afferent information about body position and ongoing movements from proprioceptors. It also receives information about movements initiated in the cerebral cortex. After integrating this and other information, the cerebellum sends efferent information to multiple sites in the brain, including the motor cortex, to coordinate ongoing movements. The cerebellum does not initiate movements, but it is essential for normal coordination of voluntary movements.

It is clear that repetition of a pattern or sequence of movements increases the ease with which those movements can be repeated (i.e., training). This indicates that a type of learning can also occur within the neural circuits regulating voluntary movements. After such learning occurs, a series of practiced movements are virtually automatic and can be done without any conscious direction. Exactly how and where this learning occurs is not known, but the basal nuclei (see Chapter 9) appear to have special importance in coordinating and enabling the automatic performance of repeated movement patterns. **Dopamine is an important neurotransmitter in certain basal nuclei, and Parkinson's disease in humans is associated with the loss of dopaminergic neurons in this area of the brain. Patients with Parkinson's disease exhibit a variety of abnormal movements, and complex movement patterns seem to be especially affected. Treatment with L-dihydroxyphenylalanine (L-dopa), a precursor of dopamine, may relieve the symptoms, but it does not prevent further neuronal loss and progression of the condition.**

All UMNs have their effects on skeletal muscle activity and movement indirectly by ultimately affecting LMN neuron activity. Because the final common pathway for all movement (reflex or voluntary) is via the LMN and because the function of UMNs is to regulate LMN activity, abnormal movements may result from dysfunction of either LMNs or UMNs regulating the activity of a specific muscle. The abnormal movement may be primarily voluntary movements, reflex-based movements, or both. By close observation of abnormal movements and with a detailed knowledge of LMNs, UMNs, and the primary functions of the sites within the CNS from where UMNs originate, clinicians can determine the type and location of dysfunctional neurons causing the abnormal movements.

Physiology of the Autonomic Nervous System

Regulation of ANS activity

The ANS functions to maintain a relatively stable internal body environment; that is, to maintain a state of homeokinesis (homeostasis). It does so by regulating the activity of cardiac muscle, smooth muscle, and glands. The distribution of ANS nerves is widespread, including all viscera. Normally the regulation of ANS activity occurs below the level of consciousness. However, emotional reactions (such as fear or excitement) and input from the cerebral cortex also affect ANS activity.

Most organs that are innervated by the ANS have both sympathetic and parasympathetic innervations, and in most cases the effects of the two divisions are antagonistic. For example, parasympathetic stimulation of the heart reduces heart rate, while sympathetic stimulation increases heart rate. The antagonistic actions are controlled to bring about appropriate overall regulation of the innervated organ. In the case of the heart, relatively high parasympathetic nerve activity to the heart in an animal at rest maintains a low resting heart rate. During rest there is little sympathetic nerve activity to the heart. To increase heart rate, such as during exercise, parasympathetic nerve activity is first reduced to permit an increase in heart rate, and sympathetic nerves to the heart are activated if a further increase in heart rate is necessary for more intense exercise.

Changes in ANS nerve activity can occur as a result of discrete reflexes. For example, the diameter of the pupil of the eye is controlled by an ANS reflex initiated by changes in the amount of light detected by the retina. The circular smooth muscle fibers of the iris constrict the pupil and are under the control of parasympathetic nerves. Changes in the amount of light reaching the retina initiate a reflex response to achieve a precise and proper pupil diameter.

Arterial blood pressure, salivary secretion, secretion of hydrochloric acid by the stomach,

urination, and defecation are among functions regulated in part by ANS reflexes. The reflex centers for various ANS reflex arcs are found throughout the CNS. For example, the brainstem has several centers regulating blood pressure, and the reflex center for urination is in the sacral region of the spinal cord. ANS reflexes may use sympathetic nerves, parasympathetic nerves, or both. For example, the ANS reflex regulation of blood pressure uses sympathetic nerves to blood vessels and both parasympathetic and sympathetic nerves to the heart.

The sympathetic division of the ANS is primarily responsible for the fight-or-flight response that is associated with fear, anxiety, rage, and other strong emotions. The outcomes of this response can be predicted by imagining what changes would favor skeletal muscle activity for either fighting or running away. Outcomes include increases in heart rate, blood pressure, blood glucose, and blood flow to skeletal muscle; dilation of airways in the lungs (e.g., bronchi); dilation of the pupils; and decreased activity of the digestive tract.

The fight-or-flight response is a short-term event characterized by high levels of sympathetic nerve activity throughout the body. This widespread sympathetic activation is not the result of a discrete reflex but is a more general sympathetic activation initiated in response to fear, anxiety, stress, and so on. The hypothalamus and amygdala in the brain appear to be especially important sites in the initiation of the sympathetic response, but it is not clear how feelings of fear, stress, and so on affect these centers to initiate the response.

In addition to widespread increases in sympathetic nerve activity, the fight-or-flight response includes an increase in the release of epinephrine and norepinephrine from the adrenal medullae. Chromaffin cells of the adrenal medullae are innervated by preganglionic sympathetic neurons (see Chapter 9), and these cells release their catecholamines when stimulated. In most species the primary catecholamine released by chromaffin cells is epinephrine. Epinephrine and norepinephrine in the circulation bind to adrenergic receptors throughout the body to amplify the general effects of increased sympathetic nerve activity. The blood levels of these catecholamines are relatively low and functionally insignificant when animals are not undergoing a strong sympathetic response.

The list of events in the fight-or-flight response includes dilation of the pupil of the eye. The control of pupil size was earlier described as also being controlled by a parasympathetic reflex based on light reaching the retina. This is an example of how circumstances may affect which division of the ANS dominates the regulation of an organ or gland. If an animal is not undergoing a strong sympathetic response, the parasympathetic nerves are the primary regulator of pupil size, but during times of intense stress, sympathetic stimulation may dilate the pupil in spite of the animal being in a brightly lit environment.

Autonomic Neurotransmitters and Their Receptors

The postganglionic neurons of the parasympathetic division of the ANS use acetylcholine as a neurotransmitter, while almost all postganglionic neurons of the sympathetic division use norepinephrine. Acetylcholine is also the neurotransmitter used by preganglionic neurons in both the sympathetic and parasympathetic divisions.

The organ response to ANS stimulation depends not only on the neurotransmitter being released but also on the type of cell membrane receptor on the cells of the organ. Muscarinic and nicotinic are the two general classes of acetylcholine receptors. Nicotinic receptors are found on skeletal muscle cells at the neuromuscular junction and in all autonomic ganglia (both sympathetic and parasympathetic), where acetylcholine is released by preganglionic neurons. Muscarinic receptors are found in most organs innervated by postganglionic parasympathetic neurons. Stimulation of muscarinic receptors brings about diverse cellular responses ranging from hyperpolarization of sinoatrial nodal cells to slow heart rate to contraction of urinary bladder smooth muscle for urination. Table 10–1 lists the organs where muscarinic receptors are found and the organ response to the stimulation of those receptors by parasympathetic nerves. More details on the precise mechanisms of these effects appear in the appropriate chapters on the different body systems. **Parasympathetic stimulation increases salivary gland secretion, stimulates gastrointestinal motility, slows heart rate, and tends to reduce cardiac output. These are often undesirable during surgery. Muscarinic receptor antagonists (such as atropine) are often used as preanesthetic agents to block peripheral muscarinic receptors and reduce these potentially harmful effects of parasympathetic stimulation.**

Adrenergic receptors, which may be stimu-

Table 10-1. Location of Muscarinic Receptors and the Effects of Stimulation by Neurotransmitters of the Autonomic Nerves

Location	Effect
Heart	
Sinoatrial node	Reduce heart rate
Atrioventricular node	Reduce impulse conduction velocity
Salivary glands	Increase secretion
Gastrointestinal tract	Increase motility of smooth muscle in wall and secretion of lining epithelium
Urinary bladder	Contract smooth muscle to empty bladder
Circular muscle of iris of eye	Constrict smooth muscle to reduce pupil
Ciliary muscle controlling lens of eye	Contract muscle for lens accommodation
Endothelial cells lining blood vessels	Stimulate release of nitric oxide to relax smooth muscle
Smooth muscle of lung airways (bronchiolar)	Contract smooth muscle to shrink airways

lated by either epinephrine or norepinephrine, also fall into two general classes, α-receptors and β-receptors. However, because of their physiologic and clinical importance, the subtypes of α- and β-receptors also must be considered. Table 10–2 lists the key subtypes of adrenergic receptors, their sites, and the effects of their stimulation. Stimulation of α_1-receptors causes contraction of smooth muscle, and stimulation of β_2-receptors causes smooth muscle relaxation. Epinephrine has a high affinity for β_2-receptors, and it is released into the circulation during a strong sympathetic response. The β_2 effects on smooth muscle of airways and blood vessels supplying skeletal muscles are appropriate for fight-or-flight.

Regeneration and Repair in the Nervous System

In mammals most neurons are fully differentiated at birth, although division of glial cells (including those that myelinate axons) continues postnatally. With very few exceptions, neurons are incapable of mitosis, and therefore nerve cells lost to injury or disease are not replaced.

Axons, however, may regenerate following injury if the neuronal cell body is healthy.

Axonal regeneration in the CNS does not usually result in recovery of function. It is believed that mature oligodendrocytes prevent regrowth and reestablishment of meaningful neuronal connections. This is why spinal cord injuries are generally irreversible. The partial recovery of function seen over time with some CNS injuries is mostly attributable to recruitment of remaining uninjured connections and to the individual's ability to learn to use those remaining connections.

Axons in the peripheral nervous system (nerves) are frequently injured by crushing (as in forced extraction of a calf during dystocia) or cutting (e.g., wire cuts). Unlike the situation in the CNS, peripheral axons are capable of considerable repair. The likelihood that a given nerve injury will undergo functional recovery is correlated with (1) how close to the nerve cell body the injury is and (2) whether or not the nerve sheath is disrupted. The more proximal a nerve injury, the less likely it is to recover. In fact, axonal injury that occurs very close to the cell body may result in death of the neuron. Axonal injuries that preserve the sup-

Table 10-2. Location of Adrenergic Receptors and the Effects of Stimulation by Neurotransmitters of the Autonomic Nerves

Receptor subtype	Locations	Effect
α_1	Vascular smooth muscle	Contracts muscle to constrict vessel
	Smooth muscle sphincters in gastrointestinal tract	Contracts muscle to constrict sphincters
	Radial muscle of iris of eye	Contracts muscle to enlarge pupil
	Smooth muscle sphincter of urinary bladder	Contracts muscle to reduce opening into urethra
β_1	Heart: sinoatrial node	Increase heart rate
	Heart: atrioventricular node	Increase impulse conduction velocity
	Heart: ventricular muscle	Increase force of contraction
β_2	Arterial vessels supplying blood to skeletal muscle	Relaxes smooth muscle to permit dilation of vessels
	Smooth muscle of lung airways (bronchiolar)	Relaxes muscle to permit airways to open
	Smooth muscle in wall of gastrointestinal tract	Relaxes muscle to reduce motility
	Liver	Increases glycogenolysis, gluconeogenesis in some species

portive tissues of a nerve (e.g., a crushing in-jury with minimal disruption of the myelin and connective tissue sheath) have a better chance of healing than those in which the epineurium is disturbed (e.g., a cut nerve). Minor injuries to peripheral nerves may regenerate at 2 to 4 mm a day, whereas more severe injuries may take many months to recover, if they recover at all.

Horses that are anesthetized or restrained in lateral recumbency should have their halter removed to avoid injury to the facial nerve. The buckles of halters are often ventral to the ear, where branches of the facial nerve are close to the skin. Facial paralysis resulting from compression of the nerve by a halter buckle may or may not be reversible, depending on the severity and duration of the compressive injury.

Dystocia, or difficult birth, is common among first-calf heifers bred to large bulls. The young cow may have difficulty passing a very large calf through the pelvic canal. Because the obturator nerve passes on the medial aspect of the body of the ilium next to the reproductive tract, it is at risk for compression by the over-sized calf. Overzealous pulling on a large calf can crush the obturator nerves bilaterally, par-alyzing the muscles that adduct the pelvic limbs. The cow so affected may become recum-bent, with pelvic limbs splayed out laterally. Recovery depends on the severity of the injury.

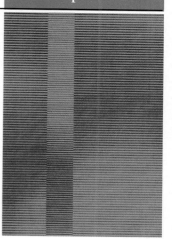

SENSE ORGANS

Sensory, or *afferent,* systems are the means by which the nervous system receives information about the external environment (*exteroception*), the internal environment (*interoception*), and the position and movement of the body (*proprioception*). The body uses sensory information to generate reflex movements (e.g., a blink of the eye when it is menaced, withdrawal of a limb from a hot surface, contraction of the bowel when it is stretched) without the participation of the conscious parts of the brain. Much (but not all) sensory information is also directed to the cerebral cortex for conscious perception.

Sensation is the conscious perception of sensory stimuli. It is impossible to know exactly what an animal (or another person, for that matter) sees, feels, hears, or smells. We infer what sensations an animal may experience by observing its reaction to various stimuli, by identifying homologies between human and animal sensory systems, and by imagining what we might feel in similar situations.

The experience of a given sensation as it is perceived at the cortical level has qualities that make it distinct from other types of sensations. This perceptual distinction defines the *sensory modality.* For example, the stimulus for the photoreceptors of the retina is light; the sensory modality that is experienced when photoreceptors are stimulated is vision. *Somatic sensation* describes modalities that arise primarily from innervation of body surfaces and musculoskeletal elements; it includes pain, touch, temperature, and position sense (proprioception). **Special senses** include **smell (olfaction), vision, taste (gustation), hearing (audition),** and **equilibrium (vestibular sensations).** Conscious sensory experiences arising from the viscera are limited primarily to pain, stretch, and pressure.

Certain animals have sensory systems that have no homology in human beings. For instance, migratory birds and some insects are able to sense geomagnetism of the earth, information they use for navigation. A number of species of fish can detect and generate electric fields. Other animals exploit the traditional sense modalities for highly specific (and expressly nonhuman) purposes. For example, cetaceans and bats both use highly modified auditory circuits for sonar navigation. In spite of growing anecdotal support, however, there remains no reliable evidence that domestic animals can sense an impending earthquake.

Sensory Receptors

Sensory experiences begin at **receptors,** specialized cells or nerve endings that detect a particular aspect of the internal or external environment. They are the mechanism by which the nervous system changes some sort of environmental energy (e.g., heat, pressure, light) into the electrical activity of neurons, a process called **transduction.**

In somatosensory systems, the receptor is a specialized peripheral terminal of the primary afferent neuron (the sensory neuron extending from the central nervous system [CNS] to the periphery); for the special senses, the receptor is usually a separate specialized neural cell that synapses with the primary afferent. As described earlier, sensory receptors may be described by the origin of the stimulus: exteroceptors (external environment), interoceptors (visceral organs), and proprioceptors (position and movement sense). They may also be described on a structural basis as **encapsulated** and **nonencapsulated** types. Nonencapsulated, or **free (naked) nerve endings** are widely distributed and are sensitive primarily to painful stimuli. Encapsulated receptors, which vary widely, are primarily concerned with touch sensations; these receptors are invested with specialized connective tis-

sue capsules that impart modality specificity to the receptor (Fig. 11–1).

The most functionally relevant classification scheme for receptors is based on the type of stimulation to which a receptor best responds. In this system, there are five general types of receptors: (1) **mechanoreceptors,** which respond to physical deformation; (2) **thermoreceptors** for both heat and cold; (3) **nociceptors,** which respond to stimuli that are potentially injurious to tissue (**noxious stimuli**); (4) **photoreceptors,** the light receptors of the retina; and (5) **chemoreceptors,** which respond to chemical changes associated with taste, smell, blood pH, and carbon dioxide concentrations in the blood. In normal circumstances, each receptor is preferentially sensitive to one type of stimulus; the unique stimulus to which a given re-

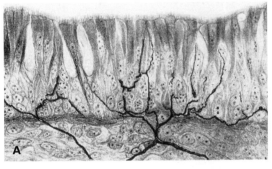

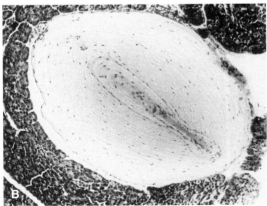

Figure 11-1. Encapsulated and nonencapsulated receptors. *A)* Naked nerve endings with Golgi stain in respiratory epithelium. These receptors transmit information about pain. *B)* Pacinian corpuscle, a type of touch receptor, has a connective tissue capsule surrounding the terminus of the primary afferent neuron.

ceptor is most sensitive is called the **adequate stimulus** for that receptor.

Receptors are specialized for transduction of environmental energy into action potentials. The adequate stimulus produces a local change in membrane potential of the receptor, a voltage change known as the **receptor potential** or **generator potential.** The receptor potential is usually depolarizing, brought about by the opening of cation channels permeable to Na$^+$ and K$^+$.

The receptor potential is a graded event that spreads passively over the local membrane of the receptor; the amplitude of the potential change and the distance along the membrane that the receptor potential travels are proportional to the strength of the stimulus. When the change in membrane potential reaches a critical level, the **threshold,** an action potential begins in the trigger zone of the sensory neuron's peripheral process. This signal is conducted along the axon into the CNS.

Many encapsulated receptors exhibit a physiologic characteristic called **adaptation.** With sustained stimulation, the receptors cease firing after their initial burst of activity. When the stimulus is withdrawn, the receptor again responds with a volley of action potentials. In doing so, the adapting receptor signals the beginning and end of the stimulus, rather than firing throughout its duration. Typically, touch receptors adapt rapidly; naked nerve endings—nociceptors—as a rule do not adapt but fire continuously throughout application of a noxious stimulus.

Somatosensation

Pain

Pain is the conscious perception of **noxious stimuli.** A noxious stimulus is one that is capable of producing tissue damage; it can be thermal, chemical, or mechanical. The receptor for noxious stimuli is the **nociceptor,** a naked (not encapsulated) nerve ending.

As a rule, axons transmitting noxious information are smaller and less myelinated than those carrying tactile or body position information. Activation of pain fibers of medium diam-

eter and myelination (so-called **Aδ fibers**) is associated with a sharp, pricking quality of pain as reported by human beings. Activation of the smallest diameter **C fibers,** which are unmyelinated, produces a dull, burning type of pain. The preponderance of C fibers in visceral sensory fibers explains the burning, aching quality of visceral pain.

As indicated in Chapter 9, a number of ascending spinal cord tracts transmit information about noxious stimuli to brain structures. In addition to projecting to the cerebral cortex for conscious perception, pain pathways typically have strong connections to autonomic centers in the brainstem and parts of the brain that produce increased mental alertness and behavioral and emotional responses to painful stimuli. These connections are responsible for producing signs of sympathetic stimulation (e.g., increased heart and respiratory rates, dilation of pupils), emotional responses, and escape behaviors (Fig. 11–2).

The ability of a given noxious stimulus to produce a perception of pain is a highly mutable property that can be modified in the periphery, in the spinal cord, and in the brainstem.

Threshold of nociceptors in the periphery is not a constant. Importantly, many substances released by injured tissues and inflammatory cells stimulate or lower the threshold of nociceptors. Thus, in damaged or inflamed tissue, stimuli that would normally be below threshold for detection may produce activity in nociceptive afferents. These events contribute to the development of **primary hyperalgesia,** a phenomenon wherein the perception of pain in injured tissues is increased. A dramatic example of this is made by sunburned human skin; the inflammation of the injured skin modifies threshold of nociceptors so that even a light touch (for instance, contact with clothing) can activate them.

Events in the dorsal horn of the spinal cord can also affect transmission of nociceptive information. Rapid, prolonged firing of action potentials in the primary afferent neuron can produce changes in the neuron on which it synapses, making it respond more vigorously to subsequent stimulation. This is called **wind-up** or **spinal facilitation of pain.**

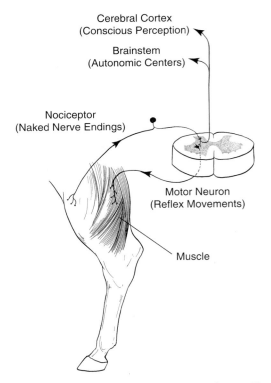

Cerebral Cortex
(Conscious Perception)

Brainstem
(Autonomic Centers)

Nociceptor
(Naked Nerve Endings)

Motor Neuron
(Reflex Movements)

Muscle

Figure 11-2. Divergence in nociceptive pathways. The primary afferent neuron brings information about painful stimuli into the CNS. From there the information produces reflex movements and goes to the brainstem to produce autonomic and other involuntary responses and to the cerebral cortex for conscious perception.

It is also known that activity in non-noxious tactile primary afferents can reduce transmission in central pain pathways, probably by activating inhibitory neurons of the dorsal horn that reduce the release of neurotransmitter from the primary afferent. This has been called the *gate control theory,* and may explain, at least in part, why vibration, massage, and acupuncture can reduce perception of pain.

Activity in spinal nociceptive pathways is also strongly influenced by descending antinociceptive systems that originate in the brainstem. The midbrain and medulla both possess a series of midline nuclei that inhibit nociception via their connections with nociceptive pathways. These nuclei use multiple neurotransmitters, most notably **endorphins,** transmitters with powerful antinociceptive properties.

Stoicism, an apparent indifference to pain, is largely determined by personality and training, among both humans and animals. High-strung individuals often exhibit exaggerated reactions to stimuli that scarcely merit attention in more laid-back individuals. Interestingly, the effectiveness of applying a twitch to a horse's upper lip as a method of restraint during mildly painful procedures has long been attributed to redirecting the horse's attention from the procedure to the moderately noxious stimulus of the twitch. Recent studies, however, have shown that the correctly applied twitch actually stimulates a release of endorphins, lowers the heart rate, and produces behavioral signs of sedation in the horse. This very old technique of restraint may actually be recruiting some of the neuroanatomic pathways postulated to be stimulated by acupuncture.

Proprioception

Proprioception is the nonvisual perception of body position. It is a complex sensory modality that is created through the input of a variety of specialized receptors called **proprioceptors.** These include **joint receptors** (providing information on tension and pressure within joints), **muscle spindles** (signaling changes in muscle length), **Golgi tendon organs** (signaling tension in tendons), and **skin mechanoreceptors** (which report contact with the environment).

The cerebral cortex uses proprioception to help formulate voluntary motor plans; pathways carrying proprioceptive information to the cortex are said to be carrying **conscious proprioception.** The same proprioceptors also deliver information to other spinal cord tracts that ascend to the cerebellum. Since the cerebellum is not involved with conscious perception, body position information in these tracts is said to be **unconscious proprioception.** The cerebellum uses proprioceptive information to adjust ongoing motor movements so that they are smooth and accurate. The information in conscious and unconscious proprioceptive pathways arises from the same peripheral receptors and primary afferent neurons; it is only the ultimate destination (and therefore use) that is different.

For the cerebral cortex and cerebellum to make effective use of feedback on body position to guide movements, the proprioceptive information must be delivered very rapidly to these brain regions. Consequently, proprioceptive tracts typically have few synapses and are composed of very large diameter, highly myelinated axons (called *Aα fibers*). In fact, the very fastest (up to 120 m/second) axons of the entire nervous system transmit proprioceptive information.

We, and presumably animals, are generally not aware of proprioception, but it is critically important in the execution of accurate, well-coordinated movements. Injury to the proprioceptive pathways results in awkward, inaccurate, uncoordinated gait and movement. The incoordination typical of proprioceptive deficits is referred to as *ataxia.*

Visceral Sensations

Visceral sensations involve structures within the body cavities. Most visceral afferent information is not available to consciousness but is instead important in directing the autonomic activity in viscera. Receptors of the viscera are confined to mechanoreceptors and chemoreceptors. The latter as a rule do not project to cortical levels, so perceived sensations are primarily limited to pain and pressure. Since unmyelinated C fibers are the predominant type of sensory fiber innervating the viscera, visceral pain has a burning, aching quality.

Remarkably, the viscera tend to be relatively insensitive to stimuli such as crushing, cutting, and thermal injury. Surgical manipulation, therefore, tends to produce very little activity in sensory systems. Visceral afferents do respond vigorously to stretch, dilation, tension, and ischemia (reduced blood flow), however. For this reason, cramping (increased muscular tension in the wall of a viscus) and stretching due to gas accumulation are quite painful. The cramping, stretching, and/or ischemia that occurs when the equine large intestine twists or is displaced can produce severe abdominal pain, called *colic,* in horses.

Referred Pain

In humans and presumably in animals, most visceral sensations are ill defined and poorly localized. Noxious stimuli originating in viscera, such as might be caused excessive dilation of a viscus, are often perceived as originating instead from a somatic region (body wall or skin), a phenomenon called **referred pain.** This perception is thought to result from the fact that information from that region of viscera converges on neurons and pathways that also convey information from somatic structures. Since we are much more familiar with sensations arising from our skin and body wall, the pain is interpreted to originate in these somatic structures.

A well-known example of referred pain comes from human medicine; pain due to ischemia of heart muscle is usually perceived as radiating across the left shoulder and down the left arm. This is *angina pectoris.* A veterinary example may be the high degree of sensitivity in the region of the sternum that some cows exhibit with traumatic gastritis caused by a wire or nail perforating the wall of the forestomach.

Chemical Senses

Chemical senses are those that detect particular molecules in the external or internal environment. Chemical senses that detect molecules outside the body include **gustation** (taste) and **olfaction** (smell). Within the body, the chemical senses include the detection of blood pH and carbon dioxide concentration. These latter afferents are associated with autonomic reflexes and do not project to the cerebral cortex for perception.

Gustation

Taste, or **gustation,** is the modality associated with dissolved substances contacting specialized receptor cells on the tongue and throat region. The receptors, simply called **taste cells,** are arranged in a group with supporting cells, a cluster that constitutes the **taste bud** (Fig. 11–3). Taste buds are not distributed evenly on the surface of the tongue; they are confined to specific forms of papillae (tiny projections), the **vallate, foliate,** and **fungiform papillae.**

Sensory nerve fibers subserving taste are distributed to the rostral two-thirds of the tongue by a branch of the facial nerve, the **chorda tympani.** Taste in the caudal third of the tongue is conveyed by fibers of the glossopharyngeal nerve. Somatic sensations (heat, cold, touch, pain) from the tongue are conveyed by a branch of the trigeminal nerve. It is likely that taste buds on areas other than the tongue (e.g., the pharynx and epiglottis) are innervated by the vagus nerve.

Traditionally, four basic taste sensations are identified. These are **sweet, salt, bitter,** and **sour.** Individual taste cells have membrane receptor physiology designed to detect the chemical substances associated with these tastes. The more complex sensory experiences that we normally associate with taste (for example, the flavors that we detect when we distinguish between an apple and a carrot) are created primarily from stimulation of olfactory (smell) receptors in combination with the basic taste modalities. For them to stimulate taste cells, chemicals must be in solution. Dissolution of

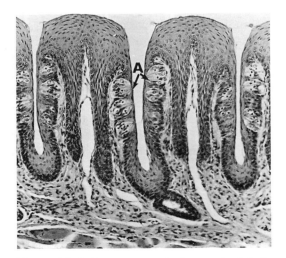

Figure 11-3. Photomicrograph of a taste bud. Individual cells include taste cells and other nonneural supportive cells. (Micrograph courtesy of Dr. Sue Kinnamon, Colorado State University, Fort Collins, CO.)

substances so that they can be tasted is an important function of saliva.

In addition to the four basic tastes, a fifth taste modality with its own specific taste cell receptor has been identified. This taste, experienced when the amino acid glutamate is present, imparts a savory quality to foodstuffs. Because this taste modality was first described by Japanese researchers, it is known by the Japanese word for savory or delicious: **umami.** It is the presence of the umami taste receptor that explains the improved flavor of foods when **monosodium glutamate (MSG)** is added.

Olfaction

Olfaction is the sense of **smell. Olfactory sensory neurons** are scattered among supporting cells throughout the olfactory mucosa in the dorsocaudal part of the nasal cavity. The apex of each olfactory neuron bears a single dendrite with a tuft of several fine hairlike projections, which are the actual receptors for the sense of smell. An axon from each olfactory neuron passes through the cribriform plate of the ethmoid bone; the mass of fine fibers thus entering the cranial vault collectively constitutes the **olfactory nerve.** These fibers synapse within the **olfactory bulb** on neurons whose central processes make up the **olfactory tracts** of the brain.

Neural connections within the olfactory parts of the brain are complex. Olfaction is the only sensory modality that is not routed through the thalamus before reaching conscious perception at a primary sensory cortex. Olfaction is also known to have profound connections to the limbic lobe, the part of the brain that generates emotional and autonomic behaviors. Smells, therefore, are uniquely capable of eliciting emotions and behaviors.

There is a subset of olfactory sensory neurons outside the olfactory epithelium in the **vomeronasal organ,** a diverticulum of the nasal cavity in the hard palate. These olfactory neurons appear to be receptors for **pheromones,** chemical substances that can influence the behavior of other individuals. Pheromones are likely especially important in reproductive behaviors. In spite of vigorous research efforts, no human pheromones have yet been unequivocally identified.

Hearing and Balance

The ear can be divided into three main parts: the external, middle, and inner ears. The *external ear* extends from the exterior as far as the *tympanic membrane* (eardrum). The *middle ear* begins at the tympanic membrane; it is an air-filled space within the temporal bone. The *inner ear* is housed entirely in the petrous temporal bone, forming an elaborate fluid-filled system of chambers and canals (Fig. 11–4, *A*).

External Ear

The part of the ear visible on the outside of the head, the *auricle,* or *pinna,* varies considerably in shape and size between and within species. Its appearance is dictated primarily by the shape and rigidity of the *auricular cartilage,* an elastic cartilage that is somewhat funnel shaped. The pinna acts as a capturing device for air pressure waves, and its shape and mobility are structurally important for sound localization. The many skeletal muscles that move the pinna are categorized as rostral and caudal auricular muscles.

A tubular extension of the pinna, the cartilaginous *external acoustic canal* (*meatus*), extends from the pinna to the tympanic membrane. The external acoustic canal is lined with a modified skin possessing few hairs and abundant sebaceous and ceruminous glands. The combined secretion of these glands is called *cerumen,* a brown waxy substance that protects the canal. A separate *annular cartilage* adjacent to the funnel-shaped base of the auricular cartilage forms most of the external acoustic canal. A third cartilage, the *scutiform cartilage,* lies medial to the auricular cartilage, embedded in the rostral auricular muscles. It functions as a fulcrum for the attached auricular muscles.

Middle Ear

The middle ear is an air-filled space, the *tympanic cavity,* lined by mucous membrane and contained within the temporal bone. In most domestic animals, the middle ear features a ventrally expanded cavity, the *tympanic bulla,* visible on the ventral surface of the skull. The middle ear is closed to the external ear canal by

the intact tympanic membrane and communicates with the nasopharynx via the *auditory tube* (formerly eustachian tube). In the horse, the auditory tube is expanded to form the large air-filled *guttural pouch* dorsocaudal to the nasopharynx. The connection between the middle ear and the pharynx is normally closed except briefly during swallowing. The opening of the auditory tube brought about by swallowing or yawning permits equalization of air pressures between middle and external ears.

Three *auditory ossicles* span the middle ear from tympanic membrane to the *vestibular (oval) window.* From superficial to deep, they are the *malleus (hammer), incus (anvil),* and *stapes (stirrup)* (Fig. 11–4). These tiny bones provide a mechanical linkage from the tympanic membrane to the vestibular window, and through them vibrations are transmitted from the former to the latter. The size and leverage of the auditory ossicles provide mechanical advantage; the energy of pressure waves striking the tympanic membrane is concentrated on the smaller vestibular window, increasing the system's sensitivity to faint stimuli.

There are also two striated muscles within the middle ear, the *m. tensor tympani* and the *m. stapedius.* These two small muscles damp vibrations of the auditory ossicles in the presence of excessively loud noises. It is persistent contraction of these muscles that produces the temporarily reduced hearing acuity notable after, for example, attending a very loud music concert.

The chorda tympani, a branch of the facial nerve, passes through the tympanic cavity. The chorda tympani carries fibers for taste from the rostral two-thirds of the tongue and also parasympathetic fibers destined for the mandibular and sublingual salivary glands. Infections of the middle ear (otitis media) can be associated with dysfunction of this nerve. Likewise, sympathetic fibers that innervate the eye pass through the tympanic cavity; diseases affecting the middle ear can produce signs of lost sympathetic innervation (**Horner's syndrome**), including a constricted pupil, sunken globe, and drooping of the upper eyelid.

In horses, cranial nerves VII and IX to XII and the continuation of the sympathetic trunk pass adjacent to the guttural pouch, separated from

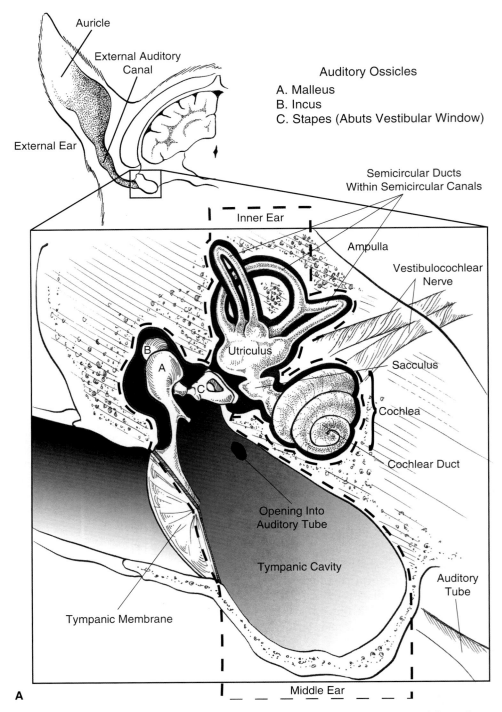

Figure 11-4. Anatomy of the hearing and vestibular apparatus. *A)* External, middle, and internal ears with surrounding temporal bone. *B)* Membranous labyrinth. Hatched regions indicate the sites of neuroepithelium, including the spiral organ of the cochlear duct, the maculae of the utriculus and sacculus, and the cristae ampullares of the semicircular ducts. (Part B reprinted with permission from Banks. *Applied Veterinary Histology.* 2nd ed. Baltimore: Williams & Wilkins, 1986.)

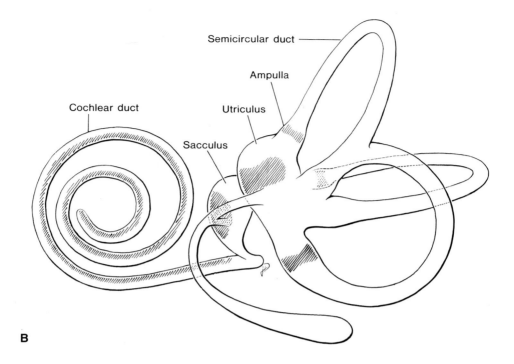

Semicircular duct

Ampulla

Cochlear duct

Utriculus

Sacculus

B

its interior only by mucous membrane. Diseases of the guttural pouch can therefore produce distinctive neurologic dysfunctions when these nerves are affected.

Internal Ear

The internal ear is housed entirely within the petrous temporal bone. It is a multichambered membranous sac (the *membranous labyrinth*) closely surrounded by a sculpted cavity of bone (the *osseous labyrinth*). The inner ear detects both sound and acceleration of the head (Fig. 11–4, *A* and *B*).

The membranous labyrinth in the internal ear is a system of fluid-filled sacs and ducts. The primary anatomic features of the membranous labyrinth are (1) two enlargements, the *utriculus* (*utricle*) and *sacculus* (*saccule*); (2) three loops attached to the utriculus, the *semicircular ducts;* and (3) the spiraled *cochlear duct.* These are filled with a fluid, the *endolymph.* The membranous labyrinth is housed in the osseous labyrinth, a similarly shaped, slightly larger excavation in the petrous temporal bone. The osseous labyrinth is filled with *perilymph.*

The inner ear may be divided into two functional parts. In one, the osseous labyrinth forms a coiled, snail shell–shaped *cochlea,* inside of which is the cochlear duct, an extension of the membranous labyrinth. The cochlear duct houses the receptors for audition. These receptors are innervated by the *cochlear division* of the vestibulocochlear nerve.

The second part constitutes the *vestibular apparatus.* Within the utriculus, sacculus, and semicircular ducts that constitute the vestibular apparatus are the receptors that detect accelerations of the head, including acceleration due to gravity. Accelerations of the head contribute to the sense of *equilibrium* or *balance.* The vestibular apparatus is innervated by the *vestibular division* of the vestibulocochlear nerve.

Physiology of Hearing

The environmental energy detected in audition is air pressure waves produced by vibration. These pressure waves can be described in terms of their *frequency,* the time between peaks of pressure waves, measured in hertz (Hz, cycles per second). Frequency determines the perceived pitch of sounds, with higher frequencies producing sounds of higher pitches. Air pressure waves are also described in terms of their *amplitude,* a property that reflects the energy and consequently the loudness of these waves. Amplitude is expressed in *decibels* (dB), the units by which loudness is measured. The decibel scale is logarithmic, so that the loudest sounds that can be heard without discomfort (around 100 dB) are a million times as energetic as the faintest audible sounds.

The cochlear portion of the osseous labyrinth resembles a snail shell (cochlea is Latin for snail). The space on the inside of the cochlea is full of perilymph, and it spirals around a central bony core, the *modiolus.* The corresponding part of the membranous labyrinth is the cochlear duct, which extends throughout the coiled length of the cochlea. The duct is stretched transversely from the modiolus to the outer wall of the bony cochlea, effectively dividing this perilymph-filled space into two: the *scala vestibuli* above and the *scala tympani* below the duct.

The scala vestibuli originates in the region of the vestibular window, and by this association, the perilymph within it receives pressure waves from the vibration of the auditory ossicles. At the apex of the cochlea the scala vestibuli is continuous with the scala tympani at a connection called the *helicotrema.* The scala tympani receives pressure waves from the fluid in the scala vestibuli (and more importantly, through vibrations of the intervening cochlear duct); these waves are dissipated at the termination of the scala tympani, the *cochlear (round) window,* which abuts the air-filled space of the middle ear.

The receptor cells of the auditory system are within the cochlear duct as components of the *spiral organ (organ of Corti)* (Fig. 11–5). The spiral organ contains the receptor cells of the internal ear, mechanoreceptors called *hair cells* for the bundle of *cilia* on their apex. The cilia of the hair cells in the spiral organ are embedded in a relatively stiff overlying membrane, the *tectorial membrane.* The walls between the cochlear duct and the scalae vestibuli and tympani are called the *vestibular* and *basilar membranes,* respectively.

Cross-sectional views of the cochlea give the impression that the components within are arrayed as repeating separate units, but they are

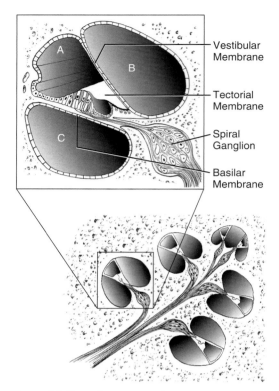

Figure 11-5. Median section of the cochlea. Expanded view shows spiral organ within cochlear duct (A), between the scala vestibuli (B) and scala tympani (C).

longitudinally continuous throughout the extent of the spiraled cochlea.

The hair cells synapse with peripheral processes of primary afferent neurons whose cell bodies lie within the *spiral ganglion.* The spiral ganglion is housed in the modiolus, and the axons of the afferent neurons within it gather to form the *cochlear nerve.* Transduction of the mechanical energy of air pressure waves into the electrical impulses of neurons in the auditory system takes place in the following manner: Air pressure waves captured by the pinna are funneled down to the tympanic membrane, and they put that membrane into vibratory motion. This motion is carried across the air-filled cavity of the middle ear by movements of the auditory ossicles. These ossicles transfer the vibrations to the vestibular window via the foot of the stapes. The perilymph in the osseous labyrinth receives the pressure waves transmitted to it by the vibrations of the vestibular window. These are carried into the cochlea by the scala vestibuli. The vestibular membrane between scala vestibuli and cochlear duct vibrates in response to the pressure waves and transfers those vibrations across the cochlear duct to the basilar membrane and underlying perilymph of the scala tympani. Movement of the basilar membrane results in movement of the hair cells in the spiral organ that rests upon it, and this produces bending of the hair cells' cilia against the more rigid tectorial membrane. It is the bending of the cilia that results in a depolarization within the hair cells. When this depolarization reaches sufficient intensity, it initiates an action potential in the primary afferents of the spiral ganglion.

The ability to discriminate one pitch from another has its basis in a number of anatomic and electrical features of the spiral organ. Most simply, the basilar membrane varies in width from the base of the cochlear duct, where it is most narrow, to the apex, where it is widest. This difference in width means that each portion of the membrane has a different frequency at which it preferentially vibrates, with the widest part of the membrane vibrating at low frequency and the narrow part at high.

The axons of the cochlear nerve enter the brainstem with the vestibular nerve at the junction of the medulla and pons and terminate in *cochlear nuclei* on the lateral side of the medulla. From this first synapse, multiple pathways produce auditory-mediated reflexes and conscious perception of sound. Auditory information destined for the cortex is distributed bilaterally in the medulla, pons, and midbrain. The pathways for conscious perception of sound continue on to the thalamic relay nucleus for audition, and from there fibers project to the *primary auditory cortex* on the lateral aspect of the cerebrum. The result of bilaterality of the pathways is that auditory information from both cochleae reaches both left and right auditory cortices.

The bilaterality of auditory representations in the brain means that for a brain lesion to produce complete deafness, it must affect both sides of the pathway. Such brain injuries are often incompatible with life; therefore, most deafness is peripheral (associated with the cochlear nerve or internal ear). In animals, incomplete loss of hearing is difficult to detect.

Disease processes that affect the ability of the tympanic membrane or auditory ossicles to transmit vibrations to the vestibular window produce *conduction deafness*. Those that affect the spiral organ or more proximal components of the auditory system (including the cochlear nerves, brainstem, and auditory cortices) produce *sensorineural deafness*. Most inherited deafness is sensorineural, brought about by degeneration of cochlear hair cells. Congenital deafness has been associated with white hair coats or the merle or piebald color genes in a variety of species, including dogs (most notably the Dalmatian), cats, and horses. In these individuals, low numbers of pigment-containing cells appear to be linked to degeneration of cochlear hair cells within a few weeks of birth.

Mechanisms of Balance

The **vestibular system** is a complex neurologic system that is concerned with maintaining a stable orientation in relation to gravity and while in motion. Its influence is widely distributed throughout the nervous system; vestibular reflexes are responsible for the position of eyes, neck, trunk, and limbs in reference to movement or position of the head.

The receptor organs of the vestibular system are housed in the part of the membranous labyrinth known as the **vestibular apparatus** (Fig. 11–4, *B*). These organs are the **maculae** of the utriculus and sacculus and the **cristae ampullares** of the semicircular ducts. Afferent information from these structures gives rise to motor reflexes that maintain stabile visual images on the retinas during movement of the head, to keep the head level with respect to gravity through neck movements, and to produce trunk and limb movements to counteract displacements of the head.

The utriculus and the smaller sacculus each posses a **macula**, a thickened oval plaque of neuroepithelium (Fig. 11–6, *A*). The maculae consist of a population of hair cells very like those of the spiral organ. These are covered by a gelatinous sheet, the **otolithic membrane**, into which project the cilia of the hair cells. The surface of the otolithic membrane is studded with

A.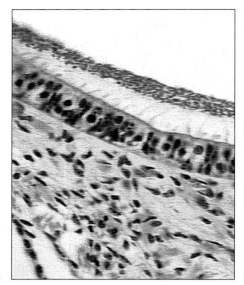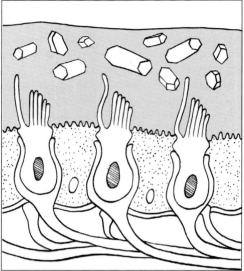

B.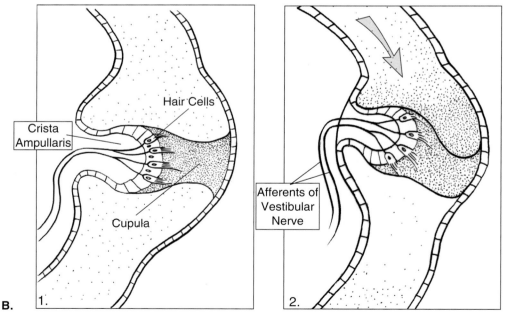

Figure 11-6. Receptor organs of the vestibular apparatus. *A)* Anatomy of the macula. Hair cells, surrounded by nonneural supportive cells, are surmounted by a gelatinous otolithic membrane in which are embedded calcium carbonate crystals called otoliths. Inertial movements of the otolithic membrane bend the cilia of the hair cells, changing their membrane potential. Inset shows photomicrograph of a macula. *B)* Anatomy of the crista ampullaris. Hair cells and supportive cells are found in a crest of tissue on one side of the ampulla. A gelatinous cupula, in which the hair cells are embedded, forms a flexible barrier across the ampulla. Inertial movements of endolymph bend the cupula (inset), bending the cilia of the hair cells.

crystals of calcium carbonate, the **otoliths,** or **statoconia,** which increase the inertial mass of the otolithic membrane. When the head accelerates in a straight line, the individual senses **linear acceleration.** The inertia of the otolithic membrane causes it to lag behind the head under conditions of linear acceleration (including the always present acceleration due to gravity); this dragging of the otolithic membrane bends the cilia of the underlying hair cells with shearing vectors dependent on the direction of acceleration.

Attached to the utriculus are three half-circular extensions of the membranous labyrinth, the semicircular ducts. The ducts lie in three planes, at approximately right angles to one another, and are designated anterior, posterior, and lateral to describe their orientation. As an extension of the membranous labyrinth, each duct is filled with endolymph and surrounded by perilymph.

One end of each duct is dilated to form an **ampulla,** within which are housed the receptor organs of the semicircular ducts (Fig. 11–6, *B*). One wall of the ampulla features a transverse ridge of connective tissue, the **crista ampullaris,** which supports a neuroepithelium of hair cells. Attached to the crista is a gelatinous **cupula;** this extends across the ampulla, forming a flexible but complete barrier to the flow of endolymph. The cilia of the hair cells are embedded in the cupula and are therefore bent by movements of it.

The semicircular ducts detect **angular acceleration** (**rotation**), and their planes of orientation roughly correspond to the X-, Y-, and Z-axes of three-dimensional space. When the head rotates, the semicircular duct lying in that rotational plane moves with it. The endolymph inside the duct, however, must overcome its inertia at the start of rotation, and as a consequence briefly lags behind the movement of the head. The flexible cupula, acting as a dam across the ampulla, bulges in response to the endolymph's push, and in doing so, bends the cilia of the embedded hair cells. With three pairs (right and left) of semicircular ducts detecting movement in the three planes of space, complex rotational movements of the head are encoded in the firing patterns of the six cristae ampullares.

Afferent neurons synapse with the hair cells of the vestibular apparatus. Their cell bodies are in the **vestibular ganglion,** and their axons constitute the **vestibular nerve,** which joins the cochlear nerve to become the eighth cranial nerve. Most axons in the vestibular nerve synapse in the large **vestibular nuclei** of the pons and rostral medulla.

Vestibular Reflexes. If there were no mechanism to keep the eyes fixed on a target when the head moved, visual images would continually slip across the retina during head movement, and focusing on the visual field would be difficult or impossible while the head was moving. The vestibular nuclei use information about acceleration to coordinate extraocular eye muscle movements with movements of the head and thereby fix the visual image in one place on the retina as long as possible. When the excursion of the moving head carries the fixed image out of visual range, the eyes dart ahead in the direction of movement to fix upon a new image. This new image is held on the retina while the head continues turning until a compensatory jump ahead is again needed. This mechanism results in a cycle of slow movement opposite the direction of turn (eyes fixed on target) followed by a rapid readjustment in the same direction as the turn. This oscillatory reflex eye movement is called **nystagmus.**

Nystagmus is a *normal* reflex, generated in response to movement of the head. Nystagmus is considered abnormal when it occurs in absence of head movement; this **resting (spontaneous) nystagmus** is a sign of vestibular disease.

Axons of some neurons in the vestibular nuclei project caudad in a motor tract that influences activity in cervical and upper thoracic spinal cord segments. These motor connections activate neck musculature and forelimb extensors, producing the **vestibulocollic reflex,** which generates neck movements and forelimb extension to help keep the head level with respect to gravity and movement.

Some fibers from the vestibular nuclei form an ipsilateral descending motor tract that extends the length of the spinal cord. This **lateral vestibulospinal tract** is part of the ventromedial motor system (See Chapter 9). Its activity has the primary effect of increasing tone in antigravity muscles (proximal limb extensors and axial muscles). This **vestibulospinal reflex** uses vestibular information to produce limb and trunk movements that counteract the displacement of the head that elicits it. This mechanism is designed to prevent falling with shifts in head position.

Animals and people with injury to one side of their vestibular system express the vestibular reflexes in the absence of appropriate stimuli. These individuals commonly have resting nystagmus, head tilt, and a tendency to lean, circle, or fall to one side.

Vision

The eye is an elaborate organ whose primary function is to collect and focus light upon the photosensitive retina. It lies within a cone-shaped cavity of the skull, the **orbit,** which houses the eyeball (**globe**) and a number of other soft tissue structures, the **ocular adnexa** (e.g., muscles, glands), that act upon the eyeball in service of its light-collecting function. Unlike the human orbit, which is a complete bony cone, the ventral portion of the orbit of domestic species is bounded by soft tissues, notably the pterygoid muscles.

Ocular Adnexa

Palpebrae. Two mobile folds of haired skin protect the anterior aspect of the eyeball. These are the eyelids, or **palpebrae.** The gap between the margins of the two palpebrae is the **palpebral fissure,** and its shape and size are controlled by the muscles of the eyelids. A layer of dense connective tissue in the palpebrae, the **tarsal plate** (**tarsus**), affords them a certain amount of rigidity. The palpebrae have thin but otherwise typical haired skin on their superficial side. This skin ends at the lid margin with a sharp transition to mucous membrane. The margin may have **cilia** (eyelashes).

Abundant modified sweat and sebaceous glands are associated with the lid margin. A row of large modified sebaceous glands, the **tarsal glands** (**Meibomian glands**), is especially clinically significant, as they commonly become in-

fected, develop tumors, or become impacted. The tarsal glands are present in both palpebrae and open into a shallow furrow near the mucocutaneous junction of the eyelid. The openings of their ducts are readily seen when the margin of the lid is everted, and the glands themselves are usually visible as yellowish-white columns under the mucous membrane on the inner surface of the lid. The tarsal glands produce an important oil layer of the tear film.

The **conjunctiva** is the mucous membrane that lines the inside of the palpebrae and the anterior surface of the eyeball (excluding the clear cornea). Diseases of the conjunctiva are the most common eye disorders. The conjunctiva is rich in mucus-producing glands, lymphocytes, nerves, and blood vessels. The very small space between the eyelids and the surface of the eye is the **conjunctival sac,** and it is into this space that eye medications are usually instilled.

Inflammation of the conjunctiva, or *conjunctivitis*, is characterized by redness and increased mucus production. *Cancer eye,* squamous cell carcinoma of the conjunctiva, is relatively common in Hereford, Holstein, and shorthorn breeds of cattle.

Domestic species possess a **nictitating membrane,** or **third eyelid.** This is a fold of mucous membrane arising from the ventromedial aspect of the conjunctival sac between the eyeball and palpebrae. It is given rigidity by a T-shaped cartilage, and it smooths the tear film and protects the cornea.

The third eyelid has at its base a serous gland, called simply the **gland of the third eyelid,** which normally contributes about 50% of the tear film. Ruminants, the pig, and laboratory rodents possess another deeper gland associated with the third eyelid. This is the **harderian gland.** It, too, contributes to the tear film.

Lacrimal Apparatus. The **lacrimal apparatus** comprises a series of serous, seromucoid, and mucous glands and the duct systems that drain their secretions from the conjunctival sac (Fig. 11–7). It provides a moist environment for the anterior surface of the eye. The **lacrimal gland** lies in the dorsolateral portion of the orbit; its secretion, together with that of the gland

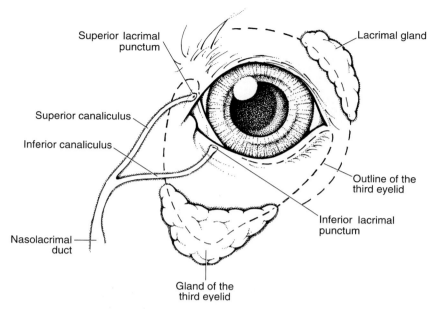

Figure 11-7. The lacrimal apparatus. The gland of the third eyelid and the lacrimal gland each contribute about 50% of the total volume of tears. The majority of the tear film is drained by the canaliculi leading into the nasolacrimal duct, which terminates within the nasal cavity. (Reprinted with permission from Smith B.J. *Canine Anatomy.* Philadelphia: Lippincott Williams & Wilkins, 1999.)

of the third eyelid, is the major contributor to the tear film. In addition to the lacrimal gland and the gland of the third eyelid, the smaller, more diffuse glands of the conjunctiva and the eyelids contribute oil and mucus to the tear film.

The tears drain from the conjunctival sac via two small openings on upper and lower palpebrae near the medial corner. These are the superior and inferior **lacrimal puncta,** which open into short ducts (superior and inferior **canaliculi**) that join one another at a small sac near the medial corner of the eye that is the origin of the **nasolacrimal duct.** The nasolacrimal duct travels through the bones of the face to open into the nasal cavity and/or just inside the nostril. Moisture on the nose of domestic animals is largely derived from the tears.

Extraocular Muscles. The globe of the eye moves by the action of seven striated muscles, designated *extraocular muscles* to distinguish

them from the intraocular muscles that lie entirely within the eyeball (Fig. 11-8).

The **m. retractor bulbi** arises lateral to the optic nerve and divides into four flat muscle bellies that insert on the equator of the eyeball in a nearly complete muscular cone. Contraction of the **m. retractor bulbi** results in retraction of the eyeball into the orbit. Also, a series of four straight muscles originate at the apex of the orbit and project to the equator of the globe, superficial to the four bellies of the **m. retractor bulbi.** They are named for their insertion on the globe: **mm. rectus dorsalis, rectus ventralis, rectus medialis,** and **rectus lateralis.**

The **m. obliquus dorsalis** (dorsal oblique m.) lies between the dorsal and medial recti muscles and tapers to a thin tendon at the level of the posterior pole of the eyeball. This tendon passes around a small cartilaginous **trochlea** of cartilage anchored to the medial orbital wall. The trochlea redirects the pull of the tendon, which inserts on the dorsal part of the eyeball. When the dorsal oblique muscle contracts, the dorsal part of the

OCULAR MUSCLES

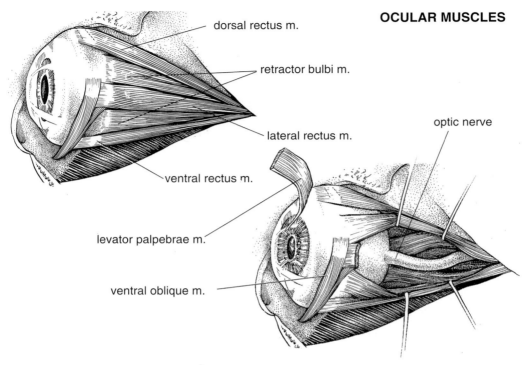

Figure 11-8. Extraocular muscles of the right eye viewed from the medial aspect.

eyeball is pulled toward the medial portion of the orbit (i.e., the left eyeball rotates counterclockwise and the right rotates clockwise).

The **m. obliquus ventralis** (ventral oblique m.) originates from a fossa in the ventral portion of the orbital rim; it runs dorsolaterad, ventral to the insertion of the ventral rectus muscle; and it inserts via two short tendons on the lateral aspect of the globe. The ventral oblique muscle rotates the globe opposite to the rotation produced by the dorsal oblique muscle.

One other muscle found within the orbit is not strictly an extraocular muscle, since it does not act on the eyeball itself. The **m. levator palpebrae superioris** is the primary lifter of the upper eyelid. It arises between the origins of the dorsal oblique and dorsal rectus muscles and inserts via a wide tendon in the connective tissue within the upper eyelid.

The **periorbita** is a cone-shaped connective tissue sheath that surrounds the eyeball and its muscles, nerves, and vessels. Like the extraocular muscles, the periorbita originates in the apex of the orbit; at the rim of the orbit, it blends with the periosteum of the facial bones. The periorbita contains circular smooth muscle that squeezes its contents and places the eyeball forward in the orbit. Adipose tissue both within and outside the periorbita acts to cushion the orbital contents. Because of its location behind the eyeball, the adipose tissue is frequently called **retrobulbar fat.**

Globe

The **eyeball** (**globe**) comprises three concentric layers: the fibrous tunic, the vascular tunic, and the nervous tunic (Fig. 11–9). The three tunics of the eyeball surround several chambers filled with either liquid or a gelatinous material. The posterior 75% of the globe is filled with an acellular gel, the **vitreous body,** and as a consequence this portion is also called the **vitreous chamber.** The lens divides it from the **anterior segment** of the eyeball. The anterior segment of the eye is filled with a fluid called **aqueous humor.**

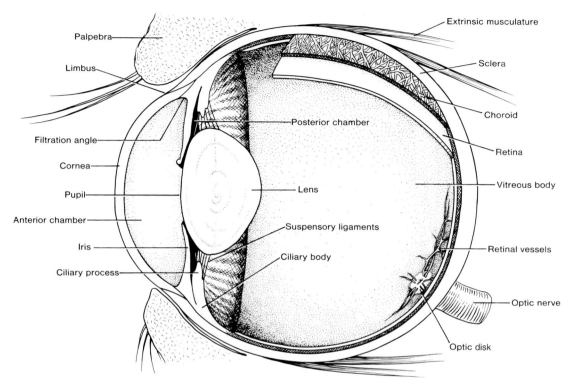

Figure 11-9. Sagittal section of a bovine eye. (Reprinted with permission from Banks W.J. *Applied Veterinary Histology*. 2nd ed. Philadelphia: Williams & Wilkins, 1986.)

Fibrous Tunic. The outer *fibrous tunic* of the eyeball is made up of a posterior opaque *sclera* and an anterior transparent *cornea.* Both are composed of very dense collagenous tissue. The sclera is white, variably tinged gray or blue; it meets the clear cornea at a transitional region called the **limbus.** The axons of the optic nerve pierce the sclera at the posterior pole of the eye, the *area cribrosa.* The tough sclera is the site of insertion for the extraocular eye muscles.

The *cornea* is the transparent anterior part of the fibrous tunic. It is the most powerful refracting layer of the eye (bends light more strongly than even the lens); its transparency and regular curvature are therefore critical elements for focusing of light on the retina. Corneal transparency is a function of (1) lack of vascular elements and cells, (2) lack of pigment, (3) relative dehydration of the collagenous tissue, (4) a smooth optical surface (provided in conjunction with the tear film), and (5) a highly regular, laminar pattern of collagen fibers that reduces light scatter. The cornea's anterior and posterior surfaces are covered with specialized epithelium, but most of its thickness is composed of collagen fibers.

Vascular Tunic. The middle tunic of the eyeball, the *vascular tunic,* or *uvea,* is composed of three parts, the choroid, ciliary body, and iris. The uvea in the posterior portion of the eye is the *choroid.* It is highly vascular and possesses multiple layers. The deepest (closest to the center of the globe) of these is the **tapetum.** The tapetum of animals is a reflective surface designed to bounce incoming light back onto the retina and enhance vision in low light. The shape and color of the tapetum are variable between species and individuals, but as a rule it is confined to the dorsal part of the posterior globe. The ventral portion of the choroid is usually not reflective. The pig and most primates lack a tapetum.

The *ciliary body* is the anterior continuation

of the uvea. It is a circumferential thickening of the vascular tunic, and it gives rise to many fine **suspensory ligaments** that support the lens. When the muscles in the ciliary muscle contract, they allow the lens to assume a more spherical shape; this increases its refractive power, a change that brings close objects into focus on the retina. This process of focusing on near objects is called **accommodation.** It is the capillaries of the ciliary body that produce the aqueous humor in the anterior segment of the eyeball.

The **iris** is the most anterior portion of the uvea and the only part of the vascular tunic normally visible in the living animal. It consists of a pigmented ring of tissue, perforated in its center by the **pupil.** The iris divides the aqueous-filled anterior segment of the eye into **anterior** (in front of the iris) and **posterior** (between the iris and lens) **chambers.** The iris controls the amount of light entering the posterior part of the eye by changing the size of the pupil. Constrictor muscles, innervated by the parasympathetic fibers of the oculomotor nerve, reduce the size of the pupil when they contract. Dilation of the pupil is accomplished by activity of the dilator muscles, innervated by sympathetic nerves.

The iris derives its color from pigmented epithelial cells primarily on the posterior surface of the iris. The typical color distribution depends on the species and is related to the coat color of the individual. In herbivores, the pigmented epithelium of the posterior surface of the iris forms nodular masses along the margin of the pupil that are visible in the anterior chamber. These are often very large in horses, in which species they are called **corpora nigra.** In cattle the same structures are usually smaller and are called **iridial granules.** Their function is unknown.

The site where the anterior surface of the iris meets the fibrous tunic is the **iridocorneal angle (filtration angle)**; there the aqueous produced by the ciliary body is reabsorbed into the venous circulation. Abnormalities here (e.g., congenital narrowing or obstruction due to inflammation) can prevent normal egress of aqueous from the anterior chamber and result in increased intraocular pressure, a condition called **glaucoma.**

Nervous Tunic. The deepest layer of the eyeball is the **internal (nervous) tunic** or **retina.** The retina develops embryologically as an outgrowth of the diencephalon and is therefore composed of neurons and glia. The light-sensitive part of the retina extends from just posterior to the ciliary body to the site at which nerve fibers exit the eyeball near the posterior pole of the globe. In clinical practice the retina is routinely viewed through the pupil with an ophthalmoscope; the portion of the retina that can be viewed in this manner is called the **fundus.**

The retina has many layers. One of these is the **photoreceptor layer,** in which are found the specialized neural receptor cells of the visual system, the **rods** and **cones.** Each photoreceptor features an external segment that consists of orderly stacks of flattened, disk-shaped plasma membrane. These are replete with **photopigment,** the molecules that are sensitive to photons of light. Photoreceptors have one of two basic shapes: either a tall cylinder or a shorter, tapering stack. The cylindrical photoreceptors are **rods,** equipped with a photopigment that renders them sensitive to very low levels of light. The tapering photoreceptors are **cones,** each expressing one of three known photopigments with sensitivity to a specific wavelength of light. Cones are, therefore, color receptors. As a rule, animals with nocturnal habits have retinas populated primarily with rods, whereas those with diurnal habits (e.g., primates and birds) have more cones, particularly in the region that receives light from the center of the visual field.

Most domestic animals have some color vision. Their retinal cones are primarily sensitive to blue and yellow wavelengths of light, with few or no red-sensitive cones. Vision in these species is probably rich in blue, green, and yellow tones. The flapping red cape wielded by the matador therefore attracts the bull by its movement, not by its color.

The photoreceptors synapse with other neurons of the retina, and visual information undergoes early neural processing within the retina. Ultimately, the axons of neurons called **ganglion cells** project to the **optic disk,** where they exit the globe and become the optic nerve.

Lens. The *lens* is a transparent proteinaceous biconvex disk suspended between the posterior chamber and the vitreous chamber. It is surrounded by an elastic *capsule* that serves as an attachment site for the suspensory ligaments at the lens's equator.

Cells of the lens are called **lens fibers,** and they are generated continuously throughout life. As these are added to the outside of the lens, older lens fibers are pushed toward the center, resulting in a lamellar arrangement of fibers, often likened to the layers of an onion.

As the animal ages, more lens fibers are added to the outside of the lens, compressing the fibers at the center. These old cells harden and after middle age begin to lose their transparency. This change is *lenticular sclerosis.* Although the sclerotic lens looks milky, lenticular sclerosis does not usually interfere with vision. More severe changes in the lens fibers can produce significant opacity that interferes with transmission of light and therefore vision. These opacities are *cataracts.* Cataracts can be congenital or can develop as a consequence of injury to the lens or metabolic disease (e.g., diabetes mellitus).

Visual Field and Light Path

The part of the environment from which light will enter the eyes and stimulate the retinas is the *visual field* (Fig. 11–10). In predators and arboreal animals, such as birds and primates (for whom accurate depth perception is essential), the eyes are placed so that the visual fields overlap to varying degrees. This region of overlap, where objects are simultaneously viewed by both eyes, is the *binocular field;* the visual cortex evaluates the slightly different view from each eye and uses the information to provide depth perception. Prey animals, on the other hand, have lateral eyes with a much smaller binocular field. Such eye placement increases the *peripheral vision* so that the combined visual field is nearly completely panoramic. Such vision is *monocular* (seen only with one eye) and therefore lacks very accurate depth cues, but the clear advantage of this wide field of view for a prey animal needs no explanation.

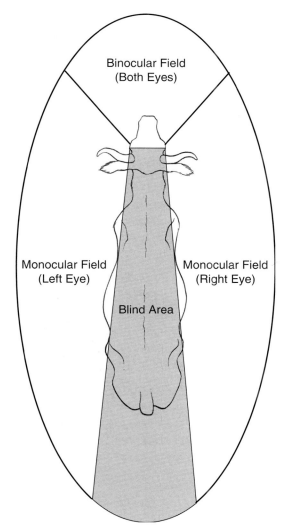

Figure 11-10. Visual fields of the ox as viewed from above. The region seen by both eyes (binocular field) is the region of best depth perception, but the nose creates a wedge-shaped blind spot directly in front of the animal. Peripheral vision (the monocular fields) creates a nearly complete circle of vision around the animal, except for about 3% directly behind.

Light traveling from the visual field to the retina passes through a series of transparent media that refract and focus it on the light-sensitive retina of the posterior part of the globe. These *dioptric media* include the cornea, the aqueous, the lens, and the vitreous body. As indicated before, the cornea is actually the most refractive medium of the eye, but the lens is the only part of the light path with the ability to change its refractive index. This property makes it the organ of accommodation for focus on near objects. Light entering the vitreous chamber of the eye is bent by the more anterior parts of the eye in such a way that the image that is focused on the retina is inverted and reversed.

The site where the ganglion cell axons leave the eye (the optic disk) has no photoreceptors and is therefore considered the **blind spot** of the retina. Dorsolateral to the optic disk is a region of the retina relatively free from large blood vessels and especially densely packed with photoreceptors (particularly cones). This is the region of greatest visual acuity, the **area centralis (macula)**.

Visual Pathways of the Brain

The electrical information generated by exposure of photoreceptors to light undergoes initial neural processing within the retina. This information ultimately leaves the eye via the optic nerve, the fibers of which are the axons of the ganglion cells of the retina. Most of the axons of the optic nerve synapse in the thalamus, and from there visual information travels to the **primary visual cortex** in the occipital lobe of the brain (the most caudal part of the cerebral cortex) for conscious perception.

A smaller subset of ganglion cell axons project to other destinations in the brain. Some reach the **rostral colliculi** of the mesencephalon, where visual stimuli induce reflex movements of the eyes and head. Others project to the **pretectal nuclei,** also in the region of the mesencephalon;

these nuclei communicate with the oculomotor nuclei to coordinate the reflex constriction of the pupils in response to light. Finally, a very small number of ganglion cell axons project to a specific group of cells of the hypothalamus, the **suprachiasmatic nucleus.** The suprachiasmatic nucleus is the biologic clock, the part of the brain that sets **circadian rhythms.** Circadian rhythms are physiologic processes that vary regularly on a daily basis; prominent circadian rhythms include sleep–wake cycles, melatonin secretion, and body temperature fluctuations. The suprachiasmatic nucleus has an intrinsic rhythmicity that closely approximates 24 hours, but the projections from the retina keeps the nucleus's cycle entrained to the actual photoperiod of the day.

Many domestic species are seasonal breeders, meaning that their reproductive cycles are determined by the season. The most powerful determinant of the onset and cessation of breeding cycles in these species is the length of the day. The retinal projections to the suprachiasmatic nucleus are the brain's record of day length, and they therefore determine the reproductive cycles via their influence on the autonomic functions of the hypothalamus. It is common agricultural practice to alter breeding behavior by exposing animals to artificial light. For instance, in the horse industry, in which an early foaling date is desirable, mares are commonly exposed to artificially increased day length in the winter so as to cause these spring breeders to begin fertile estrous cycles earlier than they would if exposed only to natural light.

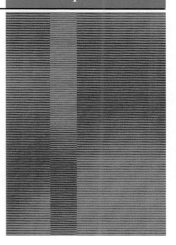

ENDOCRINOLOGY

As with the nervous system, the basic functions of the endocrine system are communication and regulation. The classic endocrine system (Figure 12–1) consists of a group of ductless glands that secrete **hormones** (chemical messengers that function in extremely small concentrations). The hormones circulate throughout the body to bring about physiologic responses. However, this classic description does not account for other types of chemical messengers involved in other types of cell-to-cell communication and regulation. For example, normal endothelial cells of blood vessels release prostacyclin, a prostaglandin (discussed later) that acts locally to inhibit the adhesion of blood platelets. This action helps prevent platelets from forming inappropriate blood clots in normal vessels. When prostacyclin diffuses away from its site of production or is washed away by blood flow, it rapidly degrades, so it has no systemic effect. A local effect such as this is termed a *paracrine* effect. Many types of compounds, including proteins, small peptides, amines (derivatives of amino acids), derivatives of fatty acids, and even a gas (nitric oxide), have been found to function as paracrine agents.

The objective of this chapter is to introduce the basic concepts of endocrinology, including the relationships between the nervous and endocrine systems. More details on specific hormones and paracrine agents, their regulation, and their actions will be given in later chapters on the specific systems that the agents affect.

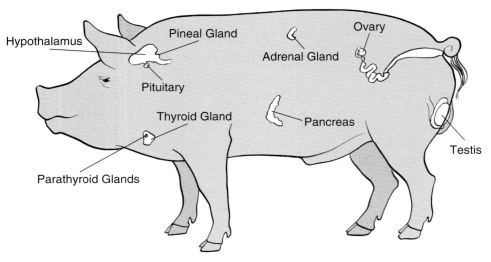

Figure 12-1. Approximate location of classic endocrine glands. Both ovary and testis are shown.

Hormones and Their Receptors

Chemical Classes of Hormones

The classic hormones can be grouped according to their chemical structure as **peptides, steroids,** or **amines.** The amines are biochemical modifications of a single amino acid, tyrosine. The synthesis of steroid hormones begins with cholesterol as a substrate. Cholesterol has carbon atoms arranged in adjoining four rings, and this ring structure is common to all steroid hormones (Fig. 12–2).

Eicosanoids

Eicosanoid is a general term for compounds that are chemical derivatives of long-chain fatty acids. **Prostaglandins, thromboxanes,** and **leukotrienes** are eicosanoids that function as chemical messengers. Arachidonic acid, a component of cell membranes, is the precursor fatty acid in most cases. While these agents are not classic hormones, they are important chemical messengers involved in the regulation of vastly different physiologic functions. In most cases, prostaglandins, thromboxanes, and leukotrienes act as paracrine agents, for they function near their

site of origin and are rapidly metabolized after entering the blood stream. This rapid metabolism in the blood is true for many paracrine agents and is a factor that contributes to their characteristic localized effect.

Prostaglandins have been isolated from nearly every tissue of the animal body, although they derive their name from the prostate gland, from which they were originally isolated. There are a number of prostaglandins. Each has a slight difference in chemical structure, and each may have multiple regulatory functions in a variety of tissues. Furthermore, one prostaglandin may have opposite physiologic effects in different organs. In general terms, prostaglandins are implicated in regulation of blood vessel diameter, inflammation, blood clotting, uterine contraction during parturition, and ovulation, among many others. Because prostaglandins are important in many reproductive functions, these substances will be revisited in Chapter 27.

Leukotrienes are similar in structure to prostaglandins, being produced from arachidonic acid via a different enzymatic pathway. There are several families of related leukotrienes, each with specific functions. Leukotrienes are produced primarily by monocytes and mast cells and are usually associated with allergic reactions. Release of leukotrienes increases vascular permeability and induces constriction of air-

Cholesterol:

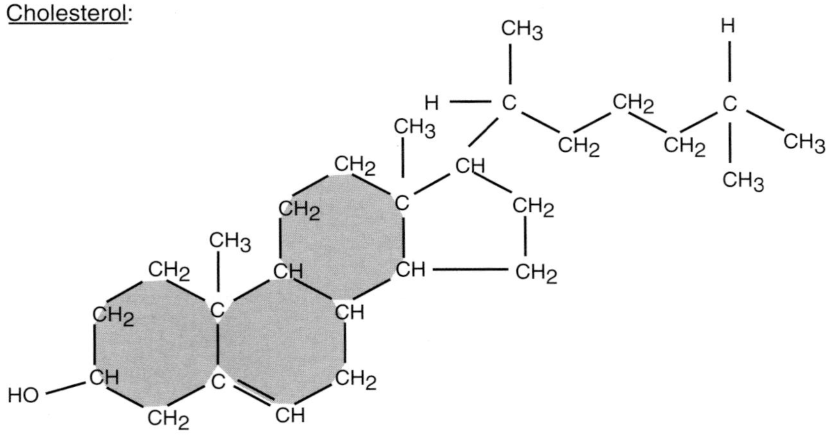

Figure 12-2. The structure of cholesterol.

ways; in humans, these substances have been implicated in producing some of the most prolonged manifestations of asthmatic attacks.

Because of the prominent role of prostaglandins as mediators of inflammation, drugs that inhibit prostaglandin synthesis are antiinflammatory. These are the *nonsteroidal antiinflammatory drugs*, or *NSAIDs*, of which *aspirin, ibuprofen*, and *acetaminophen* are widely used over-the-counter varieties. The side effects of these drugs (e.g., gastric ulceration and kidney injury) occur due to the indiscriminate inhibition of both undesirable effects (i.e., inflammation) and important desirable effects (e.g., maintenance of blood flow to stomach and kidneys). Most NSAIDs also inhibit the formation of thromboxanes, because some of the same enzymes are involved in the synthesis pathways for prostaglandins and thromboxanes. Aspirin reduces the synthesis of thromboxanes for blood clotting, and this is part of the rationale for their use in animals and people to reduce the potential for clot formation. Newer NSAIDs have been developed to inhibit only the production of prostaglandins associated with inflammation.

Hormone Receptors

Only certain specific populations of cells respond to an individual hormone. The term *target organ* is used to identify the tissue whose cells will be affected by a given hormone. Some hormones have multiple target organs, for they affect cells in several sites. For example, both skeletal muscle and liver are among the target organs for insulin. Table 12–1 lists the major endocrine glands, their hormones, and their general effects on their target organs.

Cells within target organs are capable of recognizing and responding to a given hormone, because they contain specific receptors capable of binding, or forming a chemical union, with the hormone. As described in Chapter 2, these cellular receptors may be components of the cell membrane and have a binding site exposed to the extracellular fluid or they may be contained within the cytoplasm or nucleus of cells. In either case, a receptor for a specific hormone must be present for a cell to respond to the hormone.

The presence and number of receptors within target cells may change in certain conditions. Such changes are one way that the biologic effect of a given hormone can be regulated. For example, levels of *estrogen*, a reproductive hormone, increase in circulation shortly before birth (parturition), and this stimulates an increase of *oxytocin* receptors in the smooth muscle of the uterus. The increase in oxytocin receptors prepares the uterus so that oxytocin can promote uterine contractions when released during parturition. Without the increase in oxytocin receptors stimulated by estrogen, oxytocin

Table 12-1. Major Endocrine Glands, The Hormones They Secrete, and Primary Action and Target Tissue of the Hormones

Endocrine Gland	Hormone	Action (target tissue or organ)
Hypothalamus	CRH	Stimulates ACTH release (adenohypophysis)
	GnRH	Stimulates FSH, LH release (adenohypophysis)
	GHRH	Stimulates GH release (adenohypophysis)
	GHIH	Inhibits GH release (adenohypophysis)
	TRH	Stimulates TSH release (adenohypophysis)
	Dopamine (prolactin-inhibiting hormone)	Inhibits prolactin release (adenohypophysis)
	Oxytocin and antidiuretic hormone synthesized in hypothalamus; stored, released from neurohypophysis	
Adenohypophysis (anterior pituitary)	ACTH	Stimulates cortical development, glucocorticoid release (adrenal cortex)
	FSH	Stimulates follicular development (ovary), sperm development (testes)
	LH	Stimulates ovulation, development of corpus luteum, secretion by corpus luteum (ovary), secretion of androgens (testes)
	GH	Promotes growth in immature animals; metabolic effects on carbohydrate, lipid, protein metabolism in adults
	TSH	Stimulates release of thyroid hormones (follicular cells of thyroid gland)
	PRL	Promotes lactation (mammary gland), maternal behavior (central nervous system)
Neurohypophysis (posterior pituitary)	Oxytocin	Stimulates uterine contraction, milk let-down (uterus, mammary glands)
	ADH	Conserves water, reduces urine volume (kidney); constricts vessels to raise blood pressure (arterioles)
Adrenal cortex	Glucocorticoids	Essential for normal response to stress; important roles in protein, carbohydrate metabolism (multiple organs including liver)
	Mineralocorticoids (aldosterone)	Conserve Na, eliminate K (kidney)
Adrenal medulla	Epinephrine, norepinephrine	Augments sympathetic response to stress by actions on several organs
Thyroid follicular cells	T_4, T_3	Increases oxygen consumption, ATP generation (almost all cells)
Thyroid para-follicular cells	Calcitonin	Promotes calcium retention (bone)
Parathyroid	PTH (parathyroid hormone)	Promotes increase in plasma calcium, reduction in plasma phosphate (bone, kidney)

(continued)

Table 12-1. Major Endocrine Glands, The Hormones They Secrete, and Primary Action and Target Tissue of the Hormones (*Continued*)

Endocrine Gland	Hormone	Action (target tissue or organ)
Pancreatic islets: β-cells	Insulin	Promotes glucose uptake; protein, lipid synthesis by various tissues, organs, including skeletal muscle, liver, adipose tissue
Pancreatic islets: α-cells	Glucagon	Promotes glycogenolysis, gluconeogenesis (liver)

ACTH, corticotrophin; ADH, antidiuretic hormone, also called arginine vasopressin; CRH, corticotropin-releasing hormone; FSH, follicle-stimulating hormone; GH, growth hormone; GHIH, growth hormone–inhibiting hormone; GHRH, growth hormone–releasing hormone; GnRH, gonadotropin-releasing hormone; LH, luteinizing hormone; PRL, prolactin; PTH, parathyroid hormone; TRH, thyrotrophin-releasing hormone; TSH, thyrotrophin.

release itself would not provide adequate uterine contractions for normal parturition. An increase in receptors on target cells is termed **up-regulation,** and a decrease is termed **down-regulation.**

Cellular Effects of Peptide Hormones

The receptors for peptides hormones are found in the cell membrane. Peptides cannot freely diffuse through the lipid bilayer of the cell membrane, so their receptors must be in the outer cell membrane to be available to the hormones in the extracellular fluid. As described in Chapter 2, the binding of the hormone with the membrane receptor is the first step in a series of events that brings about changes in the target cell. The subsequent events, which vary with the participating peptide hormones, include changing the permeability of membrane channels, stimulating or inhibiting the activity of membrane bound enzymes, and stimulating or inhibiting the activity of intracellular enzymes.

When enzymatic activity is increased by a hormone–receptor interaction, the intracellular concentration of that enzyme's product increases. For example, many peptide hormones activate the enzyme **adenylyl cyclase,** which increases the intracellular production of **cyclic AMP** (cAMP) by its action on adenosine triphosphate (ATP). The cAMP activates other intracellular enzymes that ultimately bring about the characteristic biologic response to the hormone

(e.g., cellular secretion, cellular contraction, protein synthesis). The term **second messenger** is a general term for the intracellular compounds, such as cAMP, that function as an intermediate in the sequence of steps leading to the biologic response. Two other common second messengers involved in the cellular response to peptide hormones are **diacylglycerol (DAG)** and **inositol triphosphate (IP$_3$).** These second messengers are formed by the action of a membrane-bound enzyme, phospholipase C, on phospholipids in the cell membrane.

Ionic calcium (Ca^{2+}) concentration in the cytosol is normally lower than that in typical extracellular fluid, but some cells accumulate even higher concentrations of Ca^{2+} within their endoplasmic reticulum. Increases in cytosolic Ca^{2+} concentrations may result from the entry of extracellular Ca^{2+} through membrane channels or by Ca^{2+} diffusing from within the endoplasmic reticulum into the cytosol through channels within the membrane of the endoplasmic reticulum. Increases in intracellular free Ca^{2+} above the typical low levels may also act as a second messenger for certain hormones. The increase in Ca^{2+} begins a series of events that ultimately results in changes in intracellular enzymatic activity and a biologic response.

In many cases the biologic response to peptide hormones is rapid and relatively quickly reversed. For example, the action of antidiuretic hormone on cells in the kidney to change their permeability to water can occur within a matter of minutes. Such rapid effects are possible because pathways leading to the biologic effects may only require activation of enzymes (proteins) that are already in the cell. When the hormone is removed or degraded, the effects are reversed by the inactivation of these enzymes.

In some cases, the biologic response to peptide hormones is longer lasting because the intracellular pathways lead to an increase in DNA transcription and the formation of messenger RNA (mRNA). In these cases, the effect is prolonged by the presence of newly synthesized intracellular proteins. The general term for agents that directly influence DNA transcription is *transcription factor*. So peptide hormones may bring about changes in transcription factors within cells.

Cellular Effects of Steroid and Thyroid Hormones

Receptors that bind steroid and thyroid hormones are found either in the cytosol or in the nucleus. Steroid and thyroid hormones are lipid soluble and can reach these intracellular receptors by diffusing into the cell through the cell membrane. The receptor with its bound hormone acts as a transcription factor for specific genes within the DNA to increase or decrease the formation of mRNA that corresponds to the specific gene. Ultimately, the change in mRNA results in a change in protein production, and this brings about the biologic response.

Biologic responses to steroid and thyroid hormones typically develop more slowly but last longer than responses to peptide hormones. In part, this is because all effects are related to changes in protein synthesis. The synthesis of new protein or the degradation of protein already present requires more time than the activation or inactivation of enzymes already present.

Negative and Positive Feedback Regulation

Assuming that adequate numbers of functioning receptors are available, the biologic effect of any hormone is directly proportional to the concentration of the hormone in the body fluids available to bind to the receptors. This concentration is primarily determined by two factors: the rate of hormone release from endocrine cells and the rate of elimination from the body fluids. In normal conditions, the concentration is typically determined by the rate of release. Peptide hormones and amines are stored in secretory granules by endocrine cells, so that they are readily available for release. Steroid hormones are not stored and must be synthesized just prior to release.

The release, and thus the plasma concentration, of most hormones is controlled by some type of *negative feedback regulation.* In this type of regulation the rising levels of the hormone bring about a biologic response that inhibits further hormone release. For example, β-cells in the pancreatic islets are directly affected by the concentration of glucose in the body fluids. An increase in glucose concentration causes the β-cells to increase their release of insulin. One effect of insulin is to promote the uptake of glucose by skeletal muscle cells. As glucose is removed from the body fluids, the stimulus for insulin release is removed, and this has a negative effect on insulin release. This negative feedback regulation of insulin release is a major factor in determining a normal plasma concentration of glucose.

The negative feedback regulation of insulin by changes in plasma glucose is a relatively simple and straightforward feedback loop. The plasma constituent, glucose, being regulated by the hormone, insulin, has a direct effect on the cells releasing the hormone. However, negative feedback loops can be quite complex and have multiple organs in the loop. Some of the more complex loops involve the hormones regulating reproduction in domestic animals and the hypothalamus, the anterior pituitary gland, and the gonads. These are discussed further in Chapters 25 and 27.

A second type of feedback regulation that is seen much less frequently than negative feedback is *positive feedback regulation.* In this case, the hormone brings about a biologic response that produces a further increase in the release of the hormone. This type of regulation is unusual, and it is not designed to maintain a stable or homeostatic level of some activity or blood constituent. One of the few examples of this type of regulation is the relationship between oxytocin release and dilation of the uterine cervix. An increase in oxytocin release is associated with dilation of the uterine cervix during parturition (details in chapters on reproduction), and oxytocin acts on the smooth muscle of the uterus to increase uterine contractions. When the cervix dilates during parturition and oxytocin is released, the contractions of the uterus move the fetus out of the uterus through the cervix. This further dilates the cervix, providing a greater stimulus for secretion of oxytocin. The overall effect is to expel the fetus when the cervix is dilated.

Hypothalamopituitary Axis

The **hypothalamus** is ventral to the thalamus in the diencephalon and forms the floor and part of the wall of the third ventricle (see Chapter 9). The **pituitary gland,** or **hypophysis cerebri,** is attached to its base by the **infundibulum,** a stalk of nervous tissue (primarily axons). Cell bodies of neurons whose axons form the infundibulum are found in the hypothalamus, and their termini abut on capillaries in the neural part of the pituitary gland (**neurohypophysis, posterior pituitary,** or **pars nervosa**). Associated with the infundibulum is a unique system of arterioles and capillaries called the **hypothalamohypophysial portal system.** This system is a true vascular portal system in that blood from a capillary network in the hypothalamus flows through portal vessels (similar to veins) to the glandular portion of the pituitary (**adenohypophysis, anterior pituitary,** or **pars distalis**), where it enters a second capillary network (Fig. 12–3). During development, the pituitary gland forms by the conjoining of a ventral outpouching of the diencephalon (the future infundibulum and neurohypophysis) and a diverticulum, **Rathke's pouch,** which arises from the nearby dorsal ectoderm of the pharynx. The cells of Rathke's pouch become the adenohypophysis.

The neurotransmitters released by hypothalamic neurons whose termini end in the neurohypophysis enter the blood and are carried to distant sites to function as systemic hormones (Fig. 12–3). These peptides are manufactured by the neuronal cell bodies within the hypothalamus, transported via axons into the neurohypophysis, and released directly into blood vessels when action potentials arrive at the telodendria.

Other hypothalamic neurons release neurotransmitters that are carried from the hypothalamus to the adenohypophysis via the hypothalamohypophysial portal system (Fig. 12–3). There, these neurotransmitters act on endocrine cells either to stimulate or to inhibit the release of other hormones (Table 12–1). While these neurotransmitters do not travel to a distant site to stimulate target cells, they are transmitted via the blood

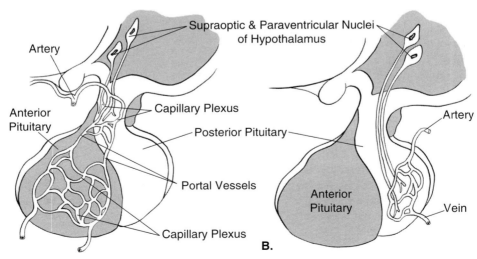

Figure 12-3. Relation between hypothalamus, neurohypophysis, and adenohypophysis. A) Drawing illustrates network of portal vessels. B) Drawing illustrates direct neural connection between hypothalamus and neurohypophysis.

from their site of origin to their site of action. Thus, these neurotransmitters may be considered hormones, but they are also referred to as inhibiting or releasing factors. All of these neurotransmitter–hormones except dopamine are small peptides, and the small peptides are rapidly degraded after passing through the hypothalamo-hypophysial portal system and entering the general circulation. The unique portal system permits the delivery of a relatively high concentration of the releasing or inhibiting factors to the adenohypophysis so that a biologic effect is possible.

The different cell types of the adenohypophysis exhibit different histologic staining characteristics, depending on the hormone they produce. As a consequence, cells are characterized as basophils, acidophils, or chromophobes, among other specific types. These endocrine cells are arranged in cords or clusters around blood-filled sinusoids, in keeping with their role as an endocrine organ. The neurohypophysis has the typical microscopic appearance of nervous tissue, consisting of unmyelinated axons and supportive glial cells.

Historically the pituitary gland was known as the master gland because of the large number of hormones secreted and their wide-ranging effects. Several hormones from the adenohypophysis stimulate distant endocrine glands to increase production of their own hormones (Table 12–1). These stimulatory adenohypophyseal hormones are often called **trophic** or **tropic hormones.**

The hypothalamus functions as a crucial interface between the nervous and endocrine systems, where sensory information is integrated and used to regulate the endocrine output of the pituitary gland. Much of this information is related the status of the internal environment in question (e.g., extracellular fluid osmolality, blood glucose concentration, body temperature and metabolic rate). Release of adenohypophyseal hormones can also be regulated through more direct negative feedback loops based on the blood concentrations of the hormones involved. The hormone produced by the target endocrine gland of a specific trophic hormone can act on (1) the hypothalamus to reduce the production of its releasing factors and (2) the adenohypophysis to reduce its release of the tropic hormone (Fig. 12–4). The tropic hormones of the adeno-

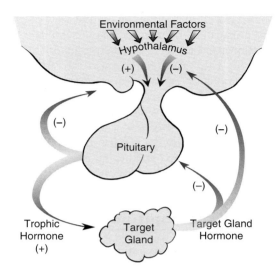

Figure 12-4. Potential feedback loops to regulate hypothalamic releasing hormones and tropic hormones from adenohypophysis. Stimulation of secretion indicated by (+) and inhibition indicated by (−).

hypophysis may also reduce hypothalamic releasing factors via a short negative feedback loop.

A synopsis of the hormones released into the general circulation by the hypophysis, the factors that regulate their release, and their general functions is presented here. Further details on these functions will be given in subsequent chapters when the function of their target organs is covered. All of these hormones are **peptide** or **protein hormones** based on their chemical structure.

Hormones of the Neurohypophysis

Two hormones, oxytocin and antidiuretic hormone, are released by the neurohypophysis.

Oxytocin is produced by the neurons of the paraventricular nucleus of the hypothalamus. When released into the blood stream by their axon terminals, it induces contraction of target smooth muscle fibers of the mammary gland and the uterus. As a result of its actions in the mammary gland, oxytocin aids in the phenomenon of milk let-down, wherein suckling stimulates ejection of milk from the duct system of the gland.

Physical stimulation of the mammary gland (e.g., suckling) is a strong stimulus to secretion of oxytocin, but it is common for other sorts of stimuli to condition a reflex release of the hormone. For example, dairy cows frequently learn to associate the milking parlor and the preparations for milking with milk let-down. Even before the mammary gland is handled in any way, oxytocin is released and milk may be seen dripping from the teats.

In the pregnant uterus, oxytocin acts on the myometrium (muscle of the uterus) to produce uterine contractions for expulsion of the fetus at parturition. Stretching of the cervix by the fetus stimulates further secretion of oxytocin, which then stimulates greater uterine contractions. Oxytocin is sometimes administered by injection at parturition to enhance uterine contractions.

Antidiuretic hormone (*ADH*) is produced by neurons of the supraoptic nucleus in the hypothalamus and released from the neurohypophysis in response to increases in blood osmolality (concentration of dissolved substances) or severe decreases in blood pressure, both of which are influenced by the animal's hydration status. The water-retaining effects of ADH on the kidney are discussed in Chapter 23. ADH also produces constriction of blood vessels, an effect that gives the hormone its other name, *vasopressin* or *arginine vasopressin* (the form found in most mammals).

Hormones of the Adenohypophysis

Growth Hormone

The release of **growth hormone** (GH), also called somatotropin or somatotropic hormone, from the adenohypophysis is regulated by hypothalamic factors that either stimulate (*GH-releasing hormone,* or *GHRH*) or inhibit (*GH release–inhibiting hormone, GHIH,* or *somatostatin*) release. GH levels are highest in young growing animals, but adult animals continue to secrete it. Increases in GH secretion in adults occur in response to a variety of stimuli, but probably the most important physiologic stim-

ulus is a reduction in plasma glucose. In adults, GH functions as a regulator of metabolism during starvation, deficits in plasma glucose, or hibernation. It acts to reduce protein breakdown and the use of glucose for energy in skeletal muscle and to increase the mobilization of fatty acids from adipose tissue.

The role of GH in the determination of body stature in growing animals was introduced in Chapter 5. As was discussed earlier, GH itself has little direct effect on cartilage proliferation and bone growth in young animals. Its growth-promoting effects are mediated by other peptides, **somatomedins** (primarily **insulinlike growth factors 1 and 2 [IGF-1 and IGF-2]**), which are released by the liver and cells in the area of growth plates in bone when stimulated by GH. The somatomedins are the direct stimulators of chondrocytes within the growth plates. Somatomedins also have negative feedback effects on the hypothalamus and adenohypophysis to regulate the release of GH.

In addition to GH, the secretion of somatomedins by the liver of young growing animals is regulated in part by nutrition. Inadequate nutrition may retard growth in part because of a suppression of somatomedin secretion. Small dogs have lower blood levels of IGF-1 than large dogs, suggesting that within a species body size and IGF-1 levels are correlated.

Excessive GH in young animals leads to **gigantism.** Increases in body size are not possible in older animals where growth plates are closed. Excessive GH (with associated IGFs) in mature animals leads to **acromegaly.** Further increases in stature are not possible in mature animals, but cartilage proliferation around joints and other skeletal locations produces enlargements in these areas and a characteristic coarseness of facial features. Affected adults also have derangements of carbohydrate and lipid metabolism (increased blood levels of glucose and fatty acids) because of the metabolic effects of excessive GH.

The amino acid sequence of GH varies among mammalian species, and thus GH produced by one species is not always biologically effective in a different species. Recombinant DNA technology has been used to produce both human recombinant GH and recombinant bovine somatotropin. The human product is used clinically to prevent certain types of human pituitary dwarfism, and the bovine product is used to increase both lactation and food efficiency.

Adrenocorticotropic Hormone

The primary target cells of **adrenocorticotropic hormone (ACTH)** are the cells of the adrenal cortex (outer region of the adrenal glands) that produce glucocorticoids. Glucocorticoids are steroid hormones that function in the regulation of metabolism (discussed later).

Adrenal Glands. The two adrenal glands are located close to the kidneys (*ad,* toward; *ren,* kidney). Shape, size, and exact location vary from one species to another. Each gland consists of an outer region, the **adrenal cortex,** and an inner region, the **adrenal medulla.** These parts of the adrenal gland come from separate embryonic precursors and have distinctly different functions, in spite of their close physical· association within a single connective tissue capsule.

The blood supply to the adrenal gland varies, but in general, small arteries enter the capsule surrounding the gland. These arteries are derived directly from the aorta or from its branches, including the renal, intercostal, and lumbar arteries. Veins from the adrenal gland drain to the caudal vena cava.

Three zones or regions of the adrenal cortex can be identified by light microscopy in most mammals, and each zone is the source of different hormones. From outermost to innermost the three layers or zones are *zona glomerulosa, zona fasciculata,* and *zona reticularis* (Fig. 12–5). All hormones secreted from all three zones are steroid hormones, so cells of all zones have ultrastructural characteristics of steroid-secreting cells.

The hormones secreted by the adrenal medulla (epinephrine and norepinephrine) are amines and are stored in secretory granules prior to release. These endocrine cells are termed *chromaffin cells* because of their affinity for chromium stains. As was described in Chapter 10 in the section on the autonomic nervous system, epinephrine and norepineph-

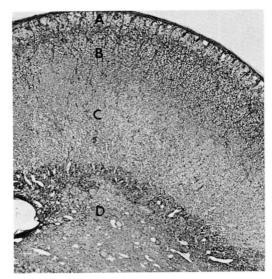

Figure 12-5. Adrenal gland of the horse. The cortical zones, zona glomerulosa (*A*), zona fasciculata (*B*) and zona reticularis (*C*), can be recognized, as can the medullary region (*D*). (Reprinted with permission from Dellman H.D. *Veterinary Histology: An Outline Text-Atlas.* Philadelphia: Lea & Febiger, 1971.)

rine are released from the adrenal medulla in times of stress, and this release is regulated via the autonomic nervous system. **A tumor of chromaffin cells is termed a *pheochromocytoma,* and this neoplasia typically results in excessive secretion of epinephrine and norepinephrine. The resulting clinical signs are those of excessive stimulation of the sympathetic nervous system (e.g., increased heart rate and blood pressure and increased metabolic rate).**

Hormones of the Adrenal Cortex. The zona glomerulosa secretes **mineralocorticoids** (primarily **aldosterone**) that function in the regulation of sodium and potassium balance. The regulation of balance is primarily accomplished by controlling of the loss of sodium and potassium in urine; more details on their specific functions are given in Chapters 18 and 23. Mineralocorticoid secretion is not regulated by ACTH but rather by the serum potassium concentration and the **renin–angiotensin system,** another group of chemical messengers discussed in more detail in Chapter 18.

Glucocorticoids (primarily **cortisol** and **corticosterone**) are the major secretory product of both the zona fasciculata and zona reticularis, and ACTH is the major regulator (stimulator) of their secretion. Without ACTH the fasciculata and reticularis both atrophy, but the glomerulosa remains intact. The inner zones of the adrenal cortex are also a source of adrenal sex hormones (androgens and estrogens), but the rates of secretion in normal adult animals are very low and not necessary for normal reproductive behavior and function.

The secretion of ACTH from the adenohypophysis is stimulated by a hypothalamic hormone, **corticotropin-releasing hormone (CRH)**, and this is the most important regulator of ACTH release. However, the regulation of CRH, hence ACTH release, is extremely complex and affected by a wide variety of stimuli. ACTH increases are considered to be a classic sign of **stress,** and plasma levels of ACTH or cortisol are often used in experimental settings to evaluate the overall stress placed on an animal by any type of physical or emotional stimulus (e.g., restraint, starvation, presence of a predator). Both ACTH and glucocorticoids have negative feedback effects on the pituitary and the hypothalamus to maintain normal resting blood levels of ACTH and glucocorticoids, but stressful stimuli can override these effects.

Glucocorticoids have many target tissues throughout the body. In general their effects on these target tissues would seem an appropriate response to counteract stressful stimuli. For example, glucocorticoids increase the rate of gluconeogenesis (glucose formation) by the liver and increase the rate of fatty acid mobilization from lipid tissue. In skeletal muscle protein synthesis is reduced and protein degradation is increased, which means that more amino acids are available for gluconeogenesis by the liver. These metabolic effects are particularly important during starvation.

Glucocorticoids are often used therapeutically to inhibit inflammatory and immune responses. The doses used for these effects produce blood levels that are much higher than those seen in normal animals, even when they are responding to stress. Such levels and effects are described as supraphysiologic or pharmacologic. Among the many components of the inflammatory process that are inhibited by glucocorticoids are the synthesis pathways for prostaglandins, leukotrienes, and thromboxanes.

Thyroid-Stimulating Hormone

The target cells for **thyroid stimulating hormone** (TSH), also called thyrotropin, are endocrine cells of the thyroid that produce and release thyroxine (T_4) and triiodothyronine (T_3) when stimulated by TSH. Both are considered amine hormones, for each consists of a linkage of two iodinated tyrosine residues (Fig. 12–6). The 3 and 4 refer to the number of iodine atoms in their molecules. These hormones are necessary for normal growth and development in young animals, and they regulate basal metabolic rate in the adult.

Thyroid Gland. The **thyroid gland** is associated with the proximal part of the trachea near the thyroid cartilage of the larynx. Its appearance varies widely among species, with the thyroid gland of most animals possessing two distinct lobes, variably connected across the midline by a strip of thyroid tissue called the isthmus. In pigs, the bulk of the gland lies primarily on the ventral aspect of the trachea rather than being clearly divided into lateral lobes. A connective tissue capsule covers the gland and gives rise to septa that divide the substance of the thyroid and support the vasculature of the gland. Arterial blood supply to the thyroid and the

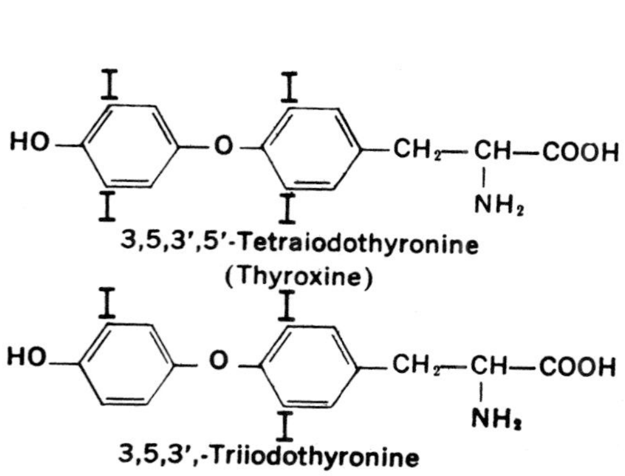

Figure 12-6. Thyroid hormones.

associated parathyroid glands (discussed later) arrives as branches of the common carotid artery.

Microscopically, the thyroid gland consists of *follicles,* spheres lined by a simple epithelium of cells that ranges from cuboidal to columnar (Fig. 12–7). Thyroid follicles are filled with the product of the follicular lining cells, a gel-like substance called *colloid,* which consists of a protein–iodine complex, *thyroglobulin.* The hormones T_3 and T_4 are stored in the colloid as iodinated tyrosine residues that are part of thyroglobulin molecules (Fig. 12–8). This type of storage is a unique among endocrine glands.

Scattered among the follicular lining cells and adjacent to them are a small subset of thyroid cells, the *C cells (parafollicular cells).* The C cells produce *calcitonin,* a peptide hormone that lowers the blood level of calcium by inhibiting the action of osteoclasts. Calcitonin release is directly regulated by the negative feedback of serum calcium concentration on C cells, not by TSH. The physiologic importance of calcitonin in the overall regulation of serum calcium concentration is minimal compared with the role of parathyroid hormone (discussed later).

Thyroxine and Triiodothyronine. Both T_4 and T_3 are biologically active (bind to thyroid

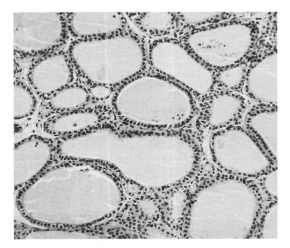

Figure 12-7. Thyroid follicles of varying sizes and shapes are filled with colloid and lined with follicular cells. (Reprinted with permission from Dellman H.D. *Textbook of Veterinary Histology.* 5th ed. Baltimore: Lippincott Williams & Wilkins, 1998.)

hormone receptors), and most of the circulating hormones are bound to plasma proteins. The T_4 and T_3 in the body fluids that are not protein bound are the biologically active molecules, but they are also subject to degradation. In many species, the plasma levels of T_4 are much higher than those of T_3 because the affinity of T_4 for plasma proteins is greater than T_3. The intracellular receptors for the thyroid hormones bind both T_4 and T_3, but they have a higher affinity for T_3. Because of the intracellular receptor affinity for T_3 and the potential for T_4 to be converted to T_3 after it enters target cells, many consider T_3 to be the more biologically important of the two hormones.

Secretion of T_4 and T_3 from the thyroid is a complex series of events that begins with the phagocytosis of thyroglobulin by follicular cells. Endocytotic vesicles containing thyroglobulin then fuse with lysosomes that contain enzymes necessary to degrade the thyroglobulin and release free T_4 and T_3 from their storage form as part of thyroglobulin molecules. The free T_4 and T_3 are then secreted into the blood (Fig. 12–8). TSH from the adenohypophysis stimulates follicular cells to synthesis thyroglobulin and to secrete T_4 and T_3 into the blood. Thus, the overall effect of TSH is to increase blood levels of the thyroid hormones.

Plasma levels of thyroid hormones are relatively stable in adult animals; unlike many other hormones, they do not show a significant diurnal rhythm. These stable levels are primarily maintained by negative feedback of T_4 and T_3 at the level of the pituitary. The thyroid hormones have direct effects on cells in the adenohypophysis to inhibit TSH synthesis and release. Thyrotrophin-releasing hormone (TRH) from the hypothalamus is always present and acts to promote TSH synthesis and release, but its levels do not respond to feedback regulation by T_4 and T_3.

Almost all tissues of the body are target tissues for thyroid hormones, for almost all have receptors for thyroid hormones. In mature animals the most general effect of thyroid hormones is to increase overall oxygen consumption and heat production. The *basal metabolic rate* is a measure of oxygen use in resting conditions, so thyroid hormones are said to increase it. The exact intracellular mechanisms responsi-

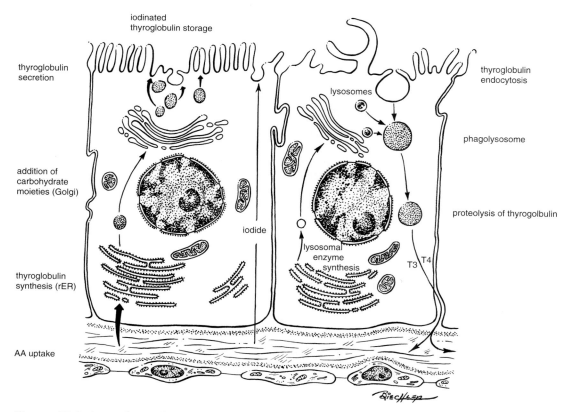

Figure 12-8. Biosynthesis of thyroglobulin (*left*) and its resorption, proteolysis, and secretion (*right*). Events are depicted in two cells, but they do occur in the same cell. (Reprinted with permission from Dellman H.D. *Textbook of Veterinary Histology*. 5th ed. Baltimore: Lippincott Williams & Wilkins, 1998.)

ble for these general effects are not known, but the effects are known as the *calorigenic action* of the thyroid hormones. The calorigenic action is associated with an overall increase in the metabolism and use of carbohydrates and lipids, which is consistent with the increased use of oxygen and heat production.

Chronic exposure of some animals to cold is associated with an increase in TSH, T_4, and T_3. The increased calorigenic effect of the thyroid hormones should work to maintain normal body temperature in the cold environment. The response to the cold appears to be a result of an increase in TRH release by the hypothalamus. The hypothalamus is known to be the reflex center for other reflexes involved with the regulation of body temperature on a short-term

basis (e.g., peripheral vasodilation or vasoconstriction).

Thyroid hormones are essential for normal growth and development in young animals. Two systems of special importance are the skeletal and nervous systems. Animals with thyroid hormone deficits (**hypothyroidism**) do not attain normal stature and have a variety of central nervous system abnormalities. In humans with severe deficits at birth, mental development remains impaired throughout life even if replacement therapy is begun when the person is 4 to 5 years of age. *Cretinism* is the term for the human condition caused by a congenital lack of thyroid hormone and characterized by arrested physical and mental development and lowered metabolic rate.

Other Endocrine Glands

Parathyroid Glands

The **parathyroid glands** are small aggregates of endocrine tissue within or near the thyroid gland. Most domestic animals have two pairs of parathyroid glands, but the exact number and location vary with the species. Commonly, one pair is visible outside the thyroid gland and is therefore designated **external parathyroids.** The second pair is often buried in the substance of the thyroid, and these are the **internal parathyroids.** The pig lacks grossly visible internal parathyroids.

The two types of parathyroid cells are chief cells and oxyphil cells (Fig. 12–9). **Chief cells** are small, usually dark cells that are associated with the production of **parathyroid hormone** (**PTH, parathormone**). The less numerous oxyphil cells are larger, with granular cytoplasm and a small, dark nucleus. These cells have been described in horses and cattle (and humans) but are not found in other domestic species. Their function is unknown, although the fact that they appear later in life has suggested that they may be senescent chief cells.

Parathyroid Hormone. Parathyroid hormone (PTH), a peptide hormone, is the major controller of the level of blood calcium and

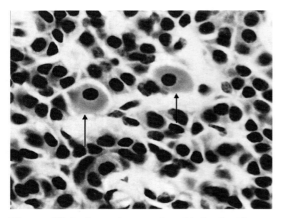

Figure 12-9. An equine parathyroid gland with two large oxyphil cells (*arrows*) among numerous chief cells. (Reprinted with permission from Dellman H.D. *Textbook of Veterinary Histology.* 5th ed. Baltimore: Lippincott Williams & Wilkins, 1998.)

phosphate. It does this by stimulating release of calcium and phosphate from bone, decreasing excretion of calcium and increasing excretion of phosphate by the kidney, and promoting the formation of active vitamin D by the kidney (discussed later). In bone, PTH acts on both osteocytes and osteoclasts to promote the release of calcium phosphate. The action of PTH on osteocytes releases calcium and phosphate from stores associated with the extracellular fluids in and around bone. PTH stimulates the degradation of bone by osteoclasts while it inhibits bone formation by osteoblasts. The overall effect of PTH is to increase blood calcium concentration and lower blood phosphate concentration by increasing its urinary excretion.

The forms of **Vitamin D** consumed in the diet or produced in the skin by the action of ultraviolet light on precursors is not the most active form of the vitamin. These forms are further metabolized in the liver to a second precursor form that is further metabolized in the kidneys to the most biologically active form. It is this final form (1,25-dihydroxycholcalciferol or **calcitriol**) that functions as the true vitamin D. PTH promotes the formation of this final metabolite within the kidney. Two major functions of vitamin D are to increase the rate of calcium absorption from the gastrointestinal tract and to reduce the loss of calcium in the urine. Thus, the overall effect of vitamin D is to retain calcium in the body.

The only significant regulator of PTH release is the concentration of ionized calcium in the blood plasma. Normally about 50% of the calcium in plasma is bound to plasma proteins (primarily albumin), and this bound calcium is not biologically active. The other 50% is unbound and exists as calcium ions. Chief cells detect decreases in the concentration of ionized calcium, and they respond by increasing their secretion of PTH. The resulting rise in plasma calcium has a negative feedback effect on further PTH secretion.

Diets insufficient in calcium are uncommon in domestic animals other than carnivores, but they can occur, especially with diets formulated primarily on grain products, which typi-

cally have high phosphorus and low calcium. In such cases, the chronically low intake of dietary calcium stimulates increased secretion of PTH to keep blood calcium levels adequate for nerve and muscle function. Calcium is removed from the bone matrix, and this decalcification can lead to bone deformities and osteoporosis. This creates the medical condition *nutritional secondary hyperparathyroidism.* In young animals, growth may be disrupted and limb and spine abnormalities may develop, a manifestation of hyperparathyroidism sometimes called *rickets.* A particular form of nutritional hyperparathyroidism commonly called *bran disease* or *bighead* is seen in horses fed excessive amounts of cereal byproducts (e.g., bran) in conjunction with calcium-poor hay. Bone tissue that has been decalcified by high levels of circulating PTH is frequently replaced with soft, bulky fibrous tissue; this is especially prominent in the flat bones of the face and mandible, giving rise to the appearance of an enlarged head. Prompt correction of the dietary imbalance may improve most symptoms (e.g., lameness) of bran disease, although the enlarged facial features are usually permanent.

Pancreatic Islets

The **pancreas** of domestic animals is a bilobed gland adjacent to the proximal part of the duodenum (small intestine). The pancreas is an important exocrine gland whose enzymatic secretions are delivered to the lumen of the duodenum by one or two ducts. Scattered throughout the substance of the pancreas are small masses of endocrine tissue called **pancreatic islets** (formerly the **islets of Langerhans**).

The pancreatic islets are clumps of pale-staining cells, arranged in irregular cords separated by capillaries (Fig. 12–10). Special stains are used to demonstrate the types of epithelial cells found in the pancreatic islets. The known number of distinct kinds of cells is still growing, but the two best characterized are the **α-cells** and **β-cells.** The β-cells are the more numerous (about 75% of all cells in the islet), and they produce the hormone **insulin.** α-Cells produce the hormone **glucagon.**

β-Cells are sensitive to increases in blood glu-

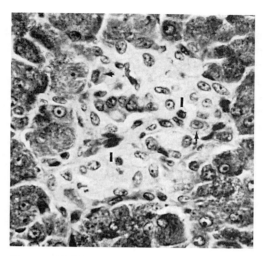

Figure 12-10. Pancreatic islet surrounded by cells of exocrine pancreas. Endocrine α-cells labeled with *arrow* and β-cells, with *I*. (Reprinted with permission from Dellman H.D. *Textbook of Veterinary Histology.* 5th ed. Baltimore: Lippincott Williams & Wilkins, 1998.)

cose (sugar), such as occur after a meal containing digestible carbohydrates, and they release insulin in response to such increases in blood glucose. Insulin lowers blood glucose by stimulating the uptake of glucose by many cells of the body, including skeletal muscle. Insulin also stimulates skeletal muscle and liver cells to synthesize **glycogen,** the storage form of glucose. It affects the metabolism of amino acids and lipids, for it stimulates protein synthesis in skeletal muscle and liver and the deposition of lipids in adipose tissue. Insulin is the major endocrine stimulus for the state of **anabolism** that exists after a meal is digested and nutrients are absorbed. When blood glucose decreases (such as during fasting), the stimulus for insulin secretion is lost and insulin levels are extremely low.

Glucagon causes liver cells to break down glycogen to release glucose, stimulates adipocytes to release fatty acids, and increases the synthesis of glucose in the liver from substrates other than carbohydrates, such as amino acids. The stimulus for glucagon release is a decrease in blood glucose to levels associated with fasting. α-Cells detect such decreases and respond by secreting glucagon in proportion to the reduction in blood glucose.

Insulin is necessary for the uptake of glucose by many cells, including skeletal muscle, which makes up most of the body mass. Without sufficient insulin, glucose accumulates in the blood after a meal, for it cannot be transported across cell membranes into cells where it can be used for fuel. The metabolic consequences of insufficient insulin (or of resistance to its effect) create the condition called *diabetes mellitus.*

Epiphysis (Pineal Gland)

The **epiphysis cerebri** (**pineal gland** or **pineal body**) is a midline structure on the dorsocaudal aspect of the diencephalon. In fish, amphibians, and some reptiles it possesses photoreceptors, and its proximity to the thin calvaria makes it literally a third eye, the function of which is thought to involve setting daily and yearly biologic cycles based on photoperiod. In mammals, including humans and domestic animals, the pineal has no photoreceptors, and its location deep inside the braincase renders it incapable of detecting photoperiods directly. The epiphysis nonetheless does receive information about light and dark cycles indirectly from a nucleus of the hypothalamus. The cells of the epiphysis, although neuronal by lineage, are secretory, and they are supported by neuroglia and receive axonal input. These specialized cells are called **pinealocytes.**

The pinealocytes manufacture serotonin and an enzyme that converts this peptide to **melatonin,** a hormone. Manufacture of melatonin exhibits a profound diurnal rhythm, with releases into the blood peaking during darkness. It is likely, therefore, to be intimately involved in regulating sleep–wake cycles. It appears, too, to be linked to reproduction, inasmuch as the onset of puberty is associated with a profound fall in production of melatonin.

Early discoveries about the link between melatonin and sleep and reproduction have spawned a wave of enthusiastic speculation about its possible use as a cure for insomnia, an aphrodisiac, a treatment for jet lag, and an antiaging drug, among others. To date, however, no controlled studies have supported any of these claims.

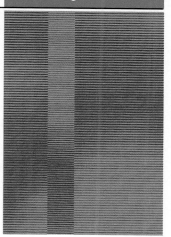

THE INTEGUMENT

Integument

The integumentary system comprises the skin with its adnexal structures (e.g., hair and glands), horns, hoofs, claws, and other modifications of the epithelial covering of the body. The skin is an important protective barrier, reducing water loss, invasion of microorganisms, and abrasive trauma. For many species, it is an important organ of thermoregulation through perspiration, control of cutaneous blood flow, and disposition of the hair coat. Modifications of the integument are used for protection (claws and horns) and provide a tough covering to the feet where they contact the ground (hoofs and footpads).

All of the components of the integument may be considered modifications of the surface epithelium, derived from the embryonic ectoderm, in conjunction with an underlying vascularized component derived from mesoderm (see Chapter 3). In fully developed skin, these become the superficial *epidermis* and deep *dermis,* respectively. Specialized integumentary structures, such as hoofs and horns, likewise have homologous superficial epithelial and deep connective tissue components.

Skin

Skin covers the outside of the animal and is continuous with mucous membranes at oral, anal, and urogenital orifices, the vestibule of the nostril, and the palpebral fissure; these sites are characterized by a **mucocutaneous junction.** Thickness of skin varies both between species and on a given individual, being generally thickest where it is most exposed (e.g., on the back) and thinner in protected regions (e.g., the groin). The skin adheres tightly to underlying structures in some locations, but in others is loosely attached to allow for considerable movement. The looseness of skin attachment is exploited by veterinarians who frequently inject medications or fluids for rehydration into the space underneath the skin (a **subcutaneous** injection).

Epidermis

The outer layer of skin, the epidermis, is an avascular stratified squamous epithelium that is nearly free of nerve endings. In most areas it can be divided into several histologic layers. They are as follows, from deep to superficial: (1) A layer of mitotically active cuboidal or columnar cells, the **stratum basale,** follows the contour of the underlying dermis, to which it is closely applied. (2) The **stratum spinosum** has a spiny appearance because of its desmosomes (intercellular bridges) connecting adjacent cells. (3) The **stratum granulosum** consists of spindle-shaped cells containing basophilic keratohyalin granules. (4) The **stratum lucidum,** which is variably present, comprises cells that are poorly stainable. (5) The **stratum corneum** consists of layers of dead, flattened cells. Presence and relative thickness of each layer is reflected in the overall thickness of the skin (Fig. 13–1).

Cells in the stratum basale undergo mitotic division, which pushes the more superficial layers still farther from the blood vessels in the

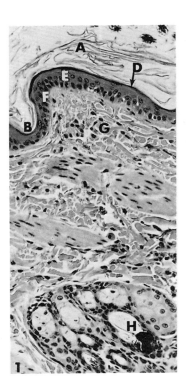
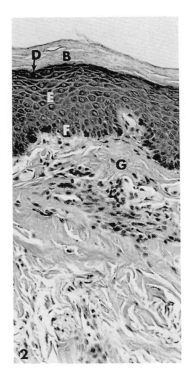
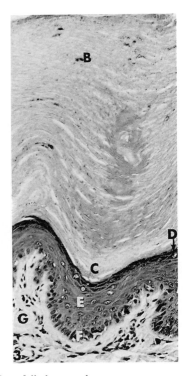

Figure 13-1. Feline skin. *1)* Hairy skin from lumbar region. Note multiple hair follicles near bottom of micrograph. *2)* Hairless skin from nose; epidermis is thicker in this region. *3)* Footpad. Epidermis is markedly thickened in this region, with most of the increase due to thickening of the stratum corneum. *A)* Flaking keratin. *B)* Stratum corneum. *C)* Stratum lucidum. *D)* Stratum granulosum. *E)* Stratum spinosum. *F)* Stratum basale. *G)* Dermis. *H)* Hair follicle. (Reprinted with permission from Dellman H. D. and Brown E.M. *Textbook of Veterinary Histology.* 2nd ed. Philadelphia: Lea & Febiger, 1981.)

underlying dermis. As distance from nutrients increases, the cells flatten and die, leaving a dense mat of their primary constituent, the fibrous protein **keratin.** The drying and hardening of the superficial cells, a process called both **keratinization** and **cornification,** renders the surface of the skin tough and resistant to drying. As the stratum basale continuously adds cells to overlying layers, the stratum corneum flakes off and is replaced. The rate at which this occurs can be influenced by trauma or disease processes. A **callus** is a local increase in thickness in response to continuous trauma.

Dermis

The epidermis forms an undulating sheet with fingerlike projections, the **epidermal pegs,** which project into the underlying connective tissue, the **dermis.** The dermis (also known as the **corium,** especially where it is associated with mod-

ifications like hoofs and horns) bears ridges and nipplelike projections (the **dermal papillae**) that interdigitate with the overlying epidermis (Fig. 13–2); these are most especially prominent in weight-bearing structures, such as footpads and hoofs. The interface between epidermal pegs and dermal papillae provides increased surface area for formation of a strong junction between these two layers. A **blister** is a local disruption of this association between layers, usually due to repeated trauma.

Arteries, veins, capillaries, and lymphatics of the skin are contained in the dermis. Sensory nerve fibers, in addition to supplying the dermis, may extend a short distance into the epidermis. Sympathetic nerves provide motor innervation to blood vessels, glands, and arrector pili muscles of hair follicles in the dermis. These structures do not receive parasympathetic innervation.

Color of skin is due to the pigment granules generated in the cytoplasm of the resident pigment cells, **melanocytes.** These cells in the stra-

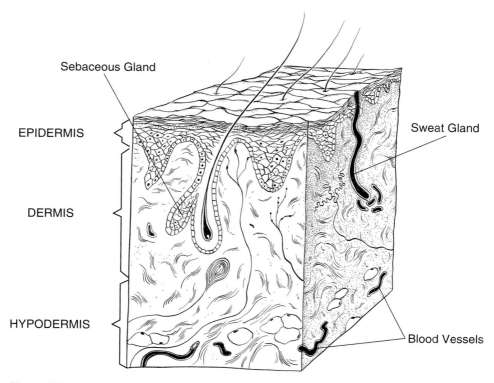

Figure 13-2. Skin anatomy.

tum basale produce the pigment, *melanin,* which is brown, yellowish-brown, or black. Packets of melanin pigment are manufactured by the melanocytes and transferred to surrounding cells of the epidermis; the same process incorporates pigment into cells that cornify into hairs. The expression of different colors in skin and hair comes primarily from the relative amount of melanin produced in the melanocytes rather than from differences in numbers of melanocytes or presence of other pigments. This expression can be influenced by certain pituitary hormones, notably melanocyte stimulating hormone (MSH) and adrenocorticotropic hormone (ACTH) (see Chapter 12).

Absence of pigment in the skin (*albinism*), which may be partial or total, arises from a genetic inability of melanocytes to manufacture pigment. Lack of pigment can render the skin more susceptible to actinic damage (i.e., cellular damage due to ultraviolet light), hence formation of carcinoma (cancer) of the skin or other exposed epithelia. *Cancer eye,* or squamous cell carcinoma of the conjunctiva of the eye, is common in white-faced cattle (e.g., Hereford) living at high elevations, where the ultraviolet component of sunlight is little attenuated.

Hypodermis

In nearly all areas of the body, a layer of loose connective tissue separates the dermis from underlying structures. This areolar connective tissue, known variously as the *superficial fascia, subcutis,* or *hypodermis,* permits movement of the skin without tearing. Where the skin is tightly attached to underlying bone or muscle, a dimple on the body surface may be seen. This is a tie, as is seen where the dermis is attached to the spinous processes of vertebrae. Variable amounts of fat, the *panniculus adiposus,* are present in the hypodermis, with species-dependent distribution and relative abundance. The panniculus adiposus is an especially notable feature of pigs; on the dorsum of the pig, it is called backfat.

Adnexa of the Skin

Hair

Hair is a defining characteristic of mammals. All common domestic mammals except the pig have abundant hair. There are three main types of hair on domestic mammals: (1) *guard hairs,* which form the smooth outer coat, (2) *wool hairs,* also called the *undercoat,* which are fine and often curly, and (2) *tactile hairs,* long stiff hairs with specialized innervation that renders them effective as organs of touch.

An individual hair arises from a modification of the epidermis, the *hair follicle* (Fig. 13–3). The follicle invaginates from the surface of the skin as a double-layered root sheath that surrounds the hair and terminates in a *hair bulb* of epidermal origin. The hair bulb surrounds a small knob of dermis called the *dermal papilla.* The *internal epithelial root sheath* intimately covers the root of the hair and is continuous with the epithelial cells covering the dermal papilla. The *external epithelial root sheath* surrounds the internal root sheath, is continuous with the epidermis, and gives rise to the sebaceous glands that are associated with hair follicles. The division of the epithelial cells covering the dermal papilla generates the hair itself. Growth and multiplication of these cells extrude the hair from the follicle, causing it to grow.

An individual hair has a *medulla* at its center, surrounded by a scaly *cortex,* outside of which is a thin *cuticle.* All parts of the hair are composed of compressed, keratinized epithelial cells. The bulk of the hair comprises the cortex, which consists of several layers of cornified cells. The amount and type of melanin in cortical cells determine whether the hair will be black, brown, or red. The cuticle is a single layer of thin, clear cells covering the surface of the cortex. The medulla may contain pigment, which has little effect on hair color, but air spaces between medullary cells are believed to give a white or silver color to the hair if the cortex lacks pigment. Wool hairs lack a medulla or have only a very small one, accounting for their fine, flexible nature.

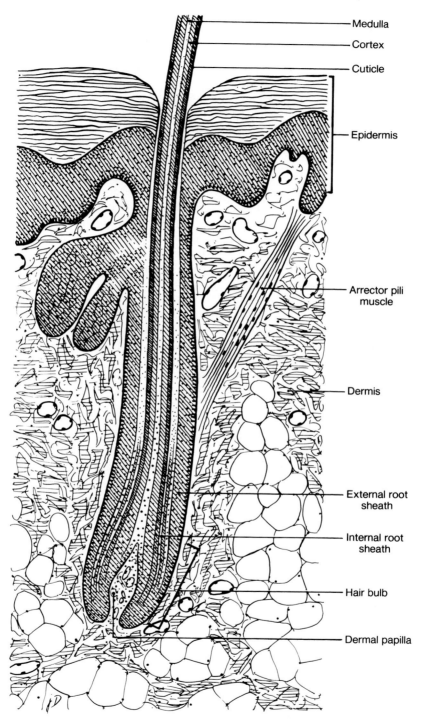

Figure 13-3. Single hair follicle. Epidermal cells adjacent to the dermal papilla give rise to the keratin of the hair. (Reprinted with permission from Banks, Applied Veterinary Histology, 2nd ed., Baltimore: Williams & Wilkins, 1986.)

Tactile hairs, used as probes or feelers, are also called **sinus hairs** because a large blood-filled sinus surrounds the deep portions of the follicle. These hairs are thicker and usually longer than guard hairs and are most commonly found on the face, around lips and eyes. These hairs are particularly well supplied with sensory nerve endings that are sensitive to the movement of the hair.

When a hair is ready to shed, the epithelial cells over the papilla stop multiplying and become cornified. The papilla atrophies, and the hair may fall out, be pulled out, or be pushed out by a new hair that develops from epithelial sheath cells in a manner similar to the hair formation just described. A seasonal shedding of the hair coat from the light coat of summer to the heavy coat of winter and back again is characteristic of most domestic species and is largely triggered by changes in the photoperiod.

The **arrector pili muscle** (plural: arrectores pilorum muscles) is a tiny bundle of smooth muscle fibers that extends from the deep portion of the hair follicle at an angle toward the epidermis (Fig. 13–3). Contraction of the muscle will straighten the hair toward 90°. This orientation increases the insulating properties of the hair coat during exposure to cold and is used by some animals during fight-or flight-reactions, presumably as a means of increasing the apparent size of the animal. The arrectores pilorum muscles are innervated by sympathetic nerves.

Glands

Sebaceous glands are classified as holocrine glands because their oily secretory product, sebum, is produced by disintegration of epithelial cells within the glands. Most of these oil-producing glands are derived from the external epithelial root sheath and empty their secretion into the hair follicle (Figs. 13–2 and 13–3). Contraction of the arrector pili muscle compresses the glands and aids in emptying them. Sebaceous glands that open directly onto the skin surface include those in the ear canal, around the anus, and in the penis, prepuce, and vulva, along with the tarsal glands of the eyelid.

Certain animals have specialized sebaceous glands, thought to be marking glands, that are characteristic of their species (Fig. 13–4). Sheep have several cutaneous pouches that are lined with sebaceous glands. These are the (1) **infraorbital pouches,** found at the medial canthus of the eye and larger in rams than in ewes, (2) **interdigital pouches** on the midline above the hoofs of all four feet, and (3) **inguinal pouches** near the base of the udder or scrotum. Goats have sebaceous **horn glands** caudal to the base of the horn (or where the horn would be in polled animals); secretion in these glands is increased during breeding season and is especially pungent in bucks. In pigs, sebaceous **carpal glands** are present on the mediopalmar aspect of the carpus in both boars and sows.

Sudoriferous glands or **sweat glands** (tubular skin glands), can be found over the entire bodies of farm animals, including the horse, cow, sheep, and pig, although in this last species they are sparse. The horse is the only farm animal that sweats readily. Tubular glands occur on the planum nasolabiale of the cow, planum nasale of the sheep, and planum nasale of the pig (all hairless areas of the nose), where they moisten these surfaces but play little role in cooling. Many modified epithelial structures, including hoofs and horns, lack sweat glands.

Horses are distinguished among domestic animals by their abundant production of sweat. Equine sweat glands, unlike those of most other species, are sensitive to circulating epinephrine, which is why a nervous horse breaks into a sweat in the absence of physical exertion. Equine sweat, moreover, is especially rich in protein; this albuminous sweat will foam when agitated by working muscles. For this reason, a hard-worked horse will lather up on the neck and shoulders and between the pelvic limbs.

The mammary gland is thought to be a modification of tubular sweat glands. Its unique importance warrants its own chapter (Chapter 29), and therefore the mammary gland is not considered here.

Modified Epidermis

Modifications of the epidermis give rise to organs such as hoofs and horns. Many of these tissues have an underlying vascularized connective tissue corium (dermis) that is very promi-

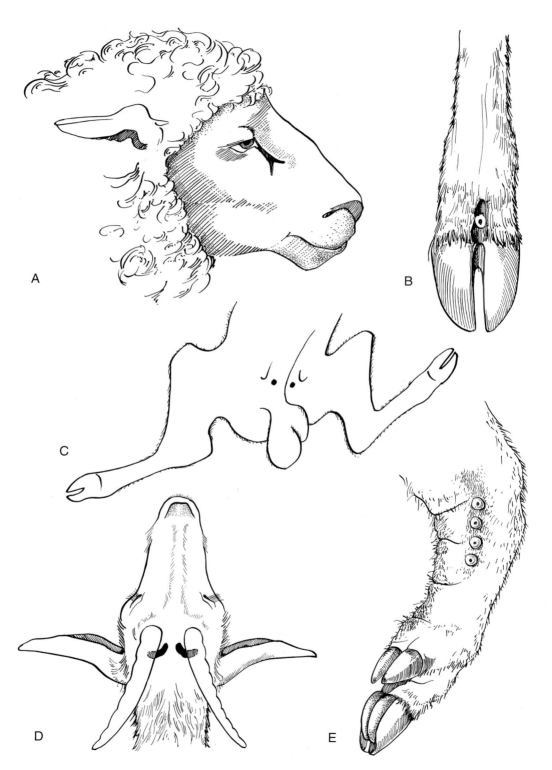

Figure 13-4. Specialized sebaceous glands. A) infraorbital pouch of the sheep; B) interdigital pouch of the sheep; C) inguinal pouch of the sheep; D) horn glands of the goat; E) carpal glands of the pig.

nently folded into papillae or laminae (sheets). In some places this corium is directly continuous with the underlying periosteum. Because it contains the blood vessels and nerves, the corium is often called the sensitive part of the hoof or horn. The insensitive portions of these structures are derivatives of the overlying epithelium. Nonetheless, it is helpful to keep in mind that the substance of the hoof wall, the horn, and other epidermal modifications is generated by the deepest layer of the epithelium (homologous to the stratum basale of skin) and not by the underlying corium.

Hoofs

Hoofed animals are **ungulates** (L. *unguis,* nail), and most common farm mammals fall in this category. A defining characteristic of ungulates is the presence of a well-developed hoof associated with the distal phalanx. Although the hoofs of pigs, ruminants, and horses differ significantly in their gross appearance, they share certain features. Like the skin from which they are derived, hoofs have an outer avascular epidermal layer and an inner vascularized dermis; the dermis of hoofs and horns is more commonly called **corium.**

Different parts of the epidermis and corium of the hoof are named for their location (Fig. 13–5). The outside of the hoof is covered by a thin, waxy layer called the **periople.** The thick **hoof wall** grows from a belt of epidermis at the **coronary band,** the region where haired skin becomes hoof. The deep side of the hoof wall is intimately connected to the underlying corium, which blends with the periosteum of the distal phalanx. The connection between hoof wall and corium is characterized by interdigitating sheets of hoof wall and corium. These are the laminae, of which there are **insensitive laminae** (part of the epidermis) and **sensitive laminae** (part of the corium). The laminae are especially elaborately developed in the equine hoof.

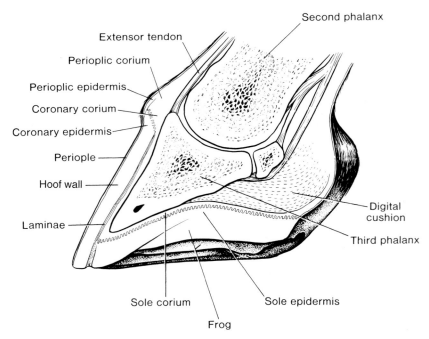

Figure 13-5. Anatomy of the equine hoof. This median section of the hoof illustrates the transition from haired skin to hoof at the coronary band and the relationship between the horny parts of the hoof and the underlying bony structures. (Reprinted with permission from Banks W.J. *Applied Veterinary Histology.* 2nd ed. Baltimore: Williams & Wilkins, 1986.)

The part of the hoof in contact with the ground features a horny **sole** (extensive in the horse, smaller in other domestic ungulates) and a softer **bulb of the hoof.** Deep to the bulb of the hoof is a shock-absorbing modification of the subcutis called the **digital cushion.** The bulb forms a large part of the palmar–plantar aspect of the feet of ruminants and pigs, in which it bears a considerable portion of the animal's weight. In contrast, the equine hoof features a keratinized V-shaped **frog,** which is more flexible than the adjacent sole of the hoof but harder than the bulbs of other ungulates.

The equine hoof is a highly specialized structure and is so important that it will be covered in depth in Chapter 14. The following is a brief overview of the anatomy of the hoofs of artiodactyls, the even-toed ungulates (Fig. 13–6).

A convenient terminology for the digits of even-toed animals is to refer to the digits by number (III and IV in ruminants and pigs), and then relate each digit to the midline of the respective foot. The **axial** side of the digit is the side closest to the midline of the foot and the **abaxial** side is the side farthest from the midline of the foot.

The hoof wall consists of a nearly vertical axial portion that reflects sharply caudad at the **toe** (tip of the hoof) to be continuous with the abaxial portion of the wall. The abaxial hoof wall is convex and the axial wall is concave, and both the axial and abaxial surfaces are continuous with the bulb of the hoof. The lateral digit bears more weight than the medial one (as a clinical consequence, most foot lameness in dairy cattle is referable to the lateral hoof). In contrast to the horse, the sole and bulb of the foot carry a great

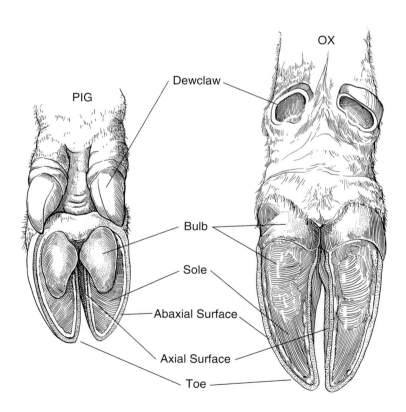

Figure 13-6. Palmar view of the feet of the pig (*left*) and the ox (*right*). The accessory digits (dewclaws) of the pig are well developed relative to those of the ox. The bulb of the porcine hoof also comprises a larger portion of the bottom of the foot. Surfaces adjacent to the midline are described as axial, whereas those toward the outside of the hoof are abaxial.

deal of weight relative to the walls and toe. The bulb of the porcine hoof is especially prominent, providing a larger proportion of the weight-bearing surface than in ruminants.

Horns

Horns of cattle and sheep are formed over the cornual process, a bony core that projects from the frontal bone of the skull (Figs. 13–7). Both male and female cattle of horned breeds have horns, although the female animal's horns are smaller. In most horned sheep and goat breeds, both males and females have them, although in a few breeds only rams or bucks are horned. Animals that lack horns naturally are **polled.**

The corium of the horn completely envelops the cornual process and blends with its periosteum. The horn itself consists of dense keratin, much like the hoof wall, and elongates from the base. A soft type of horn called the **epikeras** covers the surface of the horn at the base and extends a variable distance toward the apex of the horn. The epikeras resembles periople of the hoof.

Variations in level of nutrition of the animal are reflected in variations in rapidity of horn growth, resulting in a series of rings on the horn. These alternations in thickness of the horn may reflect seasonal stresses, notably the stress of calving in cows. The age of the animal may be estimated by counting the rings on the horn.

Dehorning can be accomplished by destroying the corium when only buttons (the small cutaneous primordium of the future horn) are present in the young animal (usually less than 8 weeks for cattle). This is most typically done by surgical removal of the button or by its destruction with a hot iron or with caustic material. For humane reasons, veterinarians administer a local anesthetic block of the cornual nerve before dehorning. After the horn has started to develop, the entire corium and cornual process must be removed along with the horn epidermis and a small amount of adjacent skin to ensure complete dehorning. If any parts are left, an irregular horn stub (a scur) may develop. Dehorning after 3 or 4 months of age risks opening the frontal sinus to the outside, as the cornual diverticulum enlarges into the bony core of the horn as the animal matures.

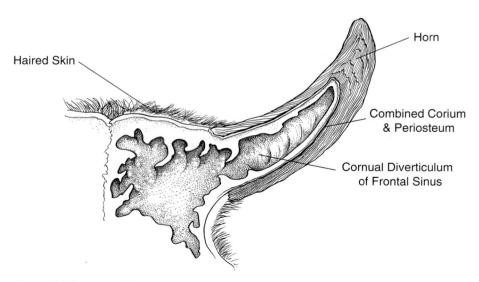

Figure 13-7. Longitudinal section of a horn. The horn is supported by a bony core, the cornual process of the frontal bone, which is invaded by a diverticulum of the frontal sinus. Periosteum and corium are blended on the surface of the cornual process.

Dewclaws

The accessory digits, commonly known as **dewclaws**, of ruminants correspond to digits II (medial) and V (lateral). Ruminant dewclaws lack well-developed phalanges; their hoofs have a wall and small bulb. Ruminant dewclaws do not bear weight and as a rule have little clinical significance. Dairymen occasionally have the medial dewclaws on the pelvic limbs removed as a prophylactic measure against injury to the udder by these horny growths. The dewclaws of pigs, like the weight-bearing digits, have three phalanges and a smaller but well-developed hoof. Porcine dewclaws occasionally make contact with the ground when the pig stands on soft surfaces.

Chestnuts and Ergots

Chestnuts are hornlike growths on the medial sides of horses' limbs. The front chestnuts are proximal to the carpus, and the hind chestnuts are slightly distal to the hocks. The chestnuts are thought to be vestigial metacarpal and metatarsal footpads.

Ergots are small projections of cornified epithelium in the center of the palmar (plantar) part of the fetlock of the horse. The tuft of hair at the fetlock hides the ergot in most instances.

Coat Color in Horses

The description of equine coat color can vary with the breed or the part of the country. The following guidelines are provided to familiarize you with some of the more common colors and the terms used to describe them, but it should be understood that legitimate disagreements will arise between knowledgeable equestrians. Most solid colors (no spots) are derived from variations on and dilutions of black, bay, gray, and chestnut.

True **black** horses are rare except in a few breeds (e.g., Shire and Percheron). The body hairs and all the points are completely black without brown or white hair intermixed. Black coats frequently bleach with prolonged exposure to sunlight, rendering them less deeply black.

The **bay** horse's body color ranges from tan through red to reddish-brown. The **points** (mane, tail, lower limbs, and ear rims) are black; the black limbs may not be apparent on individuals with extensive white markings. Horsemen add many adjectives to the basic term bay, but fortunately most of them are self-explanatory. Blood bay, red bay, mahogany bay, and sandy bay are just some examples of these terms. Very dark bays (sometimes called black bay or mahogany bay) are described as **brown** in some registries (notably the Jockey Club, which registers Thoroughbred horses).

A **gray** horse's coat has an admixture of white and darker (generally black) hairs. The skin is black. Many gray horses are dark at foaling and gradually accumulate white hairs as they age, lightening the entire coat. When the darker hairs are red, the gray may have a pink cast, and depending on the breed and the horseman's preference, these horses may be referred to as rose gray or roan (discussed later). **Dappling** is characterized by a pattern of dark and light circles in the coat with the centers lighter. Any color can be dappled, but the term is most commonly applied to gray horses.

Chestnut horses are some shade of red or brown, varying from diluted shades that are nearly yellow to a deep liver chestnut. The points on the chestnut may be the same as the body color, lighter (sometimes even flaxen), or slightly darker, but they are never black. As with *bay*, many descriptive adjectives can be added to *chestnut* to describe the color more specifically. One variation of chestnut is **sorrel,** most often encountered in reference to the quarter horse. In this breed, sorrel is used for light chestnut shades, including red chestnut, whereas the term chestnut is reserved for dark (liver) shades.

Palomino describes a light-colored body with lighter mane and tail. The most desirable palomino horses have a body color of "newly minted gold" with white mane and tail. This ideal is uncommon, though, and most palominos have body hairs in some less golden shade of yellow. All palominos' manes and tails are white or cream. Strong dilutions of palomino can be nearly white in appearance. These diluted horses, described as **cremello,** often arise from palomino × palomino crosses.

A **buckskin's** body color is yellow or gold,

and points are black. Many buckskins also carry **dun** markings (discussed later), most prominently the dorsal stripe. Some purists insist that true buckskins *must* have dun markings, that horses without the dorsal stripe are a variety of bay, but this is not a widely held conviction.

The term **dun** has been used loosely to describe a variety of diluted colors, but a more restrictive (and more common) use limits the term to mean colors that are characterized by the **dun markings.** These line-backed duns always have a dark **dorsal stripe** running from the mane to the base of the tail. Other, less universal markings include a shoulder bar, transverse stripes on the caudal aspect of the forearm and sometimes the hock (so-called zebra stripes), and concentric darker rings on the forehead (cobwebbing). There are many shades of dun, described by a variety of adjectives (e.g., yellow dun, red dun). One notable variety of dun is called **grullo** (grew'yoh) or **grulla** (grew'yuh) (masculine and feminine, respectively). Grullos have black points, and the body is a slate color, often with a bluish cast.

Roan hair coats are composed of dark hairs mixed evenly with white hairs over most of the body. Unlike grays, roans do not lighten with age, although the seasonal variation in a given roan's appearance may be considerable. The specific terms used to describe roans depend on the background color into which the white hair is mixed. The roan pattern on black horses, for instance, may be described as blue roan; on bay as red roan; on the sorrel coat as strawberry roan.

The defining characteristic of the **pinto** is large, irregular patches of white against a solid color. This pattern can take one of two basic forms, *overo* or *tobiano*. Distinguishing between these two patterns can be difficult, and in fact, some individuals have characteristics of both. The **tobiano** is a white horse splashed with darker spots. White patches extend over the midline of the back, and the head is solid colored, although there may be white facial markings. Generally, all four limbs are white. Spots are usually smooth-edged and rounded. The **overo** is a colored horse splashed with white. White rarely extends over the midline of the back. Generally at least one and often all four limbs are the dark color. The head and face are often broadly marked with white. The markings are irregular and splashy. A further set of descriptors used to describe pinto coat patterns distinguishes between black and white (**piebald**) and brown and white (**skewbald**) pintos. Overo and tobiano refer to pattern distribution, while skewbald and piebald refer to color combination.

A **Paint** is fundamentally a Quarter Horse with pinto coloration. The Paint Horse Association registers only horses with Paint or Quarter Horse lineage. A Paint may be double-registered as a pinto, but not all pintos are registrable as Paints.

The **Appaloosa** is also distinguished by its characteristic coat pattern. The Nez Perce Indians of northeastern Oregon and northern Idaho, particularly in the region of the Palouse River, whence the breed derives its name, used selective breeding to develop the Appaloosa. In addition to the classic spotted hair coat, three distinctive pigmentation patterns are common in Appaloosas: (1) the sclera of the eye is white, (2) skin is mottled black and white (this is most obvious around lips, eyes, and genitalia), and (3) hoofs are striped vertically in black and white. The most striking thing about the Appaloosa is, of course, its showy, spotted hair coat (although not all registered Appaloosas have spots!). This may assume many patterns, each of which is described with specialized terms by aficionados of the breed. Many Appaloosas feature a solid body color with a white and/or spotted blanket over the hips and loins. White horses with dark spots over the entire body are **leopard Appaloosas.**

Wool

As the name implies, **wool** is composed of the wool hairs, or undercoat, of animals bred for their ability to produce usable fiber. The hair coat of important wool-producing breeds characteristically lacks any appreciable guard hairs, so that the fleece is soft and curly, made up of long, fine hairs. The grade of wool is related to the fiber diameter, crimp (a reference to the waviness), and length of the fibers, with fine, wavy, long fibers being most desirable. Prior to processing, the wool has an oily feel imparted by **lanolin,** a product of cutaneous sebaceous glands. Lanolin is sometimes called wool grease or wool wax. It is removed from the fiber when the fleece is cleaned and used in a variety of ointments, emollients, and skin products.

Most commercial wool is acquired from sheep, with the merino and the rambouillet be-ing the most commercially important breeds. Angora and cashmere goats and camelids (camels, llamas, and alpacas) are also used for wool. The long, fine wool of the Angora goat is called mohair, whereas that of the cashmere goat is used to make cashmere wool.

ANATOMY AND PHYSIOLOGY OF THE FOOT OF THE HORSE

The foot of the horse is a highly modified single digit, adapted for rapid running across grasslands. The structures from the carpus (which horsemen frequently call the knee) distad in the thoracic limb of the horse correspond to the wrist and hand of humans. These structures comprise the *manus,* and an examination of the bony components will reveal the same basic plan for both species: two rows of carpal bones, a single fully formed metacarpal bone for each digit (of which there is only one in the horse), and three phalanges within each digit. Likewise, the hock and more distal structures in the equine pelvic limb are homologous to the ankle and foot of humans; these constitute the *pes.* From the cannon bone distad, the equine manus and pes are nearly identical, except in a few details of blood supply and innervation. In common usage, the term *foot* is used to describe both manus and pes (Fig. 14–1). Among domestic horses, most lameness is referable to the foot (and most of these are associated with the forefoot, which bears more weight).

The hoof, presented in general terms in the preceding chapter, is only one part of the complex that is the equine foot. This chapter discusses the detailed anatomy of the hoof and the other components of the foot, along with the specialized ligamentous apparatus (stay apparatus and reciprocal apparatus) characteristic of the limbs of *Equidae.*

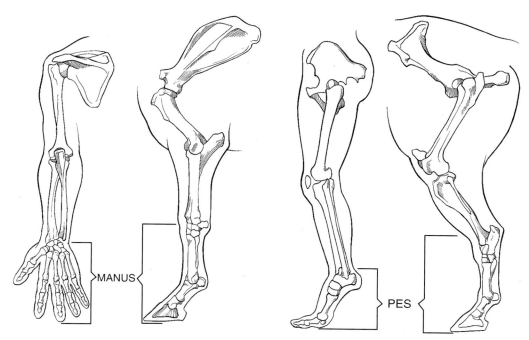

Figure 14-1. Comparative anatomy of human and equine limbs. In the thoracic limb, the manus comprises the carpus and elements more distal (corresponding to the human wrist and hand). In the pelvic limb, the pes includes the tarsus and elements more distal (the human ankle and foot). The horse therefore stands on a single digit, homologous to the human finger or toe.

Structure of the Foot

Bones and Cartilages

Anatomy of the carpus and tarsus are discussed in Chapter 6. In the thoracic limb, the large metacarpal III (**cannon bone**) and medial (II) and lateral (IV) metacarpal bones (**splints**) articulate proximally with the carpus, and the cannon bone articulates distally with the proximal phalanx and two proximal sesamoid bones. Similarly in the pelvic limb, metatarsals II to IV articulate proximally with the tarsus, and the cannon bone (metatarsal III) articulates distally with the proximal phalanx and the two proximal sesamoid bones. As a rule, metatarsal III is somewhat longer and rounder in cross-section than metacarpal III.

The three phalanges include (1) the **proximal phalanx** (**long pastern bone**), (2) the **middle phalanx** (**short pastern bone**), and (3) the **distal phalanx** (**coffin bone**) (Fig. 14-2). The proximal phalanx articulates with the cannon bone at the **fetlock** (metacarpophalangeal and metatarsophalangeal joints) and with the middle phalanx at the **pastern** (proximal interphalangeal joint). Middle and distal phalanges articulate at the **coffin joint** (distal interphalangeal joint).

The two **proximal sesamoid bones** lie at the palmar/backplantar surface of the fetlock. The single **distal sesamoid** (**navicular**) **bone** lies at the palmar or plantar aspect of the coffin joint.

The distal phalanx features medial and lateral palmar/plantar processes to which are attached rhomboidal **ungual cartilages** (formerly collateral cartilages) (Fig. 14–3). The dorsal margins of these cartilages extend proximal to the hoof, where they are palpable under the skin near the heels of the foot. Flexibility of the ungual cartilages probably aids in pumping blood away from the foot.

Trauma (by either direct injury or chronic heavy work) may ossify the ungual cartilages; this produces a condition called *sidebone*

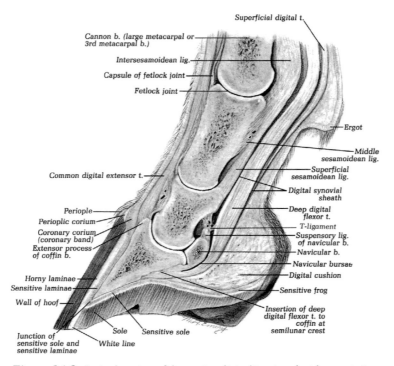

Figure 14-2. Sagittal section of the equine digit. (Reprinted with permission from Miller L. J. and Van Hoosen N. *Horseshoeing Theory and Hoof Care.* Philadelphia: Lea & Febiger, 1977.)

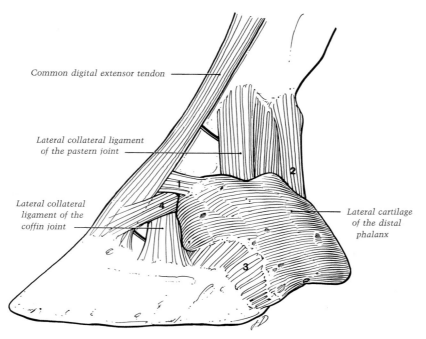

Figure 14-3. Lateral view of the equine digit. The ungual cartilage (lateral cartilage of distal phalanx) is stabilized by four ligaments. (Reprinted with permission from Stashak T.S. *Adam's Lameness in Horses.* 5th ed. Baltimore: Lippincott Williams & Wilkins, 2002.)

(Fig. 14–4). Lameness may or may not accompany sidebone. Penetrating injury in the region of the coronary band may lead to infection of the ungual cartilage and the development of chronic draining tracts. This is called *quittor.*

Cornified Tissues

The hoof is a cornified modification of epidermis, under which lies a vascular layer, the corium (Fig. 14–5). The region where hairy skin changes to

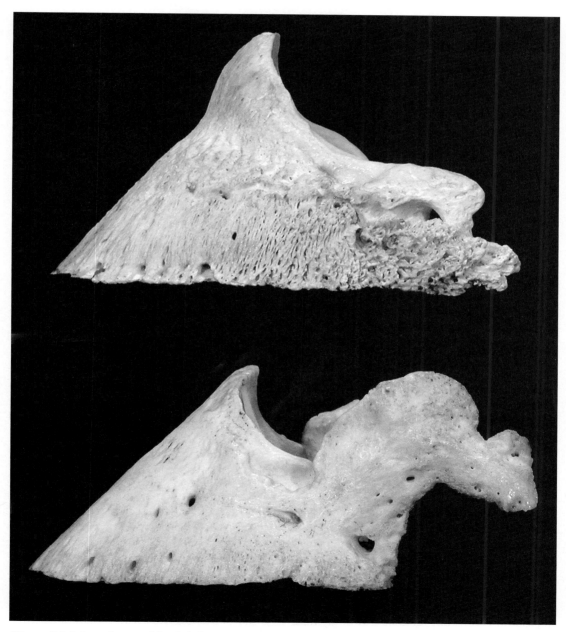

Figure 14-4. Lateral views of distal phalanges. *Top,* Normal distal phalanx. *Bottom,* Ossification of ungual cartilage seen as an irregular bony projection from the palmar process of this phalanx. This condition is known as sidebone. (Photo supplied by A. Fails. Colorado State University, Fort Collins, CO)

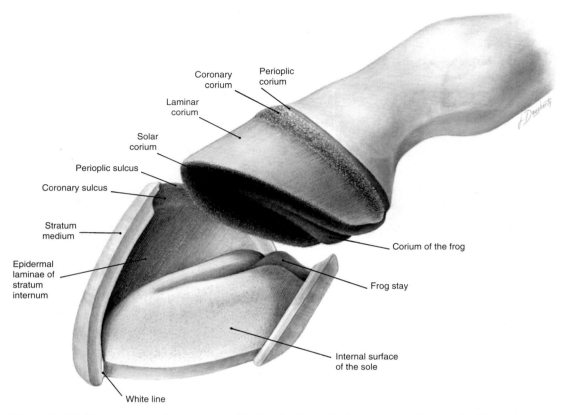

Figure 14-5. Dissected view of the relation of the hoof to the underlying corium. (Reprinted with permission from Stashak T.S. *Adam's Lameness in Horses.* 5th ed. Baltimore: Lippincott Williams & Wilkins, 2002.)

hoof is the **coronary band** (or coronet). The **hoof wall** is the portion of the hoof that is visible when the horse is standing. It is divided into a **toe** in front, medial and lateral **quarters** on the sides, and medial and lateral **heels** behind that turn sharply forward at the **angles** to be continued by the **bars** on the bottom of the hoof (Fig. 14–6).

Pigmentation of the germinating layer of epidermis determines the color of the hoof wall. White hoofs are found where the hair at the coronary band is also white, and dark hoofs are associated with dark hair in this area. The widely held conviction that black hoofs are stronger than nonpigmented (white) hoofs has no scientific basis but remains a strongly held belief with much anecdotal support.

A thin band of **perioplic corium** at the coro-

nary band is associated with the layer of epidermis that produces the thin, waxy **periople** (**stratum tectorium**) on the surface of the hoof wall. A wider band of **coronary corium** underlies the portion of the epidermis that generates the bulk of the hoof wall (often called the **stratum medium**). The coronary corium features very prominent papillae that interdigitate with the coronary epidermis; hoof wall produced by epidermis adjacent to these papillae assumes a tubular configuration. This **tubular horn** can be distinguished from surrounding **intertubular horn** on microscopic examination. Both contribute to the stratum medium (Fig. 14–7).

The periosteum on the convex surface of the distal phalanx blends with longitudinal leaves of corium called the **laminar corium,** which, because it is well innervated, is often called the **sensitive laminae** of the hoof. The sensitive

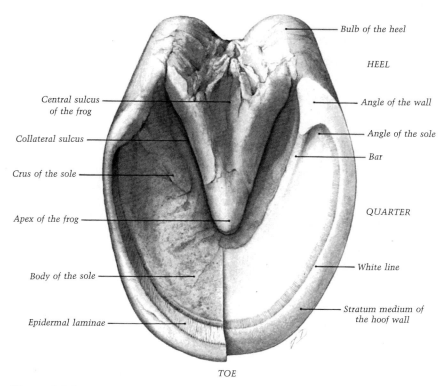

Central sulcus of the frog

Collateral sulcus

Crus of the sole

Apex of the frog

Body of the sole

Epidermal laminae

Bulb of the heel

HEEL

Angle of the wall

Angle of the sole

Bar

QUARTER

White line

Stratum medium of the hoof wall

TOE

Figure 14-6. Gross anatomy of the ground surface of the equine hoof. The right side of this hoof is shown freshly trimmed. (Reprinted with permission from Stashak T.S. *Adam's Lameness in Horses.* 5th ed. Baltimore: Lippincott Williams & Wilkins, 2002.)

laminae interdigitate with epidermal laminae (Figs. 14–7 and 14–8), which, because they are not innervated, are described as **insensitive laminae.** The large surface area afforded by the thousands of interdigitating laminae creates a strong connection between the distal phalanx and the hoof wall. Most of the weight of the horse is transferred by the laminae to the hoof wall rather than directly to the sole of the foot.

Inflammation of the laminae is *laminitis.* Because the hoof is a relatively closed space, such inflammation is extremely painful. Laminitis of sufficient severity can result in detachment of insensitive from sensitive laminae, so that the intimate association between hoof wall and distal phalanx is lost (Fig. 14–9). In such a case, the distal phalanx may rotate downward, and the hoof wall grows abnormally, producing an irregular flared wall and up-curled toe. This chronic condition is *founder.*

The hoof wall reflects sharply at the heels, turning back toward the center of the sole to become right and left **bars.**

The **sole** of the foot is a concave keratinized plate that attaches to the palmar–plantar surface of the third phalanx. It includes the entire ground surface of the foot not occupied by the wall or the frog (discussed later). Normally, the concavity of the sole allows the wall and frog to bear most of the weight and wear (Fig. 14–6).

Where the outer margin of the sole meets the inner margin of the wall, a narrow, light-colored mark appears that is known as the **white line.** This is where the epidermal laminae of the hoof wall come into wear as the hoof wall elongates. The white line is useful as a landmark for driving nails in shoeing. A properly directed nail started at or outside the white line will not touch any sensitive structures of the foot.

The *frog* (cuneus unguis) is a specialized, wedge-shaped pad near the heels of the foot

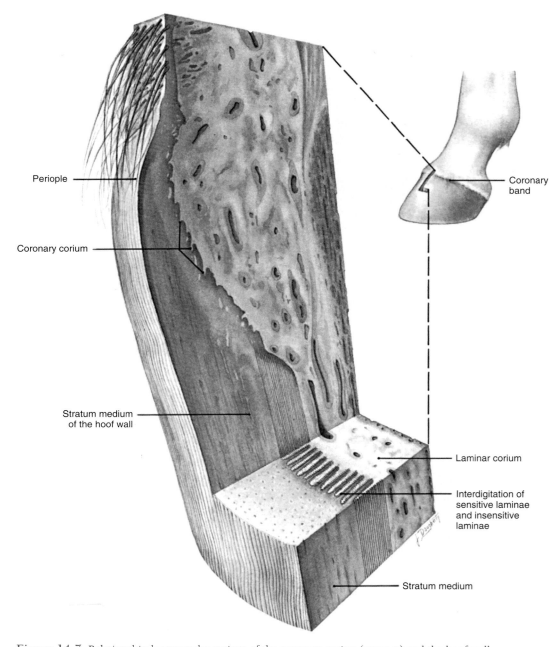

Periople

Coronary corium

Stratum medium
of the hoof wall

Coronary
band

Laminar corium

Interdigitation of
sensitive laminae
and insensitive
laminae

Stratum medium

Figure 14-7. Relationship between the corium of the coronary region (coronet) and the hoof wall. *Insert,* The gross location of this section. Note the cross-sectional appearance of the laminae. (Reprinted with permission from Stashak T.S. *Adam's Lameness in Horses.* 5th ed. Baltimore: Lippincott Williams & Wilkins, 2002.)

(Fig. 14–6). The horn of the frog is relatively pliable, and the compression of the frog against the ground is important for return of blood from the foot. Deep grooves (***collateral sulci*** or ***paracuneal sulci***) demarcate the sides of the frog from adjacent sole, and a single ***central sulcus*** corresponds to a spine of tissue called the ***frog stay*** on the dorsal (deep) side of the

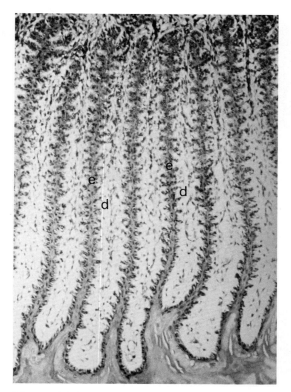

Figure 14-8. Photomicrograph of a cross section of equine fetal hoof in the region of the laminae. Epidermal laminae (*e*) interdigitate with dermal laminae (*d*). (Reprinted with permission from Stashak T.S. *Adam's Lameness in Horses*. 5th ed. Baltimore: Lippincott Williams & Wilkins, 2002.)

frog (Fig. 14–5). Deep to the frog is the ***digital cushion,*** a thick wedge of fibrofatty tissue (Fig. 14–2).

Tendons

No muscle bellies extend below the carpus or tarsus in the mature horse. The tendons of several muscles in the thoracic and pelvic limbs continue into the foot, where each tendon inserts on one or more phalanges, as described in Chapter 7 (see Figs. 7–8 and 7–10).

The common digital extensor tendon passes down the dorsal aspect of the metacarpus and over the fetlock and inserts on the extensor process of the distal phalanx. The long digital extensor tendon has the same course and insertion in the pelvic limb.

In the thoracic limb, the lateral digital extensor tendon inserts on the proximal end of the proximal phalanx after pursuing a course lateral to the common digital extensor tendon. In the pelvic limb, the lateral digital extensor tendon merges with the tendon of the long digital extensor muscle and through it inserts on the extensor process of the distal phalanx.

The tendon of the deep digital flexor muscle (in both thoracic and pelvic limbs) passes down the palmar/plantar side of the cannon bone and crosses the fetlock; it inserts on the palmar/plantar portion of the distal phalanx. In this course, it passes over the proximal and distal sesamoid bones.

The superficial digital flexor tendon passes distad on the cannon bone just superficial to the deep digital flexor tendon, with which it shares a synovial sheath. Distal to the fetlock the superficial digital flexor tendon divides into two branches, which pass on each side of the deep digital flexor tendon and insert at the proximal end of the middle phalanx and the distal end of the proximal phalanx.

Strain of the flexor tendons can result in tendonitis. The inflammation produces a convex profile to the normally straight tendons. This *bowed tendon* is most commonly seen in horses used at speed (e.g., racehorses) (see Fig. 7–9).

Ligaments

The ligaments of the foot include the ***medial*** and ***lateral collateral ligaments*** of fetlock, pastern, and coffin joints. These are the typical ligaments found in any ginglymus joint. In addition, a specialized structure, the ***suspensory ligament,*** runs parallel to the cannon bone on its palmar/plantar aspect. In animals with more than one digit, this structure usually has a considerable amount of muscle; in such animals, it lies between adjacent metacarpals or metatarsals and is therefore called the interosseous muscle.

The suspensory ligament is found between the cannon bone and the deep digital flexor tendon (Fig. 14–10). It attaches proximally to the proximal end of the cannon bone and to the distal row of carpal or tarsal bones. It passes

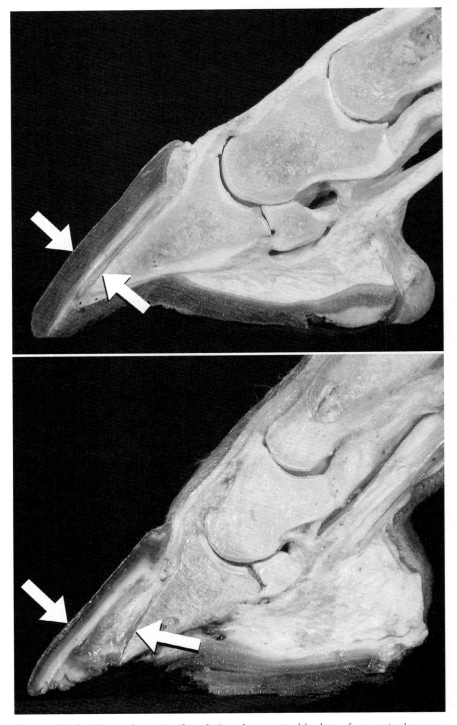

Figure 14-9. Chronic laminitis (founder) is characterized by loss of congruity between epidermal and dermal laminae. The distal phalanx is rotated away from the hoof wall by the distractive force of the deep digital flexor tendon. *Top,* Normal hoof in sagittal section. *Arrows* emphasis the parallel surfaces of the hoof wall and distal phalanx. *Bottom,* Hoof with chronic laminitis and rotation of the distal phalanx. (Photo supplied by A. Fails. Colorado State University, Fort Collins, CO)

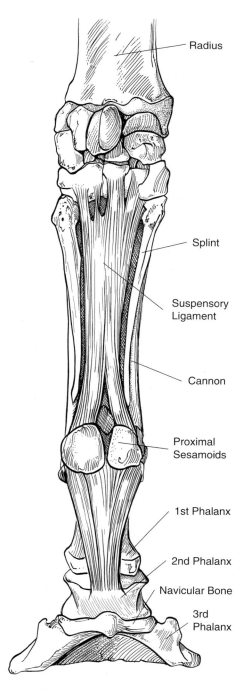

- Radius
- Splint
- Suspensory Ligament
- Cannon
- Proximal Sesamoids
- 1st Phalanx
- 2nd Phalanx
- Navicular Bone
- 3rd Phalanx

Figure 14-10. Palmar view of the equine foot, illustrating the elements of the suspensory ligament and proximal sesamoids. The suspensory ligament and the ligaments of the proximal sesamoids form a continuous ligamentous band that passes from the carpus and proximal metacarpus to the proximal and middle phalanges. This part of the stay apparatus is the most important support for the fetlock joint.

down between the splint bones on the palmar/plantar surface of the cannon bone in the horse.

Upon reaching the fetlock, the suspensory ligament divides into several branches. The main continuation of the suspensory ligament attaches to the proximal sesamoid bones and the ligaments that bind these two bones together. In addition, medial and lateral bands (***extensor slips*** or ***extensor branches***) extend to the dorsal side of the fetlock to attach to the tendon of the common digital extensor muscle. This attachment occurs in the region of the proximal phalanx. The suspensory ligament acts as a strong supportive mechanism for the fetlock, discussed below with the stay apparatus.

The proximal sesamoid bones form a critical physical connection between the suspensory ligament and three sets of ***sesamoidean ligaments*** that connect the proximal sesamoid bones with the middle and proximal phalanges. Together, this set of structures provides a relatively inelastic band that supports the fetlock (discussed later in the section on the stay apparatus). The proximal sesamoids are also linked by a broad ligament, the ***palmar* (*plantar*) ligament.** This ligament forms a smooth depression between the sesamoid bones, covered by synovium for frictionless movement of overlying flexor tendons. The proximal sesamoids are further stabilized by **medial** and **lateral collateral sesamoidean ligaments** to the distal end of the cannon bone and proximal end of the proximal phalanx and by two **short sesamoidean ligaments** attaching them to the proximal phalanx.

The sesamoidean ligaments that connect the proximal sesamoids to more distal structures include, from superficial to deep, a **straight sesamoidean ligament,** two **oblique sesamoidean ligaments,** and a pair of **cruciate sesamoidean ligaments** (Fig 14–11). Their names describe their gross appearance; the straight ligament attaches to the middle phalanx and the others, to the proximal phalanx. As a group, these ligaments are often called the distal sesamoidean ligaments, but as this name sounds as though they are associated with the distal sesamoid (navicular) bone, it is probably best avoided.

The distal sesamoid bone (navicular bone) has a number of ligaments associated with it. **Medial** and **lateral collateral ligaments** attach the navicular to the distal phalanx, and an ad-

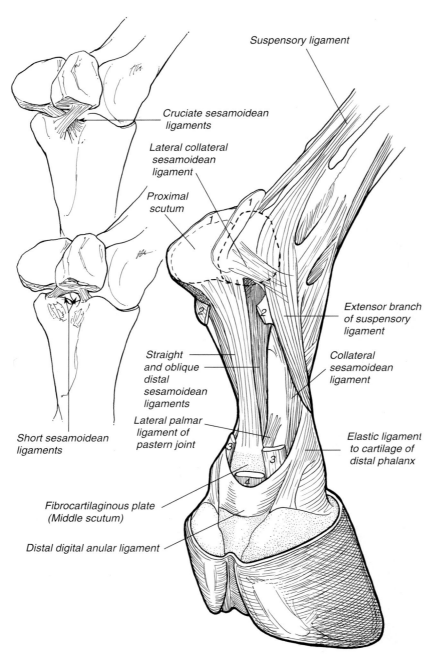

Figure 14-11. Sesamoidean ligaments. Broken lines indicate the positions of the proximal sesamoid bones. Numbers indicate the cut stumps of the (*1*) palmar annular ligament of the fetlock, (2) proximal digital annular ligament, (3) superficial digital flexor tendon, and (4) deep digital flexor tendon. (Reprinted with permission from Stashak T.S. *Adam's Lameness in Horses.* 5th ed. Baltimore: Lippincott Williams & Wilkins, 2002.)

ditional unpaired ligament (***impar ligament***) extends from the distal sesamoid to the solar surface of the distal phalanx. The proximal face of the navicular bone is connected to the middle phalanx and the deep digital flexor tendon by the ***T ligament*** (Fig. 14–2).

The many ligaments and tendons of the equine digit are bound together with a number of encircling annular ligaments. These are reasonably discrete thickenings of the local deep fascia. The ***palmar/plantar annular ligament*** arises from the proximal sesamoids and wraps around the palmar/plantar aspect of the fetlock, where its collagenous fibers blend with the flexor tendon sheath. The ***proximal digital annular ligament*** is more distal, forming a supportive sleeve on the palmar/plantar aspect of the pastern. Finally, the ***distal digital annular ligament*** forms a sling around the deep digital flexor tendon near the insertion of the superficial digital flexor tendon, holding the deep digital flexor tendon close to the pastern (Fig. 14–11).

Synovial Structures

The tendons of the superficial and deep digital flexor muscles share a synovial sheath that has its most proximal extent some 5 to 8 cm above the fetlock and that extends distad to the middle of the middle phalanx. The ***navicular bursa*** lies between the navicular bone and the deep digital flexor tendon. Inflammation of this bursa is one component of ***navicular disease***.

Navicular disease is a common cause of fore-limb lameness in Quarter Horses and Thoroughbreds. A variety of pathologies are described with navicular disease, and not every affected horse shows all of them. These include erosion of the articular cartilages of the navicular bone, bursitis of the navicular bursa, adhesions between the deep digital flexor tendon and navicular bone, and erosions or necrosis of the navicular bone. There is a hereditary component to the disease, probably related to a certain conformational type, often described as a heavy horse on small feet with upright pasterns, which expose the navicular bone and associated struc-tures to excessive concussive forces. Improper trimming of the hoof, so that the toe is left too long and heels overshortened, increases the stress on the deep digital flexor tendon and may aggravate a predisposition to navicular disease.

The structure of the synovial joints between the phalanges and between the cannon and proximal phalanx is typical (see Chapter 6). The joint cavity of the fetlock is especially voluminous to accommodate the wide range of motion in this ginglymus joint. Part of the joint cavity extends proximad between the cannon bone and suspensory ligament. Accumulation of excess synovial fluid within this ***palmar (plantar) recess*** may be associated with the trauma of hard training. This produces a visible distension of the recess called ***wind puffs*** or ***wind galls***.

Function

The primary function of the foot can be summed up in the word ***locomotion***. A highly adapted aid to efficient locomotion, the foot absorbs concussion, stores energy in its elastic tissues, and provides leverage for muscles that insert on the bones within it. A secondary function of the equine foot is standing support. The famous ability of horses to sleep while standing owes itself primarily to the ligamentous structures of the foot and other more proximal parts of the limb.

Concussion and Storage of Energy

A large part of the mechanism for absorbing concussion depends on angulation of the joints of the limbs at the time of impact and immediately following contact of the foot with the ground. The muscles, tendons, and ligaments act as springs that absorb the shock of impact by permitting some flexion of the shoulder and elbow and hyperextension of fetlock, pastern, and coffin joints. Some of the energy of the foot striking the ground is stored as ligamentous and tendinous structures stretch; this energy is released as the foot leaves the ground. The rebound of ligaments and tendons straightens the joints and aids in lifting the foot, so that very little energy is expended on these parts of gait.

The hoof and its contents absorb concussion because of the elasticity of the hoof wall, ungual cartilages, digital cushion, and frog. As the frog strikes the ground, both the digital cushion and the frog are compressed, widening and thinning them. Pressure on the bars, the ungual cartilages, and the wall spreads the heels and forces blood out of the vascular bed of the foot. The direct cushioning effect of the frog and digital cushion is enhanced by the resiliency of the wall and the hydraulic shock-absorbing effect of the blood in the hoof. At the same time the hoof is spread by frog pressure, blood is forced out of the vascular structures of the foot, which not only absorbs concussion but also pumps blood out of the foot and into the veins of the leg against gravity. This pumping action of the foot is an important means of returning venous blood from the foot to the general circulation.

Horses confined to a stall for extended periods are often deprived of the pumping benefits of the active foot, with the result that tissue fluid accumulates in the distal limb. This gives the appearance of swelling, which horsemen call *stocking up*, in the pasterns, fetlocks, and sometimes even more proximal. The swelling, however, is not due to inflammation, is not painful, and very quickly resolves when the horse is encouraged to exercise for a time.

Flexibility of the hoof is also an important consideration in correct shoeing. For most purposes, the shoe should be nailed only as far back as the quarters so that the heels are free to expand over the top of the shoe. For the same reason, most farriers apply shoes that are slightly

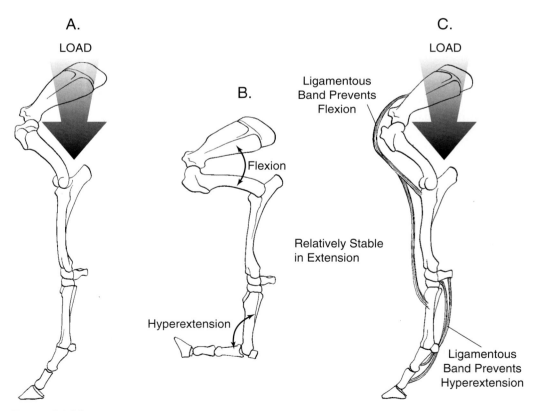

Figure 14-12. When the appendicular skeleton is loaded with weight (*A*), the joints tend to collapse (*B*). The stay apparatus is a series of ligamentous bands that cross the joints and passively prevent this collapse (*C*).

wider in the heel than the foot to which they are affixed. By this means, the expanding heels of the hoof are able to spread and still maintain contact with the shoe.

Stay Apparatus

Ligamentous structures that store and release energy during locomotion are also found proximal to the foot. These elements of the **stay apparatus** are also the elements of the limb that permit the horse to stand with minimal physical effort.

To understand the function of the stay apparatus, it is necessary to keep several concepts central: (1) Ligaments, while elastic, do not stretch nearly as much as muscle. Tendons, because they connect with muscles, offer much less resistance to stretch than do ligaments. (2) When joints are loaded (i.e., bearing weight), they tend to collapse. (3) To keep joints from collapsing with minimal muscular effort, ligamentous straps must be cross the joint to counteract the tendency to fold during weight bearing (Fig 14–12).

Thoracic Limb Stay Apparatus

The thoracic limb is in part affixed to the trunk by the fan-shaped *m. serratus ventralis,* extending from the scapula to the ribs. This muscle is characterized by a thick, tendinous layer that is capable of supporting the trunk without contraction of the muscle fibers. The weight of the trunk is thereby supported effortlessly by a slinglike structure composed of right and left *mm. serrati ventrales* (see Fig. 7–7); by this construct, much of the weight of the horse is transferred to the thoracic limbs.

When bearing weight, the shoulder joint tends to flex, and the fetlock, pastern, and coffin joints tend to hyperextend, while the carpus and elbow are relatively stable when loaded in the extended position. Components of the stay apparatus cross all of these joints, counteracting their tendency to collapse under load (Fig. 14–13).

The extensor surface of the shoulder is crossed by the tendon of origin of the *m. biceps brachii,* a very broad, partly cartilaginous tendon that is continuous with a very dense fibrous

band running through the length of the muscle belly. This fibrous band is continuous with the tendons of insertion, including the lacertus fibrosis, a substantial band that blends into the deep fascia of the *m. extensor carpi radialis.* This feature of the *m. biceps brachii* creates a continuous ligamentous connection from the scapula through the length of the brachium, across the elbow, and to the proximal metacarpus via its connection with the tendon of the *m. extensor carpi radialis.* It is this band of connective tissue that will, without muscular effort, counteract flexion of the shoulder when the limb is bearing weight. This same continuous band, through its connection with the *m. extensor carpi radialis,* contributes further to the stability of the carpus in extension.

The elbow is surprisingly stable when fully extended and loaded. The *m. triceps brachii,* the primary extensor of the elbow, probably contributes to this stability by maintaining a slight amount of tone, even when the horse is dozing on his feet.

The rest of the stay apparatus is primarily concerned with holding the fetlock and to a lesser extent pastern and coffin joint in a physiologic position. Without a ligamentous check on the palmar aspect of these joints, the fetlock would drop to the ground and the toe would point upward, with the sole off the ground when the limb was loaded.

The primary support of the fetlock and pastern joints comprises the suspensory ligament, the proximal sesamoid bones, and the ligaments of the proximal sesamoid bones. Recall that these structures form a continuous ligamentous connection between the palmar aspect of the carpus or proximal metacarpus distal to the proximal and middle phalanges.

The tendons of both digital flexor muscles offer additional support to the fetlock and pastern joints, and the tendon of the deep digital flexor muscle resists hyperextension of the coffin joint. Remember, though, that muscle tends to stretch easily. These digital flexors can support the distal joints without muscular effort because they both feature accessory ligaments, ligamentous connections between more proximal bones and the insertions of the tendons.

The superficial digital flexor muscle possesses a ligamentous head that attaches to the

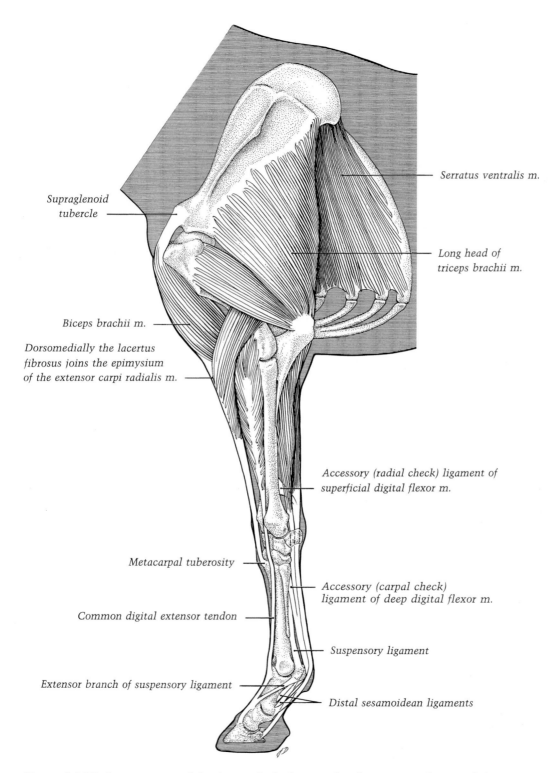

Figure 14-13. Stay apparatus of the thoracic limb. (Reprinted with permission from Stashak T.S. *Adam's Lameness in Horses.* 5th ed. Baltimore: Lippincott Williams & Wilkins, 2002.)

caudal aspect of the distal radius and joins the muscle's tendon near the carpus. This ***accessory ligament of the superficial digital flexor muscle*** is commonly known as the **radial** or **proximal check ligament,** and its presence creates a continuous, ligamentous band from the radius to the insertion of the tendon on the proximal and middle phalanges. This provides additional support to fetlock and pastern.

The deep digital flexor muscle also features an accessory ligament, this one attaching to the caudal part of the carpal joint capsule and blending with the muscle's tendon just distal to the carpus. This ***accessory ligament of the deep digital flexor muscle*** is more commonly called the **carpal** or **distal check ligament.** It creates a continuous ligamentous band that extends from the carpus to the distal phalanx, supporting all of the joints in the digit.

Injury to the flexor tendons produces some dropping of the fetlock as some of the resistance to hyperextension is lost. If injury includes the deep digital flexor tendon, the toe is likely to come off the ground, as this tendon is the only one resisting hyperextension of the coffin joint. The most devastating injuries, however, involve the suspensory ligament and/or the proximal sesamoid bones. Fractures of the proximal sesamoids are the most common of all fractures in the forelimb. If the fractures are complete (transverse fractures of both sesamoids), or if the suspensory ligament is transected, the ligament loses its connections to the phalanges, and the fetlock will drop to the ground. Such an injury is often irreparable and may necessitate destruction of the horse.

Pelvic Limb Stay Apparatus & Reciprocal Apparatus

Distal to the tarsus, the stay apparatus in the pelvic limb is more or less identical to that of the thoracic limb (Fig. 14–14). The ***accessory ligament of the deep digital flexor muscle*** (***tarsal check ligament***) arises from the plantar aspect of the tarsus and proximal metatarsus; this accessory ligament is rather long and very slender and may even be absent in some individuals. The superficial digital flexor muscle of the pelvic limb is nearly entirely tendinous and

therefore needs no accessory ligament to create a continuous band from origin (caudal distal femur) to insertion on proximal and middle phalanges. Furthermore, the tendon of the superficial digital flexor muscle inserts on the tuber calcanei, providing, in effect, a check ligament at this point.

For the pelvic limb to support weight without collapsing, the stifle and hock must be prevented from flexing. This is accomplished by one mechanism to lock the stifle in extension and a second mechanism (the ***reciprocal apparatus***) that guarantees that the hock will always flex and extend in unison with the stifle. The reciprocal apparatus provides that as long as the stifle is locked in extension, the hock will be likewise.

Recall that the equine patella features a hook-shaped medial parapatellar cartilage and three patellar tendons that insert on the tibial tuberosity (Fig. 6–6). During movement, the patella glides up and down the femoral trochlea as the quadriceps muscle contracts and relaxes, respectively. When the horse stands at rest, however, the patella is drawn proximad so that the parapatellar cartilage and medial patellar tendon are hooked over the large medial ridge of the trochlea. In this position, the stifle is held in extension without muscular effort. Typically, the horse activates this mechanism in one pelvic limb, resting the other with the toe on the ground; horsemen sometimes refer to this posture as standing hip-shot.

The hock and stifle normally flex and extend in unison because of the reciprocal apparatus, a combination of ligamentous structures connecting the femur with the tarsus and metatarsus (Fig. 14–15). On the cranial aspect of the crus, the ***peroneus tertius,*** an entirely ligamentous structure, extends from the region of the lateral femoral condyle to insertions on the tarsus and proximal metatarsus. In doing so, it forms a relatively unstretchable band across the extensor surface of the stifle and the flexor surface of the tarsus. On the caudal aspect of the crus, the superficial digital flexor muscle, which is also entirely tendinous, arises from the distocaudal femur and inserts on the calcaneus and digit. This forms a ligamentous connection that crosses the flexor surface of the stifle and extensor surface of the tarsus. As shown in Figure

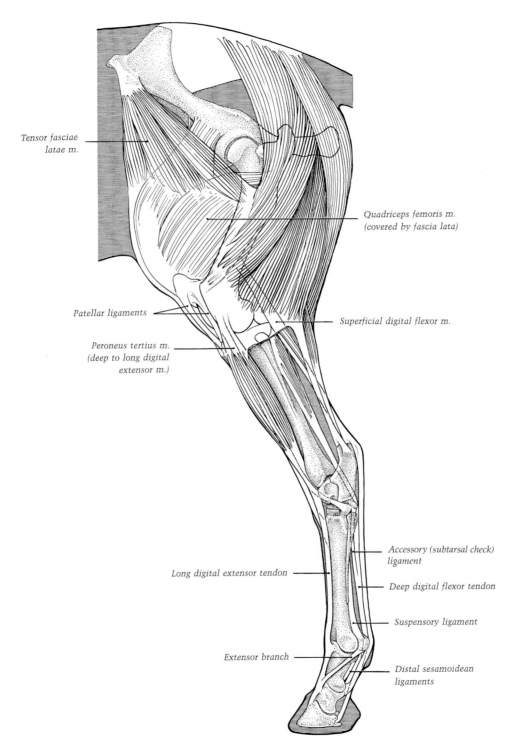

Tensor fasciae
latae m.

Quadriceps femoris m.
(covered by fascia lata)

Patellar ligaments

Superficial digital flexor m.

Peroneus tertius m.
(deep to long digital
extensor m.)

Accessory (subtarsal check)
ligament

Long digital extensor tendon

Deep digital flexor tendon

Suspensory ligament

Extensor branch

Distal sesamoidean
ligaments

Figure 14-14. Stay apparatus of the pelvic limb. (Reprinted with permission from Stashak T.S. *Adam's Lameness in Horses.* 5th ed. Baltimore: Lippincott Williams & Wilkins, 2002.)

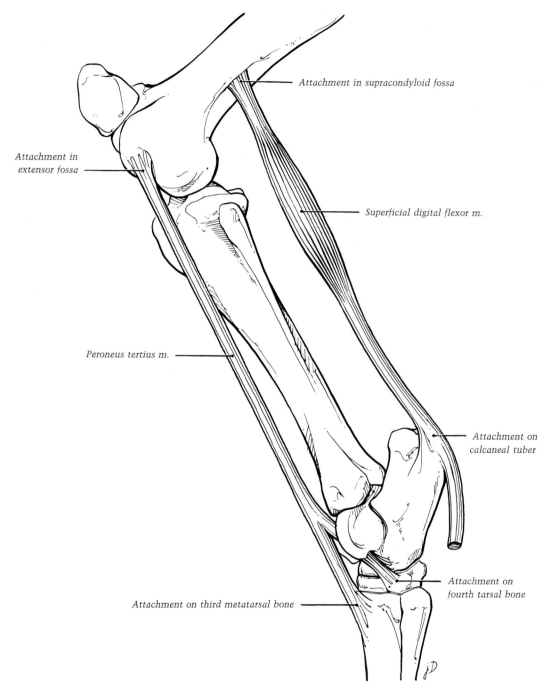

Attachment in supracondyloid fossa

Attachment in extensor fossa

Superficial digital flexor m.

Peroneus tertius m.

Attachment on calcaneal tuber

Attachment on fourth tarsal bone

Attachment on third metatarsal bone

Figure 14-15. Reciprocal apparatus. (Reprinted with permission from Stashak T.S. Adam's Lameness in Horses. 5th ed. Baltimore: Williams & Wilkins, 2002.)

14–16, these elements create a parallelogram of ligaments, wherein the change in angle in the stifle is accompanied by a similar change in the tarsus.

In *upward fixation of the patella,* the patella locks above the medial ridge of the femoral trochlea at inappropriate times. The condition may be due to conformational abnormalities or a neuromuscular disorder. The affected animal exhibits a sudden extension of stifle (and hock) that may be intermittent or persistent. Treatment entails transection of the medial patellar ligament, which prevents the patella from becoming fixed over the ridge.

Can horses sleep standing up? Yes and no. Sleep is divided into five stages, numbered I through V, distinguished on the basis of neural and skeletal muscle activity. Stages I through IV are a continuum of increasing depth of sleep, with I and II indicating light sleep (drowsing) and III and IV indicating deep sleep. Stage V is what is described in humans as REM (rapid eye movement) sleep. This is the part of sleep most usually associated with dreaming. One of the defining characteristics of REM sleep is that other than eye and respiratory muscles, all skeletal muscles are in a state of flaccid paralysis. Horses are awake about 19 hours of a day and spend about 2 hours each in light and slow-wave sleep, during which they can stand with only the most minimal of muscle tone, thanks to the stay apparatus. Horses normally have REM sleep for only about an hour a day, but because REM sleep is associated with paralysis of voluntary muscles, horses must lie down during that time.

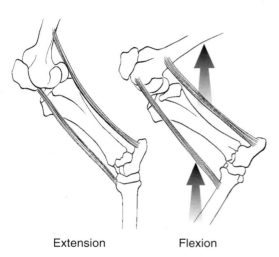

Extension   Flexion

Figure 14-16. The change in the angle in the stifle is accompanied by a similar change in the hock.

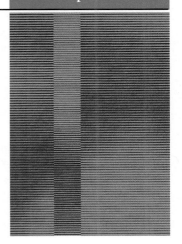

BLOOD AND OTHER BODY FLUIDS

Single-celled organisms that live in seawater have an external environment that provides all of the needs of the organisms, such as food, disposal of excreted wastes, and relatively constant conditions for maintenance of life. As the complexity of organisms increases, the problem of supplying each cell with a proper environment becomes more acute. Higher forms of animals have developed circulating blood, and the fluids derived from it, as a means of maintaining a relatively constant environment for all cells.

Blood

Most of the functions of blood are included in the following list:

1. Distribution of nutrients absorbed from the digestive tract
2. Transport of oxygen from the lungs to cells throughout the body
3. Transport of carbon dioxide from metabolizing cells to the lungs
4. Transport of waste products from metabolizing cells to the kidneys for excretion
5. Transport of hormones from endocrine glands to target cells
6. Assist in body temperature control by transporting heat from deeper structures to the surface of the body
7. Assist in maintaining a constant pH of body fluids by providing chemical buffers

8. Assist with the prevention of excessive loss of blood from injuries by providing proteins and other factors necessary for blood coagulation
9. Assist with the defense of the body against disease by providing antibodies, cells, and other factors of body defense (see Chapter 16)

Blood consists of cells and other cell-like formed elements suspended in a fluid called *plasma.* Some of its functions are specific to individual cells; for example, erythrocytes are primarily responsible for the transport of oxygen. Other functions, such as assisting with body defense, involve a variety of blood cells and other plasma components. **Blood volume** is the total amount of blood in an animal's body, including formed elements and plasma. Typical values given as a percentage of body weight are 7–9%. Lean, muscular, athletic animals tend to have higher percentages than animals with more body fat. (Specific gravity is an index, or ratio, of the weight of a substance to the weight of an equal volume of water. A specific gravity greater than 1 means that an equal volume of the substance weighs more than water, at 1 g/mL. Blood and plasma have slightly higher specific gravities than water, primarily because of the blood cells and proteins, but the slight difference is usually disregarded when estimating blood or plasma volumes based on body weight.)

A large number of *plasma proteins* are suspended in the plasma, and electrolytes (e.g., Na^+, K^+, and Cl^-) and other substances (e.g., glucose and urea) are dissolved in the plasma. While there are some minor species differences (e.g., adult ruminants typically have slightly lower values for blood glucose than other mammals), the values in Table 15–1 are typical normal ranges for the major chemical constituents of mammalian plasma.

Plasma is a subdivision of a larger body fluid compartment known as *extracellular fluid,* or *ECF* (see Chapter 2). *Interstitial fluid,* fluid outside of cells but not within vessels, is the other subdivision of the ECF compartment. The primary difference between interstitial fluid and plasma is that plasma contains a much higher concentration of proteins that cannot easily diffuse through the walls of capillaries.

Formed Elements of Blood and Hematopoiesis

The formed elements of the blood include *erythrocytes* (red blood cells), *leukocytes* (white blood cells), and *platelets.* Because erythrocytes and platelets both lack nuclei, they are not typical cells (see Plate II).

Hematopoiesis is the formation and development of all formed elements of blood (erythrocytes, leukocytes, and platelets), and all of these have a common ancestor, *pluripotent stem cells* (see Chapter 3 and Fig. 15–1). Pluripotent stem cells can replicate to provide more pluripotent stem cells or give rise to more differentiated

Table 15-1. Representative Values for Selected Constituents of Typical Mammalian Plasma

Constituents	Units of Measurement	Typical Range
Sodium	mEq/L	135–155
Potassium	mEq/L	3.0–5.5
Chloride	mEq/L	95–110
Bicarbonate	mEq/L	22–26
Total protein	g/dL	6–8
Albumin	g/dL	3–4
Blood urea nitrogen	mg/dL	10–25
Creatinine	mg/dL	1.0–1.5
Glucose	mg/dL	70–100

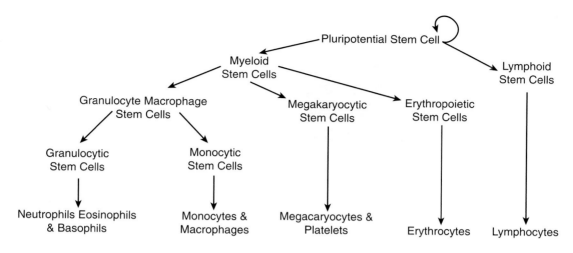

Figure 15-1. Summarized pathways to illustrate origin of blood cells and platelets.

stem cells that are committed to develop along one of two specific paths, **myeloid** and **lymphoid.** Figure 15–1 is an abbreviated family tree for blood cells and platelets, with the mature cells and platelets listed at the bottom of the maturation pathways. It is abbreviated in that several immature forms between the stem cells and the mature forms have been omitted. In theory, with enough time for an adequate number of cell divisions, a single pluripotent stem cell could repopulate a depleted bone marrow with additional pluripotent stem cells and give rise to mature erythrocytes, leukocytes, and platelets.

During early experimental studies on hematopoiesis, individual immature cells were isolated from bone marrow and maintained in cell culture. These studies demonstrated that in the right conditions, certain individual cells would form in vitro colonies that contained immature and mature cells of a specific cell line. The most undifferentiated cells that could form the cells of a specific lineage were termed **colony-forming units** (CFUs). More current literature uses the stem cell terminology, but for example, a myeloid stem cell is equivalent to a colony-forming unit—granulocytic, erythrocytic, monocytic, and megakaryocytic (CFU-GEMM).

Obviously, the proliferation and differentiation of bone marrow stem cells must be highly regulated. For example, the generation of eryth-

rocytes should increase in response to blood loss after hemorrhage, while the generation of leukocytes should increase in response to an infection. A large variety of circulating chemical messengers have been found to regulate the proliferation and differentiation of bone marrow stem cells. The general term for such agents is **hematopoietin.** An individual hematopoietin may stimulate committed cells within development pathways to give rise to specific blood cells or may have a more general effect by stimulating less committed stem cells. For example, **erythropoietin** is the hematopoietin that stimulates a specific increase in erythrocyte production, and **interleukin-2** stimulates increases in the production of several leukocytes. More information on individual hematopoietins is provided in later sections of this chapter and in Chapter 16. Based on the CFU terminology, hematopoietins have also been described as **colony-stimulating factors.**

Erythrocytes

Erythrocytes (Gr. *erythro-,* red; *-cyte,* cell) range from about 5 to 7μm in diameter. They are biconcave disks with a thick circular margin and a thin center (Fig. 15.2). The biconcave shape provides a relatively large surface area for gas exchange across the cell membrane. Eryth-

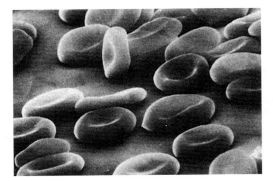

Figure 15-2. Red blood cells as seen by scanning electron microscopy. (Reprinted with permission from Cohen B.J. and Wood D.L. *Memmler's The Human Body in Health and Disease.* 9th ed. Philadelphia: Lippincott Williams & Wilkins, 2000.)

rocytes have no nuclei and few organelles. Total erythrocyte counts are expressed as number of cells per microliter of whole blood, and most domestic animals have about 7 million per microliter (Table 15–2). (Total leukocyte and platelet counts are also expressed per microliter of blood.)

The protein **hemoglobin** is the major intracellular constituent of erythrocytes. Hemoglobin is a complex molecule containing four amino acid chains (**globin portion**) held together by noncovalent interactions. Each amino acid chain contains a **heme** group (red porphyrin pigment), and each heme group contains an atom

of iron. Hemoglobin concentration is measured in grams per 100 mL of blood, and typical values for normal hemoglobin concentrations range from about 11 to 13 g/100 mL in domestic mammals.

Hemoglobin functions in the transport of both **oxygen** and **carbon dioxide.** Oxygen binds to the ferrous iron in the heme group to form **oxyhemoglobin** (HbO_2); this process is termed **oxygenation** (not oxidation). The amount of oxygen that can be bound is proportional to the amount of iron present, with one molecule of oxygen combining with each atom of iron. Because of the binding to hemoglobin, blood can contain about 60 times as much oxygen as would be dissolved in a similar quantity of water in the same conditions. Carbon dioxide also binds to hemoglobin at a different site on the molecule. Carbon dioxide binds to α-amino groups of peptide chains to form **carbaminohemoglobin.**

Binding of oxygen and carbon dioxide to hemoglobin is readily reversible. Blood arriving at the lungs from the peripheral circulation contains carbaminohemoglobin and is exposed to air with a relatively high concentration of oxygen and a relatively low concentration of carbon dioxide. In the lungs, carbon dioxide dissociates from carbaminohemoglobin, resulting in the formation of hemoglobin, which can bind oxygen to become oxyhemoglobin. When the blood containing oxyhemoglobin returns to the peripheral tissues that are relatively deficient in oxygen, the bound oxygen is released

Blood Element	Horse	Cow	Dog	Chicken
			Table 15-2. Representative Values for Blood Cell and Platelet Numbers per Microliter of Blood in Selected Domestic Animals		
Erythrocytes	8–11[a]	6–8[a]	6–8[a]	2.5–3[a]
Total leukocytes	8–11[b]	7–10[b]	9–12.5[b]	20–30[b]
Neutrophils	4–7[b]	2–3.5[b]	6–8.5[b]	5–10[b]
Lymphocytes	2.5–4[b]	4.5–6.5[b]	2–3.5[b]	11–18[b]
Monocytes	400–500	350–500	450–600	2–3[b]
Eosinophils	200–500	150–500	200–500	600–2,000
Basophils	<100	<100	<100	200–900
Platelets	150–450[b]	300–500[b]	300–500[b]	25–40[b]

[a]Millions
[b]Thousands

to the tissues. Carbon dioxide can then bind to hemoglobin to continue the cycle.

Methemoglobin is a true oxidation product of hemoglobin that is unable to transport oxygen because the iron is in the ferric (Fe^{3+}) rather than the ferrous (Fe^{2+}) state. Certain chemicals, such as nitrites and chlorates, produce methemoglobinemia (methemoglobin in the blood). **Nitrate poisoning** has been reported in cattle grazing on highly fertilized plant growth. In these cases, nitrates in the plants are converted to nitrites in the rumen and cause the formation of methemoglobin when absorbed into the blood.

Carboxyhemoglobin is a more stable compound formed when carbon monoxide combines with hemoglobin. The affinity of hemoglobin for carbon monoxide is 210 times that of its affinity for O_2. The carboxyhemoglobin is unable to carry oxygen, and the animal essentially suffocates, although the blood is typically cherry red.

Erythropoiesis and Degradation of Erythrocytes.
Erythrocyte formation, called **erythropoiesis,** is regulated by the hormone **erythropoietin,** a glycoprotein hormone that is released from specific cells of the kidneys in response to reduced oxygen delivery. For example, when animals move from low altitudes to high altitudes, where less oxygen is available, erythropoietin release is increased. Erythropoietin acts on stem cells in the bone marrow to increase the production of erythrocytes. The increase in erythrocyte number is not immediate (requires some days) because mature erythrocytes must be formed from stimulated stem cells before release from the bone marrow. The larger number of erythrocytes increases oxygen delivery to the kidneys, and this has a negative feedback effect on erythropoietin release. It is via this feedback that a stable rate of erythrocyte production is maintained.

Recombinant human erythropoietin (rhEPO) has been used in appropriate clinical cases to stimulate erythrocyte production in both humans and animals. However, an antibody response to the human molecule occurs in more than 25% of animals, and these antibodies neutralize endogenous erythropoietin as well as the rhEPO. The inappropriate use of rhEPO has been reported in normal human athletes in an attempt to increase their exercise capacity. The potential for abusive use in animal athletes also exists.

Mature erythrocytes of mammals have no nuclei. Immature forms in the bone marrow do have nuclei, but these are lost during the latter stages of development. The appearance of large numbers of nucleated erythrocytes in the circulation is an indication that immature forms are being inappropriately released from the bone marrow. In birds and reptiles, nuclei normally persist in the red cells throughout the life of the cells.

Typically, erythrocytes circulate for only 3 to 4 months after their release from the bone marrow. The removal and recycling of senescent erythrocytes is one function of a group of specialized cells, the **monocyte–macrophage system** (formally known as the reticuloendothelial system). The macrophages of this system are found fixed or in residence in several sites throughout the body but are especially prevalent in the spleen and liver. These macrophages are derived from circulating monocytes; hence the name of the system. The macrophages phagocytize intact erythrocytes or cellular debris and hemoglobin that are released when erythrocytes disintegrate in the blood. The macrophages degrade the globin portion of hemoglobin and release the resulting amino acids into the circulation. Iron is removed from the heme portion and released into the blood, where it is transported in combination with a protein, **transferrin.** Cells that require iron have cell membrane receptors that bind transferrin, and this is the means by which cells can take up iron from the circulation. This includes hematopoietic cells in the bone marrow, which have the highest metabolic need for iron on a daily basis. Iron from the circulation also accumulates in the liver in a retrievable storage form, **ferritin.**

After the protein and iron are removed from hemoglobin, a green pigment, **biliverdin,** remains. This is reduced to **bilirubin** (a yellowish pigment), which is transported to the liver in combination with blood albumin. The liver conjugates it; then it passes to the gallbladder in the bile and finally to the intestine, where most of it is reduced to **bilinogens.** These are either excreted in the feces (giving the brown color to feces), or reabsorbed into the blood and then excreted in the urine as **urobilinogen.** The reduction in the intestine is accomplished by resident microorganisms.

Clinical Conditions and Procedures Involving Erythrocytes. *Icterus (jaundice)* is a syndrome characterized by a yellowish discoloration of skin, mucous membranes, and/or sclera. It results from accumulation of bilirubin in the blood and may be caused by liver damage, by occlusion of the bile ducts, or by an increased rate of erythrocyte destruction. In case of either liver damage or blockage of the bile ducts, the bile pigments are not secreted into the intestine but are resorbed into the circulatory system, causing icterus. When blood damage is excessive, as in some parasitic blood diseases, such as **anaplasmosis,** the bile pigments are liberated into the blood faster than the liver can conjugate and secrete them, and icterus results.

Hemolysis is the breakdown of erythrocytes and the release of hemoglobin. Bacterial toxins, snake venoms, blood parasites, and hypotonic solutions can cause so much hemolysis that the hemoglobin in plasma produces a reddish color, and the condition is called **hemoglobinemia.** The hemoglobin can then be excreted in the urine, and this is termed **hemoglobinuria (red water).** Hemolysis can also be produced in a blood sample by physically disrupting the erythrocytes (e.g., forceful and rapid expulsion of blood from a syringe).

Hemagglutination is clumping of erythrocytes. Erythrocytes have membrane proteins that act as antigens, and agglutination results if erythrocytes with specific antigens are added to a solution containing appropriate antibodies. **Blood typing** is a general term describing the procedures used to identify the antigen or antigens in a given blood sample. Clumping may occur during transfusions of blood within the same species, such as between humans, if blood of the wrong type (i.e., containing the wrong combination of antigens) is used. At least seven blood types have been identified in horses, and

it is desirable to ensure that there is adequate matching of types before attempting transfusions between horses. Blood typing has also been done in cattle and dogs, but usually a single transfusion can be done between two cattle or between two dogs with little difficulty. However, repeated transfusions can be problematic, because the initial transfusion may provide unmatched antigens that stimulate the formation of antibodies. Blood types are inherited in all species, and they are often used to establish and monitor pedigrees.

Anemia (Gr. *an-,* without; *-emia,* blood) results if either the number of functional erythrocytes or the quantity of hemoglobin per unit of blood is below normal. Anemia may be due to deficient blood formation, as with diseases of the bone marrow, kidney disease with inadequate production of erythropoietin, or poor nutrition, including dietary deficiency of iron, copper, vitamins, or amino acids. Anemia may also be caused by accelerated loss or destruction of erythrocytes, such as with hemorrhage or parasites.

The **hematocrit** (packed cell volume) is the percentage by volume of whole blood that is erythrocytes. Routine hematocrit determinations require a glass tube treated to inhibit blood clotting (hematocrit tubes). Hematocrit tubes containing blood are centrifuged until the blood cells are packed in the lower end (Fig. 15–3). Hematocrits typically range from 35 to 45 for most mammalian species and are generally considered to be an indicator of the total erythrocyte count.

Hemoconcentration is a decrease in the fluid component of blood with a resulting increase in the ratio of cells to fluid. It is indicated by an excessively high erythrocyte count (**polycythemia**) or a high hematocrit. Reductions in plasma volume may result from inadequate water intake or excessive loss of fluids from the body, such as with vomiting or diarrhea.

Platelets

Blood **platelets,** also called **thrombocytes,** are fragments of **megakaryocytes,** large cells formed and residing in the bone marrow. Thrombocytes are the smallest of the formed elements in the blood at 2 to 4 μm. They are surrounded by a

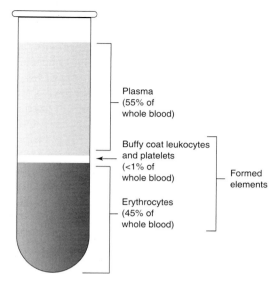

Figure 15-3. Layering of blood components in an anticoagulated and centrifuged blood sample. (Reprinted with permission from Porth, C.M. *Pathophysiology.* 5th ed. Philadelphia, Lippincott, 1998.)

plasma membrane and contain some organelles but not nuclei. Thrombocytes range from 150,000 to 500,000 per microliter of blood in most mammalian species (Table 15–2). The appearance of platelets in a stained smear may be considerably different from their actual appearance in circulating blood, where they are oval disks. In smears they may appear as circular disks, star-shaped fragments, or clumps of irregular shape.

Platelets reduce loss of blood from injured vessels. By adhering to vessel walls and to each other in the area of the injury, platelets may form a plug upon which a *thrombus* (clot) forms to occlude the opening in the vessel and prevent further blood loss. Substances released by platelets and lodged on their surface membranes stimulate clotting and help cause local constriction of the injured blood vessel (described in more detail later in this chapter).

Leukocytes

Leukocytes or white blood cells (Gr. *leuco,* white) differ considerably from erythrocytes in that they are nucleated and are capable of in-

dependent movement to exit blood vessels (see Plate II,[a]). Leukocytes may be classified as either *granulocytes* or *agranulocytes* based on the presence or absence of cytoplasmic granules that stain with common blood stains, such as Wright's stain. These stains contain an acid dye, eosin, which is red, and a basic dye, methylene blue, which is bluish. Granulocytes are named according to the color of the stained granules (i.e., *neutrophils,* which have granules that stain indifferently; *eosinophils;* and *basophils*). The nuclei of granulocytes appear in many shapes and forms, leading to the name *polymorphonuclear leukocytes* (Gr. *poly,* many; *morpho,* form). However, the term is commonly used to indicate neutrophils, because they are normally the most prevalent granulocyte. Monocytes and lymphocytes are the two types of agranulocytes.

Neutrophils. Neutrophils, a first line of defense against infection, constitute a large percentage of the total leukocyte number (Table 15–2). Upon tissue injury or microbial invasion, neutrophils rapidly accumulate within the interstitial fluids of the injured or invaded area. The active movement of neutrophils and other leukocytes out of intact blood vessels and into the interstitial fluid is *diapedesis.* Chemical messengers known as *chemotactic factors* attract neutrophils to these sites. *Chemotactic factor* is a general term for a variety of compounds that are capable of attracting neutrophils and in some cases other leukocytes. These factors may be produced by invading microorganisms, by leukocytes after interacting with microorganisms, or by damaged tissue.

Neutrophils are phagocytes; they engulf invading bacteria to destroy them. The destruction involves the action of enzymes in the intracellular granules of the neutrophils and cell membrane–bound enzymes that are activated when phagocytic vesicles are completely formed. During phagocytosis neutrophils may also release enzymes that contribute to the local inflammation. In the process of responding to the potential infection, many of the attracted neutrophils are destroyed. **Pus,** the semiliquid material that results from the collective responses to a microbial invasion, may contain neutrophils and cellular debris. An *abscess* is an accumulation of pus that has been isolated by the formation of surrounding connective tissue.

Neutrophilia is an increase in the number of circulating neutrophils in the blood that occurs with bacterial infections. Circulating neutrophils can increase as a result of an immediate release of existing neutrophils from the bone marrow and an increase in neutrophil production. **Neutropenia** refers to an abnormally low number of circulating neutrophils. The word endings -*philia* and -*penia* can be combined with the root names of the other leukocytes to indicate similar conditions (e.g., eosinophilia is an increase in eosinophils).

Eosinophils. *Eosinophils* contain red-staining cytoplasmic granules. Normally eosinophils are less than 10% of total leukocytes (Table 15–2), but they may increase in number with allergic conditions and parasitism. Eosinophils are ameboid and somewhat phagocytic. Their primary function seems to be the regulation of allergic responses and tissue responses to parasites. They act by removing antigen–antibody complexes, which stimulate allergic responses, and by inhibiting some of the mediators of allergic responses, such as **histamine.**

Basophils. *Basophils* contain blue-staining granules and are rarely seen in normal blood. The granules of basophils contain multiple compounds including **heparin,** which prevents blood clotting, and **histamine,** which relaxes smooth muscle of blood vessels and constricts smooth muscle in airways. Cells that are very similar but distinct, **mast cells,** are found in many sites throughout the body but are especially prevalent in connective tissue below an epithelial lining exposed to the external environment (e.g., dermis, wall of airways, and wall of gastrointestinal tract). Basophils and mast cells release the contents of their granules during allergic responses, and these chemicals contribute to the characteristic tissue responses. The release of the granules is mediated in part by the binding of specific antibodies and the associated allergen (antigen).

Monocytes. *Monocytes* are the largest of the circulating leukocytes. They are phagocytic and develop into even larger **macrophages** when they exit vessels and enter the tissues. Like neutrophils, monocytes are attracted by chemotactic factors to areas of tissue injury and microbial invasion. In addition to phagocytosis of tissue debris and microbes, macrophages have a major role in the overall initiation and regulation of inflammatory and immune responses. During their response to tissue injury or microbial invasion, macrophages release numerous chemical messengers that coordinate the function of other cells responding to injury or invasion. Macrophages also function in the processing of antigens, a necessary step in the initiation of an immune response. These functions are discussed in more detail in Chapter 16.

Lymphocytes. In most species, **lymphocytes** are the second most prevalent circulating leukocyte after neutrophils, but they are more prevalent than neutrophils in ruminants (Table 15–2). Based on their functions, three general types or groups of lymphocytes have been identified (B lymphocytes, T lymphocytes, and NK, or natural killer cells), but these types cannot be identified by differences in appearance. In blood smears, lymphocytes vary in size, with a relatively large nucleus surrounded by a small amount of cytoplasm (Plate II, Chapter 1). Lymphocytes function in specific immune responses and immune surveillance, and these functions are discussed in Chapter 16.

Differential White Blood Cell Counts. Differential counts indicate the percentage of each type of white cell in the blood sample (Table 15–2). The various types of leukocytes have different functions and respond differently to various types of infections or diseases, so differential counts can be useful for diagnosis. Differential counts taken over time can also be used to evaluate the response of an animal to infection or disease. A differential count is made by spreading a drop of whole blood thinly on a glass slide to form a blood smear. The smear is dried and stained with a blood stain, such as Wright's stain. After staining is complete, the slide is examined with a microscope and the number of white cells of each kind is tabulated until a predetermined total number of white cells has been counted. The number counted is usually a multiple of 100, and the percentage of each leukocyte type observed in a given sample of blood is called the differential leukocyte count or differential white cell count. In reference laboratories, both total red and white cell counts are semiautomatically determined by sophisticated laboratory equipment.

Plasma and Serum

When a sample of blood is treated with an ***anticoagulant*** to prevent clotting and permitted to stand in a tube undisturbed, the cells gradually settle to the bottom, leaving a straw-colored fluid above. This fluid portion of the blood is plasma. When blood is allowed to clot, the cells are trapped in a meshwork of clotting proteins, leaving a yellow fluid, the ***serum.*** Essentially, serum is plasma minus the plasma proteins responsible for producing the clot.

Plasma is about 92% water and 8% other substances. The kidneys are responsible for maintaining constant proportions of water and other constituents of the plasma by the selective filtration and resorption of water and other substances from the blood plasma. The total osmolality of plasma at normal body temperature is about 290 mOsm/kg. Osmolality is a measure of the number of osmotically active particles (not the mass of the particles) per unit of solute. The two predominant particles in plasma are sodium and chloride ions (Table 15–1), and these contribute the most to the total osmolality of plasma or serum.

The plasma proteins consist of two major types: ***albumin*** and ***globulins.*** Albumin is the most prevalent plasma protein and is the predominant protein synthesized by the liver. Many small compounds and electrolytes (e.g., calcium ions) bind to albumin and circulate in plasma in this bound form. This prevents their rapid loss in the urine. Because albumin and other large proteins do not readily pass through capillary walls, they also provide an effective osmotic force to prevent excessive fluid loss from capillaries into the interstitium.

The globulins in serum or plasma may be classified according to their migration (separation) by electrophoresis. ***α-Globulins*** and ***β-globulins*** are classes that are synthesized in the

liver. Members of these classes have a variety of functions, including transport in a manner similar to albumin, body defense (see Chapter 16), and blood clotting. Many of the globulin proteins are inactive precursors of enzymes or substrates for enzymes involved in blood clotting (discussed later in this chapter).

The ***γ-globulins*** are synthesized by cells of the immune system. Most of the known circulating antibodies are included in the γ-globulin fraction. The γ-globulin content of the blood therefore increases following vaccination and during recovery from disease. ***Immune serum*** or ***hyperimmune serum*** can be produced by repeatedly inoculating an animal with a specific antigen. Serum from that animal can then be injected into an animal susceptible to the same disease to provide passive protection for as long as the antibodies remain in the susceptible animal. This provides merely temporary immunity.

Blood pH

A typical pH range for blood is 7.35 to 7.45, just slightly on the alkaline side of neutral. The pH of blood is kept within rather narrow limits by a variety of mechanisms that include contributions by the kidneys (see Chapter 23) and the respiratory system (see Chapter 19). Several chemical buffer systems in the plasma also contribute to the control of blood pH. The most important of these is the bicarbonate buffer system, and the bicarbonate ion is the base in this system. The bicarbonate ion is the second most prevalent anion in plasma (Table 15–1). In acidosis or acidemia the blood pH is abnormally low, and in alkalosis or alkalemia the pH is abnormally high.

Hemostasis and Coagulation

Hemostasis, the stoppage of bleeding, may involve three basic reactions: (1) constriction by the smooth muscle of the injured vessel to reduce the opening, (2) formation of a platelet plug to occlude the opening, and (3) clot formation to complete occlusion of the opening. Injuries to vessels do not require the formation of a clot (***coagulation***) if hemostasis can be achieved by the first two reactions.

Platelets and the Endothelium

When a vessel is injured and the endothelial cell lining is damaged so that the underlying connective tissue is exposed, platelets adhere to collagen and other proteins in the connective tissue. This **platelet adhesion** results from binding between platelet cell membrane proteins and the connective tissue. The cell membrane of adhered platelets undergoes alterations, and secretory granules are also released. These two events stimulate other platelets to adhere to those already present. The collection of platelets forms a **platelet plug** that may be sufficient (together with local vasoconstriction) to occlude extremely small openings in damaged vessels and bring about hemostasis. **Platelet aggregation** is the term applied to the overall sequence of events responsible for the formation of the platelet plug.

Platelet aggregation is also subject to regulation by two different eicosanoids, **thromboxane A$_2$** (TXA$_2$) and **prostacyclin** (PGI$_2$). TXA$_2$ is a stimulant of platelet aggregation, while prostacyclin inhibits platelet aggregation. The primary source of TXA$_2$ in the area of a damaged vessel is adhered platelets that increase their synthesis of TXA$_2$ after adhesion. The primary source of prostacyclin is intact, undamaged endothelial cells. As the platelet plug grows and extends to areas where endothelial cells remain intact, the local concentration of prostacyclin generated by undamaged endothelial cells acts to stop the growth of the platelet plug. TXA$_2$ and **serotonin** (also released by adhered platelets) are both vasoconstrictors, stimulating smooth muscle contraction to assist with hemostasis.

Aspirin inhibits the formation of eicosanoids by binding to and inhibiting cyclooxygenase, an enzyme necessary for their synthesis. TXA$_2$ and prostacyclin are both eicosanoids, so aspirin initially reduces the formation of both. However, platelets do not have nuclei and cannot synthesize new enzymes, while nucleated endothelial cells can synthesize additional cyclooxygenase. Because of these differences in the two cells types, treatment with aspirin at an appropriate dose and an appropriate schedule preferentially reduces thromboxane synthesis by platelets. This is the basis for the use of aspirin when it is desirable to reduce the tendency for blood coagulation (e.g., humans with cardiac diseases and animals with heartworms.)

Some of the substances released by aggregating platelets and some of the cell membrane components exposed by aggregated platelets act to promote coagulation. Thus, with larger sites of injury, more platelets aggregate and more stimulants of clotting are present in the local area. Coagulation is initiated when the local concentration of these substances reaches some critical level. Platelets are required for normal coagulation in response to vascular damage. Clotting may also be stimulated outside of the body when a foreign surface, such as the glass surface of a test tube, induces the same reactions as exposure to collagen.

Intrinsic and Extrinsic Coagulation Pathways

The ultimate product of blood coagulation is a relatively solid gel plug (clot or **thrombus**). This plug may be red or somewhat clear. The color varies with the number of erythrocytes and other blood cells trapped in the clot. Erythrocytes and leukocytes are not necessary for coagulation, and they may or may not be present in a clot.

A clot is relatively solid because of interlacing strands of **fibrin** (a protein polymer) that are covalently cross-linked. Trapped within this network are other blood components (e.g., platelets, leukocytes, erythrocytes), but the key element is the fibrin. Thus, the most basic explanation of coagulation is that it is a series of biochemical reactions to produce and stabilize a protein polymer, fibrin.

The series or chain of biochemical reactions that links initial vascular damage to a stabilized fibrin network is the **intrinsic clotting pathway,** or **intrinsic cascade** (Fig. 15–4). It is intrinsic because all substances necessary for the cascade are present in the circulation. This pathway includes several proteolytic enzymes (**clotting factors**) normally in the plasma in an inactive form. When one of these inactive forms con-

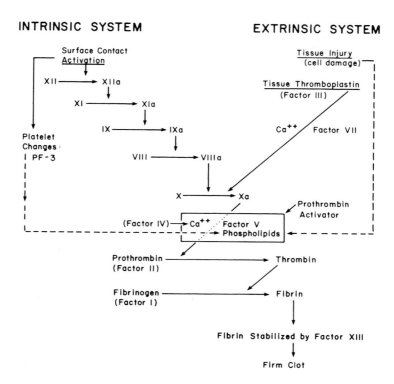

INTRINSIC SYSTEM　　　　　　　　**EXTRINSIC SYSTEM**

Figure 15-4. Extrinsic and intrinsic pathways leading to the generation and stabilization of fibrin that forms the framework of a blood clot. PF-3 refers to factors associated with the cell membranes of platelets.

verts to an active form, it activates the next enzyme in the cascade. This type of cascade allows for amplification at multiple steps so that many molecules of fibrin can be generated as the result of the activation of one initial molecule. As shown in Figure 15–4, the first step in the intrinsic cascade is the activation of factor XII. This occurs when inactive factor XII comes in contact with collagen at a site of tissue damage. The factor numbers refer to the sequence in which they were discovered, not the sequence of their involvement in the cascade. The numbered factors have also been identified by common name (Table 15–3).

Coagulation can also be initiated when a protein from interstitial fluid (***tissue factor*** or ***tissue thromboplastin***) forms an active complex with an inactive plasma protein, factor VII (Fig. 15–4). Tissue thromboplastin increases in interstitial fluid in the area of cellular injury and is apparently released from injured cells. The

factor VII–tissue factor complex activates factor X. Factor X is a component of the intrinsic cascade, so from this point on the pathway to fibrin formation and linkage is the same as in the intrinsic cascade. The cascade that is initiated by tissue thromboplastin is the ***extrinsic cascade,*** or ***extrinsic pathway.*** The final product of both the extrinsic and intrinsic cascades is a fibrin clot, and some clotting factors are common to both. The only differences are some of the factors found in the early steps of the cascades (Fig. 15–4).

Calcium ions are required as cofactors at various steps in both cascades (Fig. 15–4), and several anticoagulants used to prevent blood clotting outside the body do so by binding calcium ions. These include sodium citrate, potassium citrate, ammonium citrate, and ethylenediaminetetraacetic acid (***EDTA***). EDTA is usually in the form of a sodium or potassium salt.

Clot formation at the site of injury reduces

Table 15-3. International nomenclature of coagulation factors with synonyms.

Factor[a]	Synonyms
I	Fibrinogen
II	Prothrombin
III	Tissue thromboplastin
IV	Calcium
V	Proaccelerin; labile factor
VII	Proconvertin; stable factor
VIII	Antihemophilic globulin; antihemophilic factor A
IX	Christmas factor; antihemophilic factor B
X	Stuart-Power factor
XI	Plasma thromboplastin antecedent; antihemophilic factor C
XII	Hageman factor
XIII	Fibrin stabilizing factor

[a]International nomenclature.

blood loss and occludes the opening in the damaged vessel. This tends to remove stimuli necessary for continuation of coagulation by covering the exposed collagen and preventing the entry of tissue fluid into the vessel. The undamaged endothelial cells adjacent to the damaged area also secrete prostacyclin, an inhibitor of platelet adhesion and aggregation. If coagulation continued unchecked beyond the site of injury, blood vessels throughout the body would be occluded inappropriately, and blood flow would be halted. Two additional plasma proteins, **protein C** and **antithrombin III,** prevent coagulation from continuing inappropriately. Protein C circulates in an inactive form that is activated by **thrombin.** Thrombin forms as part of both the intrinsic and extrinsic pathways and is also responsible for one of the final steps in both, the production of fibrin from fibrinogen (Fig. 15–4). Thus, as formation of thrombin by the coagulation pathways promotes clot formation, thrombin also restrains the process so that it does not become uncontrolled. Antithrombin III is also inactive by itself, but when bound to **heparin** (present on normal endothelial cell membranes), the heparin–antithrombin III combination inactivates

thrombin. Here again, the presence of intact, healthy endothelial cells acts to prevent or halt coagulation.

In many cases, the damage to small vessels can be repaired so that normal blood flow can again occur. These repair mechanisms include removal of the clot and proliferation of endothelial cells to reestablish normal vascular lining. A key element in clot removal is the activation of the fibrinolytic system. This system is similar to the clotting cascade in that an inactive plasma protein or proenzyme, **plasminogen,** is activated to **plasmin,** which converts fibrin to soluble fragments. There appear to be several different pathways by which plasminogen can be activated to plasmin, but these are not as well understood as the activation of clotting factors. However, the presence of fibrin may stimulate several of these pathways. It seems that as fibrin is generated, it also begins to initiate its own ultimate destruction. Plasminogen is also activated by **tissue plasminogen activator,** an enzyme secreted by normal, intact endothelial cells.

The majority of the plasma factors for both the coagulation and fibrinolytic cascades are synthesized in the liver, and this synthesis is vitamin K dependent. Vitamin K is a lipid-soluble essential vitamin whose normal intestinal absorption requires bile salts. If the liver is diseased or the bile duct is obstructed, the resultant lack of bile in the gut reduces the absorption of lipids and vitamin K. Bacteria in the mammalian intestine also synthesize absorbable vitamin K.

Dicumarol **is a toxic form of a general class of compounds known as** *coumarins.* **Dicumarol, found in spoiled sweet clover hay or silage, inhibits the clotting of blood. It is antagonistic to vitamin K and reduces the synthesis of vitamin K–dependent clotting factors. Among these is prothrombin.** *Sweet clover poisoning* **is the hemorrhagic condition resulting from excessive dicumarol ingestion. Clinical signs are related to reductions in the ability of blood to clot. Small cuts or bruises may result in bleeding that is difficult to stop.** *Warfarin* **is another coumarin and vitamin K antagonist that is used commercially in rodent poisons.**

Lymph

Normally there is very little net egress of fluid as blood flows through capillaries. Recall that the capillaries are relatively impermeable to plasma proteins, and these generate an effective osmotic force to retain fluid within the vessels. However, there is a relatively small net loss of both protein and fluid from capillaries. These are normally taken up by a system of small **lymphatic** vessels, and the resultant fluid is **lymph.**

Lymphatic vessels begin as blind-ending vessels similar in structure to capillaries, and these join to form larger vessels resembling veins. The direction of lymph flow is from small lymphatics to large ones. The largest of the lymphatic vessels join with large veins just cranial to the heart, and here all lymph returns to the blood. **Edema** is an abnormal accumulation of fluid within the interstitial space. Blockage of lymphatic vessels can produce edema within the area normally drained by those lymphatics.

Lymph is a clear, colorless liquid somewhat similar to blood plasma, from which it is derived. Lymph usually contains numerous lymphocytes, inorganic salts, glucose, proteins, and other nitrogenous substances. Neutrophilic leukocytes are not normally present in great numbers except during acute infections.

Lymph derived from the intestine during digestion may contain large quantities of lipids, giving it a milky appearance. This milky lymph, called **chyle,** results from the absorption of lipids into the **lacteals,** the small lymphatics of the intestine.

Serous Fluids

Serous fluids in the body cavities include peritoneal, pleural, and pericardial fluid. Normally these fluids are present as a thin film that reduces friction between apposed surfaces. Inflammation or infection of the serous membranes causes increased production of serous fluids. Examples are **pleuritis** (pleurisy), **peritonitis,** and **pericarditis.**

Chapter 16

BODY DEFENSES AND THE IMMUNE SYSTEM

Introduction

Body defense is protection against injury; *immunity* is protection against foreign microorganisms or the harmful effect of antigenic substances (antigens). *Antigens* are molecules that can stimulate an immune response directed at that specific molecule, and in most cases antigens are either components of foreign cells or secretions by microorganisms. While the ability to mount immune responses is part of the body's defenses, it is not the only means by which the body is defended. A number of *nonspecific defenses,* general defense mechanisms that do not need to recognize specific antigens to be effective, also protect the body against injury.

Foreign refers to cells or substances that are not self. *Self* refers to cells and substances that are normal components of an animal's body and that normally do not elicit an immune response. The ability to differentiate between foreign and self is a critical function of the immune system. *Autoimmune* disorders occur when the immune system erroneously identifies self tissues or antigens as foreign and mounts an inappropriate immune response. The immune system must also be able to identify and eliminate self cells that have changed so that they may be harmful. The identification and elimination of these altered cells is protection against the development of cancers.

The *immune system* can be defined as all of the structures and cells involved in providing immune protection. This is not an anatomically defined system, as cells of this system can be found throughout the body in many tissues. Lymphocytes are the primary cell type involved in an immune response, and the wide distribution of lymphocytes throughout the body provides them ready access to invading microorganisms and newly introduced antigens. Lymphocytes are not a uniform group of cells, and the different subtypes of lymphocytes have specific roles in the overall generation and regulation of an immune response. However, in general, the primary responses are production of circulating antibodies (**humoral response**), generation of lymphocytes capable of removing the potentially harmful cell (**cellular response**), or both.

Inflammation can be defined as the response of tissues to injury. The classic signs of *acute inflammation* (swelling, pain, heat, and redness) are produced as a result of the injury and the tissue response. ***Chronic inflammatory responses*** may not demonstrate these classic signs. The desired outcome of the response to injury is complete repair with the restoration of tissues to their original state. Obviously this may or may not be possible, depending on the severity and type of injury and the ability of tissues to respond. While the effects of injury produce local changes that initiate an inflammatory response, cells attracted to the area of injury (e.g., leukocytes and macrophages) also participate in inflammatory responses.

Nonspecific Defenses

Epithelia that cover surfaces exposed to the external environment function as protective barriers to prevent entry of injurious agents, such as microbes and chemicals. This barrier function can be enhanced by epithelial secretions, such as hydrochloric acid in the stomach and nonspecific antimicrobial agents in saliva (e.g., lysozyme). Physical disruption of the barrier or loss of epithelial function can provide an entryway for injurious agents to reach the body fluids and possibly spread.

When microbes or injurious agents penetrate an epithelial barrier, their presence and any tissue damage that they produce initiate a response, inflammation. The initial phases of this response are immediate and similar regardless of the type or identity of the microbe or agent. Thus, these are **nonspecific responses,** or **innate responses.** The terms **nonspecific immune response** and **innate immune response** have also been used. A **specific** or **acquired immune response** entails identification of the specific microbe or agent and development of a response directed at that specific agent.

Local tissue phagocytes (macrophages) are among the first cells to respond during a nonspecific response; they attempt to engulf and destroy any foreign microbe or substance. The primary mode of destruction is by intracellular fusion of phagocytic vesicles with enzyme-containing lysosomes. An accumulation of neutrophils in the area is another component of the rapid nonspecific response. Recall that neutrophils are attracted to an area of injury and inflammation by chemotactic factors and that chemotactic factors may include substances released from damaged cells and by the invading microbes. Chemotactic factors are also released by tissue macrophages as part of their response to foreign microbes.

The release of chemotactic factors by responding macrophages is one example of a general scheme by which nonspecific and specific immune responses are regulated. That is, many of the cells participating in the response secrete chemical messengers that affect the function of other responding cells. In this example, macrophages already responding secrete chemical agents that act as chemotactic factors to attract neutrophils. In this way, higher levels of macrophage activity in response to greater numbers of microbes can promote the accumulation of greater numbers of neutrophils.

Cytokine is the general term applied to all chemical messengers (primarily proteins) that regulate cells involved in any immune response. Responding cells produce many of the cytokines, but other cell types also secrete them. More than 100 compounds have been classified as cytokines, which provides some insight to the complexity of these responses. The various cytokines that function as chemotactic factors are collectively termed **chemokines.** Interleukin-1 is a specific cytokine that also functions as a *pyrogen* (an agent that produces fever). The pyrogen effect of interleukin-1 is but one example of a systemic effect of a cytokine that is unrelated to cells of the immune system. Many of the systemic changes characteristic of a diseased animal are produced by cytokines leaving a site of inflammation and entering the general circulation.

Specific chemokines also attract more macrophages to areas of inflammation. Since macrophages are derived from circulating monocytes, part of this effect requires that monocytes migrate from vessels and develop into tissue macrophages. The monocyte response is slower than that of neutrophils, so an accumulation of inflammatory cells that is primarily neutrophils is characteristic of an acute inflammatory response. An accumulation of macrophages is more characteristic of a chronic inflammatory response.

Another characteristic of an acute inflammatory response is increases in local blood flow and in movement of fluid and plasma protein into the interstitial space. Agents that affect blood vessels in the local area of inflammation bring about these changes. Locally produced agents include eicosanoids (see Chapter 12) that are produced by a variety of cell types.

Plasma proteins delivered to a site of inflammation include **complement** (also known as **complement proteins**). These are a group of plasma proteins that are normally inactive in circulation (similar to the clotting factors), but some can be activated by the presence of certain polysaccharide components of the outer coverings of bacteria. The activated complement proteins can activate other complement proteins (similar to the clotting cascades). The activated complement proteins have a number of effects that contribute to the local nonspecific response. These include (1) leukocyte chemotaxis, (2) direct attack on bacteria by increasing the permeability of their cell walls, (3) stimulation of **histamine** release from mast cells, and (4) **opsonization.** Opsonization is the facilitation of engulfment by phagocytes, and any agent that can perform this facilitation is termed an **opsonin.** The local release of histamine causes a further increase in blood flow and accumulation of interstitial fluid and plasma proteins by its actions on blood vessels.

One unique aspect of viral infections is that viruses can replicate only within cells. Viruses must enter cells of the animal's body and use the cell's own synthetic processes to form new viruses to infect other cells. Two types of nonspecific defense mechanisms function to prevent viral infection and replication. **Interferons** are polypeptides produced and secreted by cells containing viruses, and almost all types of cells produce interferons after being infected by viruses. Interferons are a means by which an infected cell can prevent further spread of the viral infection, because they act on other cells in the area to prevent viruses from using the synthetic pathways of newly infected cells to produce new viruses. Viruses may enter cells protected by interferons, but they cannot replicate within protected cells. Interferons are not specific for individual viruses, so interferons produced in response to infection by one virus will protect against infection by a different virus.

Natural killer (NK) cells are a specific type of lymphocyte that can recognize and destroy cells infected with viruses. This recognition does not appear to be based on viral antigens, so it is not specific for any given virus. The NK cells destroy the infected cell by the secretion of substances known as **perforins** and **granzymes** while in direct contact with the infected cell. These secretions act on the cell membrane and enter the infected cell to destroy it. While NK cells act in a nonspecific manner, their numbers are normally relatively low and are only increased during a specific immune response.

Specific Immune Response

Innate immune responses lack **specificity** and **memory,** two important characteristics of specific immune responses. Immunologic specificity means that the response is directed at a specific antigen, while immunologic memory refers to the ability to have a fast, amplified response after an initial exposure to an antigen. These characteristics are extremely important, for they are the theoretical basis for **vaccinations.** Vaccination is essentially induction of a specific immune response and immunologic memory by planned exposure to an antigen in a manner that does not produce disease.

Lymphocytes are the essential leukocytes that develop a specific immune response. Their functions in this response include (1) antigen recognition, (2) antibody production, (3) cytotoxic attack on infected cells, (4) immunologic memory, and (5) regulation of the specific immune response. An individual lymphocyte does not perform all of these functions, but rather subpopulations or subtypes of lymphocytes are responsible for different aspects of the specific immune response. In an attempt to generalize a very complex process, this chapter describes the specific immune response by considering the different types of lymphocytes and the roles that each has in the overall response.

B Lymphocytes

B lymphocytes (*B cells*) are the lymphocyte subtype associated with the production of antibodies or the humoral component of a specific immune response. The first step in the humoral response is recognition of a foreign antigen by B cells. This occurs when an antigen (usually a protein as either a free molecule or a molecule on the surface of a cell membrane or a cell wall) binds to specific cell membrane receptors on a selected subpopulation of B cells. This subpopulation of B cells (a *clone*) is the only group of B cells with a membrane receptor capable of binding the antigen, and it is stimulated to proliferate. The process by which a particular subpopulation of B cells increases in number is termed *clonal selection.*

For clonal section to be effective, each animal must have a ready supply of lymphocytes with unique membrane receptors (i.e., proteins) capable of binding every potential antigen that may be encountered throughout the life of the animal. These lymphocytes with their unique membrane proteins must develop in utero or early in life for the animal to be *immunocompetent* (i.e., capable of mounting a specific immune response). Protein synthesis in developing lymphocytes appears to have some unique aspects that permit synthesis of the necessary tremendous variety of membrane protein. A later section of this chapter has more on B cell development.

As the number of B cells in a selected clone increases during a mature immune response, some of the B cells begin to differentiate into *plasma cells.* Plasma cells can synthesize and secrete antibodies specific for the antigen that stimulated the development of the selected clone. Thus, each plasma cell secretes only one antibody. Other B cells in the selected clone develop into *B memory cells* (Fig. 16–1). These cells remain in the body for extended periods (years or perhaps throughout life). Since these cells developed from a clone specific for a given antigen, the ready supply of them means that the next time this specific antigen is encountered (e.g., a second infection or exposure after a vaccination), the immune response can be accelerated and amplified.

The development of B memory cells and plasma cells and the secretion of antibodies are modulated by numerous cytokines. Cytokines, as the chemical messengers (proteins) secreted by a variety of cells in response to injury or microbial invasion, modulate the activity of cells of the immune system. One cell type that secretes cytokines essential for a normal humoral response is the *helper T cell* (Fig.16–1). T cells are another of the general classes of lymphocytes, and helper T cells are a specific subtype of T cells. The characteristics and functions of helper T cells are described later in this chapter.

Immunoglobins

Immunoglobulin is a general term for a protein that can bind to an antigen; it includes both antibodies (circulating immunoglobulins) and those found in the cell membranes of B cells. Immunoglobulins fall into five major classes based on their chemical and functional characteristics (Table 16–1). Immunoglobulin (Ig) G is the predominant circulating immunoglobulin. IgG has a variety of functions, including (1) binding free circulating antigens to reduce their potential for harm (neutralization) and promote their removal by phagocytes, (2) binding antigens associated with bacterial cell walls and promoting their phagocytosis, (3) binding antigens and activating complement to promote inflammation and destruction of harmful microbes, and (4) acting as an agglutinin to clump particulates so that they can be more effectively phagocytized. IgG does not actually destroy any

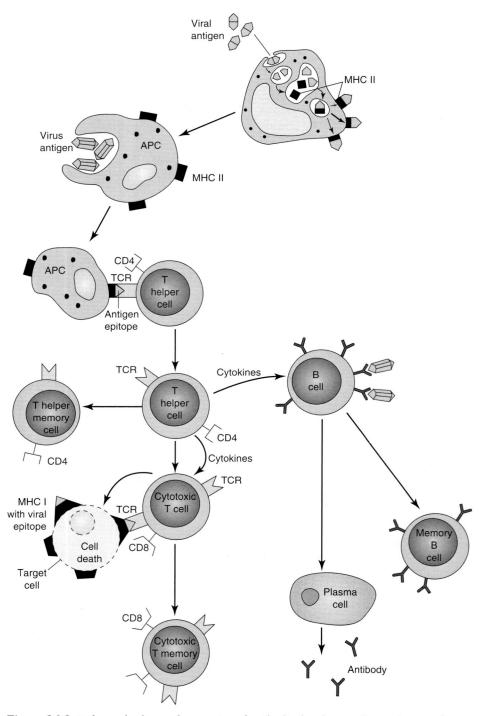

Figure 16-1. Pathways leading to the secretion of antibodies by plasma cells, production of memory cells, and generation of cytotoxic cells. Viral particles are used as an example of an antigen source. Viral epitope refers to the portion of the virus that is recognized as an antigen. TCR refers to the T-cell receptor that is capable of interacting with cell membrane proteins on other cells that are presenting antigens, and APC refers to antigen-presenting cell. (Reprinted with permission from Porth C.M. *Pathophysiology.* 5th ed. Philadelphia: Lippincott, 1998.)

Table 16-1. Classes and Characteristics of Immunoglobulins

Class	Characteristics
IgG	Antiviral, antitoxin, antibacterial. Main immunoglobulin in circulation. Activates complement; binds to macrophages.
IgA	Major immunoglobulin in body secretions to protect mucous membranes and epithelial surfaces.
IgE	Binds to mast cells and basophils as part of allergic reactions. Responds to parasitic infestations.
IgM	Associated with early immune responses. Forms natural antibodies, such as those associated with blood cell antigens.
IgD	Found on B lymphocytes and needed for maturation of B cells.

Adapted from Porth, C.M.: *Pathophysiology.* 5th ed. Philadelphia, Lippincott, 1998.

harmful substance or agent; it promotes destruction or removal indirectly.

IgE is the class of immunoglobulins associated with most allergic responses. When an *allergen* (an agent capable of inducing an allergic response) is first encountered, specific IgE is produced and incorporates into the cell membrane of mast cells. When the same allergen is again encountered, the allergen binds to the specific IgE on the mast cells, and this stimulates the mast cells to release their secretory granules containing **histamine** and produce *leukotrienes.* These agents bring about many of the cell and tissue responses characteristic of allergies.

T Cells and Cell-Mediated Immunity

T cells are the type of lymphocyte associated with the component of an immune response known as **cell-mediated immunity**. Whereas the humoral response involves antibodies that can have their effect at sites distant from their site of production, the cell-mediated immune response requires that the responding T cells be in contact with the cells bearing the foreign antigen. As with B cells, T cells have various subtypes, each with its specific functions. The subtypes include cytotoxic T cells, helper T cells, memory T cells, and NK T cells (Fig. 16–1). NK T cells and helper T cells are introduced earlier in this chapter.

As with the humoral response, antigen recognition initiates the cell-mediated response. However, antigen recognition by T cells requires that the antigenic material be presented as part of a complex on the cell membrane of other immune cells. This complex consists of the antigenic material and intrinsic cell membrane proteins known as **major histocompatibility complex** (MHC) proteins.

The genes that code for MHC proteins are found on a single chromosome, and MHC proteins are continuously synthesized in all cells of an animal's body except for erythrocytes, which do not have nuclei and are not capable of protein synthesis. After synthesis, MHC proteins enter the outer cell membrane so that a portion is exposed to the exterior. As MHC proteins prepare for insertion in the cell membrane, they form complexes with antigenic materials found within the cell. When the complex enters the membrane, the antigen is exposed to the exterior. The exposed antigen is then in a position to be recognized by T cells.

Cell membranes hold two major classes of MHC proteins, class I and class II (Fig. 16–1). Class I MHC proteins are found in all cells except for erythrocytes. Class I MHC proteins continuously present potential antigenic materials on the surface of all cells. These materials include peptides and other antigenic materials normally produced in cells, as well as antigenic materials produced as a result of an abnormality in cell function. If a foreign cell (i.e., not self) is introduced into an animal's body, the antigenic material presented by its class I MHC proteins is unique for that foreign cell and differs from endogenous self cells. When viruses infect normal cells and alter their synthetic pathways, they change the antigenic materials presented by the class I proteins of the infected cell. By recognizing these new antigens, T cells recognize foreign or infected cells, allowing initiation of a cellular immune response directed at cells bearing the foreign antigen.

Only selected cell types have class II MHC proteins. These include lymphocytes, free and fixed macrophages, microglia in the central nervous system, and a population of cells in the spleen and lymph nodes known as *dendritic cells.* Cells that contain class II MHC proteins are termed *antigen-presenting cells* (APCs), for they process and present antigens derived from foreign material or microbes (Fig. 16–1). These antigens are derived from microbes or material that the APCs take up by phagocytosis or pinocytosis. APCs process materials in phagocytic or pinocytic vesicles to produce antigens that are complexed to class II MHC proteins and inserted into the APC cell membrane.

As with B cells, clones of T cells exist that are specific for a given antigen, and the process of antigen recognition permits a specific clone to be selected. However, the selection and activation of T cells also requires interaction between the MHC proteins holding the antigenic material and other proteins in the cell membranes of the various T cells known as *cluster of differentiation markers (CD markers).* These marker proteins determine the interactions that are possible for the different types of T cells. Helper T cells have CD4 markers (Fig. 16–1), which interact with class II MHC proteins, and cytotoxic T cells have CD8 markers, which interact with class I MHC proteins. Thus, helper T cells can recognize antigenic material presented by APCs, and cytotoxic T cells can detect foreign antigenic material presented by almost any type of cell (Fig. 16–1).

After recognizing antigens presented by APCs, the selected helper T cells are activated by interactions between other of their membrane proteins and membrane proteins found in the APCs. This interaction (*costimulation*) leads to full helper T activation. The activated helper T cells multiply and produce a subset to serve as memory cells (*memory T_H cells*). A major function of the other activated helper T cells is to secrete cytokines to promote and amplify all aspects of the innate and specific immune responses. This includes attraction and stimulation of additional macrophages and NK cells, promoting the action of cytotoxic T cells, and promoting the development of selected B cells. A key cytokine produced by helper T cells to stimulate macrophages, NK cells, cytotoxic cells, and B cells is *interleukin-2.*

Costimulation by cells presenting the specific antigen to selected cytotoxic T cells is also required for full activation of those cytotoxic T cells. The activated cytotoxic T cells also undergo a series of cell divisions to provide increased numbers of the selected clone and also produce a subset to serve as memory cells (*memory T_C cells*). Activated cytotoxic cells (killer cells) destroy cells bearing the antigen for which they were selected. Physical contact and binding between the cells bearing the antigen and the cytotoxic T cells are required for the destruction (Fig. 16–1). Secretions from the cytotoxic T cells, including perforin to disrupt the cell membrane of the antigen-bearing cells, accomplish the destruction.

Lymphocyte Origin, Development, and Residence

Just as all lymphocytes are originally derived from pluripotent stem cells that subsequently became lymphoid stem cells in the bone marrow (Fig. 15–1), the three general classes of lymphocytes (B cells, T cells, and NK cells) are all derived from lymphoid stem cells.

The differentiation of lymphoid stem cells to the types of mature lymphocytes begins early during embryonic development. Cells destined to become T cells leave the bone marrow and travel to the *thymus,* where secretions called *thymic hormones* act on them. These are not classic hormones, for they are local to the thymus, and lymphocytes must come to the thymus to be acted on. The thymic hormones guide the further development of the lymphocytes to become T cells. As part of the development in the thymus, only T cells capable of recognizing foreign antigens are selected to survive. The selected T cells that leave the thymus populate lymphoid structures throughout the body, including tonsils, lymph nodes, the spleen, and collections of lymphocytes in the intestinal wall. These structures are responsible for producing T cells in adult animals (discussed later).

Lymphoid stem cells destined to become B cells also undergo differentiation during embryonic development. In birds, lymphoid cells destined to become B cells leave the bone marrow and travel to the bursa of Fabricius, which is similar to the thymus but associated with the intestinal tract. Here the cells undergo maturation and selection similar to what happens to pre–T cells in the thymus. Mature B cells leaving the bursa in birds also populate peripheral lymphoid structures, and it is these structures that produce B cells in adult birds. An organ that is the functional equivalent to the bursa has not been identified in mammals. It is thought that B cells mature in the bone marrow in mammals and leave the marrow to populate the peripheral lymphoid structures. As with T cells, the peripheral lymphoid structures produce B cells in adult animals. The development of NK cells probably occurs in a manner similar to that for B cells.

Active and Passive Immunities

Active immunity is a state of immunity to a specific antigen achieved by the response of one's own immune system. Active immunity may include both humoral and cell-mediated responses. Passive immunity is a state of temporary immunity achieved by the transfer of immunoglobulins or T cells from an animal with active immunity to another that has not encountered the antigen involved. Passive immunity is a temporary state because the immunoglobulins and/or T cells are degraded or destroyed over time.

Immunological Surveillance

NK cells and cytotoxic T lymphocytes (killer cells) both recognize and destroy cells with foreign antigens in their cells membranes. *Cancer cells* have surface antigens that are not present in normal cells and thus can be recognized as foreign. It is believed that cancer cells routinely develop in the body but are soon recognized and destroyed by the killer cells that recognize the abnormal antigens. This recognition and destruction are termed *immunological surveil-*

lance. Clinically evident cancers develop when this surveillance is inadequate.

Lymphatic System

The **lymphatic system** includes the lymphoid tissues (e.g., lymph nodes and nodules and the spleen) and the lymphatic vessels distributed throughout the body (Fig. 16–2). It drains tissue fluid (called **lymph** within the lymphatic system) and is a framework for the circulation, production, and maturation of immune cells. The tissue fluid–draining function of the lymphatic system augments the venous circulation and therefore assists in the control of interstitial fluid pressures. The lymphatic system is also an important component of immunologic defense of the body, as movement of lymph brings microorganisms and other foreign substances into contact with immune cells.

Lymphoid tissue consists of accumulations of lymphocytes trapped in the spaces between fibers of reticular connective tissue. The lymphoid tissue may be scattered diffusely in some regions (as is commonly found in mucous membranes), may appear as nodules (as in the intestinal submucosa), or may be encapsulated to form specific organs, including lymph nodes, the spleen, thymus, and tonsils. The lymphatic vessels and tissues are arranged so that tissue fluid is exposed to aggregates of immune cells, which scrutinize the fluid for foreign cells and substances, thereby assisting in the control of infection.

Lymphatic Vessels

The lymphatic vessels constitute a one-way pathway that parallels the venous system and eventually empties into the cranial vena cava or some of its tributaries. The smallest lymphatics begin blindly between tissue cells as **lymphatic capillaries,** which collect the tissue fluid not absorbed by the venous system. When the tissue fluid enters the lymphatic vessels, it is known as **lymph,** which consists of fluid originally derived from the blood, a variety of blood cells, and sometimes microbes. Lymphatic vessels carry lymph back to the great veins of the heart.

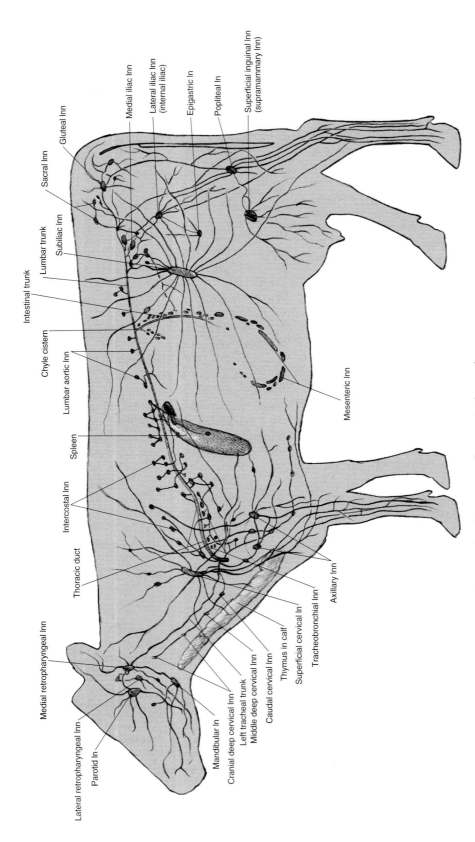

Figure 16-2. The lymphatic system of the cow. (Reprinted with permission from McCracken et al.: *Spurgeon's Color Atlas of Large Animal Anatomy*. Baltimore, Lippincott Williams & Wilkins, 1999.)

Medial iliac lnn

Lateral iliac lnn (internal iliac)

Epigastric ln

Popliteal ln

Superficial inguinal lnn (supramammary lnn)

Gluteal lnn

Sacral lnn

Lumbar trunk

Subiliac lnn

Intestinal trunk

Chyle cistern

Lumbar aortic lnn

Spleen

Intercostal lnn

Thoracic duct

Medial retropharyngeal lnn

Lateral retropharyngeal lnn

Parotid ln

Mandibular ln

Cranial deep cervical lnn

Left tracheal trunk

Middle deep cervical lnn

Caudal cervical lnn

Thymus in calf

Superficial cervical ln

Tracheobronchial lnn

Axillary lnn

Mesenteric lnn

Lymph Nodes

Lymph nodes are discrete knots of lymphoid tissue scattered along the course of lymph vessels (Fig. 16–3). Lymph nodes filter the lymph and act as one of the first defenses against infection by harboring lymphocytes, plasma cells, and macrophages.

Each lymph node is surrounded by a connective tissue capsule that sends numerous connective tissue **trabeculae** into the substance of the node. The node is roughly divided into **cortex, paracortex,** and **medulla,** with large numbers of lymphocytes and macrophages in all three. Lymphocytes in the cortex are arranged in nodules. Dark-staining groups are **primary nodules,** and light-staining groups are **secondary nodules.** Secondary nodules are areas of rapid B cell proliferation, and for that reason their cores are called **germinal centers.** The paracortex, deep to the cortex, is populated primarily with T lymphocytes and dendritic cells.

Lymphocytes in the medullary portion of the lymph node are arranged in **medullary cords** rather than nodules. These tend to be primarily accumulations of **plasma cells.**

Immediately deep to the capsule of the node is a space, the **subcapsular sinus,** that communicates with other sinuses of the cortex and medulla. Lymph delivered by afferent lymph vessels enters the subcapsular sinus and is slowly filtered through the cortex and medulla, to emerge finally at the **hilus** of the node, where blood vessels and nerves enter and the efferent lymphatic vessels emerge, carrying the lymph that has percolated through the node. This arrangement is ideally suited for the presentation to immune cells of antigens collected in the tissue fluid.

Oddly enough, the porcine lymph node's his-

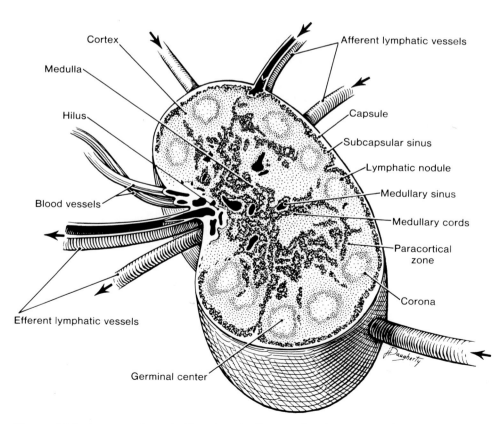

Figure 16.3. Anatomy of a typical lymph node. (Reprinted with permission from Banks W.J. *Applied Veterinary Histology*. 2nd ed. Baltimore: Williams & Wilkins, 1986.)

tologic architecture is a reverse of that seen in other species, with the nodules found in central regions and medullary cords on the periphery of the node. Flow of lymph likewise is reverse, with afferents entering at the hilus and percolating through the lymphatic tissue to emerge at the capsule.

Lymph nodes are scattered throughout the body, and in general their number and location are fairly consistent within a given species (Table 16–2). For convenience, groups of related nodes are often called a **lymphocenter.** The condition of the lymph node often reflects the health of the area from which it receives lymph. If a specific area is infected, the lymph nodes in that area tend to enlarge as the germinal centers begin producing additional lymphocytes in response to the antigens delivered to the node. For example, a horse with **strangles,** a bacterial infection of the nasal cavity and pharynx, frequently shows enlargement of the mandibular

and retropharyngeal lymphocenters. The lymph nodes at these locations receive their afferent vessels from the nasal cavity, mouth, and pharynx.

Neoplastic (cancerous) cells may spread throughout the body by way of the lymphatic channels; this is **metastasis.** When a tumor (cancer) is removed surgically, it may also be necessary to remove the regional lymph nodes draining the cancerous area to prevent further spread of the condition if it is suspected that neoplastic cells have infiltrated the nodes. The meat inspector uses his or her knowledge of the lymphatic system to determine whether a given part of a carcass should be condemned. An enlarged node may indicate infected or cancerous tissue in the region of the body draining to the node and necessitate condemnation of all or part of the carcass.

Hemal nodes are small dark red or black nodes in cattle and sheep, usually in the dorsal

Table 16-2. Selected Lymph Nodes (Lymphocenters) of Cattle

Name of Node	Location
Mandibular	Intermandibular space
Parotid	Rostroventral to external meatus of ear
Retropharyngeal	Dorsal to pharynx
Deep cervical	Dorsolateral to trachea, divided into cranial, middle, & caudal groups
Superficial cervical (formerly prescapular)	Cranial to shoulder joint
Axillary	On medial aspect of shoulder near brachial plexus
Mediastinal	Within the mediastinum, divided into cranial, middle, and caudal groups
Intercostal	Between ribs near thoracic vertebrae
Sternal	Deep surface of sternum
Bronchial	Associated with major bronchi
Lumbar	Group of nodes around aorta at level of last thoracic and first few lumbar vertebrae
Iliosacral	Group of nodes around terminus of abdominal aorta
Celiac	Group of nodes around origin of celiac a.
Cranial mesenteric	Group of nodes around origin of cranial mesenteric a.
Subiliac (formerly prefemoral)	Cranial to thigh in flank region
Superficial inguinal (scrotal or mammary)	Bulls, cranial to external inguinal ring; cows, dorsocaudal part of udder
Ischiatic	Group of nodes lateral to sacrotuberous ligament
Popliteal	Caudal to stifle joint

parts of abdominal and thoracic cavities. They resemble lymph nodes but are found on the course of small blood vessels and have blood within their sinuses.

Spleen

The **spleen** is a lymphoid organ associated with the circulatory system. It is attached to the stomach either directly by connective tissue, as in the ruminants, where it adheres closely to the rumen, or by the gastrosplenic ligament. The splenic capsule is thick and rich in elastic fibers and smooth muscle cells. Extensions of the capsule, trabeculae, penetrate into the interior of the organ, forming a connective tissue framework. The shape of the spleen varies considerably from one species to another, being long and thin in the pig, oblong in cattle, and sickle-shaped in the horse.

The parenchyma (substance) of the spleen consists of **red pulp** and **white pulp.** The red pulp has a dark red appearance because it is engorged with blood. The white pulp is lighter colored, as it is composed largely of lymphatic nodules, which are constructed much like the follicles of lymph nodes. Both B and T lymphocytes are found in abundance in the white pulp. The association of blood capillaries with the white pulp ensures that blood will be exposed to populations of immune cells.

In addition to important immunologic functions, the spleen functions as a storage area for red blood cells, so the size of the spleen varies from time to time even within a given individual, as well as from species to species, depending on the number of red blood cells in the spleen at a given time. The spleen is also an important site where senescent (old and worn-out) red blood cells are removed from the circulation, broken down, and their iron stored. These blood-related functions are associated with the red pulp of the splenic parenchyma. Although the spleen is a useful organ, it is not essential in the adult, as all of its functions can be carried on by other organs. The spleen can be removed (**splenectomy**) without significant impairment to a mature animal.

Thymus

The **thymus** is an organ of immature animals, undergoing involution at puberty, although never completely disappearing. It lies cranial to the heart, with portions extending along the trachea craniad into the ventral neck. The connective tissue components of the thymus form a loose areolar network that divides the organ into grossly visible lobules. Histology reveals distinct cortex and medulla, both of which consist of accumulations of lymphocytes (in this location called **thymocytes**); it is within the thymus that embryonic lymphocytes undergo differentiation and leave to populate the many other lymphatic tissues of the body.

Tonsils

In the most traditional sense, a **tonsil** is an unencapsulated aggregate of lymphatic nodules associated with the pharyngeal mucosa. These aggregates lack afferent lymphatic vessels, instead relying on their proximity to the epithelial surface to make contact with antigens. Many tonsils are characterized by deep invaginations on their epithelial surfaces called **crypts,** which presumably increase the surface area for contact with lymphatic tissue. Although the word tonsil is usually reserved for the lymphatic organs associated with the pharynx, identical histological elements are found in the mucous membranes of the prepuce and vagina and in the submucosa of the intestinal tract.

ANATOMY OF THE CARDIOVASCULAR SYSTEM

The cardiovascular system consists of the *heart* and a system of vessels for distribution of the blood to the tissues of the body and to the lungs for exchange of gases. Whether or not the blood is oxygenated, vessels that carry blood away from the heart are called *arteries,* and vessels that carry blood toward the heart are called *veins.* Circulation to the lungs (*pulmonary circulation*) is functionally and anatomically separate from circulation to the rest of the body (*systemic circulation*). Conceptually, it is therefore useful to regard the heart as two separate pumps housed within the same organ; one is a low-pressure pump that directs blood returning from the body to the lungs (i.e., the pulmonary circulation), and the other is a high-pressure pump that distributes blood to the systemic circulation.

Heart

The heart is a cone-shaped hollow muscular structure. The **base** is directed dorsad or craniodorsad and is attached to other thoracic structures by large arteries, veins, and the pericardial sac. The **apex** of the heart is directed ventrad and is entirely free within the pericardium. In the living animal, the right side of the heart is on the right side of the body but oriented more cranial than the left side, which is left and somewhat caudal (Fig. 17–1).

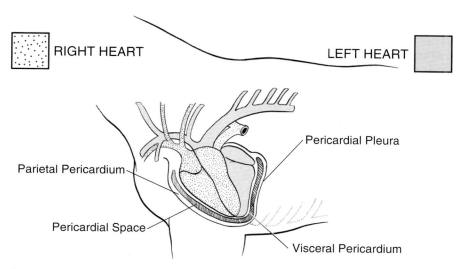

Figure 17-1. Orientation of the heart within the thorax. The right side of the heart lies more cranial than the left. The surface of the heart is covered with visceral pericardium, which the pericardial space separates from the parietal pericardium. The pericardial pleura is most superficial and is attached to the parietal pericardium by the fibrous pericardium. These three layers constitute the pericardial sac.

Pericardium

The heart is partially surrounded by a serous membrane called the **pericardium.** The pericardium, like other serous tissues (the pleura and peritoneum), creates a closed cavity (the **pericardial space**) that contains only a small amount of fluid for lubrication. The heart is invaginated into the pericardium much like a fist thrust into an inflated balloon (see Fig. 1–9). This arrangement results in two distinct layers of pericardium. The inner layer, which is intimately adherent to the outer surface of the heart, is called **visceral pericardium,** or **epicardium.** The outer layer, called **parietal pericardium,** is continuous with the visceral layer at the base of the heart and is reinforced by a superficial fibrous layer (the **fibrous pericardium**), which in turn is covered by a layer of mediastinal pleura (also called pericardial pleura) (Fig. 17–1). The parietal pericardium, fibrous pericardium, and mediastinal pleura together form the **pericardial sac,** which is grossly identifiable as a thin but tough tissue surrounding the heart.

In cattle, only the diaphragm separates the heart in the thoracic cavity from the reticulum in the abdominal cavity. Sharp metallic objects (most commonly, bits of wire) that are swallowed often accumulate in the reticulum. The contractions of this organ can cause these foreign bodies to penetrate the adjacent diaphragm and the pericardial sac, resulting in an infection of the sac called hardware disease. **The tissues of the pericardium thicken, and fluid builds up within the pericardial sac, which leads to heart failure in affected cattle. Hardware disease is usually prevented by administering a magnet by mouth; the magnet, which tends to remain in the reticulum, gathers swallowed metallic objects and prevents them from migrating through the wall of the forestomach.**

Cardiac Anatomy

The heart wall consists of three layers: an outer serous covering called **epicardium,** an inner endothelial lining called **endocardium,** and a thick muscular layer called **myocardium.**

The epicardium is the same as the visceral layer of pericardium. The endocardium is a layer of simple squamous endothelial cells that lines the chambers of the heart, covers the heart valves, and is continuous with the lining of the blood vessels. The myocardium consists of cardiac muscle, described in Chapter 8.

The heart is divided into right and left sides, which correspond to the low-pressure (pulmonary circulation) and high-pressure (systemic circulation) systems mentioned earlier. Each side has two chambers: an **atrium,** which receives blood by way of large veins, and a **ventricle,** which pumps blood from the heart through a large artery (Fig. 17–2). The atria are thin-walled chambers, each of which features an appendage called an **auricle.**

The myocardium of the ventricles, which pump blood back into vascular beds, is much thicker than that of the atria. The wall of the left ventricle is also thicker than that of the right; blood ejected from the left side during its contraction is under higher pressure than that ejected from the right ventricle. The right ventricle does not quite reach the apex of the heart, as the apex is formed entirely by the more muscular left ventricle. The myocardium between the two chambers is the **ventricular septum.**

Between the atrium and the ventricle of each side is the **atrioventricular valve,** or **A-V valve** (Fig. 17–2). The left A-V valve is occasionally called the **bicuspid valve,** because in humans it has two distinct flaps, or cusps. Another more commonly used synonym is **mitral valve,** because of its imagined resemblance to a bishop's miter, or two-sided hat. The right A-V valve is also called the **tricuspid valve** because in humans it has three flaps or cusps. The valve leaflets are attached to the inner wall of the ventricle at the junction of atrium and ventricle. The free margin or margins of the cusp are tethered to the ventricular wall by fibrous cords called **chordae tendineae.** The chordae tendineae attach to small muscular protrusions called **papillary muscles** that project into the lumina of the ventricles. These chordae tendineae, which resemble strings on a parachute, prevent the valve from everting into the atrium when the ventricle contracts and closes the A-V valve by forcing blood against the ventricular side of the valve (Fig. 17–3, A).

Each ventricle's outflow tract features a **semilunar valve** that assures blood flows only from the ventricle into the artery and not in the opposite direction. The semilunar valves have three cuplike leaflets, with convex side facing the ventricle (Fig. 17–3, B). The **aortic valve** is at the junction of the left ventricle and aorta.

The **pulmonary valve** is at the junction of the right ventricle and pulmonary trunk.

Blood returning to the heart from the systemic circulation is delivered to the right atrium by the **cranial** and **caudal venae cavae** (Fig. 17–4). From the right atrium, this deoxygenated blood passes through the right A-V valve into the right ventricle. From the right side, the right ventricle wraps around the cranial side of the heart and terminates as the funnel-shaped **conus arteriosus.** The conus arteriosus is the origin of the pulmonary trunk, from which it is divided by the pulmonary valve.

Just distal to the pulmonary valve, the pulmonary trunk divides into right and left **pulmonary arteries,** carrying blood to the respective lungs.

The **pulmonary veins** return blood from the lungs to the left atrium. From the left atrium, blood passes through the left A-V valve into the thick-walled left ventricle. The left ventricle pumps the blood past the aortic valve into the **aorta.** The aorta and its branches carry oxygenated blood to all parts of the body, including the heart and lungs (Fig. 17–4).

Vessels

Blood Vessels

Blood vessels resemble the branching of a tree in that the arteries start as large vessels and divide into smaller and smaller branches. The smallest arteries are **arterioles,** which are continuous with the smallest blood vessels, **capillaries.** Capillaries again unite to form small **venules** that unite to form larger and larger veins. The largest veins empty into the atria of the heart.

Arteries are tubular structures that carry blood away from the heart. Like all blood vessels, they are lined with endothelium. The walls of arteries tend to be thick and elastic, properties that are important in maintaining blood pressure. Smooth muscle in the walls of smaller arteries controls the diameter of these vessels.

Capillaries are tiny tubes composed almost entirely of endothelium, a continuation of the simple squamous epithelium that lines the heart

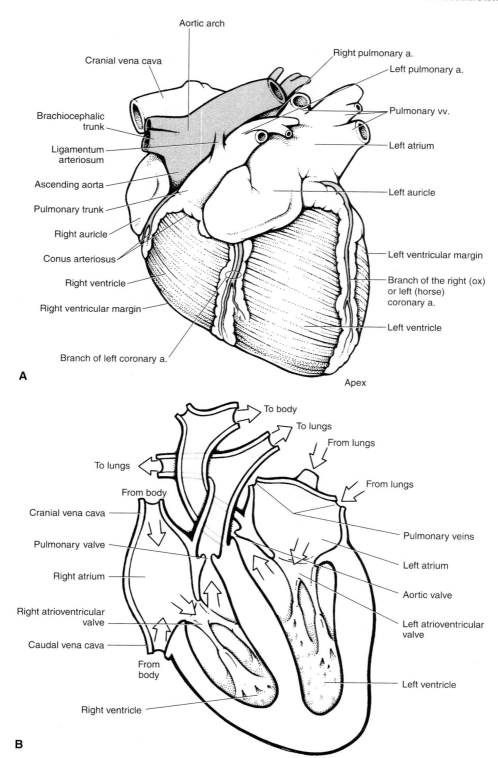

Figure 17-2. *A)* Left lateral view of the heart. *B)* Internal anatomy of the heart. *Arrows* depict the direction of blood flow. (Adapted with permission from Smith B.J. *Canine Anatomy.* Baltimore: Lippincott Williams & Wilkins, 1999.)

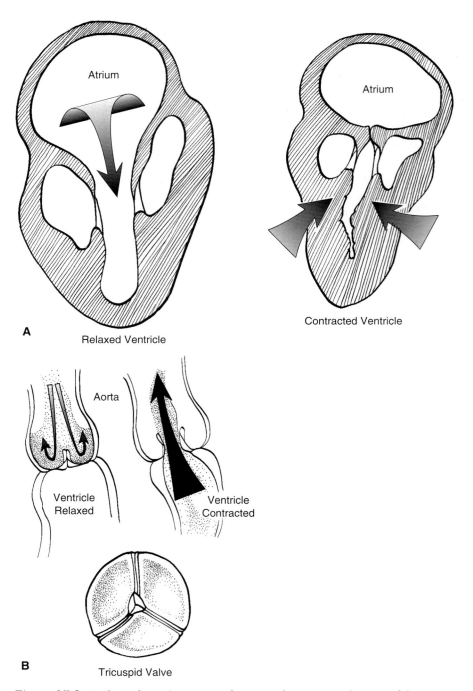

Figure 17-3. Cardiac valves. *A)* Function of an A-V valve. During relaxation of the ventricle (*left*), the valve leaflets open to allow blood to flow from the atrium into the ventricle (*arrow*). During ventricular contraction (*right*), valve leaflets are forced closed. The chordae tendineae prevent the margins of the valve from everting back into the atrium. *B)* A semilunar valve. Viewed from above, the valve consists of three cuplike leaflets. During relaxation of the ventricle, back-pressure of blood in the vessel closes the valve. When the ventricle contracts, leaflets part and blood flows through the valve (*arrow*).

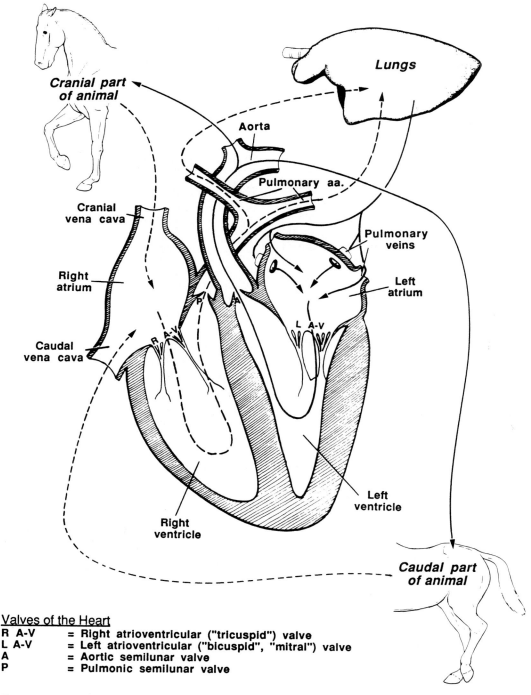

Valves of the Heart

R A-V	= Right atrioventricular ("tricuspid") valve
L A-V	= Left atrioventricular ("bicuspid", "mitral") valve
A	= Aortic semilunar valve
P	= Pulmonic semilunar valve

Figure 17-4. Flow of blood through the heart. *Broken lines* indicate deoxygenated blood in the pulmonary circulation. *Solid arrows* indicate oxygenated blood in the systemic circulation. Blood flowing into the brachiocephalic trunk supplies primarily the cranial half of the animal, whereas that flowing into the main continuation of the aorta (arch and then thoracic aorta) supplies the caudal half of the animal.

and blood vessels. These thin-walled vessels are only large enough in diameter to accommodate a single file of erythrocytes. The wall acts as a selectively permeable membrane that permits water, oxygen, and nutrients to leave the blood for tissue cells and permits waste products from tissue cells to enter the blood. Much of the fluid that passes out of the capillaries into tissue spaces again returns to the blood by passing back through the capillary walls. Some fluid remains in the tissues, and excess fluid normally is removed by lymph vessels.

Capillaries unite to form venules, which merge into larger and larger veins. Veins are larger in diameter than the arteries they parallel and have much thinner walls. Venous blood pressure is typically quite low. Movement of body parts, whose muscles squeeze blood back toward the heart, assists flow of blood through the veins. Valves, usually consisting of two cusps each, are scattered at irregular intervals throughout the venous and lymphatic systems. A valve frequently is present where two or more veins unite to form a larger vein. The valves ensure a unidirectional flow of venous blood toward the heart.

Lymphatic Vessels

The walls of capillaries are thin enough to permit fluid as well as nutrients and gases to escape into spaces between tissue cells. Some of this extracellular fluid (ECF) does not reenter capillaries or veins directly but is picked up by thin-walled lymphatic vessels. Lymphatic vessels resemble veins in that they contain numerous valves permitting flow only toward the heart. The smallest lymphatic vessels are blind capillary-sized structures that begin in intercellular spaces, where they accumulate extracellular fluid. Fluid within the lymphatic vessels, called **lymph,** is transported to larger and larger lymph vessels and finally emptied into the cranial vena cava or one of its tributaries. The **tracheal trunks,** two large lymph vessels draining the head and neck, usually terminate in the jugular veins. Lymph from the caudal half of the body is delivered to the large **thoracic duct** (of which there may be one or two), which traverses the thoracic cavity adjacent to the aorta to empty its lymph into the cranial vena cava.

Movement of lymph is driven largely by gravity or changing pressures of adjacent structures. For example, contraction of a muscle applies pressure to the adjacent lymphatic vessels and forces the lymph farther toward the heart, since the valves prevent backflow. The lymph is filtered by nodular structures called lymph nodes (see Chapter 16) scattered along the course of most lymphatic vessels.

Pulmonary Circulation

The pulmonary circulation is the part of the vascular system that circulates the blood through the lungs (Fig. 17–5). Deoxygenated blood is delivered into the pulmonary system by contraction of the right ventricle. After passing into the pulmonary trunk, blood enters the right pulmonary artery to go to the right lung and the left pulmonary artery to go to the left lung. Each pulmonary artery subdivides into **lobar arteries** going to individual lobes of the lungs. The lobar arteries again subdivide many times, finally forming arterioles that supply the extensive capillary beds of the lungs, where gaseous exchange takes place (see Chapter 19). After the blood passes through the capillary bed of the lungs, it enters venules, which combine to form pulmonary veins. These pulmonary veins, after leaving the lungs, deliver oxygenated blood to the left atrium, completing the pulmonary circulation.

As gases are exchanged, the color of the blood changes from the bluish color of deoxygenated blood to the bright red of oxygenated blood. In the adult the pulmonary circulation is the only place where deoxygenated blood is found in arteries (which, by definition, carry blood away from the heart) and oxygenated blood is found in veins (returning blood to the heart).

Systemic Circulation

Systemic circulation refers to the movement of oxygenated blood to all areas of the body and the return of deoxygenated blood to the heart (Fig. 17–5). The following descriptions of the blood vessels of the systemic circulation are based mainly on the horse (Fig. 17–6). Animals having different digestive systems, such as ru-

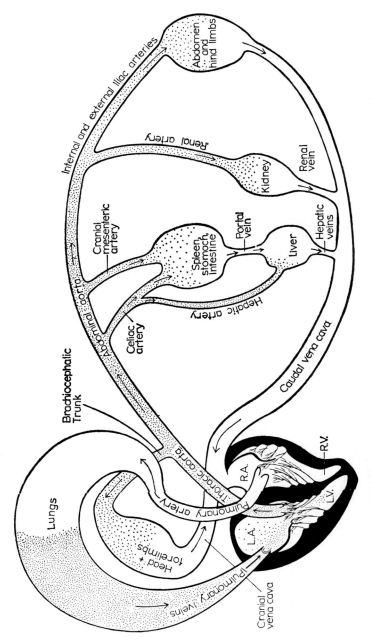

Figure 17-5. General scheme of important vascular beds in the adult animal. *Stippling* indicates high oxygenation; in this diagram the left atrium and ventricle are depicted on the left. Note the hepatic portal system associated with the viscera.

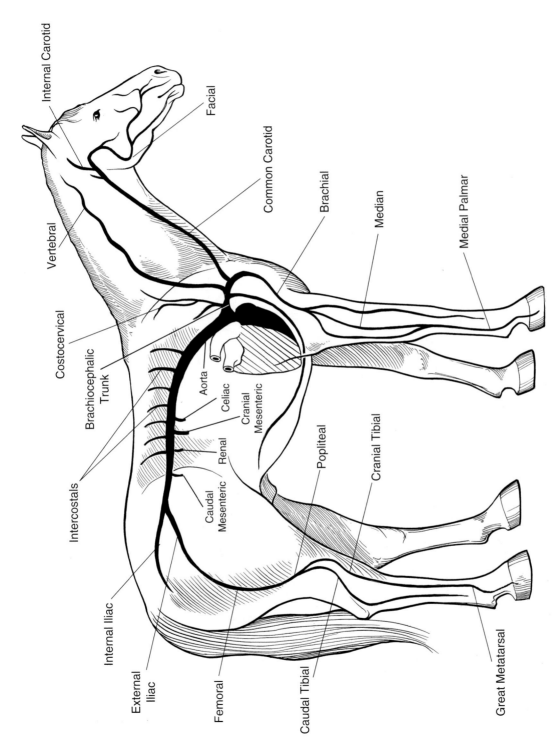

Figure 17-6. Main arteries of the horse.

Internal Carotid

Facial

Common Carotid

Brachial

Median

Medial Palmar

Vertebral

Costocervical

Brachiocephalic Trunk

Aorta

Celiac

Cranial Mesenteric

Renal

Caudal Mesenteric

Poptiteal

Cranial Tibial

Intercostals

Internal Iliac

External Iliac

Femoral

Caudal Tibial

Great Metatarsal

minants, and those having more than one digit per limb of course have a somewhat different arrangement of arteries and veins in association with their specific anatomy.

Aorta

Aortic Arch. The left ventricle receives oxygenated blood from the left atrium and pumps the blood throughout the systemic circulation by way of the largest artery, the *aorta.* The aortic valve, at the junction of the left ventricle and aorta, prevents backflow of blood from the aorta into the left ventricle when the ventricle relaxes.

Two large vessels arise from the aorta immediately distal to the aortic valve. These are the right and left *coronary arteries,* and they are the arterial blood supply for the myocardium. Most of the venous blood from the myocardium is returned to the right atrium by way of the *coronary veins,* which empty directly into the right atrium by way of the *coronary sinus,* adjacent to the opening of the caudal vena cava.

After emerging from the base of the heart, the *aortic arch* courses dorsad and then caudad, just ventral to the bodies of the thoracic vertebrae. The aorta continues as the *thoracic aorta* until it passes through the aortic hiatus of the diaphragm to become the *abdominal aorta.* Arteries that supply the head, neck, and thoracic limbs branch from the aortic arch.

In horses and ruminants, the aortic arch gives rise to a single large *brachiocephalic trunk,* whose many branches distribute blood to the cranial half of the animal. The precise pattern of the main arterial branches is species dependent, but the following generalities can be made: (1) The main blood supply to the thoracic limbs arises as right and left *subclavian arteries.* (2) The right and left *costocervical trunks* provide arterial blood to regions of the neck and cranial thoracic wall. (3) Right and left *common carotid arteries,* a main source of blood for the head and brain, arise from a single *bicarotid trunk.*

Thoracic Aorta. The *thoracic aorta* passes caudad just ventral to the vertebral bodies. As it does so, pairs of segmental arteries arise from its dorsal aspect to supply the thoracic wall and

epaxial muscles. Each of these *dorsal intercostal arteries* enters the corresponding intercostal space, giving off a *spinal branch* that enters the vertebral canal to supply the spinal cord and spinal nerve roots. The continuation of the dorsal intercostal artery follows the caudal border of each rib ventrad. Other branches of the thoracic aorta supply parts of the esophagus, lungs, and diaphragm.

Abdominal Aorta. The aorta is called the *abdominal aorta* after it passes through the *aortic hiatus* of the diaphragm. Ventral to the last few lumbar vertebrae, it terminates by dividing into two *external iliac arteries* (supplying the pelvic limbs) and two *internal iliac arteries* (supplying the gluteal and perineal region). Some species have a *median sacral artery,* a small midline continuation of the aorta that continues ventral to caudal vertebrae as the *median caudal artery.* The accompanying *median caudal vein* (tail vein) at this site is often used for collection of blood from adult cattle.

The abdominal aorta features paired *lumbar arteries* arising from its dorsal side, supplying the abdominal wall and epaxial muscles and giving off *spinal branches* that supply the spinal cord and spinal nerve roots of the lumbosacral region. Paired visceral branches provide arterial blood to the kidneys (*renal arteries*) and gonads (*testicular* or *ovarian arteries*). Three unpaired visceral branches supply nearly all the abdominal viscera. These are, from cranial to caudal, the *celiac, cranial mesenteric,* and *caudal mesenteric arteries.*

The *celiac artery* arises shortly after the aorta passes through the diaphragm. This is a large unpaired artery that supplies the stomach (*gastric artery*), the spleen (*splenic artery*), and the liver (*hepatic artery*). The exact branching pattern of this artery depends to a great extent upon the type of stomach; the ruminant has a much more complex distribution of the celiac artery than do animals with a simple stomach.

Immediately caudal to the celiac artery is the *cranial mesenteric artery.* This large, unpaired artery branches into a number of smaller arteries that supply blood to most of the small intestine and much of the large intestine. The number and distribution of the branches of the cranial mesenteric artery vary among species.

The caudal part of the large intestine and the rectum receive blood from a relatively small unpaired artery, the **caudal mesenteric artery.**

Arterial Distribution to the Head

Most of the structures of the face, head, and cranial neck are supplied by the right and left **common carotid arteries,** each of which runs craniad in a connective tissue sheath with the vagosympathetic trunk of the same side (Fig. 17–7, *A*). This **carotid sheath** lies in a groove dorsolateral to the trachea. Branches of the common carotid arteries supply the thyroid gland and larynx. In the region of the larynx, the common carotid artery gives off the **internal carotid artery,** a primary source of blood for the brain. The continuation of the common carotid artery is the **external carotid artery,** whose many branches supply the face, tongue, and structures of the oral and nasal cavities. The *facial artery* is convenient for taking a pulse as it passes across the mandible.

The internal carotid arteries or their derivatives enter into an anastomotic ring of vessels on the base of the brain called the **cerebral arterial circle** (formerly circle of Willis) (Fig. 17–7, *B*). The cerebral arterial circle gives rise to arteries that supply the cerebral hemispheres and rostral parts of the brainstem. More caudal parts of the brainstem and the cerebellum receive most of their blood supply from branches of the **basilar artery.** This single ventral artery is formed by the joining of right and left **vertebral arteries.** The robust vertebral arteries ascend from their origin in the thoracic inlet, run alongside the cervical vertebrae, enter the foramen magnum of the skull, and there coalesce into the basilar artery (coursing rostrad) and the **ventral spinal artery** (running caudad).

Arterial Distribution to the Thoracic Limb

The right and left subclavian arteries follow the same course on each side of the body, and each gives off similar branches. Within the thorax each subclavian artery gives off a number of branches that supply blood to the caudal part of the neck, much of the thoracic wall, and the dorsal part of

the shoulder. The subclavian artery passes cranial to the first rib on the respective side, passing into the axilla (armpit) of the thoracic limb, where it is called the **axillary artery.** The axillary artery enters the limb, becoming the **brachial artery** in the region of the brachium and then the **median artery** as it continues distal to the elbow. The largest terminal branch of the median artery in the horse is the **medial palmar artery,** which passes distad in the metacarpus to the fetlock, where it divides into medial and lateral **digital arteries.** In ruminants, the median artery is continued in the manus as the **palmar common digital artery** (Fig. 17–8).

Arterial Distribution to the Pelvic Limb

The internal iliac arteries are the most medial terminations of the abdominal aorta. Each internal iliac artery and its many branches supply the region of the pelvis, the hip, and much of the genitalia.

The external iliac arteries branch to caudoventral parts of the abdominal wall and structures of the inguinal region (prepuce, scrotum, and/or mammary gland), then continue into the pelvic limbs as the **femoral arteries.** The femoral artery descends on the medial aspect of the limb, giving branches to the large thigh muscles. The femoral artery continues in the region of the caudal part of the stifle joint as the **popliteal artery.** After a very short course, the popliteal artery divides into **cranial** and **caudal tibial arteries.** The caudal tibial artery supplies the muscles of the crus, or true leg. The cranial tibial artery is larger; it passes forward between the tibia and fibula and descends on the cranial side of the crus to the hock. Where this vessel lies on the flexon suface of the hock, it is referred to as the dorsal pedal artery. In horses, it continues distad as the dorsal (great) metatarsal a. III, running in the groove between the cannon bone and lateral splint. Ultimately, it passes to the plantar aspect of the distal cannon bone by crossing laterad, deep to the splint bone. At the equine fetlock it divides into medial and lateral **digital arteries,** the primary blood supply to the foot. In ruminants, the dorsal pedal artery continues distad on the dorsal aspect of the pes; the plantar side is supplied by a continuation of

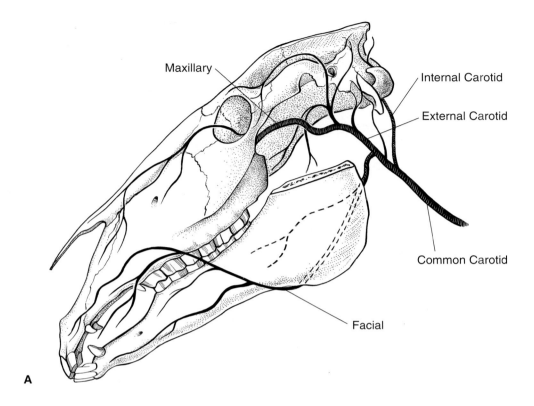

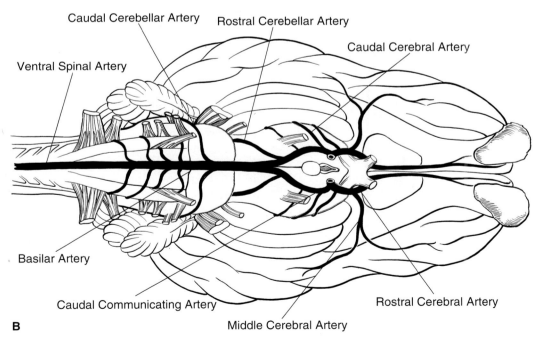

Figure 17-7. Blood supply to the head and brain. *A)* The common carotid artery branches into a large external carotid artery supplying most of the head and the internal carotid artery, which enters the skull to supply the brain. *B)* Ventral view of the brain. Internal carotid arteries enter the cerebral arterial circle.

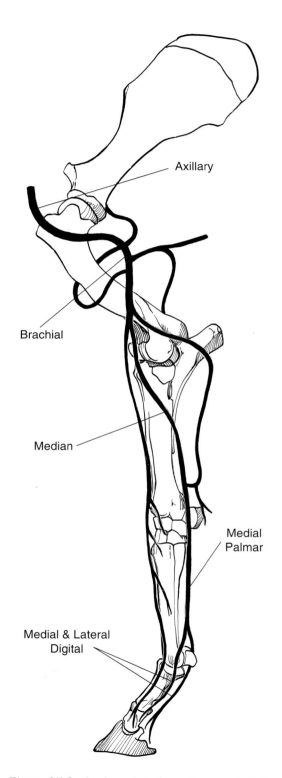

Figure 17-8. Blood supply to the equine thoracic limb medial view.

the **saphenous artery,** a medial branch of the femoral artery (Fig. 17–9).

Veins

With some notable exceptions, veins accompany arteries of the same name. These satellite veins are always larger than their respective arteries and frequently more numerous. For example, the brachial artery carrying blood to the forearm and digit may be accompanied by two or more brachial veins returning the blood to the heart. Often veins are more superficial (closer to the skin) than their respective arteries. As indicated earlier, nearly all systemic veins eventually drain into either the cranial vena cava or caudal vena cava.

Cranial Vena Cava

The cranial vena cava drains the head, neck, thoracic limbs, and part of the thorax. Tributaries to the cranial vena cava include the **jugular veins** (internal and external), **subclavian veins,** and **vertebral veins.** The external jugular veins drain the face and much of the head, while the internal jugular veins, if present, along with the vertebral veins, drain most of the blood from the brain. Each subclavian vein receives venous blood from the same areas that are supplied by the subclavian artery and its branches (shoulder, neck, and thoracic limbs). The azygos vein (the word *azygos* derives from Greek words meaning *unpaired*) lies adjacent to the vertebral column, receiving the segmentally arranged intercostal veins. In horses, the **right azygos vein** empties at the junction between cranial vena cava and right atrium. Ruminants sometimes have both right and left azygos veins but more usually have a single **left azygos vein,** which empties directly into the right atrium with the coronary sinus.

Caudal Vena Cava

The caudal vena cava is formed in the abdomen by the junction of the paired **internal iliac veins** and **external iliac veins.** These drain the gluteal and perineal regions and the pelvic limbs, re-

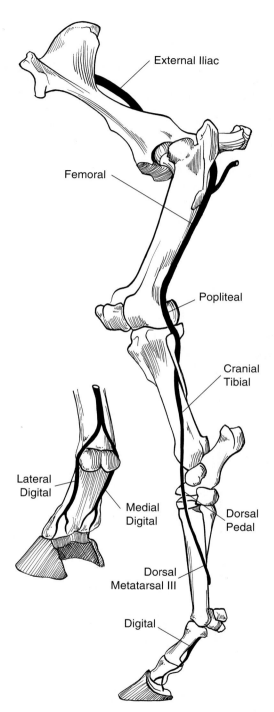

External Iliac

Femoral

Popliteal

Cranial
Tibial

Lateral
Digital

Medial
Digital

Dorsal
Pedal

Dorsal
Metatarsal III

Digital

Figure 17-9. Arteries of the pelvic limb in the horse. Primary arterial supply to the pes of the horse is the dorsal metatarsal artery III.

spectively. The caudal vena cava also receives *lumbar veins, testicular* or *ovarian veins, renal veins,* and various others from structures associated with the body walls. Just caudal to the point at which the caudal vena cava passes through the **caval foramen** of the diaphragm, it receives a number of short **hepatic veins** directly from the liver.

Portal System

A **portal system** is one in which a vessel divides into capillaries, recombines to form another vessel, and then redivides into a second capillary bed. The hypothalamohypophysial portal system was described in Chapter 12 in relation to the pituitary gland. In birds and in some reptiles and amphibians, part of the venous blood returning from the pelvic limbs enters the kidneys to form a renal portal system.

In the **hepatic portal system,** blood that has perfused the capillary beds of the viscera is brought to the liver by a single large vein, the **portal vein,** and there is redistributed into a second capillary bed within the substance of the liver (Fig. 17–5).

Tributaries to the portal vein include the **gastric vein** from the stomach, the **splenic vein** from the spleen, the **mesenteric veins** from the intestines, and the **pancreatic veins** from the pancreas. The portal vein enters the liver and immediately breaks up into smaller and smaller branches in the liver, finally ending in the **sinusoids** (capillary network) of the liver. Here the blood comes into direct contact with cells of the liver. After being acted upon by the liver cells (see Chapter 21), the blood passes from the sinusoids of the liver into the liver's venous system and eventually empties into the caudal vena cava.

Fetal Circulation

Throughout gestation, the fetus depends on the dam for the nutrients, water, and oxygen needed for growth and for the elimination of carbon dioxide and other waste products of fetal metabolism. During fetal development, the lungs are collapsed and not aerated, and the pulmonary vascular beds have high resistance to blood flow. The fetal circulation therefore bypasses these pulmonary capillary beds. Immediately after birth, however, the newborn needs to direct its blood through the pulmonary vessels for oxygenation. The heart and circulatory system are arranged in such an ingenious way that cardiopulmonary circulation just moments after birth is profoundly different from that exhibited just prior to the first breath (Fig. 17–10).

Because it is exchanging gas, supplying nutrients, and removing metabolic waste products, the placenta must necessarily receive a large proportion of the fetus's circulating blood.

It does so via two large **umbilical arteries,** extending from the caudal end of the abdominal aorta through the umbilical cord to the placenta. After passing through the placental capillaries, the blood is returned to the fetus by a single **umbilical vein,** which passes into the substance of the liver. Most of the highly oxygenated blood returning from the placenta in the umbilical vein is delivered into the caudal vena cava via a fetal bypass, the **ductus venosus.**

Associated with the heart are two features that allow blood to bypass the pulmonary circulation. During cardiogenesis, the wall be-

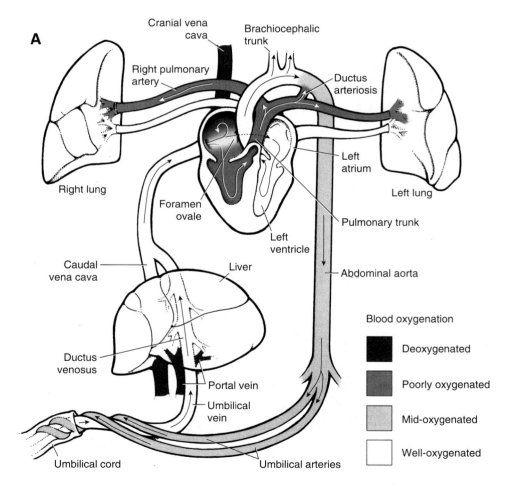

Figure 17-10. Transition between fetal (*A*) and adult (*B*) circulation. Fetal modifications include the foramen ovale, ductus arteriosus, umbilical vessels, and the ductus venosus. After birth, the ductus arteriosus and ductus venosus collapse and become ligamentous, the foramen ovale closes, and the umbilical vessels become round ligaments. (Reprinted with permission from Smith B.J. *Canine Anatomy.* Baltimore: Lippincott Williams & Wilkins, 1999.) (*continued*)

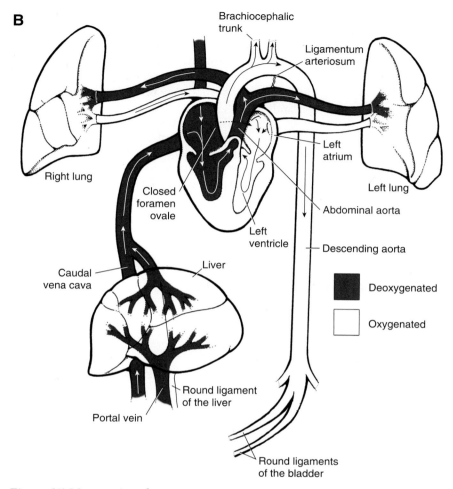

B

Figure 17-10—*continued*

tween the two atria develops a flutter valve. This aperture is called the ***foramen ovale,*** and its structure is such that the blood entering the right atrium (well oxygenated, as a goodly portion of it is returning from the placenta) finds the one-way flutter valve of the foramen ovale a convenient passageway from right to left atrium. This is one way blood bypasses the fetal lungs.

Second, blood flowing from the right ventricle into the pulmonary trunk bypasses the pulmonary arteries through the ***ductus arteriosus,*** which connects the pulmonary trunk and the aorta. In the fetus, the pressures in the right side of the heart are greater than those of the left side, since relatively little blood is returning from the lungs to the left side. As a result, the pres-

sure is higher in the pulmonary trunk than the aorta, and blood therefore passes across the ductus arteriosus from the trunk to the aorta, bypassing the pulmonary circulation.

At birth, when the neonate takes its first breath and inflates its lungs, the resistance in the pulmonary capillary bed falls precipitously. The increase in oxygenation of the newborn's blood constricts the ductus arteriosus. Within a few minutes, this formerly large vessel has shrunk drastically. Within the first week of life, it closes completely, becoming a fibrous band, the ***ligamentum arteriosum,*** identifiable grossly between the pulmonary trunk and the aorta.

These changes abruptly increase blood flow

to the now low-resistance pulmonary capillary beds. This abrupt increase in flow to the lungs produces a dramatic increase in blood returning to the left atrium, and as a consequence, pressures in the left side of the heart increase markedly. Greater blood pressure in the left atrium squeezes shut the foramen ovale, and blood no longer flows between the two atria.

A ductus arteriosus that fails to close is a *patent ductus arteriosus (PDA)*. In PDA, the conduit between the low-pressure pulmonary trunk and the high-pressure aorta persists, and blood passes from the aorta into the pulmonary circulation. This overperfuses the pulmonary capillary beds and increases the amount of blood returning to the left atrium, which dilates (is stretched). The left A-V valve is often affected by left atrial dilation in such a way as to allow regurgitation of blood. The overdistension of the left atrium is compounded, and pulmonary congestion may result.

Other modifications of circulation outside of the heart and great vessels take place at birth. One of the most obvious changes is that the placenta loses its role as oxygenator and provider of nutrients. The vasculature associated with it (umbilical arteries and veins) collapses and converts into fibrous cords (***round ligaments***) that are sometimes identifiable grossly in the adult.

Chapter 18

PHYSIOLOGY OF THE HEART AND CIRCULATION

Basic Design and Function of the Cardiovascular System

The ***cardiovascular system*** consists of the heart and the many vessels through which blood flows. While the actual anatomy of the system makes it difficult to appreciate easily, the basic design of the system is a continuous loop of branching vessels with two pumps in the loop (Fig. 18–1). The loop design can be best understood by tracing the path of a single erythrocyte as it travels. When the erythrocyte is pumped out of the left side of the heart, it enters the aorta and passes into the systemic circulation. (The ***systemic circulation*** is a subdivision of the cardiovascular system consisting of all vessels associated with all organs other than the parts of the lungs where exchange of gases (oxygen and carbon dioxide) takes place.) When blood returns from the systemic circulation, it enters the right side of the heart. The right side of the heart pumps blood into the pulmonary circulation. (The ***pulmonary circulation*** consists of vessels associated with the parts of the lungs where the exchange of gases takes place.) From the pulmonary circulation, blood reenters the heart on the left side, and from here it is pumped out into the systemic circulation to begin the loop again. The loop design means that all components of the system must function together in a highly coordinated and integrated fashion to maintain blood flow throughout the system. For example,

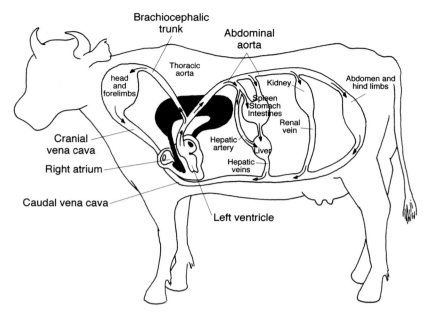

Figure 18-1. General design of cardiovascular system illustrating the systemic and pulmonary circulations. Pulmonary circulation is shown in black. (Reprinted with permission from Reece W.O. *Physiology of Domestic Animals.* 2nd ed. Baltimore: Williams & Wilkins, 1997.)

if the right side of the heart cannot pump an adequate amount of blood into the pulmonary circulation, the left side of the heart will not receive enough blood to maintain flow into the systemic circulation.

Blood flows through the vessels of the cardiovascular system because of a driving force generated by the contraction of the heart. A measurement of this driving force is the **hydrostatic pressure,** or **mean blood pressure,** in vessels. (Chapter 2 explains hydrostatic pressure.) Blood flows from a point of high mean pressure to a point of low mean pressure. In the systemic circulation, mean blood pressure is higher in the arteries than in the capillaries and higher in the capillaries than in the veins, from which blood reenters the right side of the heart (Fig. 18–1). A series of one-way valves described in Chapter 17 regulates blood flow though the heart.

The driving force of blood pressure is necessary to overcome the **vascular resistance** provided by the blood vessels. Any tube offers a resistance to the flow of liquid through it. The resistance (R) to flow through a **single tube** depends on the **length** (L) of the tube, the **radius** (r) of the tube, and the character of the fluid

flowing through the tube (viscosity, η). The resistance increases with the length of the tube, decreases as the radius of the tube increases, and increases with the **viscosity** of the fluid. While all three factors can affect resistance, changes in the radius have the largest effect, as shown in the following formula. (Poiseuille first described this formula and the mathematical relations between these factors.)

$$R = \frac{8\eta L}{\pi r^4}$$

According to this formula alone, the vessels with the smallest radius, the capillaries, would have the greatest resistance. This is true for a single vessel, but it is not true when considering the total combined resistance for the different types of vessels in the systemic circulation. Rather, the vessels on the arterial side of the circulation just before the capillaries have the greatest combined resistance. The total resistance at the level of the capillaries is less because of the extensive branching in capillary networks. Branching of vessels tends to lower resistance, and the extensive branching of capillaries in their networks is responsible for a relatively low resistance at this point in spite of the small diameter of an individual capillary. The type of arterial vessel found just outside of a capillary network (before the extensive branching) is an **arteriole,** and these vessels contribute most to the **total vascular resistance** in the systemic circulation.

Transport is the ultimate function of the cardiovascular system. Blood is the transport medium; the heart provides the force for moving blood (i.e., pump function) around the circulation; and vessels provide a path for the movement and permit exchange between blood and interstitial fluids at the level of the capillaries. The rate of transport and exchange is usually determined by the rate of blood flow through the capillaries.

Cardiac Cycle

The **cardiac cycle** is one complete cycle of cardiac contraction and relaxation (heartbeat). The events of the cardiac cycle occur in a specific sequence, and for descriptive purposes, the continuous cycle is divided into phases or periods marked by different events. Figure 18–2 illustrates the changes in blood pressures and volumes in the left atrium, left ventricle, and aorta during the cardiac cycle and identifies some phases of the cycle. The sequence of changes in blood pressures and volumes in the right atrium, right ventricle, and pulmonary trunk are similar and occur in the same sequence, but the magnitude of pressure changes in the right ventricle and pulmonary trunk are much lower. The unique characteristics of the pulmonary circulation are discussed in Chapter 19.

Diastole (dilation, from Gr. *dia,* apart; *stello,* place or put) refers to the relaxation of a chamber of the heart just prior to and during the filling of that chamber. **Systole** (contraction, from Gr. *syn,* together; *stello,* place) refers to the contraction of a chamber of the heart that drives blood out of the chamber. The adjectives *atrial* and *ventricular* can be used with *diastole* or *systole* to describe the activity of specific cardiac chambers (e.g., atrial systole refers to atrial contraction). However, *diastole* and *systole* are also classically used to describe the two most general phases of the cardiac cycle (Fig. 18–2),

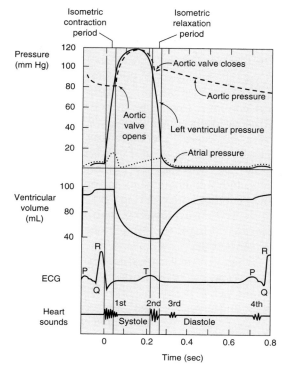

Figure 18-2. Timing of various events of the cardiac cycle. (Reprinted with permission from Porth C.M. *Pathophysiology.* 5th ed. Philadelphia: Lippincott Williams & Wilkins, 1998.)

which are based on the activity of the ventricles. So when the heart is said to be in systole or the **systolic phase** of the cardiac cycle, it is usually understood that this refers to ventricular systole.

Two distinct heart sounds can be heard during each cardiac cycle in all domestic species, and these are typically described as lub (first sound, or S_1) and dub (second sound, or S_2). These sounds are separated by a short interval and followed by a longer pause. The pause increases with slower heart rates. These sounds are used clinically to divide the cardiac cycle into systole and diastole. The first sound marks the beginning of systole, and the second sound marks the beginning of diastole (Fig. 18.2).

Systole

As the ventricles begin their contraction, blood pressure increases in them. Almost immediately the pressure within each ventricle exceeds the pressure within their respective atria, and the pressure differences force the A-V valves closed. The first heart sound is associated with closure of the right and left A-V valves (Fig. 18–2).

The ventricles continue to contract and pressure continues to increase during the early part of systole. At this point in the cycle, all four heart valves are closed, and all remain closed until pressure in the ventricles exceeds that in the arterial vessels that they supply (aorta for left ventricle and pulmonary trunk for right ventricle). The period of systole during which all valves are closed is the **isovolumetric contraction period,** because during it the volume of each ventricle remains constant.

When ventricular pressures exceed those in their respective arterial vessels, the semilunar valves open to permit ejection of blood. There is no sound associated with the opening of the semilunar valves. An initial **rapid ejection phase** of systole is followed by a reduced ejection phase, during which ventricular and arterial pressures fall (Fig. 18–2).

The elasticity of the aorta and pulmonary trunk maintains blood pressure in these vessels even though the ventricles begin to relax. When the blood pressures in these vessels are greater than the pressures in their associated ventricles, the pressure differences close the semilunar valves. The second heart sound is associated with closure of the aortic and pulmonary valves, and this sound is used to mark the end of systole and the beginning of diastole (Fig. 18–2).

Stroke volume is the volume of blood ejected from each ventricle during a single cardiac cycle. Normally the stroke volumes for the right and left ventricles are the same. If these are not equal, blood tends to accumulate in either the systemic or pulmonary circulation.

Diastole

At the beginning of diastole, both the semilunar and A-V valves are closed, so the initial phase is termed **isovolumetric relaxation.** When ventricular relaxation reaches the point that atrial blood pressures exceeds ventricular blood pressures, the pressure differences open the A-V valves. While the A-V valves are closed during systole and early diastole, blood continues to

flow into the right and left atria from the systemic and pulmonary circulations, respectively. The accumulation of blood within the atria increases atrial blood pressure. When the A-V valves open, much of the accumulated blood flows rapidly into the ventricles. Most ventricular filling occurs during this period prior to any atrial contraction (Fig. 18–2).

Blood continues to flow into the atria throughout diastole, and because the A-V valves are open, blood flows directly through the atria into the ventricles. As mentioned earlier, diastole is the phase of the cardiac cycle that lengthens most with slow heart rates, so slow heart rates provide a long period for ventricular filling.

Atrial contraction (atrial systole) occurs during ventricular diastole, forcing an additional volume of blood into the ventricles, but this amount is relatively small (perhaps 15%) compared to the volume already in the ventricles.

The volume of blood in each ventricle at the end of diastole is the **end-diastolic volume (EDV).** During systole each ventricle ejects only a percentage of its EDV (Fig. 18–2), typically 40–60%. The percentage of the EDV that is ejected is the **ejection fraction.**

Heart Sounds and Murmurs

The first and second heart sounds are associated with valve closures, but turbulent blood flow and vibrations of large vessels induced by the closures are believed to be the actual causes of the sounds. Third and fourth heart sounds may be heard in some normal horses and cattle with relatively slow heart rates. The third sound is associated with the rapid ventricular filling phase after the initial opening of the A-V valves, and the fourth sound is associated with atrial contractions (Fig. 18–2).

Heart murmur is a general term for any abnormal heart sound. Abnormalities in heart valves are a common cause of murmurs. Murmurs may occur when a valve fails to close completely (valvular insufficiency) and blood flow goes in the wrong direction at the wrong time. Murmurs may also occur when a valve fails to open completely (valvular stenosis) and blood is forced through a smaller than normal opening.

Echocardiography

Echocardiography is the use of ultrasound to image the heart and associated structures. It is a noninvasive procedure that provides dynamic images permitting visualization of structures in the heart as it contracts and relaxes. This provides much more information on cardiac function than can be obtained with a single static image, such as a radiograph.

Electrical Activity of the Heart

Like skeletal muscle, contraction of each cardiac muscle cell requires an action potential on the cell membrane, and the action potential brings about the release of calcium from intracellular stores (Fig. 18–3a). The calcium binds to regulatory proteins on the thin filaments, and movement of the regulatory proteins permits an interaction between actin and myosin to bring about contraction (see Chapter 8). However, unlike skeletal muscle, each cardiac muscle cell is not innervated by a motor neuron that is responsible for eliciting an initial action potential. In the heart, the initial action potential occurs spontaneously in a specialized group of myocardial cells found in the **sinoatrial (SA) node** of the heart, from which the action potential is propagated around the heart to bring about contraction of all cardiac muscle cells. The cell-to-cell propagation in the heart is possible because the intercalated disks provide an electrical connection between myocardial cells (Fig. 1–6).

Sinoatrial Node and Heart Rate

Figure 18–3b shows a series of action potentials from SA node cells. A unique feature of the electrical activity of these cells is that the resting membrane potential is unstable. This instability permits SA node cells to depolarize spontaneously to threshold, where an action potential is generated. The SA node (Fig. 18–4) is termed the **pacemaker** of the heart because each action potential that spontaneously develops in the SA node is propagated around the heart to stimulate action potentials in all myocardial cells and produce a contraction.

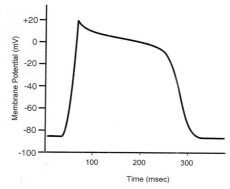

Figure 18-3a. Action potential of cardiac muscle contractile cell. Electrically-gated calcium channels in cell membrane are open during the prolonged plateau phase of the action potential to permit calcium ions to enter from the extracellular fluid. The entering calcium stimulates the release of more calcium from the sarcoplasmic reticulum. The initial depolarization phase involves electrically-gated sodium channels, and potassium channels are involved with membrane repolarization.

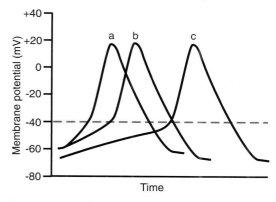

Figure 18-3b. Three sinoatrial cell membrane potentials and action potentials. Threshold voltage shown by *dotted line*. Resting potentials are unstable. Potential B is without neural stimulation; potential A represents sympathetic stimulation; and potential C represents parasympathetic stimulation. (Reprinted with permission from Rhoades R.A. and Tanner G.A. *Medical Physiology*. Boston: Little, Brown, 1995.)

Both sympathetic and parasympathetic nerves innervate the SA node. By their actions on cells in the SA node, sympathetic nerves increase the rate of spontaneous action potentials and parasympathetic nerves reduce the rate (Fig. 18–3b). This is the means by which sympathetic stimulation increases heart rate and parasympathetic stimulation reduces heart rate. Parasympathetic nerves continuously inhibit the SA node in the heart of a resting animal, and this constant inhibition is responsible for the resting heart rate. During light exercise or with excitement, the parasympathetic inhibition is reduced first to permit an increase in heart rate. With greater excitement or more intense exercise, sympathetic stimulation increases, further increasing heart rate. Highly trained athletic animals, such as racing thoroughbreds, have relatively high levels of parasympathetic stimulation to their hearts at rest.

Atrioventricular Node and Other Specialized Conductive Cells in the Heart

The **atrioventricular node** (A-V node) and the **common bundle,** or **bundle of His,** are also myocardial cells specialized for conducting action potentials. The A-V node is in the intraatrial septum, and the common bundle extends from the A-V node into the ventricle through the fi-

brous connective tissue of the **cardiac skeleton.** The cardiac skeleton separates the cardiac muscle of the atria and ventricles, so the only direct electrical connection is through the A-V node and common bundle. The common bundle divides into several branches that rapidly propagate action potentials throughout the ventricle (Fig. 18–4). The individual cells that make up these branches are the **Purkinje fibers.**

Cells of the A-V node are specialized to conduct action potentials more slowly than other myocardial cells. This characteristic allows enough time for the atria to depolarize completely and contract before action potentials spread into the ventricles to stimulate their contraction. The atrial contraction completes the filling of the ventricles so that ventricular contraction can eject a larger volume. The slow conduction through the A-V node is A-V node delay. Sympathetic and parasympathetic nerves that increase and reduce conduction velocity respectively also innervate the A-V node.

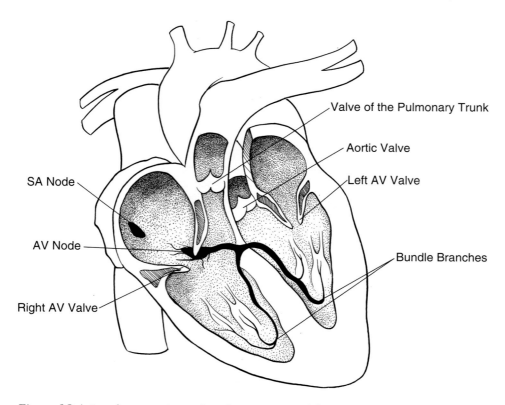

Figure 18-4. Impulse generation and conduction system of the mammalian heart.

Electrocardiography and Arrhythmias

Electrocardiography is the recording of electrical activity on the surface of the body that reflects the electrical activity in the heart. Recording electrodes are placed on the surface of the body at specific sites, and the recorded electrical activity reflects the summated electrical activity of the heart. Because of the specificity of the sites for the placement of electrodes, the patterns of electrical activity associated with a cardiac cycle are predictable, and comparisons can be made between animals. The **lead** is a specific combination of sites where the recording electrodes are placed on the body. An **electrocardiogram** is the actual recording.

Figure 18–5 shows a typical lead II (or limb lead II) electrocardiogram recorded from a dog. Major waves are P, Q, R, S, and T. The P wave is associated with atrial depolarization. The QRS complex is associated with ventricular depolarization, and the T wave is associated with ventricular repolarization. The period between the P and Q waves is associated with A-V node delay. On a typical recording from a normal dog, the waves range from 1 to 2 mV and 0.2 to 0.3 seconds. Differences in wave shape and size among species are due to normal differences in the pattern of conduction of action potentials around the heart.

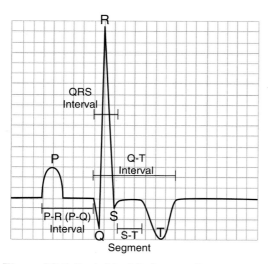

Figure 18-5. Typical lead II electrocardiogram.

Arrhythmia is a general term for any abnormality in cardiac electrical activity, including rate, rhythm, and the propagation of action potentials around the heart. Some apparently normal, healthy animals have a high incidence of cardiac arrhythmias in certain conditions. For example, it is fairly common for racing thoroughbreds to have an apparent abnormality in A-V node conduction at rest. This is characterized by a reduction in or inhibition of the conduction of action potentials through the A-V node. These disappear with exercise. A likely cause is a relatively high parasympathetic neural input to the heart at rest that damps A-V node conduction. The relatively high parasympathetic input is normally reduced with exercise.

Cardiac Output and Its Regulation

Cardiac output (**CO**) is the volume of blood pumped by a ventricle of the heart into its vessel per unit time, and it is the product of heart rate (HR) and stroke volume (SV): CO = HR × SV. The values for CO refer to the output of a single ventricle, but the outputs of the right and left ventricles should be equal. The regulation of HR is via autonomic nervous system regulation of the SA node, as described earlier, and this is one means by which CO is regulated. However, SV, the other determinant of CO, is also subject to change and regulation. The two major factors that can change SV are ventricular filling and cardiac contractility.

Ventricular Filling and Stroke Volume

Figure 18–6 illustrates the relation between end-diastolic volume (EDV) and the SV of the subsequent ventricular contraction. SV increases as EDV increases until an optimal EDV is reached. After that point, further increases in EDV are associated with reductions in SV. The cellular basis for this relation is not fully understood, but stretching of cardiac muscle appears to induce changes in the physical relationship between thin and thick filaments and in the affinity of regulatory proteins for calcium ions. These changes are associated with

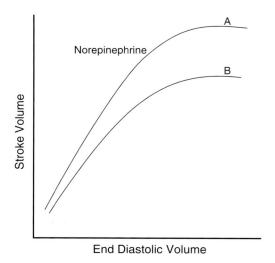

Figure 18-6. Relation between end-diastolic volume (EDV) and stroke volume (SV) in a normal heart with (A) and without (B) sympathetic stimulation.

stronger contractions until the muscle is over-stretched. The relation between stretching of cardiac muscle and force of contraction is known as the **Frank-Starling curve** or Frank-Starling law of the heart. In normal resting animals, the Frank-Starling curve is less than optimal, so increases in EDV can produce increases in SV and CO.

Ventricular filling depends on filling pressure (the blood pressure in the veins and cardiac atria that force blood into the ventricles), time for filling, and ventricular compliance (the ease with which the ventricle relaxes during filling). The filling pressure in turn depends on blood volume and constriction of the smooth muscle in veins (venoconstriction). An increase in blood volume or venoconstriction tends to increase filling pressure and EDV. Slow heart rates provide more time for filling and tend to increase EDV. Decreases in ventricular compliance tend to reduce ventricular filling, because more pressure is required to distend the ventricle during filling.

The **cardiac preload** is the force on the heart muscle prior to contraction, and one measure of it is the amount that cardiac muscle is stretched prior to contraction. In intact animals, ventricular filling pressure and EDV are used as indicators of preload.

Cardiac Contractility and Stroke Volume

The contraction force generated by individual myocardial cells can also be changed by a mechanism that is independent of the length to which cardiac muscle is stretched prior to contraction. This phenomenon is a change in **cardiac contractility;** it typically results from the direct action on myocardial cells of a hormone, neurotransmitter, or drug. Agents that can elicit changes in cardiac contractility are **inotropes.**

Norepinephrine and epinephrine are **positive inotropes,** because both increase cardiac contractility. Norepinephrine and epinephrine both bind to β-adrenergic receptors on myocardial cells, and subsequent to this binding, both elicit increases in the availability of intracellular calcium in stimulated myocardial cells. The increased calcium, as well as other changes in intracellular metabolism brought about by the β-adrenergic receptor stimulation, promotes an increase in the force of contraction. Other inotropes use different membrane receptors, but the intracellular events usually involve calcium availability or the affinity of intracellular proteins for calcium.

An indicator of myocardial contractility in the intact heart is the percentage of the EDV that is ejected during ventricular systole (i.e., **ejection fraction**). A typical value for ejection fraction in a resting animal is 40%. With sympathetic stimulation, this increases (Fig. 18–6), while with primary cardiac diseases it may reduce to 15–20%.

Structure and Function of Blood Vessels

Microscopic Structure of Blood Vessels

A single layer of endothelium, a simple squamous epithelium, lines all vessels. Capillaries are essentially endothelial tubes, but they differ notably among themselves in cell-to-cell junctions and the structure of individual endothelial cells. Tight junctions connect the endothelial cells of some capillaries, and this forms a relatively impermeable barrier to non–lipid-soluble particles. Other capillaries appear to be quite porous because of openings in the endothelial cells themselves, and these are found where high rates of capillary exchange occur.

A wall with three layers, or tunics, characterizes all types of veins and arteries. From innermost to outermost, these layers are the *tunica interna* (intima), *tunica media,* and *tunica externa* (adventitia) (Fig. 18–7). The tunica interna consists of the lining endothelium, a subendothelial layer primarily consisting of connective tissue, and in some cases, an **internal elastic membrane.** The internal elastic membrane consists of elastin and is especially prominent in large arteries.

The tunica media of all veins and arteries contains smooth muscle. Arteries have a much thicker tunica media than veins of a corresponding size, and this characteristic can be used to differentiate between the two types of vessels.

Elastic arteries are a special type whose tunica media contains concentric elastic laminae. The elastic properties of this type of artery permit vascular expansion and contraction during the various phases of the cardiac cycle. The aorta is an elastic artery that expands to increase its volume during ventricular systole and then rebounds during ventricular diastole to maintain relatively high arterial blood pressure. Arteries whose tunicae mediae consist primarily of smooth muscle are **muscular arteries.** An **external elastic membrane** is the outermost layer of the tunica media, but it is often difficult to visualize by light microscopy. **Arterioles,** the smallest of arteries, are found where arteries empty into a branching capillary network.

Some veins, and especially those in limbs below the level of the heart, have flaplike valves that consist of folds of the tunica interna. The fold forms a cuplike pocket with the free edge of

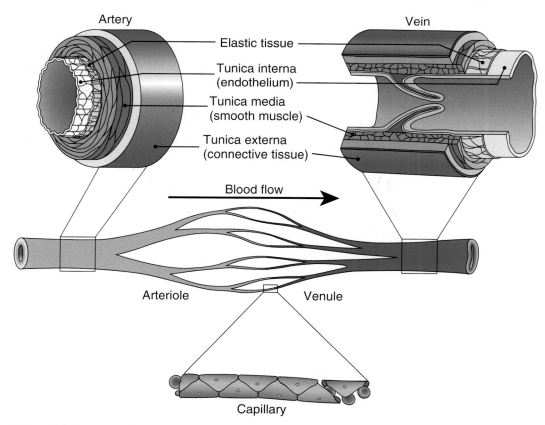

Figure 18-7. Section of small blood vessels showing the structure of their walls. A venous valve is also shown. (Reprinted with permission from Cohen B.J. and Wood D.L. *Memmler's The Human Body in Health and Disease.* 9th ed. Baltimore: Lippincott Williams & Wilkins, 2000.)

the fold directed toward the heart (Fig. 18–7). These one-way valves promote the flow of venous blood toward the heart when the vein is compressed.

Function of Blood Vessels

The arterial side of the circulation provides a ready supply of blood under relatively high hydrostatic pressure. Because of their relatively thick walls, arteries are not very compliant (i.e., do not distend easily with increases in pressure), so arterial pressure remains high as the heart pumps blood into the arteries. The arterioles at the end of the branching arterial network function as on-off valves to regulate the rate of blood flow from the arteries into capillary networks. **Sympathetic vasoconstrictor nerves** innervate the smooth muscle in the wall of most arterioles, and this is one mechanism by which blood flow is regulated. However, the degree of constriction of arteriolar smooth muscle is also subject to regulation by a large number of **vasoactive** agents, some locally produced (paracrine) and some that arrive via the systemic circulation. The paracrine agents (e.g., lactic acid, carbon dioxide, and adenosine) are typically vasodilators; they increase blood flow to the local area. Production of these agents increases when metabolism by cells in the local area increases, providing a means to match metabolic rate with blood flow. That is, an increase in metabolism brings about an increase in blood flow. The process by which local mechanisms regulate local blood flow is **autoregulation.**

Capillaries are the site of exchange between blood and the interstitial fluid that surrounds all cells. In most cases, this exchange is by simple diffusion (i.e., substances move down their concentration gradients). Gases (oxygen and carbon dioxide) and other lipid-soluble substances freely diffuse though capillary walls, but substances that are not lipid soluble, such as glucose, must diffuse through pores in the capillary wall. Exchange by diffusion does not necessarily require the movement of fluid between the capillary and the interstitial space. Oxygen, for example, can diffuse down its concentration gradient from the plasma to metabolizing cells as blood flows in a capillary past the cells. As stated earlier, the rate of capillary exchange is primarily governed by the rate of blood flow into the capillaries. In resting tissues, blood flow occurs only through a small percentage of the total capillaries at any one time. As metabolism and blood flow increase, the percentage of capillaries being perfused increases.

Typically there is a small net loss of fluid from the plasma as it flows through most capillary networks. This fluid is recovered via the lymphatics and ultimately returned to the blood where lymphatics enter large veins near the heart. A small number of plasma proteins are similarly lost from capillaries and returned via the lymph.

The forces that govern fluid movement at the capillary level are important clinically in that imbalances in these forces contribute to **edema,** an abnormal amount or collection of fluid in the interstitial space. The primary factor that forces fluid out of a capillary into the interstitial space is the blood pressure in the capillary. The primary force that tends to keep fluid in capillaries is the **effective osmotic force** (pressure) generated by plasma proteins, primarily albumin. This pressure is also termed **oncotic pressure.** Plasma proteins generate an effective osmotic force because the protein concentration in the interstitial fluid is much lower than that of plasma. At the arterial end of a capillary, the blood pressure is higher than the oncotic pressure, so some fluid is lost from the capillary, while at the venous end of a capillary the oncotic pressure is higher, so some fluid moves into the capillary (Fig. 18–8). A slight imbalance between fluid loss and fluid gain by the capillaries gives rise to a net loss and provides fluid for lymph formation.

Like arteries, veins have smooth muscle in their walls, but the walls of veins are much thinner and more compliant. The compliance of venous vessels permits relatively large changes in the volume of blood in the veins with minimal changes in venous blood pressure. Thus, the venous side of the circulation functions as a low-pressure reservoir of blood. Constriction of venous smooth muscle promotes an increase in blood flowing back to the heart and an increase in cardiac filling pressure. This contributes to increases in cardiac output and the ability to perfuse capillaries for exchange.

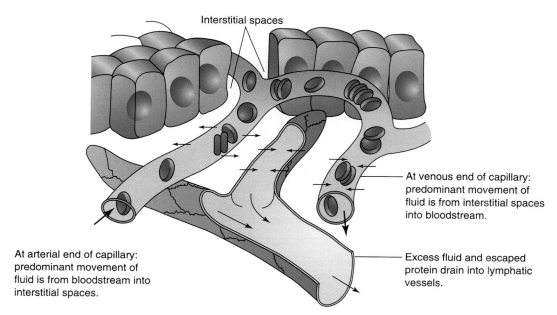

Interstitial spaces

At venous end of capillary:
predominant movement of
fluid is from interstitial spaces
into bloodstream.

At arterial end of capillary:
predominant movement of
fluid is from bloodstream into
interstitial spaces.

Excess fluid and escaped
protein drain into lymphatic
vessels.

Figure 18-8. Fluid exchanges through capillary wall and the formation and removal of interstitial fluid. (Reprinted with permission from Porth C.M. *Pathophysiology*. 5th ed. Philadelphia: Lippincott Williams & Wilkins, 1998.)

Regulation of Arterial Blood Pressure and Blood Volume

Arterial blood pressure is a function of cardiac output (CO) and *total peripheral vascular resistance* (TPR), usually written as MAP = CO × TPR, where MAP is mean arterial pressure. To understand the basis for this function, recall that arteries are relatively noncompliant and function as a reservoir of blood under pressure. The pressure depends on the amount of blood being pumped into the reservoir (CO) and the rate at which blood is permitted to flow out of the reservoir (Fig. 18–9). Recall also that the resistance of the arterioles, which contribute the most to the total vascular resistance, regulates the rate of blood flow out of the arteries. Thus, the level of cardiac function and the degree of arteriolar constriction are the two determinants of MAP. Changes in MAP can be brought about by changes in cardiac function, the degree of arteriolar constriction, or some combination of these determinants. Any chemical regulator (e.g., hormone or paracrine agent)

or neural reflex that affects cardiac activity or the smooth muscle of arterioles has the potential to alter blood pressure. The large number of therapeutic agents used to treat high blood pressure in humans and animals, and the different mechanisms by which these agents have their effects, illustrate the diversity of factors that can alter blood pressure.

In normal animals, blood volume and arterial blood pressure are directly related. Increases or decreases in blood volume tend to produce similar changes in cardiac output and therefore in arterial blood pressure. In light of this relation and the goal of biologic systems to maintain homeostasis, it is predictable that decreases in blood pressure elicit physiologic responses designed to increase blood volume and increases in blood pressure elicit responses designed to reduce blood volume. The organs primarily responsible for bringing about changes in blood volume are the kidneys. Thus, blood volume regulation by the kidneys is one factor in the ultimate determination of arterial blood pressure. Many of the chemical agents and neu-

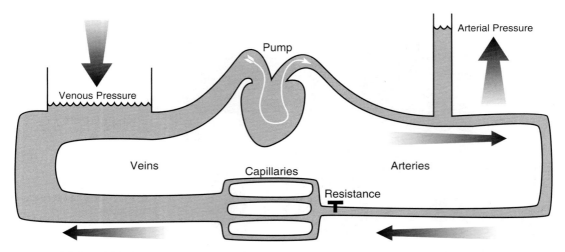

Figure 18-9. Model of circulatory system with pump supplying low compliance vessels (arteries), off-on valve vessels regulating outflow from arteries (arterioles), and low-pressure compliant vessels (veins) returning fluid to the pump. Height of fluid columns in arteries and veins indicates relative pressures in these vessels. Filling of the pump depends in part on the venous pressure.

ral reflexes that regulate mean arterial pressure by their action on the heart and blood vessels also affect the ability of the kidneys to regulate blood volume by altering the rate of urine formation.

This chapter discusses only some of the major regulators of arterial blood pressure and blood volume and for didactic purposes will classify these as neural reflexes, circulating (humoral) agents, and paracrine (locally produced) agents. This classification is a generalization; there are many subtle interactions among these classes that will not be explored in this text.

Neural Reflexes

The **arterial baroreceptor reflexes** are the neural reflexes primarily responsible for the short-term or immediate regulation of arterial blood pressure. Neural receptors in the aorta and carotid arteries respond to changes in arterial pressure in these vessels, and this information is relayed to reflex centers in the brainstem. The efferent nerves for these reflexes are the **autonomic nerves** to the heart and the **sympathetic vasoconstrictor nerves** to both arterioles and veins. Decreases in arterial blood pressure bring

about adjustments in these efferent nerves to increase heart rate, increase cardiac contractility, and promote arteriolar vasoconstriction and venoconstriction. The overall effect tends to increase both CO and TPR, so that blood pressure can be restored to its original level. Increases in arterial blood pressure above some original level should elicit reductions in cardiac activity and relaxation of the vessels. Inhibition of vasoconstrictor and venoconstrictor nerves is the mechanism by which the reflex permits relaxation of the vascular smooth muscle.

Neural receptors in the atria of the heart respond to changes in the volume of blood filling the atria, and afferent information from these receptors is relayed to brainstem reflex centers. The primary efferents involved in these reflexes are the sympathetic nerves to the kidneys. Increases in atrial filling bring about reductions in sympathetic nerve stimulation of the kidneys, and this permits an increase in the urinary excretion of sodium chloride and water. This tends to reduce blood volume and therefore cardiac filling, cardiac output, and blood pressure. Reductions in atrial filling bring about increases in sympathetic nerve activity to the kidneys. This reflex also affects the secretion of renin from the kidneys (discussed later).

Humoral Agents

Renin is an enzyme released from the kidneys, and its release is regulated in part by sympathetic nerve activity to the kidneys and arterial blood pressure in the vessels perfusing the kidneys. Increases in renal sympathetic nerve activity and/or reductions in arterial blood pressure to the kidneys elicit increases in renin secretion. Renin acts on a plasma protein substrate to produce a peptide, angiotensin I, which an enzyme converts to **angiotensin II**. Angiotensin II constricts vascular smooth muscle, so it tends to increase TPR and arterial blood pressure. Angiotensin II also reduces the urinary loss of sodium chloride and water by its action on tubules in the kidney and by promoting the release of **aldosterone** from the adrenal cortex. The overall biologic effect of angiotensin II is to increase arterial pressure and blood volume.

At rest, the plasma levels of epinephrine and norepinephrine are relatively low, so their effects on cardiac function and vascular smooth muscle are relatively minor. However, plasma levels can increase significantly in highly stressed animals or in response to severe reductions in blood pressure or blood volume. In these conditions, circulating epinephrine and norepinephrine promote increases in cardiac function and constrict vascular smooth muscle.

Atrial natriuretic peptides (ANPs) are released from the atria of the heart in response to increases in blood volume and atrial filling. ANPs promote an increase in the urinary excretion of sodium and water by a direct action on tubules in the kidney. ANPs also reduce TPR by relaxing arteriolar vascular smooth muscle that is constricted by vasoconstrictor agents.

Paracrine Agents

Endothelial cells lining many blood vessels produce and release **nitric oxide,** a local vasodilator. Nitric oxide release by endothelial cells is subject to regulation by a variety of agents, and the importance of its overall role in the regulation of TPR in normal animals is controversial. **Bacterial endotoxins are lipopolysaccharide components of the bacterial cell wall that are released when the cell is lysed. These endotoxins stimulate macrophages throughout an animal's body to produce and release unusually large amounts of nitric oxide. General overproduction of nitric oxide causes widespread vasodilation and a severe drop in arterial blood pressure. These cardiovascular changes are part of a clinical syndrome, *endotoxic* or *septic shock.***

Endothelial cells also secrete a peptide, **endothelin,** that constricts vascular smooth muscle of arterioles. As with nitric oxide, a variety of agents (e.g., angiotensin II and norepinephrine) are known to stimulate endothelin release. Interestingly, circulating vasoconstrictors tend to increase the release of this locally produced vasoconstrictor.

Cardiovascular Function During Exercise and Hypovolemia

Increases in cardiac output and rate of blood flow to skeletal muscle are needed during exercise to meet the increased metabolic needs of the active skeletal muscle. Several of the cardiovascular adjustments during exercise are learned responses or behavior responses that begin just prior to or at the initiation of exercise. These are apparently initiated by the cerebral cortex, involve autonomic nerves, and include an increased heart rate and vasodilation of arterioles supplying skeletal muscle. Increased circulating levels of epinephrine may also contribute to these changes. After exercise has begun, appropriate vasodilation of arterioles supplying active skeletal muscles is primarily maintained by local metabolites produced by the active muscles. Typically, the increase in cardiac function is greater than the degree of vasodilation, so arterial pressure rises slightly. Vascular resistance increases in other organs whose metabolism is not increased during exercise, and this prevents an increased blood flow to these organs. During exercise, the increased cardiac output (increased heart rate and contractility) is maintained by sympathetic stimulation of the heart. This sympathetic stimulation is primarily maintained by the mechanisms originating in the cerebral cortex and by reflexes based on afferent information originating in the exercising skeletal muscle.

Hypovolemia is abnormally decreased circulating fluid volume (i.e., blood volume). It can occur rapidly, as a result of hemorrhage, or slowly, as a result of dehydration. Reduced blood volume results in reduced cardiac filling pressure and ventricular filling (i.e., reduced end-diastolic volume). Without adequate filling, SV falls, and therefore cardiac output can be insufficient to maintain capillary perfusion throughout the body. A severe reduction in cardiac output drastically lowers blood pressure, eliciting a strong response by the baroreceptor reflex. An accelerated heart rate is part of this response. The reduced cardiac output and the intense peripheral vasoconstriction resulting from the reflex response both contribute to the characteristic blanching of mucus membranes. The reduced stroke volume is the major cause of weakening of the pulse.

Chapter 19

THE RESPIRATORY SYSTEM

Upper Respiratory Tract

Oxygen is a vital requirement of animals. An animal may survive for days without water or for weeks without food, but life without oxygen is measured in minutes. Delivering oxygen and removing carbon dioxide (the product of cellular respiration) are the two major functions of the respiratory system. The processes involved with these functions related to gases include ventilation (movement of air in and out of the lungs), gas exchange between air and blood in the lungs, gas transport in blood, and gas exchange between blood and cells at the level of the tissues.

Secondary functions of the respiratory system include assistance in the regulation of the pH of the body fluids, assistance in temperature control, and phonation (voice production). The role of the respiratory system in the regulation of the pH of blood and other body fluids is closely associated with the ability of the respiratory system to remove carbon dioxide. If carbon dioxide accumulates in the blood because the respiratory system cannot remove it, blood pH falls; this is ***respiratory acidosis.*** Blood pH rises if the respiratory system removes more carbon dioxide than is appropriate and blood levels of carbon dioxide are lower than normal; this is ***respiratory alkalosis.*** The changes in carbon dioxide and pH are closely linked because of the chemical reaction shown in the equation below. The bicarbonate ions and water molecules for this reaction are readily available in body fluids.

$$H_2O + CO_2 \leftrightarrow H^+ + HCO_3^-$$

The respiratory system consists essentially of the lungs and the passages that conduct air into and out of the lungs. These passages include the nostrils, nasal cavity, pharynx, larynx, trachea, and bronchi.

Nose

The **nose** of domestic animals comprises the parts of the face rostral to the eyes and dorsal to the mouth. The **external nares** (nostrils) are the external openings of the respiratory tract (Fig. 19–1). Their size and shape, highly variable among domestic farm animals, are largely dictated by the **nasal cartilages** that form this most rostral end of the respiratory tract. In addition

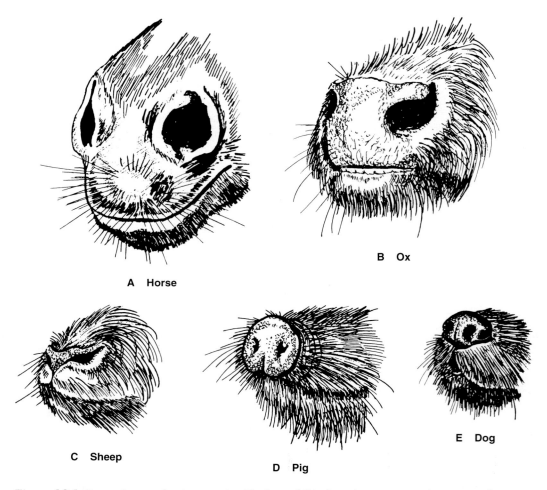

A Horse

B Ox

C Sheep

D Pig

E Dog

Figure 19-1. External nares of various species. The horse (A) lacks a planum, its nose being instead covered with fine hair. The ox (B) possesses a nasolabial planum, and the small ruminants (C) and dogs (E) have a nasal planum. The pig's external nose (D) features a rostral planum that is supported by a rostral bone. (After Nickel R., Schummer A., and Seiferle E. *Lehrbuch der Anatomie der Haustiere.* Berlin: Paul Parey, 1960.)

to these hyaline cartilages, the pig also possesses a *rostral bone* in the tip of its flat, disklike nose. This is presumably an adaptation to the rooting habits of the pig.

The lateral aspect of the nose is covered with typical hairy skin, which contains both sebaceous and sweat glands. The hairless region of the most rostral parts of the nose in species other than the horse contains no sebaceous glands but does have numerous sweat glands, which keep the region around the nostrils moist. This area is the *planum nasale* in the sheep and goat, *planum rostrale* in the pig, and *planum nasolabiale* in the cow. The grooves and bumps in the plana are distinctive enough to allow nose prints to be used for positive individual identification.

The *nasal cavity* is separated from the mouth by the hard and soft palates and separated into two isolated halves by a median *nasal septum.* The rostral part of the septum is cartilaginous, whereas the most caudal part is created in part by a plate of bone. Each half of the nasal cavity

communicates with the nostril of the same side rostrally and with the pharynx caudally by way of the *choanae* (caudal nares).

The nasal cavity is lined with mucous membrane that covers a number of scroll-like *conchae* (turbinate bones) arising from the bones of the lateral wall (Fig. 19–2). The two major conchae (*dorsal concha* and *ventral concha*) occupy rostral parts of the nasal cavity; caudal parts are filled with *ethmoidal conchae.* The vascular mucous membrane covering these conchae helps to warm and humidify inspired air. The mucous membrane investing the ethmoidal conchae is the *olfactory epithelium.* It contains the sensory endings of the olfactory nerve (cranial nerve I), which mediates the sense of smell.

The actual air space of each half of the nasal cavity is partitioned by the conchae into nasal meatuses (Fig. 19–3). The *dorsal nasal meatus* is between the dorsal concha and the roof of the nasal cavity. The *middle nasal meatus* is between the two conchae. The *ventral nasal mea-*

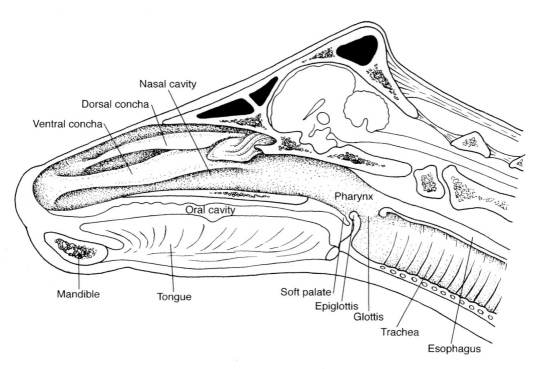

Figure 19-2. Median section of the bovine head with nasal septum removed. (Reprinted with permission from Reece W.R. *Physiology of Domestic Animals.* 2nd ed. Baltimore: Williams & Wilkins, 1997.)

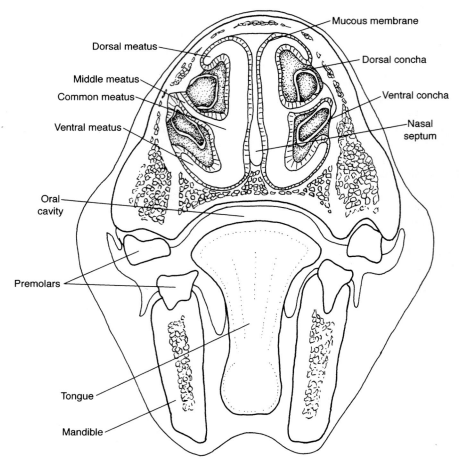

Figure 19-3. Transverse section through the nasal cavity of the horse, illustrating meatuses created by conchae. (Reprinted with permission from Reece W.R. *Physiology of Domestic Animals.* 2nd ed. Baltimore: Williams & Wilkins, 1997.)

tus is between the ventral concha and the floor of the nasal cavity. The **common nasal meatus** communicates between the others and is adjacent to the nasal septum. A nasogastric tube introduced through the nostrils into the nasal cavity and advanced into the esophagus for administration of medications is directed through the ventral nasal meatus.

Paranasal Sinuses

Many of the cranial bones contain air-filled cavities, *paranasal sinuses,* that communicate with the nasal cavity. These sinuses probably provide some protection and insulation to the head. Although there are some species differences, all farm animals have **maxillary, frontal, sphenoidal,** and **palatine sinuses** in the bones of the same name (Fig. 19–4). Several upper cheek teeth project into the maxillary sinus, which may be infected by diseased teeth. The frontal sinus is especially capacious. In horned cattle, an extension of the frontal sinus, the **cornual diverticulum,** extends well into the bony core of the horn. Dehorning of animals older than 3 or 4 months of age usually exposes the interior of the frontal sinus and predisposes it to infection.

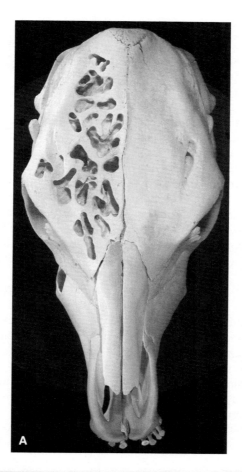

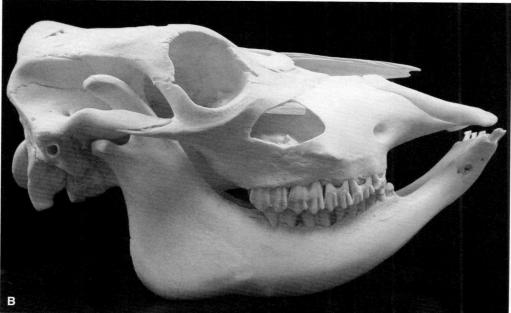

Figure 19-4. Paranasal sinuses of the ox demonstrated by sculpting of bones. A) frontal sinus, B) maxillary sinus.

Pharynx

The **pharynx** is a common soft tissue conduit for food and air, lying caudal to the oral and nasal cavities. Openings into the pharynx include the two caudal nares (choanae), two auditory tubes from the middle ears, the oral cavity, the larynx, and the esophagus. The walls of the pharynx are supported by striated muscles whose actions assist in deglutition (swallowing) and phonation. In normal circumstances, foodstuffs and liquids are directed into the esophagus from the mouth (and vice versa during rumination) with a coordinated movement that excludes these substances from the airways.

Larynx

The **larynx** is the boxlike gatekeeper to the entrance of the trachea. It is held rigid by a series of paired and unpaired cartilages that are moved relative to one another by striated laryngeal muscles. The larynx's primary function is to regulate the size of the airway and to protect it by closing to prevent substances other than air from entering the trachea. It is capable of increasing the diameter of the air passageway during forced inspiration (as during heavy exercise) and closing the opening during swallowing or as a protective mechanism to exclude foreign objects. Secondarily, the larynx is the organ of **phonation** (vocalization), hence its common name, voice box. Contraction of muscles in the larynx changes the tension on ligaments that vibrate as air is drawn past them; this vibration produces the voice.

Five mucous membrane–lined cartilages make up the larynx in most domestic animals (Fig. 19–5). The unpaired, spade-shaped **epiglottic cartilage (epiglottis),** which lies just caudal to the base of the tongue, is mostly elastic cartilage. During deglutition, movements of the tongue and larynx fold the epiglottis caudad so that it covers the entrance into the larynx.

The **thyroid cartilage** resembles a taco shell, consisting of two parallel plates, the **laminae,** on each side, joined on the ventral midline. In the human, the thyroid cartilage, or Adam's apple, projects from the ventral aspect of the neck. The laminae of the thyroid cartilage have processes that articulate with other cartilages and give attachment to a number of muscles.

The **cricoid cartilage** is shaped like a signet ring, with the broad portion dorsal. The cricoid cartilage articulates with the thyroid cartilage and the two arytenoid cartilages (discussed later) cranially and attaches to the first cartilaginous ring of the trachea caudally.

The paired **arytenoid cartilages** are irregular in shape, with processes that vary between species. The arytenoid cartilages of all species have a ventral **vocal process,** to which is attached the **vocal ligament** (vocal cord). The vocal ligaments mark the division between the **vestibule,** the laryngeal space cranial to them, and the **infraglottic cavity,** the space caudal to them (Fig. 19–5). The slitlike gap between the two vocal ligaments is the **glottis.** Movement of the arytenoid cartilages changes the tension and angle of the vocal ligaments, closing the glottis or adjusting the pitch of the voice as the ligaments vibrate.

Nonruminants also possess a **vestibular** (ventricular) **ligament** cranial to the vocal ligament. An outpocket of mucous membrane between the two ligaments forms a blind pouch called the **lateral ventricle.**

The vagus nerve (cranial nerve X) innervates the muscles (motor) and the mucous membranes (sensory) of the larynx. Most of the muscles receive their motor innervation from the **recurrent laryngeal nerve,** which for embryological reasons arises from the vagus in the thorax and must return craniad along the trachea to reach the larynx. This very long course of the axons in the recurrent laryngeal nerve (from the brainstem, where the neuronal cell bodies reside, down the neck into the thorax and back up the neck to the larynx) makes them susceptible to trauma and metabolic diseases.

Injury to the recurrent laryngeal nerve results in paralysis of most of the laryngeal muscles. Paralysis of the muscle that abducts the arytenoid cartilages and thereby increases the diameter of the glottis (the dorsal cricoarytenoid muscle) results in a condition in horses called *roaring*. A horse that is a roarer cannot expand the glottis during forceful inspiration and consequently has difficulty bringing sufficient air into the lungs when exercising. The flaccid vocal ligament flutters as air moves rapidly past

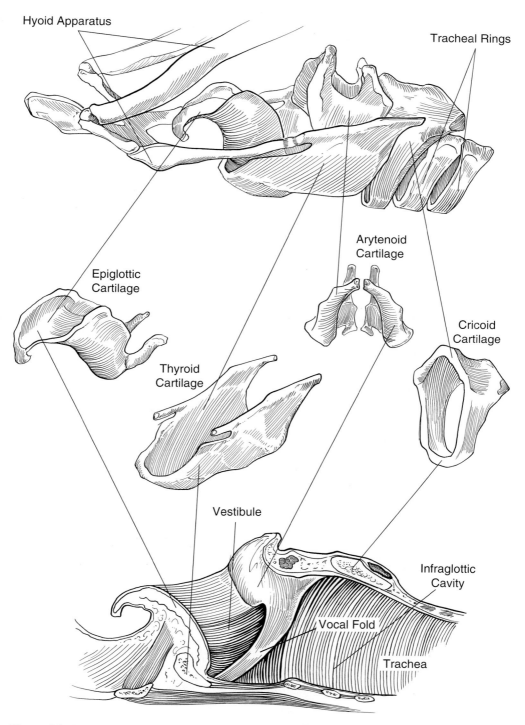

Figure 19-5. Larynx of the horse. *A*) lateral view of the assembled larynx, which is attached rostrally to the hyoid apparatus and caudally to the trachea. *B*) Individual cartilages of the equine larynx. *C*) Internal anatomy of the larynx.

it, generating a loud, hoarse sound. Roaring usually is due to unilateral damage to the left recurrent laryngeal nerve, as this nerve's course is somewhat longer than that of the right recurrent laryngeal nerve.

Trachea and Bronchi

The *trachea* extends from the caudal end of the larynx to the bronchi (Fig. 19–6). It is formed by a series of **C**-shaped hyaline *tracheal cartilages* that provide cross-sectional rigidity to resist collapse but are joined one to another by elastic *annular ligaments* that permit the trachea considerable flexibility to follow movements of the neck. The dorsal side of the trachea is completed by connective tissue and the *m. trachealis,* a smooth muscle whose tone affects the diameter of the trachea.

The trachea passes caudad as far as the base of the heart, where it divides into two *principal bronchi,* one for each lung (Fig. 19–6). The ruminants and pig have an additional *tracheal*

bronchus arising cranial to the principal bronchi; it supplies the cranial lobe of the right lung. The principal bronchi branch into secondary (also called lobar), then tertiary bronchi, subsequent branches becoming smaller and smaller. The walls of these bronchi are supported by cartilaginous plates. When the airways divide to the extent that they are less than 1 mm in diameter, the cartilage disappears, and these airways are called **bronchioles.** The bronchiole eventually branches into several *alveolar ducts,* which terminate in clusters of air sacs, the *alveoli.* It is here that the exchange of gases with the blood takes place. Some terminal bronchioles have alveoli in their walls, hence are called *respiratory bronchioles* (Fig. 19–7).

Thorax

The thorax is bounded cranially by the first pair of ribs, the first thoracic vertebra, and the cranial part of the sternum. This ring of skeletal elements is the *thoracic inlet.* The dorsal part of

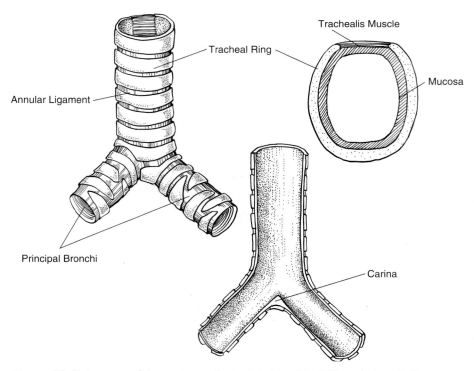

Figure 19-6. Anatomy of the trachea and principle bronchi. *A)* Ventral view. *B)* Transverse section.

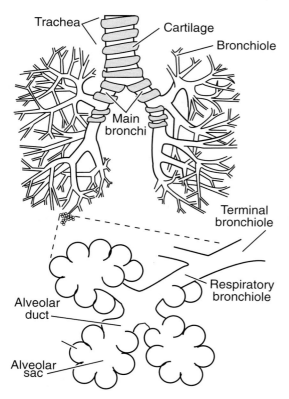

Figure 19-7. Respiratory tree consists of a series of highly branched tubes that become narrower, shorter and more numerous as they penetrate the deeper parts of the lungs. (Reprinted with permission from Rhoades R.A. and Tanner G.A. *Medical Physiology*. Boston: Little, Brown, 1995.)

Lobes of the lungs are defined by the lobar (secondary) bronchi. The lobes are grossly distinguishable in most species by deep fissures in the ventral part of the lung. In ruminants and the pig, the left lung is divided into *cranial* (apical) and *caudal* (diaphragmatic) *lobes,* with the cranial lobe having a further division into cranial and caudal parts. The right lung in these animals is divided into four lobes: cranial and caudal lobes as on the left, plus a *middle lobe* between these and a ventrocaudal *accessory lobe* near the midline (Fig. 19–8). A more or less distinct gap between lobes along the ventral margin of the lungs is usually identifiable. This is the *cardiac notch,* and it tends to be larger on the right side. At the cardiac notch, the heart makes contact with the thoracic wall, a fact that is exploited for echocardiogram imaging (wherein the ultrasound device is applied to the thoracic wall, where no lung tissue intervenes between it and the heart) and pericardiocentesis (introducing a needle through the body wall to sample fluid from the pericardial sac).

Both right and left lungs of the horse have cranial and caudal lobes, distinguished by the cardiac notch. The right equine lung also has a small accessory lobe.

After an animal has taken one breath, the lungs always retain a significant volume of air, even in pathologic conditions of collapsed lung. In the fetus, however, the lungs are nearly the consistency of liver, contain no air, and sink in water. Whether the lungs will sink or float in water is a standard test to determine whether a newborn animal was born dead, in which case the lungs sink, or drew at least one breath, in which case the lungs float.

Pleura

The thoracic cavity is lined by a serosa, the *pleura.* The smooth surfaces of the pleura are lubricated with a scant amount of serous fluid, facilitating frictionless movement of the lungs during respirations. The pleura is attached to the bony and muscular elements of the thorax by *endothoracic fascia,* a thin connective tissue layer.

The pleura consists of two separate sacs, one

the thorax is defined by the thoracic vertebrae and epaxial muscles, and the ventral part, by the sternum. The ribs and costal cartilages, linked by intercostal muscles, create the lateral walls. The overall shape of the thorax is that of a cone with the apex at the thoracic inlet. The base of the cone is covered by the dome-shaped diaphragm.

Lungs

Each **lung** is conical, with the base resting against the cranial side of the diaphragm and the apex in or close to the thoracic inlet. The medial aspect of each lung features an indentation, the **hilus,** where the principal bronchus, pulmonary vessels, lymphatics, and nerves enter the lung.

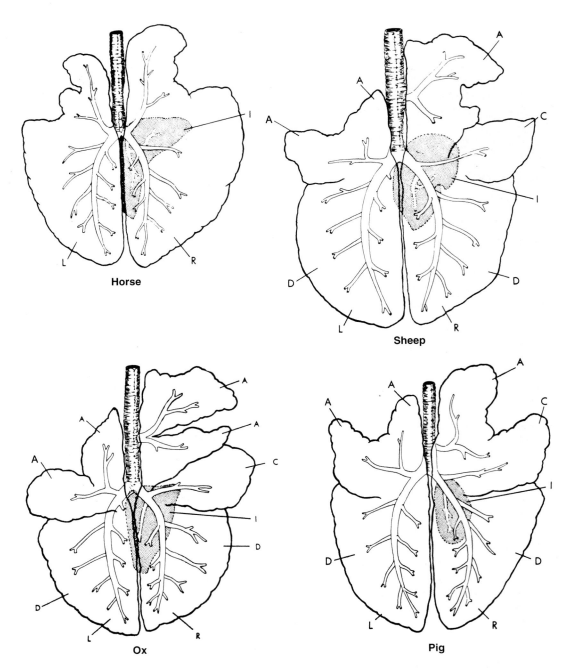

Figure 19-8. Lungs of horse, sheep, ox, and pig. L, left; R, right; A, cranial (apical); C, middle (cardiac); D, caudal (diaphragmatic); I, accessory (intermediate). (After Nickel R., Schummer A., and Seiferle E. *Lehrbuch der Anatomie der Haustiere*. Berlin: Paul Parey, 1960.)

surrounding each lung. The pleura that lines the thorax is the *parietal pleura,* and the pleura that covers the lungs is the *visceral pleura.* The pleural cavity, between parietal and visceral pleurae, is a potential space only. This pleural cavity normally contains nothing except a small amount of serous fluid; conditions that introduce fluid or gas (e.g., pus, blood, air) into the pleural space compress and may collapse the lung associated with that space.

The junction of the two pleural sacs near the midline of the thorax forms a double layer called the *mediastinum* in which are found the heart, great vessels, esophagus, and other midline structures. The caudal vena cava and right phrenic nerve (nerve innervating the right side of the diaphragm) are enclosed in a distinct fold of pleura, the *plica venae cavae.* The mediastinum of cattle is thick and forms a complete barrier between the right and left pleural cavities. In horses, parts of the mediastinum are thin, and openings between the two cavities either occur naturally or are readily created. For this reason infections or air in one pleural space may stay unilaterally contained in cattle, whereas they spread rapidly to involve both sides in the horse.

Physiology of Respiration

Ventilation

Ventilation is the process by which air is moved in (*inspiration*) and out of (*expiration*) the lungs. *Alveolar ventilation* is a more specific term that refers to the movement of air into and out of alveoli. Alveoli are the primary site of gas exchange in the lungs, so alveolar ventilation is the critical component of this function.

Panting is a mechanism to dissipate heat. Panting is characterized by an increased ventilatory rate but with a reduced **tidal volume** (volume of air moved during each breath). Alveolar ventilation increases minimally in panting animals, because the increase in air movement is primarily in the upper airways that are not sites of gas exchange. These airways are considered to be **anatomic dead space.** *Physiologic dead space* includes the anatomic dead space and any alveoli in which normal gas exchanges cannot occur.

As described earlier, there is no physical connection between the visceral and parietal pleural surfaces (except at the hilus), and the closed pleural cavity between them is a potential space filled with a small amount of fluid. The hydrostatic pressure in the pleural cavity is always slightly negative relative to **atmospheric pressure** (Fig. 19–9), and this small negative pressure exerts a pulling force to keep the lungs expanded. Enlargement of the thoracic cavity during inspiration reduces the already negative pressure in the pleural cavity, which further expands the lungs (Fig. 19–9).

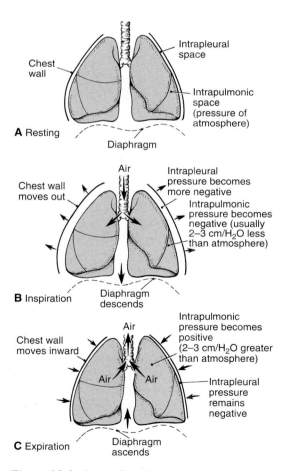

Figure 19-9. Phases of ventilation. *A,* No air movement (resting). *B,* Air moves from the atmosphere to the intrapulmonic space (inspiration). *C,* Air moves from the intrapulmonic space to the atmosphere (expiration). (Reprinted with permission from Bullock B.L. *Pathophysiology.* 4th ed. Philadelphia: Lippincott, 1996.)

During inspiration, air moves in through the upper airways and down to the alveoli because of a hydrostatic pressure gradient (i.e., atmospheric pressure) between the outside air and the air passages in the lungs (*intrapulmonic pressure*). This gradient is generated by lung expansion. Expansion increases the volume of the air passages in the lungs but reduces the pressure in them. The inverse relationship between volume and pressure of a gas is expressed as *Boyle's law.* Figure 19–9 illustrates the changes in intrapulmonic and intrapleural pressures during inspiration and expiration. The negative (inspiration) and positive (expiration) values for intrapulmonic pressures are relative to atmospheric pressure (760 mm Hg at sea level), so negative pressure is less than atmospheric and positive is greater than atmospheric.

Enlargement of the thoracic cavity is accomplished by contraction and flattening of the dome-shaped *diaphragm* and a forward and outward movement of the rib cage by the contraction of appropriate thoracic muscles. These are skeletal muscles innervated by somatic motor nerves. After inspiration, the pressure in the pleural cavity remains at its lowest point until expiration begins and the thoracic cavity begins to return to its original volume.

Expiration in a resting animal is a passive process that does not require muscle contraction. Relaxation of the muscles contracted during inspiration permits the intrinsic elastic properties of the lungs and the thoracic wall to recoil to their original volume. The return to the original volume increases the intrapulmonic pressure so that it is greater than atmospheric, and air is forced out of the lungs.

Forced expiration is an active process that forces more air from the lungs than would occur during a normal passive expiration. Forced expiration requires contraction of abdominal muscles to force viscera against the diaphragm and contraction of other muscles to pull the ribs caudad. Both of these actions reduce the size of the thoracic cavity and permit recoil of the lungs to a smaller volume than typical for resting expiration. This causes a further increase in intrapulmonic pressure and forces more air out than would occur with passive expiration. Even with the most forceful expiration, a *residual volume* of air still remains in the lungs. *Vital capacity* is the maximal amount of air that can be expired after a maximal inspiration.

Both the upper airways and the air passages in the lungs resist airflow through them. Similar to a blood vessel, the resistance of an air passage to airflow is inversely proportional to its diameter. Most of the air passages in the lungs have smooth muscle in the walls, and the constriction or relaxation of this smooth muscle determines the resistance to airflow. Much of this smooth muscle has β_2-adrenergic receptors that produce smooth muscle relaxation when stimulated. Sympathetic stimulation during exercise reduces resistance to airflow and promotes alveolar ventilation.

Airway smooth muscle constricts in response to stimulation by *histamine* or *leukotrienes.* These substances are released during allergic reactions from mast cells around airways. The resulting increase in airway resistance makes it more difficult to move air, and a more forceful skeletal muscle contraction is needed to move a given volume of air. This greatly increases the work of breathing. *Heaves* is a condition in horses that is characterized by labored or difficult breathing, and one potential cause is chronic exposure to environmental allergens, which results in chronic obstructive airway disease. The chronic need for increased skeletal muscle force may induce visible hypertrophy of the abdominal muscles (heave line).

Surface tension, a property of fluids, results from the cohesive forces that tend to pull or hold the molecules of a fluid together. An example is the tendency of a layer of fluid on a flat surface to come together and form a bubble rather than remaining as a thin, flat layer. A thin layer of fluid lines the microscopic alveoli. The surface tension of this fluid tends to draw the walls of alveoli together and collapse them. The alveolar fluid contains the *pulmonary surfactant,* a combination of substances that reduces surface tension. The reduction in surface tension promotes alveolar stability and makes alveolar expansion during inspiration easier. **Production of pulmonary surfactant does not begin until late in gestation. Neonates born prematurely may have insufficient amounts of surfactant, which results in labored breathing.**

A soft rustling sound associated with air movements in normal animals may be heard with a stethoscope. Abnormal lungs, for example lungs with abnormal amounts of fluid in the airways, may produce exaggerated sounds termed **rales. Pleuritis** (pleurisy), or inflammation of the pleura, may produce a rasping sound because of the roughened surfaces rubbing together. **Hydrothorax** (fluid in the pleural cavity) may also result from pleuritis.

Gas Exchange

The oxygen and carbon dioxide concentrations in air can be described in two ways: **partial pressures** and **percentages.** Room air is approximately 21% oxygen and 0.3% carbon dioxide. The primary component of room air is the inert gas nitrogen (about 78%). The partial pressure of an individual gas in a mixture of gases is the product of the percentage of the individual gas in the mixture and the total **barometric** or atmospheric pressure. Thus, at sea level, where atmospheric pressure is 760 mm Hg, the partial pressure of oxygen in room air is approximately 160 mm Hg.

The partial pressure of an individual gas in a mixture is one factor that determines the amount of the gas that will dissolve in a liquid (such as blood plasma). The partial pressure of a gas in a mixture can be viewed as the driving force that moves molecules of an individual gas from the air into the liquid when the liquid is exposed to a gas mixture. Thus, because partial pressures depend on both total atmospheric pressure and the percentages of individual gases, both of these factors also determine the amount of an individual gas that can be dissolved in a liquid. The unit of measurement of the amount of a gas dissolved in a liquid is also millimeters of mercury.

Gas Exchange in the Lungs. Gas exchange between the blood and alveolar air in the lungs occurs across the walls of alveoli. At its thinnest point, the alveolar wall barrier between blood plasma and alveolar air consists of the endothelial cell of pulmonary capillaries, a type I squamous epithelial cell lining the alveoli, and a fused basement membrane contributed by both cells (Fig. 19–10). Gases readily move back and forth across this very thin and fragile structure. **Any abnormality that thickens this barrier (e.g., pulmonary edema with an accumulation of extracellular fluid in the alveolar wall) can greatly reduce the efficiency of exchange. Oxygen exchange is usually affected first because its solubility is much less than that of carbon dioxide.**

Exchange begins as soon as blood enters a pulmonary capillary from pulmonary arterial vessels and continues until equilibrium between alveolar air and plasma is reached. Figure 19–11 shows typical values for partial pressures of oxygen and carbon dioxide in alveolar air and a pulmonary capillary. Plasma entering pulmonary capillaries from the pulmonary arteries contains the highest concentration of carbon dioxide and the lowest of oxygen. Because of the continuous gas exchange in the pulmonary capillaries, alveolar air contains less oxygen and more carbon dioxide than inspired air (PO_2 of 160 mm Hg and PCO_2 of 0.23 mm Hg for inspired air).

To be most efficient, the rate of pulmonary artery blood flow into an area of the lung must

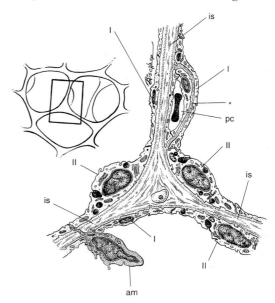

Figure 19-10. Electron micrograph of interalveolar septa of rat showing the blood–air barrier (*A*). The alveolar airspace (*B*) is lined by the squamous alveolar epithelial cell (*C*). The capillary containing red blood cells (*D*) is lined by endothelial cells (*E*). Leukocyte (*F*). (Reprinted with permission from Dellmann H.D. *Textbook of Veterinary Histology.* 4th ed. Philadelphia: Lea & Febiger, 1993.)

be balanced with the rate of air movement in and out of the alveoli in the same area. To appreciate the importance of this balancing, consider an extreme case in which one lung is collapsed so that air movement is impossible, but the collapsed lung receives the same amount of blood flow as the inflated normal lung. The lack of airflow in the collapsed lung means that any alveolar air is stagnant and contains high levels of carbon dioxide and low levels of oxygen. Gas exchange in the collapsed lung does not occur, and levels of oxygen and carbon dioxide are the same as those entering. The blood exiting the collapsed lung mixes with an equal volume of blood from the intact lung, so that blood reentering the heart from the pulmonary circulation is deficient in oxygen and has an excess of carbon dioxide.

Within the lungs, a unique type of vascular mechanism functions at the level of small arterial blood vessels to balance blood flow and airflow. This mechanism, **local hypoxic (low oxygen) vasoconstriction,** produces local vasoconstriction in response to low levels of alveolar oxygen (such as with poor alveolar ventilation). The vasoconstriction reduces blood flow into the area of poor ventilation and shunts blood into better-ventilated areas of the lungs. It is not clear how low levels of alveolar oxygen are detected and what vasoactive agent or agents are responsible for the vasoconstriction.

The hypoxic vasoconstriction mechanism operates well on a local basis to redirect blood flow into different areas of the lungs. However, when both lungs are exposed to low oxygen levels, such as at high altitudes, the mechanism produces a general increase in vascular resistance throughout both lungs. *Pulmonary hypertension* (high pulmonary circulation blood pressure) results, and the right side of the heart must work harder to pump blood through the lungs. Right heart failure with peripheral edema can result if the right heart cannot compensate for the increased resistance. A syndrome with pulmonary hypertension, right heart failure, and peripheral edema resulting from exposure to high altitude is recognized in cattle as *brisket disease,* in which edema collects in the pendulous brisket.

Gas Exchange in the Tissues. Cells in peripheral tissues consume oxygen and produce carbon dioxide during normal metabolism. This maintains relatively low oxygen and high carbon dioxide concentrations (partial pressures) in the extracellular fluid around capillaries. As arterial blood enters capillaries, partial pressure gradients promote the diffusion of oxygen out of the blood to the interstitial fluid and carbon dioxide to diffuse from the interstitial fluid into the blood (Fig. 19–11).

Gas Transport in Blood

Both oxygen and carbon dioxide dissolve in plasma, and the partial pressures of each are a measure of the amount dissolved. However, the quantity of each gas that is transported as a dissolved gas is very small compared with the amounts of each transported in other forms in the blood. Only 1.5% of the total oxygen and 7% of the carbon dioxide are dissolved.

Most oxygen in the blood (98.5%) is found chemically bound to hemoglobin in erythrocytes (see Chapter 15). Figure 19–12, *A* illustrates the relation between the partial pressure of oxygen and the **percent saturation of hemoglobin** by oxygen. At partial pressures of oxygen normally found in alveolar air (about 100 mm Hg), hemoglobin is almost completely saturated with oxygen (i.e., hemoglobin molecules cannot bind any additional oxygen). Normally the hemoglobin in erythrocytes is almost completely saturated with oxygen as blood passes through the pulmonary capillaries. At partial pressures of oxygen typically found in venous blood (40 mm Hg) a great deal of hemoglobin still has oxygen bound to it (Fig. 19–12A).

Several factors affect the ability of hemoglobin to bind chemically with oxygen. An increase in temperature, a reduction in pH, or an increase in the concentration of carbon dioxide reduces the ability of hemoglobin to bind oxygen. These factors alter the relation between hemoglobin saturation and the partial pressure of oxygen so that the saturation is less for any given partial pressure. Figure 19–12, *B* illustrates the effect of lowering pH on hemoglobin saturation, and the effects of increases in temperature or carbon dioxide are similar. High

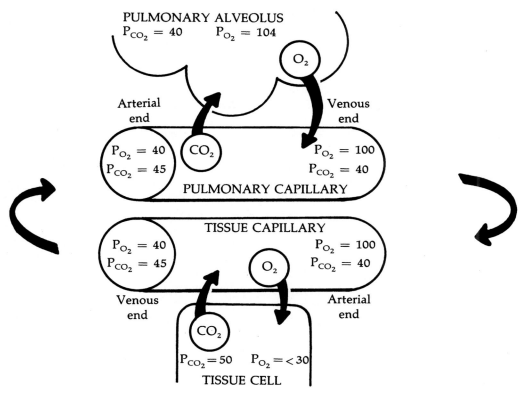

Figure 19-11. Direction of diffusion of oxygen (O_2) and carbon dioxide (CO_2), as shown by *arrows*. Values for gases in alveolar air and in fluids (plasma and intracellular fluid are expressed in millimeters of mercury). Note changes in values as blood flows from arterial to venous end of the two types of capillaries. (Reprinted with permission from Reece W.R. *Physiology of Domestic Animals.* 2nd ed. Baltimore: Williams & Wilkins, 1997.)

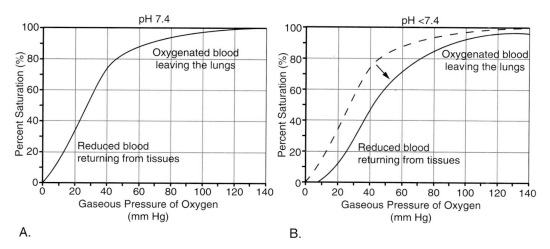

Figure 19-12. *A)* An oxygen–hemoglobin dissociation curve that illustrates the percent saturation of hemoglobin by oxygen at different partial pressures of oxygen. *B)* Effect of lowering the pH from 7.4 to 7.2 on the oxygen–hemoglobin dissociation curve.

temperature, low pH, and high carbon dioxide occur in tissues with high metabolic rates (e.g., exercising skeletal muscle). The effects of these factors on the relation between hemoglobin and oxygen is useful, because more oxygen is liberated from hemoglobin and delivered to the metabolizing cells when blood passes through such areas.

Almost all of the carbon dioxide (93%) that enters the blood in the systemic circulation diffuses into erythrocytes. Some of the carbon dioxide (23%) chemically combines with the hemoglobin in the erythrocytes to form **carbaminohemoglobin.** When the erythrocytes carrying the carbaminohemoglobin reach the pulmonary capillaries in the lungs, the reaction is reversed so that the carbon dioxide can diffuse into alveoli to be expired. Most (70%) of the carbon dioxide that enters the erythrocytes is converted to carbonic acid under the influence of the enzyme **carbonic anhydrase.** The carbonic acid rapidly dissociates into a hydrogen ion and a **bicarbonate ion** in the erythrocyte. The hydrogen ion is buffered by hemoglobin in the erythrocyte, and the bicarbonate ion leaves the erythrocyte and enters the plasma. It is in this form (bicarbonate ion in plasma) that most carbon

dioxide is transported from the peripheral tissues by the blood to the lungs (Fig. 19–13). Within the lungs, the reactions are reversed so that carbon dioxide can be reformed and be expired from the alveoli.

Control of Ventilation

Contraction and relaxation of skeletal muscle generates the forces to move air in and out of the lungs. Although the skeletal muscles of respiration can be consciously controlled, as illustrated by voluntarily holding the breath, normal ventilation is almost entirely reflexive.

The respiratory reflex centers consist mainly of three bilateral groups of nerve cells in the brainstem that have a definite effect on respiration when stimulated electrically. One of these, the **medullary rhythmicity** area, is responsible for setting respiratory rate, and it consists mainly of an **inspiratory center.** Neurons in this center are tonically active, firing at an inherent rhythmic rate by regular variations of their membrane potentials. Expiratory neurons are also in this area; however, they do not discharge spontaneously and so are normally active only during a forced expiration.

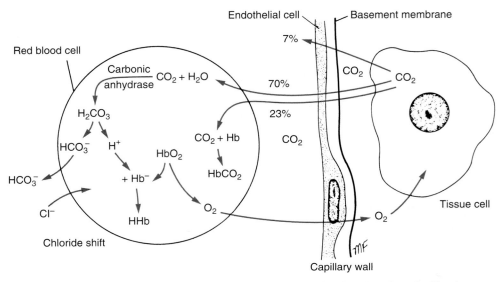

Figure 19-13. Gas exchange in systemic tissues and transport of carbon dioxide in the blood. Note that 70% of carbon dioxide is transported as bicarbonate ions. Hb = hemoglobin. (Reprinted with permission from Snell R.S. *Clinical Histology for Medical Students.* Boston: Little, Brown, 1984.)

Stimulation of the inspiratory center leads to contractions of the diaphragmatic and intercostal muscles via neural connections through the spinal cord and phrenic and intercostal nerves, respectively. Feedback circuits between the inspiratory center and the other two neural centers relax these muscles and allow for passive expiration. The interplay among these three centers provides for regular intermittent rhythmic breathing at rates appropriate for each species during *eupnea* (normal quiet breathing).

The tonic activity of the inspiratory center is regulated by neural input from a variety of sites. In resting animals, the most important neural input is from **central chemoreceptors** in the medulla of the brainstem. These receptors respond to hydrogen ion concentration changes in the interstitial fluid of the brain and stimulate the inspiratory center to increase ventilation when the hydrogen ion concentration increases. Because carbon dioxide from the blood readily diffuses into the interstitial fluids of the brain and in body fluids is in equilibrium with carbonic acid, an increase in blood carbon dioxide increases the hydrogen ion concentration in the brain and stimulates ventilation. The effects of changes in blood carbon dioxide on ventilation are so pronounced that blood carbon dioxide is considered to be the most important regulator of ventilation in most conditions.

Animals sometimes *hyperventilate* (breathe abnormally rapidly) during the induction of general anesthesia because they are excited. As a result of the hyperventilation, their blood carbon dioxide may be significantly reduced. The low blood carbon dioxide concentration means that the primary stimulus for normal ventilation is lost. These animals may undergo a period of *apnea* (cessation of breathing) until blood carbon dioxide levels are restored by metabolism.

Another group of chemoreceptors the carotid and aortic bodies also provides neural input to the inspiratory center. These **peripheral chemoreceptors** detect changes in arterial blood hydrogen ion concentration and oxygen content. Increases in hydrogen ion concentration or reductions in blood O_2 content initiate neural inputs to increase ventilation. However, the effects of these peripheral chemoreceptors are less pronounced than those of the central chemoreceptors, so changes in blood hydrogen ion concentration or oxygen content must be severe to override the effect of blood carbon dioxide.

Further regulating the inspiratory center and breathing rhythmicity is a reflex arc involving stretch receptors in the lung parenchyma, visceral pleura, and bronchioles. These receptors are stimulated as the lung inflates during inspiration, and afferent impulses are transmitted up the vagus nerves into the brainstem, where the inspiratory center is inhibited. This is the **Hering-Breuer reflex,** which reinforces the action of the other center to limit inspiration and prevent overdistension of the lungs.

Chapter 20

ANATOMY OF THE DIGESTIVE SYSTEM

Organization of the Digestive System

The *digestive system* (*digestive tract*) consists of a muscular tube lined with mucous membrane that is continuous with the external skin at the mouth and at the anus. Its primary functions are ingestion, mastication, digestion and absorption of food, and elimination of solid wastes. The digestive system reduces the nutrients in the food to molecular compounds that are small enough to be absorbed and used for energy and for building other compounds to be incorporated into body tissues.

Elements of the digestive system are the mouth, pharynx, esophagus, forestomach (ruminants), glandular stomach, small intestine, large intestine, rectum, and the accessory glands (salivary glands, liver, and pancreas).

Caudal to the diaphragm, the components of the digestive tract lie within the abdominal and pelvic cavities. Here they are invested with a simple squamous epithelium that is also called a *mesothelium* or *serosa*. Within these body cavities, the serosa is identified as *peritoneum*. Like the pleura within the thoracic cavity, it is named according to the structures to which it is applied: where it lies directly on the organ, it is called *visceral peritoneum,* and where it invests the abdominal wall, it is *parietal peritoneum* (see Figure 1–9).

Parietal and visceral peritonea are continuous with one another through reflections of the serosa that attach the organs to the body wall. These attachments collectively constitute the **mesenteries,** and they are named for the organ they suspend (discussed later). Blood vessels, lymphatics, and nerves travel within the mesenteries, reaching the organs through them.

The wall of the digestive tract comprises four layers, or tunics. These are, from within outward: (1) the **tunica mucosa,** (2) the **tunica submucosa,** (3) the **tunica muscularis,** and (4) the **tunica serosa,** or **tunica adventitia** (Figure 20–1).

The **tunica mucosa** is the layer closest to the space (the **lumen**) inside the digestive tract. It has three histologic layers. The innermost layer consists of a stratified squamous epithelium from the mouth to the level of the glandular part of the stomach; from this point to the anus, the epithelium is of the simple columnar type. Un-

derlying the epithelium of the tunica mucosa are a layer of connective tissue and a variably present smooth muscle layer.

The **tunica submucosa** is a layer of loose connective tissue in which are found blood vessels and nerves. In some locations, glands of the digestive tract can be found in the submucosa, as can lymphatic nodules.

As motility is important to the function of the digestive system, the **tunica muscularis** is generally well developed. In the horse, the cranial two-thirds of the tunica muscularis of the esophagus is striated muscle; in the pig, all but the most distal end of the esophagus is striated; and in ruminants, the entire esophagus has striated muscle. From this point, the muscle cells are smooth (involuntary) and are generally arranged in two layers. The deeper layer has

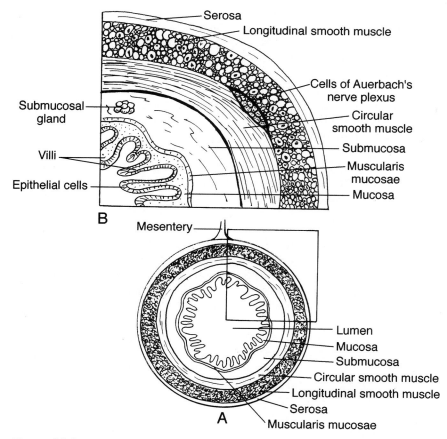

Figure 20-1. Layers of a typical segment of gut. (Reprinted with permission from Reece W.O. *Physiology of Domestic Animals.* 2nd ed. Baltimore: Williams & Wilkins, 1997.)

fibers that encircle the gut, and the more superficial muscle layer assumes a longitudinal arrangement.

The outermost tunic consists of the visceral peritoneum and scant connective tissue underlying it. This is the **tunica serosa.** The thoracic and cervical parts of the esophagus are not suspended directly within a body cavity (the thoracic esophagus is surrounded by the tissues of the mediastinum) and therefore do not have a tunica serosa. Instead, the surrounding connective tissue in these locations constitutes a **tunica adventitia.**

Mouth

The mouth is used primarily for holding, grinding, and mixing food with saliva but may also be used to manipulate the environment (through grasping of objects) and as a defensive and offensive weapon.

The entrance into the mouth is defined by the **lips** (**labia**), the appearance and mobility of which vary among species. The external parts of the lips are covered by typical haired skin, which changes to mucous membrane at the **mucocutaneous junction** of the labial margins. The upper lip of small ruminants is deeply grooved with a midline **philtrum.** Lips are densely innervated by sensory fibers, making them very sensitive tactile organs. The lips of sheep, goats, and horses are soft and flexible and aid in picking up food, whereas those of cattle and hogs are stiffer and less mobile.

The small space between the teeth and lips is the **oral vestibule.** The **oral cavity proper** lies deep to the teeth and is occupied primarily by the tongue. The oral cavity ends at a narrowing (the **isthmus of the fauces**) near the base of the tongue, where the digestive tract continues as the pharynx.

The dorsal wall of the oral cavity comprises the **hard palate** rostrally and the **soft palate** caudally. The hard palate is formed by horizontal elements of the incisive, maxillary, and palatine bones, and its thick mucous membrane covering is characterized by prominent transverse folds called **palatine rugae.** The soft palate is a musculomucosal sheet that extends toward the base of the epiglottis (see Chapter 19). The equine soft palate is exceptionally long, and the horse is uniquely unable to actively lift the soft palate so as to permit passage of air from the oral cavity to the larynx. For this reason, horses are obligate nose breathers, breathing through the mouth only when the soft palate is displaced dorsad from its normal position ventral to the epiglottis.

Teeth

Teeth are arranged in two **dental arcades,** one associated with the mandible and one, with the incisive and maxillary bones. Farm animals typically have a gap in each arch between the front teeth (incisors) and the cheek teeth (see Figure 4–4); such a physiologic gap is a **diastema.** The bit of the bridle lies in the horse's diastema.

Mammals typically exhibit **heterodonty.** That is, they have various types of teeth that are specialized for different aspects of prehension and mastication. All domestic animals also are **diphyodont.** This means they develop a set of **deciduous teeth** (also called baby teeth or milk teeth) that fall out and are replaced with **permanent teeth.** As growing teeth emerge from the gums, they are said to **erupt.** When their occlusal (grinding) surfaces meet those of the teeth in the opposing arcade, they are said to have **come into wear.** Eruption times of teeth are consistent enough to permit accurate aging of young animals by observing their dentition. The age of animals with a full set of permanent teeth can be estimated through examination of the wear patterns of the occlusal surfaces.

A tooth is anchored by its **root** in a socket of bone called an **alveolus.** A connective tissue, the **periodontium** (also called periodontal membrane), firmly attaches the root to the surrounding bone in a specialized joint, the **gomphosis** (see Chapter 6). The **crown** is the part of the tooth visible above the mucous membrane of the gum. Some teeth have a short crown separated from the root by a distinct **neck.** These teeth, of which ruminant incisors are an example, are described as **brachyodont** (Greek *brachy,* short). In contrast, equine incisors and cheek teeth have a tall, straight crown with no dis-

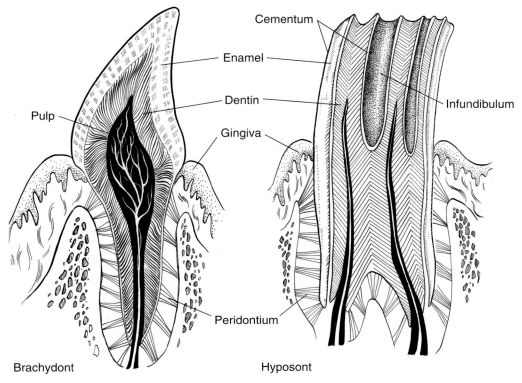

Figure 20-2. Anatomy of typical brachyodont (*left*) and hypsodont (*right*) teeth.

cernible neck. These teeth are described as **hypsodont** (Gr. *hypsi,* high) (Figure 20–2).

Most of the tooth's substance is made up of a mineralized substance called **dentin** (sometimes spelled **dentine**), with a **dental cavity** at its center. The connective tissues, nerves, and blood vessels of the tooth reside in this cavity and constitute the **dental pulp.**

Superficial to the dentin is a layer of **enamel,** a white layer consisting of inorganic crystals. Enamel is the hardest substance in the body. It also is irreplaceable, as the cells that generate it (ameloblasts) are lost following formation of the tooth. Only the crowns of brachyodont teeth are covered with enamel, whereas nearly the entire hypsodont tooth has a layer of enamel, with only a small, short region of the tooth's root lacking this layer. The enamel of hypsodont teeth is thrown into prominent folds on the grinding surfaces of these teeth, where they

form characteristic crests (**cristae enameli**) and cups (**infundibula**).

Cementum is a thin, bonelike layer on the surface of the tooth. It covers only the root of the brachyodont tooth but extends from the root to cover the crown of the hypsodont tooth.

The front teeth are called **incisors,** and in dental formulas, they are designated by the letter I. The incisors are numbered starting from the midline. The first pair of incisors is called I1, or centrals; the next pair I2, or first intermediates; next I3, or second intermediates; and the last and most lateral pair of incisors is called I4, or corners. In the nonruminants, only one pair of intermediate incisors is found. Ruminants lack incisors in the upper dental arcade. Instead, the mucous membrane in this region is modified into a dense, keratinized **dental pad,** against which the lower incisors abut when the jaws are closed. Permanent incisors are preceded by a like number of deciduous teeth.

Canine teeth (abbreviated C) are also called eyeteeth, bridle teeth, tusks, and tushes. Ruminants lack canine teeth, and although they can be well developed in stallions, they are small or absent in mares and geldings. The canine teeth of pigs are large, especially in boars, and in this species they are usually called tusks. Porcine tusks are described as *open rooted,* meaning that they continue to grow throughout life. The lower tusk is generally much larger than its partner in the upper arcade. In pigs, the permanent canines are preceded by analogous deciduous teeth; in the horse, the deciduous canines are often absent or so small that their crowns do not erupt.

Cheek teeth comprise *premolars* (P) and *molars* (M), which in herbivores are morphologically similar. Only premolars are preceded by deciduous teeth; the molars have no precursors. In the pig, the molars are larger than the premolars and have a flatter occlusal surface, in keeping with their grinding function.

The first premolar of horses is often absent, and when present, it is almost always seen only in the upper (maxillary) arcade. Unlike the other equine cheek teeth, the first upper premolar is very small and does not come into wear. This tooth is called the *wolf tooth,* and some horsemen prefer to have it removed because of the perception that it may make unwanted contact with the bit.

In the young horse, only a small part of each cheek tooth is visible, as most of the crown lies developed but unerupted beneath the gum (Figure 20–3). Throughout the horse's life, these teeth continue to erupt, so that they maintain their intraoral height even as they are worn down by the coarse forage the horse eats. Equine cheek teeth are not open rooted; no new dental tissues are created after the tooth is initially formed. They

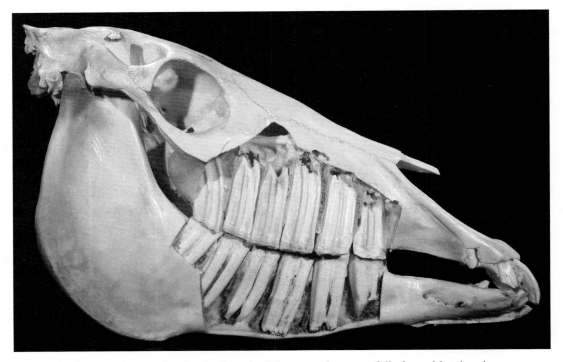

Figure 20-3. Hypsodont teeth. The cheek teeth of the young horse are fully formed but largely within the bones of the face and mandible. The teeth slowly erupt over the life of the horse as the crowns are worn by chewing of coarse feedstuffs.

are instead described as slowly erupting. Because of this phenomenon, horses are prone to develop sharp, elongated ridges of enamel on their cheek teeth. These are variously called *points* and *hooks*, and they may cause the horse considerable pain if they cut the soft cheeks, tongue, and gums. For this reason, it is considered good husbandry to file down the points and hooks periodically, a procedure called *floating the teeth* that is done with a special rasp called a *float.*

Deciduous and permanent dental formulas for domestic farm animals are shown in Tables 20–1 and 20–2.

Tongue

The *tongue* consists of a mass of muscle covered by mucous membrane. It is divided into a free *apex* at the rostral end, a meaty *body,* and a caudal *root* adjacent to the pharynx. The entire tongue is mobile through its muscular attachments to the hyoid apparatus and mandible. The muscles of the tongue (*intrin-*

sic muscles) have fibers oriented in longitudinal, perpendicular, and transverse directions, permitting the tongue a wide range of movements. This is particularly evident in the ox, which uses its tongue as a prehensile organ (Fig. 20–4).

The tongue is covered with keratinized stratified squamous epithelium. The surface is characterized by a large number of projections, the *papillae,* that are particularly well developed on the dorsal surface (Figure 20–5). Filiform, fungiform, and vallate papillae are found in all domestic animals, and foliate papillae are present in the horse, pig, and dog but not in ruminants. Ruminants additionally have large conical papillae. The filiform and conical papillae do not bear taste buds (cells specialized for gustation; see Chapter 11), but all other types of papillae do. Taste buds may also be found on the epiglottis, larynx, pharynx, and soft palate.

The *filiform papillae* look somewhat hairlike. In the ox, they consist of a connective tissue core covered by a highly cornified epithelial layer. These papillae are shorter and softer in

Table 20-1. Formulas and Eruption of Deciduous Teeth

Deciduous Teeth	Horse			Ox			Sheep			Pig		
Formulas	3	0	3	0	0	3	0	0	3	3	1	4
	3	0	3	4	0	3	4	0	3	3	1	4
Eruption of Incisors												
DI 1	birth to 1 week			birth to 2 wk			birth to 1 wk			2–4 wk		
DI 2	4–6 wks			birth to 2 wk			birth to 1 wk			1.5–3 mo		
DI 3	6–9 mo			birth to 2 wk			birth to 1 wk			birth or before		
DI 4				birth to 2 wk			birth to 1 wk					
Eruption of Canines												
										before birth		
Eruption of Premolars												
DP 1				birth to few days			usually before birth			3.5–6.5 mo		
DP 2	birth to 2 wk			birth to few days			usually before birth			7–10 wk		
DP 3	birth to 2 wk			birth to few days			usually before birth			1–3 wk (upper)		
										1–5 wk (lower)		
DP 4	birth to 2 wk									1–4 wk (upper)		
										2–7 wk (lower)		

Table 20-2. Formulas and Eruption of Permanent Teeth

Permanent Teeth	Horse				Ox				Sheep				Pig			
Formulas	3	1	3–4	3	0	0	3	3	0	0	3	3	3	1	4	3
	3	1	3	3	4	0	3	3	4	0	3	3	3	1	4	3
Eruption of Incisors																
I 1	2.5 yr				1.5–2 yr				1–1.5 yr				1 yr			
I 2	3.5 yr				2–2.5 yr				1.5–2 yr				16–20 mo			
I 3	4.5 yr				3 yr				1.5–3 yr				8–10 mo			
I 4					3.5–4 yr				3.5–4 yr							
Eruption of Canines																
	4–5 yr												9–10 mo			
Eruption of Premolars																
P 1	5–6 mo				2–2.5 yr				1.5–2 yr				12–15 mo			
P 2	2.5 yr				1.5–2.5 yr				1.5–2 yr				12–15 mo			
P 3	3 yr				2.5–3 yr				1.5–2 yr				12–15 mo			
P 4	4 yr												12–15 mo			
Eruption of Molars																
M 1	9–12 mo				5–6 mo				3–5 mo				4–6 mo			
M 2	2 yr				1–1.5 yr				9–12 mo.				8–12 mo			
M 3	3.5–4 yr				2–2.5 yr				1.5–2 yr				18–20 mo			

the horse than in other domestic animals, giving the tongue of the horse its velvety feel. Interspersed amongst the filiform papillae are *fungiform papillae,* so called because of their resemblance to a tiny mushroom.

Foliate papillae resemble the foliage or leaves of plants. They are found in the horse and pig (and only rarely in cattle) on the lateral margin adjacent to where the root of the tongue is connected to the soft palate by a mucous membrane fold, the *palatoglossal arch.*

Vallate papillae are large, circular projections surrounded by a deep groove. These papillae are arranged in a **V** shape on the caudal part of the tongue and demarcate the morphologic division between the body and the root of the tongue.

The body of the ruminant tongue has a prominent dorsal bulge, the *torus linguae,* which is thickly covered with prominent *conical papillae.* Similar cornified projections cover the inside of the lips.

Pharynx

The *pharynx* (pl. *pharynges*) is the common passage for food and air, caudal to oral and nasal cavities, lined by mucous membrane and surrounded by muscles. The pharynx can be arbitrarily divided into nasal (*nasopharynx*), oral (*oropharynx*), and laryngeal (*laryngopharynx*) portions, so named for their association with these regions.

The muscles of the walls of the pharynx are responsible for the orderly directing of air, food and liquids in such a way that air from the nasal cavity is directed into the ventral larynx and food and liquids are directed into the dorsal esophagus. Thus the paths of air and swallowed substances must cross in the pharynx; pharyngeal dysfunction can have severe consequences for the airway, which must be protected from foodstuffs (Fig. 20–6).

The *pharyngeal recess* in the horse is a median niche at the caudodorsal angle of the na-

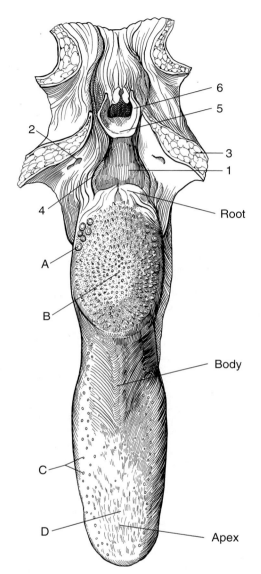

Figure 20-4. Tongue of the ox, dorsal view. The pharynx and soft palate are transected and reflected laterad. *A*) Vallate papillae. *B*) Torus linguae with conical papillae. *C*) Fungiform papillae. *D*) Filiform papillae. *1*) Oropharynx. *2*) Tonsillar crypt. *3*) Cut surface of soft palate. *4*) Palatopharyngeal arch. *5*) Epiglottis. *6*) Opening into larynx. (After Nickel R. et al. *Lehrbuch de Anatomie der Haustiere.* Berlin: Paul Parey, 1960.)

sopharynx. The pig has a ***pharyngeal diverticulum*** that opens into the dorsal wall of the pharynx near the beginning of the esophagus.

Care must be exercised not to enter this diverticulum while passing a stomach tube or giving medications via a balling gun.

Tonsils

Tonsils are more or less circumscribed aggregations of lymphatic nodules found in association with the mucous membranes of the mouth and pharyngeal region. The histologic organization of tonsils is described in Chapter 16.

In humans, each of two obvious ***palatine tonsils*** lies in a pocket on the lateral wall of the pharynx ventral to the soft palate and adjacent to the base of the tongue (these are readily seen with a mirror as elongate nodules on each side of your throat). In the horse, ox, and sheep these palatine tonsils are in about the same relative position, within the submucosa and completely covered by mucous membrane. In other words, the tonsils do not project into the pharynx at all in these animals. The ruminant palatine tonsil features a deep cleft, the ***tonsillar crypt,*** that increases the surface area through which the lymphatic tissue may come in contact with antigens (Fig. 20–4). In the pig the palatine tonsils lie in the substance of the soft palate.

The ***lingual tonsils*** consist of accumulations of lymphatic nodules in the base of the tongue. These tonsils are most prominent in the horse, ox, and pig.

The ***pharyngeal tonsil*** is an accumulation of lymphoid tissue in the submucosa of the dorsal pharyngeal wall of all domestic animals. Enlargement of the pharyngeal tonsil of humans creates the condition commonly called adenoids.

The openings of the auditory tubes (see Chapter 11) in the nasopharynx feature aggregations of lymphatic nodules, the ***tubal tonsils.***

Esophagus

The ***esophagus*** is a muscular tube extending from the pharynx to the stomach just caudal to the diaphragm. The end adjacent to the pharynx is kept closed by the *m. cricopharyngeus,* which passes from its origin on the cricoid car-

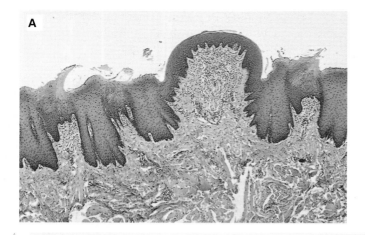

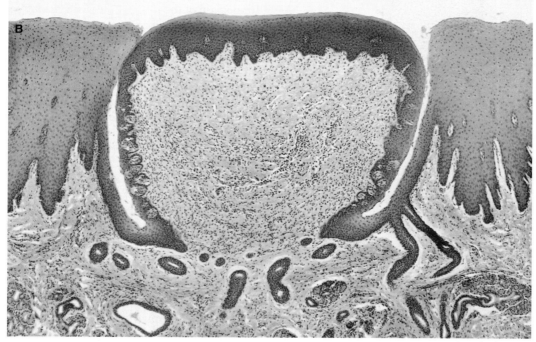

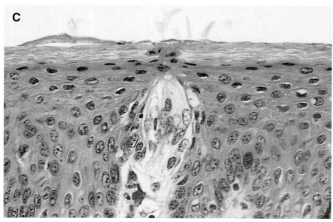

Figure 20-5. *A*) Fungiform and filiform papillae of the caprine tongue. The keratinized filiform papillae have no taste buds. *B*) Vallate papilla of the caprine tongue. Note the deep groove adjacent to the papilla; taste buds occur in the mucosa of the papilla of this groove. *C*) Higher magnification of a taste bud from an equine fungiform papilla. (Reprinted with permission from Bacha, Jr. W.J. and Bacha L.M. *Color Atlas of Veterinary Histology*. Baltimore: Lippincott Williams & Wilkins, 2000.)

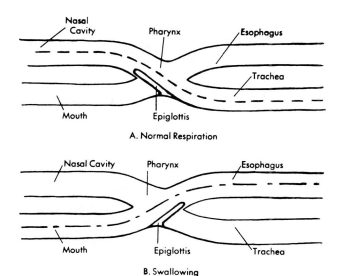

Figure 20-6. Relationship of pharynx and mouth to larynx and esophagus during (*A*) normal respiration and (*B*) swallowing.

tilage over the dorsal aspect of the proximal esophagus. While not in the strictest sense a sphincter muscle, the action of the *m. cricopharyngeus* makes it function as a sphincter for this end of the esophagus.

From the pharynx, the esophagus passes dorsal to the trachea and usually inclines somewhat to the left in the neck in the midcervical region. It again passes dorsal to the trachea when it enters the thorax and continues caudad between the trachea and the aorta through the mediastinum to pass through the diaphragm at the **esophageal hiatus.** Within the abdominal cavity, the esophagus joins the stomach.

The mucosa of the esophagus is thrown into prominent longitudinal folds that permit considerable cross-sectional dilation of the lumen to accommodate the passage of a bolus of food. The epithelium is of the stratified squamous type, being more or less keratinized in accordance with the roughness of the usual feedstuff.

The tunica muscularis of the esophagus consists of two layers that cross obliquely in the proximal esophagus, assume a spiral configuration in the midesophageal region, and form an inner circular and an outer longitudinal layer in the more distal parts. The muscle changes from striated to smooth in the caudal third of the esophagus in the horse and just cranial to the diaphragm in the pig; it is striated throughout

its length in the ruminants. Esophageal muscles, both striated and smooth, are innervated by the vagus nerve.

Nonruminant Stomach

In nonruminants (horse and pig), the stomach is just caudal to the left side of the diaphragm. It is sometimes described in these species as a **simple stomach.** The old term *monogastric* is discouraged because it perpetuates the misconception that ruminants possess more than one stomach, although the ruminant actually has a single stomach with multiple compartments.

The simple stomach is grossly subdivided into the cardia (entrance), fundus, body, and pyloric region (outflow); the pyloric region features a dense, palpable sphincter muscle called the pylorus that controls gastric emptying into more distal parts of the digestive tract (Fig. 20–7).

The esophagus joins the stomach at the **cardia,** a part of the stomach so named because of its proximity to the heart. The walls surrounding the cardia (where the lumen of the esophagus becomes continuous with that of the stomach) feature a thickening of the muscle that constitutes a functional sphincter. This muscle is especially well developed in the horse, where

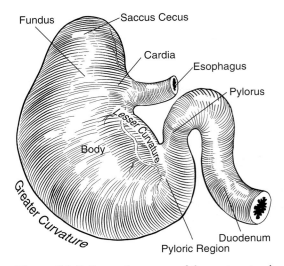

Figure 20-7. External anatomy of the equine simple stomach.

its strength and configuration make it difficult or impossible for the horse to vomit.

The cardia and pylorus are quite close together, giving the stomach a **J** shape. This arrangement results in a very short concave side between the cardia and pylorus, known as the *lesser curvature,* and a much longer convex side, the *greater curvature.* The large bulge near the cardia is the *fundus.* In the horse, the fundus is enlarged to create a blind sac, the *saccus cecus,* the mucosa of which is stratified squamous, and nonglandular. The porcine stomach features a similar albeit smaller outpocketing called the *gastric diverticulum;* the mucosa of this feature of the pig stomach is of the typical glandular, columnar type.

The *body* of the stomach is the expansile part that is defined externally by the greater curvature. The size of the gastric body is determined largely by the degree of filling. It narrows as the stomach arcs ventrad and to the right, becoming the *pyloric region.* A very strong sphincter, the *pylorus,* regulates the outflow of the stomach in this region. In the pig (and in the equivalent region of the ruminant stomach), the pylorus features a muscular and fatty enlargement, the *torus pyloricus.* Its function is unknown.

The tunica muscularis of the stomach features three discontinuous layers of smooth muscle: an outer longitudinal, a middle circular, and an inner oblique layer.

The lumen of the simple stomach features several histologically distinct regions whose names are similar to the gross parts of the stomach but that unfortunately do not directly correspond to these (Fig. 20–8). Immediately surrounding the cardia is an area of stratified squamous epithelium called the *esophageal region.* This nonglandular region is limited in swine but is expanded in the horse, in which it lines the saccus cecus. It is the esophageal region of the stomach that is so markedly expanded in ruminants, where it lines the forestomach.

Exclusive of the esophageal region, the mucosa of the simple stomach is glandular. Grossly, the mucosa here is thrown into prominent *gastric folds* that allow the stomach volume to expand to accommodate meals. On the microscopic level, the columnar epithelium of the tunica mucosa undulates in deep infoldings that create depressions called *gastric pits.*

A transition from the stratified squamous epithelium of the esophageal region to columnar epithelium in the glandular part of the stomach demarcates the beginning of the *cardiac gland region.* This transition is grossly obvious in the horse, where it is called the *margo plicatus.*

The *cardiac glands* that give this region its name are short, branched tubular glands whose major secretory product is mucus. The equine cardiac gland region is small, but it covers nearly half of the interior of the porcine stomach.

The *fundic gland region* lines much of the interior of the stomach (and certainly more than just the fundus). The typical gland is the *fundic gland* (also called the *gastric gland proper*). Fundic glands are simple tubular glands that open into the gastric pits, where they discharge their secretions.

The *pyloric gland region* corresponds more or less to the pyloric region of the simple stomach. The pyloric glands are histologically similar to the cardiac glands, and like them, they secrete mucus.

Enteroendocrine cells are scattered throughout the mucosa of the glandular stomach. These secrete hormones that affect the secretory and

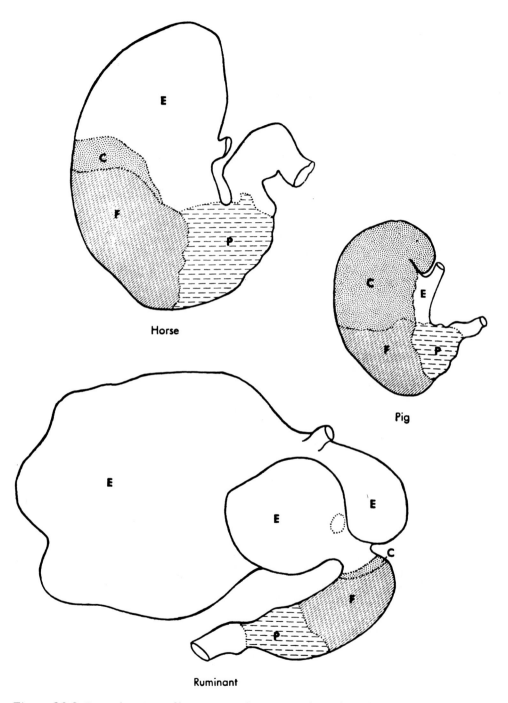

Figure 20-8. Stomach regions of horse, pig, and ruminant. *E)* Esophageal region; *C)* cardiac–gland region; *F)* fundic gland region; *P)* pyloric gland region.

muscular activity of the gut and its accessory organs (e.g., liver and pancreas).

Ruminant Stomach

The ruminant stomach is actually a single stomach modified by marked expansion of the esophageal region into three distinct and voluminous diverticula, the **rumen, reticulum,** and **omasum,** collectively known as the **forestomach (proventriculus).** These are lined with nonglandular stratified squamous epithelium and comprise a series of chambers where food is subjected to digestion by microorganisms before passing through the digestive tract to the smaller glandular portion of the stomach in the ruminant, the **abomasum.** The stomach of the ox is shown in Figures 20–8 and 20–9.

Ruminoreticulum

Because of their functional and anatomic relatedness, the reticulum and rumen are often collectively called the **ruminoreticulum.** The cardia (opening of the esophagus) is about the level of the middle of the seventh intercostal space, and it opens into the dorsal space that is common to both the rumen and reticulum. The mucosa in the region of the cardia forms two heavy muscular folds that together create a groove extending from the cardia to omasum. This is the **sulcus ruminoreticularis** (sometimes called the esophageal or reticular groove). In nursing ruminants, the act of suckling initiates a reflex contraction of the muscular walls of the sulcus, transforming it from a groove to a tube that connects the cardia with the omasum. By this reflex, swallowed milk bypasses the ruminoreticulum and is instead delivered to the more distal parts of the stomach; this ensures that the milk will not be allowed to sour in the forestomach.

The **reticulum** is the most cranial compartment of the forestomach. Its mucosa is thrown up into intersecting ridges that give the reticulum its common name, the "honeycomb." The location of the reticulum immediately caudal to the diaphragm places it opposite the heart, with only the muscular diaphragm between, so any foreign objects such as wire or nails that accumulate in the reticulum may be driven into pleural and pericardial spaces by the reticulum's muscular activity (hardware disease; see Chapter 17).

The reticulum and the **rumen** (colloquially known as the paunch) are divided ventrally by a thick, muscular **ruminoreticular fold.** The rumen extends from this fold to the pelvis and almost entirely fills the left side of the abdominal cavity; its capacity depends on the size of the individual but in adult cattle ranges from 110 to 235 L.

The rumen is subdivided internally into compartments by muscular **pillars,** which correspond to grooves visible on the exterior of the rumen (Fig. 20–9). **Right** and **left longitudinal pillars** (corresponding to right and left longitudinal grooves on the exterior) together with **cranial** and **caudal pillars** (externally, cranial and caudal grooves) form a nearly complete constricting circle in the horizontal plane. These divide the rumen into **dorsal** and **ventral sacs.** The dorsal sac is the largest compartment. The dorsal sac is continuous cranially with the reticulum over the ruminoreticular fold, so that the two compartments share a dorsal space.

Caudally the dorsal sac is further subdivided by the **dorsal coronary pillars,** which form an incomplete circle bounding the **dorsal blind sac.** The caudal part of the ventral sac forms a diverticulum, the **ventral blind sac,** separated from the rest of the ventral sac by the **ventral coronary pillars.**

As in the rest of the forestomach, the mucous membrane lining the rumen is a nonglandular, stratified squamous epithelium. The most ventral parts of both sacs of the rumen contain numerous feathery papillae up to 1 cm long, but papillae are almost entirely absent on the dorsal part of the rumen.

Omasum

The **omasum** is a spherical organ filled with muscular laminae that lie in sheets, much like the pages of a book (giving the omasum its colloquial name, "book stomach"). The stratified squamous mucous membrane covering the laminae is studded with short, blunt papillae

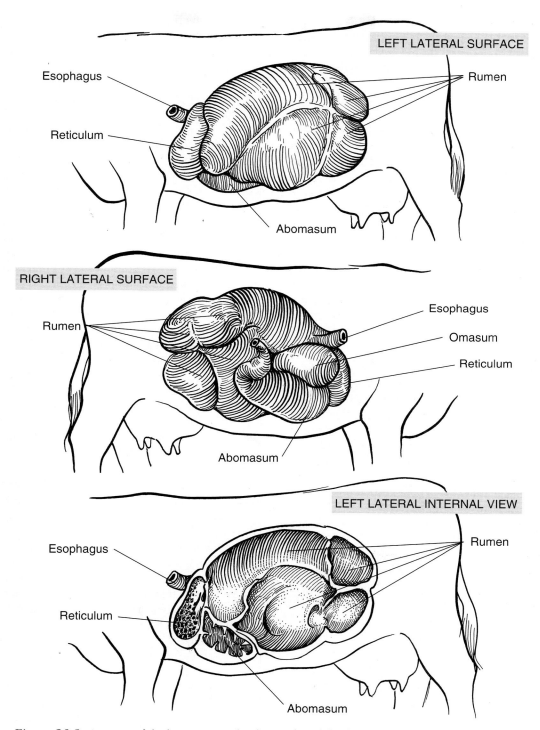

LEFT LATERAL SURFACE

Esophagus

Rumen

Reticulum

Abomasum

RIGHT LATERAL SURFACE

Rumen

Esophagus

Omasum

Reticulum

Abomasum

LEFT LATERAL INTERNAL VIEW

Rumen

Esophagus

Reticulum

Abomasum

Figure 20-9. Anatomy of the bovine stomach. *A*) View from left. *B*) View from right, *C*) Internal anatomy of the ruminoreticulum as viewed from the right.

that grind roughage before it passes distally into the abomasum. Each lamina contains three layers of muscle, including a central layer continuous with the tunica muscularis of the omasal wall.

The omasum lies to the right of the ruminoreticulum, just caudal to the liver, and in the ox makes contact with the right body wall. The omasum of the sheep and goat is much smaller than the bovine omasum and normally is not in contact with the abdominal wall. Food enters the omasum at the reticulo-omasal orifice, between the laminae, and goes on to the omasoabomasal orifice. At the junction of the omasum and abomasum are folds of mucous membrane, the **vela abomasica,** which may act as a valve to prevent return of material from the abomasum to the omasum. Activity of the omasum is probably related to sorting of foodstuffs so that small particles are passed on to the abomasum and coarser materials are returned to the reticulum.

Abomasum

The **abomasum** (true stomach) is the first glandular portion of the ruminant digestive system (Fig. 20–8). Its proximal portion is ventral to the omasum, and its body extends caudad on the right side of the rumen. The pylorus demarcates the muscular junction of the stomach and small intestine, and like the porcine pylorus, it features an enlarged torus pyloricus.

The epithelium of the abomasum consists primarily of two glandular regions, equivalent to the fundic gland region (region of the proper gastric glands) and the pyloric gland region. The cardiac gland region in the abomasum is confined to a very small area adjacent to the omasoabomasal orifice.

Small Intestine

The **duodenum** is the first of three divisions of the small intestine (Figs. 20–10 to 20–12). It is closely attached to the right side of the dorsal body wall by a short mesentery, the **mesoduodenum.** The duodenum arises at the pylorus of the stomach and receives ducts from the pancreas and liver in this region. It passes

caudad on the right side of the abdominal cavity toward the pelvic inlet, then crosses to the left side caudal to the root of the great mesentery (discussed later) and reflects craniad to join the jejunum. The mesentery becomes considerably longer at this **duodenojejunal flexure,** and the duodenum is attached at this site to the descending colon by a serosal ligament, the **duodenocolic fold.**

The transition between duodenum and the next portion of the small intestine, the **jejunum,** is defined by the marked increase in the length of the supporting mesentery. The jejunum is the longest part of the small intestine (e.g., as much as 28 m in the horse). Histologically, the jejunum is similar to the duodenum, although lymph nodules at the mucosal–submucosal junction may be more numerous.

The **ileum** is the short last part of the small intestine. It is distinguished from the jejunum by a fold of mesentery between it and the cecum. This **ileocecal fold** is found on the side of the intestine opposite the attachment of the mesentery (the **antimesenteric** side). The lumen of the ileum communicates with that of the large intestine at the **ileal orifice;** this junction is found in the right caudal part of the abdominal cavity in all species. The ileal epithelium features numerous goblet (mucous) cells, and aggregates of lymph nodules in this region are more abundant than in other parts of the small intestine. Their especially prominent arrangement in the ileum has led to the use of the term **Peyer's patches** to distinguish them.

The mesenteries that suspend the small intestine from the dorsal body wall can be named according to the part of the intestine supported, that is, **mesoduodenum, mesojejunum,** and **mesoileum.** The mesoduodenum is generally short, so the location of the duodenum is relatively fixed. The mesenteries supporting jejunum and ileum, on the other hand, are long and fanlike, so that many meters of intestine are connected to a small region of the dorsal body wall. The mesojejunum and mesoileum are often collectively called the **great mesentery,** and the narrow stalk by which they are attached to the body wall and through which blood vessels, nerves, and lymphatics reach the intestines is commonly called the **root of the**

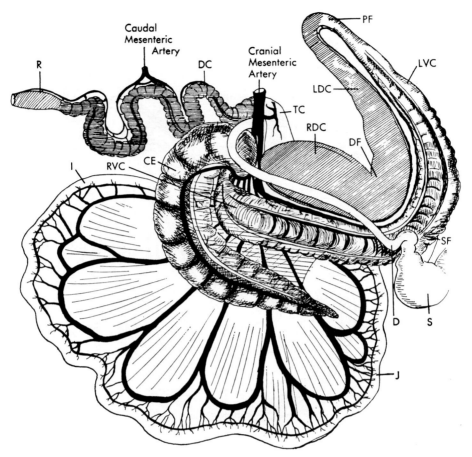

Figure 20-10. Gastrointestinal tract of the horse. *S*) Stomach; *D*) duodenum; *J*) jejunum; *I*) ileum; *CE*) cecum; *RVC*) right ventral colon; *SF*) sternal flexures; *LVC*) left ventral colon; *PF*) pelvic flexure; *LDC*) left dorsal colon; *DF*) diaphragmatic flexure; *RDC*) right dorsal colon; *TC*) transverse colon; *DC*) descending colon: *R*) rectum. (After Nickel R., Schummer A., and Seiferle E. *Lehrbuch der Anatomie der Haustiere.* Berlin: Paul Parey, 1960.)

great mesentery. The length of the great mesentery permits considerable mobility of the intestinal mass.

Large Intestine

The large intestine consists of the **cecum,** a blind sac, and the **colon,** which consists of *ascending, transverse,* and *descending* parts. The descending colon terminates as the **rectum** and **anal canal.**

There is considerably more variation in the large intestine from one species to another than in the small intestine (Figs. 20–10 to 20–12). Most of this variation results from modifications of the ascending colon. The transverse colon forms a short connection that runs transversely from distal ascending colon to proximal descending colon; it is invariably found running from right to left sides of the abdomen, just cranial to the root of the great mesentery. The descending colon is generally relatively straight, running caudad on the left side of the abdomen to the pelvic cavity, where it terminates as the rectum.

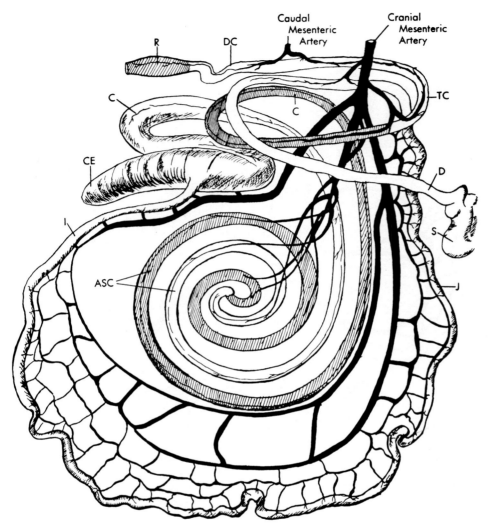

Figure 20-11. Gastrointestinal tract of the ox. *S*) Stomach (abomasum; forestomach not shown). *D*) duodenum. *J*) jejunum. *I*) ileum. *CE*) cecum, *C*) proximal loop and distal loop. *ASC*) ansa spiralis. *TC*) transverse colon. *DC*) descending colon *R*) rectum. (After Nickel R., Schummer A., and Seiferle E. *Lehrbuch der Anatomie der Haustiere.* Berlin: Paul Parey, 1960.)

Ruminants

In the ruminant (Fig. 20–10) the cecum is about 12 cm in diameter, and when full, its blind end projects as far caudad as the pelvic inlet. Cranially, the cecum is continuous with the colon.

The proximal part of the colon is the *ascending colon.* It is modified into a series of three loops in the ruminant. The **proximal loop (ansa proximalis)** forms an **S** shape that leads to the **spiral loop (ansa spiralis)**. The spiral colon forms an orderly spiraling mass on the left face of the great mesentery. The first portion of the spiral colon coils toward the center of the mesentery (centripetally), reverses direction at the central flexure, then spirals away from the center (centrifugally). The last part of the ascending colon, the **dis-**

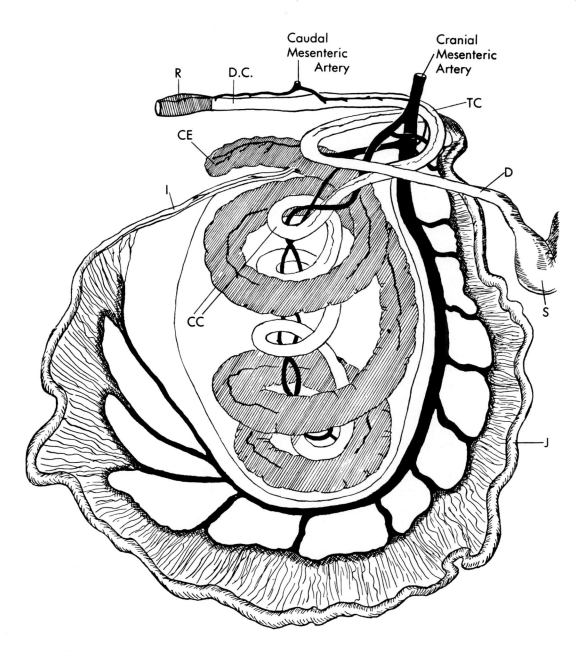

Figure 20-12. Gastrointestinal tract of the pig. *S)* Stomach; *D)* duodenum; *J)* jejunum; *I)* ileum; *CE)* cecum; *CC)* ansa spiralis (coiled colon); *TC)* transverse colon; *DC)* descending colon; *R)* rectum. (After Nickel R., Schummer A., and Seiferle E. *Lehrbuch der Anatomie der Haustiere*. Berlin: Paul Parey, 1960.)

tal loop (*ansa distalis*) connects the spiral colon with the **transverse colon.** The transverse colon crosses from right to left, cranial to the cranial mesenteric artery, which supplies the small intestine, the cecum, and the ascending colon, and continues caudad as the **descending colon** to the rectum. An **external anal sphincter** of striated (i.e., voluntary) muscle and an **internal anal sphincter** of smooth muscle characterize the walls of the most distal part of the gastrointestinal tract as it opens to the exterior of the animal at the **anus.**

The arrangement of the intestinal tract of the sheep and goat is similar to that of the ox. In small ruminants, however, the last centrifugal loop of the ansa spiralis lies much closer to the jejunum than in the ox.

Pig

The porcine cecum (Fig. 20–12) is a moderately large (1.5–2.2 L) blind sac that projects cranioventrad near the midline. The dorsal end of the cecum is continuous with the colon at the ileocecocolic junction, where the entrance of the ileum marks the division between the cecum and colon. Unlike those of most domestic species, the bulk of the porcine cecum lies to the left of midline, with its junction with the colon ventral to the left kidney.

The ascending colon of the pig, like that of the ruminant, presents a spiral arrangement of coils, although in the case of the pig the **spiral loop** is arranged in a cone shape rather than in a flat plane. The transverse colon continues from its junction with the distal end of the spiral loop, passes forward, then crosses to the left side of the abdomen. The bowel continues caudad as descending colon to the rectum. As in other animals, the rectum terminates at the anus.

Horse

The horse has the largest and most complex large intestine of any of the domestic animals (Fig. 20–10). The equine diet of grasses necessitates the assistance of microbes for digestion of celluloses, but unlike that of ruminants, the

horse's digestive system defers this fermentation until ingested food reaches the cecum. For this reason, horses are often called **postgastric fermentators.**

The cecum in the horse is a comma-shaped structure extending from its **base** in the right side of the pelvic inlet to the floor of the abdominal cavity, where the **apex** lies just caudal to the diaphragm near the xiphoid cartilage of the sternum. The ileum enters the cecum near its base at the **ileal orifice.** The cecum is the primary site of fermentation in the horse, and its average capacity is about 33 L.

The ascending colon of the horse is highly modified and extremely capacious, for which reason it is commonly referred to as the **great colon.** The proximal part leaves the cecum and passes craniad along the right ventral abdominal wall toward the sternal part of the diaphragm, where it turns sharply to the left and proceeds caudad along the left ventral abdominal wall toward the pelvic inlet. These first parts of the large colon are known respectively as the **right ventral colon,** the **sternal flexure,** and the **left ventral colon.** They are arranged like a horseshoe, with the toe forward and the branches directed caudad on either side of the apex of the cecum.

At the pelvic inlet, the left ventral colon turns sharply dorsad to form the **pelvic flexure.** The colon then continues craniad as the **left dorsal colon,** located just dorsal to the left ventral colon. As it approaches the diaphragm (just dorsal to the sternal flexure), it bends to the left as the **diaphragmatic flexure** and then continues a short distance caudad as the **right dorsal colon.** The right dorsal colon turns again to the left and crosses the midline in front of the root of the great mesentery as the transverse colon.

The descending colon in the horse (also called the **small colon** to distinguish it from the great colon) is the direct continuation of the transverse colon. The descending colon is arranged in undulations within the mesocolon, much like the small intestine in the mesentery. The small colon, however, is somewhat larger in diameter than the small intestine. The small colon is usually located near the middle of the caudal part of the abdominal cavity. It terminates within the pelvic cavity as the rectum.

Peritoneal Features

The parietal and visceral peritonea are continuous with one another at double folds of serosa called mesenteries (see above). In some locations, visceral peritoneum reflects off one region of the gut, spans a short distance, then merges onto the surface of nearby structures. Although these double folds of peritoneum are typically very thin, in this configuration they are sometimes referred to as ligaments. Some examples include the *falciform ligament,* which tethers the liver to the ventral midline; the *renosplenic ligament,* spanning between the left kidney and spleen; and the *hepatoduodenal ligament,* connecting the liver and proximal duodenum.

Omentum refers to those parts of the peritoneum connecting the stomach with other structures. It is divided into a *lesser omentum,* extending from the lesser curvature of the stomach to the liver, and the *greater omentum,* which is attached to the greater curvature of the stomach (and the comparable portion of the ruminant stomach). The greater omentum spreads like an apron from the stomach to cover most of the ventral aspect of the mass of intestine.

Accessory Digestive Organs

In addition to the numerous small glands located in the walls of the stomach and intestine, accessory glands include the salivary glands, the pancreas, and the liver.

Salivary Glands

The salivary glands of domestic farm animals comprise three pairs of well-defined glands as well as scattered lobules of salivary tissue (minor salivary glands). The chief salivary glands are the parotid, mandibular, and sublingual (Fig. 20–13). The minor salivary glands include labial, buccal, lingual, and palatine glands.

The *parotid salivary gland* is located ventral to the ear in relation to the caudal border of the mandible. In most animals, the *parotid salivary duct* passes ventrad and craniad on the deep face of the caudal part of the mandible, and crosses the cheek superficially just cranial to the masseter muscle. The duct then passes

dorsad to penetrate the mucous membrane of the cheek near the third or fourth maxillary cheek tooth.

The *mandibular salivary gland* is usually located ventral to the parotid gland, just caudal to the mandible. The mandibular salivary duct passes forward along the medial side of the mandible to open ventral to the tongue on the *sublingual caruncle,* a small hillock of mucous membrane located on the floor of the mouth.

The *sublingual salivary gland* is located deep to the mucous membrane along the ventral side of the lateral surface of the tongue near the floor of the mouth. Numerous ducts pass directly from the gland to open into the floor of the mouth just ventrolateral to the tongue. With the exception of the horse, the sublingual salivary gland also has a monostomatic portion that empties at the sublingual caruncle on the floor of the mouth by way of a single sublingual duct that runs parallel to the mandibular duct.

The salivary glands are classified as serous, mucous, or mixed. Serous glands secrete a watery clear fluid, as compared with mucous glands, which secrete mucus, a viscous material that acts as a protective covering for the surface of mucous membranes. A mixed gland produces both mucous and serous fluids. The parotid salivary gland secretes primarily a serous saliva; mandibular and sublingual glands are classified as mixed glands in domestic farms animals. Most of the minor salivary glands have a mucous secretion.

Pancreas

The pancreas is a compound gland that has both endocrine and exocrine portions. The exocrine portion of the pancreas produces sodium bicarbonate and digestive enzymes, which pass through the pancreatic ducts to empty into the duodenum close to the opening of the bile duct.

The endocrine portion of the pancreas consists of isolated groups of pale-staining cells scattered throughout the gland. These areas are called the *pancreatic islets* (formerly islets of Langerhans). They produce the hormones that pass directly into the bloodstream (see Chapter 12), most notably glucagon and insulin, which are the primary regulators of blood sugar levels.

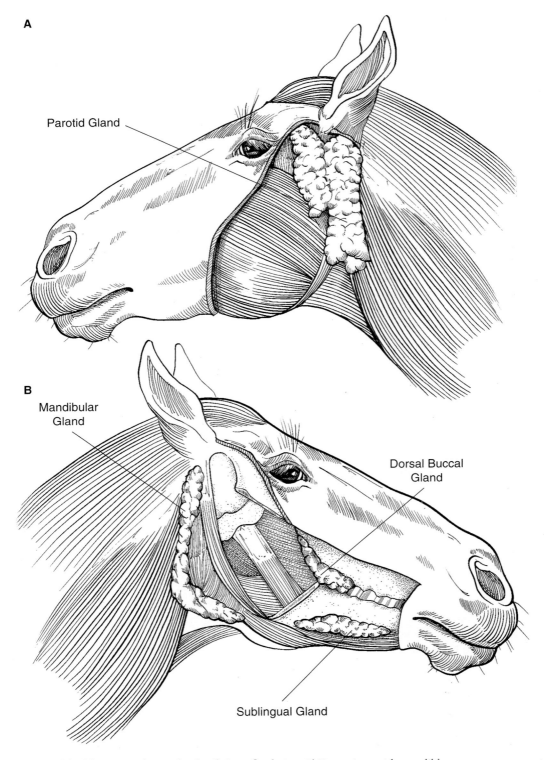

Figure 20–13. Major salivary glands. *A)* Superficial view. *B)* Deep view, with mandible cut away.

Grossly, the **pancreas** is an irregularly lobulated organ that lies adjacent to the proximal duodenum and frequently abuts the stomach, the caudal vena cava, and caudal part of the liver as well. The pancreas has the appearance of aggregated nodules, loosely connected to form an elongated gland lying parallel to the duodenum. The developing pancreas arises as two diverticula of the embryonic duodenum, and therefore always begins as a bilobed organ connected to the lumen of the gut by two ducts. During organogenesis in many species, the duct systems of the two lobes intermingle and one of the two original connections to the gut lumen is lost, so that a single duct is the normal condition of the adult in these species. The disposition of ducts of the pancreas is shown in Table 20–3.

In those species that possess it, the **pancreatic duct** opens onto a small elevation within the duodenum in common with the bile duct from the liver. This is the **major duodenal papilla**. A short distance away, a smaller **minor duodenal papilla** marks the location of the **accessory pancreatic duct**. As small ruminants lack the accessory pancreatic duct, they also lack the minor duodenal papilla.

The first branches of these ducts within the pancreas are **interlobular ducts,** so-called because they run between lobules of the pancreas. Interlobular ducts branch into **intralobular ducts** that enter individual lobules and give rise to **intercalated ducts,** which enter the **acini** (sometimes called alveoli).

Liver

The **liver** is the largest gland in the body, constituting 1–2% of total adult body weight. It varies somewhat in number of lobes and precise intraabdominal location from one species to another. However, the liver is always located immediately caudal to the diaphragm (in contact with it) and tends to be located on the right side, particularly in ruminants, in whom the large reticulorumen pushes everything else to the right.

Individual liver lobules of the pig are encircled by rather heavy connective tissue septa, which give a lobulated, "cobblestone" appearance to the surface of the porcine liver. This appearance is less distinctive in other domestic species. Liver tissue is usually a reddish brown, although accumulation of fat (whether due to a high fat diet or pathology) can give it a pronounced yellow tinge.

The liver receives two blood supplies. To provide oxygen and nutrients, arterial blood from the **hepatic artery,** a branch of the celiac artery, enters the side of the liver adjacent to the viscera, called the **porta** (Latin: gate). This is the **nutrient blood supply.** The porta also receives the large **portal vein,** which carries blood to the liver from the stomach, spleen, pancreas, and intestines. The liver performs metabolic and immunologic functions on this blood returning from the gastrointestinal tract, and so the blood of the portal vein constitutes the **functional blood supply.** Portal blood is detoxified and modified within the **sinusoids** (capillaries) of the liver and then leaves the liver by way of the short **hepatic veins** that empty into the caudal vena cava.

All domestic animals except the horse have a **gallbladder** for storage of bile. The liver's digestive secretion, **bile,** leaves the liver through **hepatic ducts,** which join the **cystic duct** from the gallbladder to form the **common bile duct,** which then passes to proximal duodenum into the lumen of which it opens in common with the pancreatic duct on the major duodenal papilla (see above).

Table 20-3. Species Variations in Pancreatic Ducts

Species	Pancreatic Duct	Accessory Pancreatic Duct
Horse	+	+
Ox	Usually absent	+
Pig	−	+
Small ruminants	+	−

Microscopically, the morphologic unit of the liver is the **hepatic lobule,** a polygonal cylinder of liver cells (the **hepatocytes**) in the center of which is a **central vein** (Fig. 20–14). At the angles on the periphery, where adjacent hepatic lobules meet, are the **portal triads,** consisting of branches of the hepatic artery and portal vein (interlobular vessels), an interlobular bile duct, and lymphatics. These communicate with the spaces between sheets, or laminae, of hepatocytes in the hepatic lobule; the spaces are the **hepatic sinusoids,** and they are characterized by the lack of a basal lamina and numerous fenestrations in the endothelium, allow free egress of blood constituents that then bathe the hepatocytes. Blood (both arterial and portal) flows from the portal canal, through the sinusoids, and is gathered by the central vein, the smallest tributary of the hepatic veins. In and around the sinusoids are fixed macrophages, which in this location are called **Kupffer cells.**

Between adjacent rows of liver cells is a tiny **bile canaliculus,** which is little more than a tube formed by grooves in the surfaces of the apposed liver cells. Bile produced by the hepatocytes is carried toward the periphery of the hepatic lobule by the bile canaliculi to the interlobular bile ducts located at the portal canal (notice that this net flow is opposite the direction of blood flow).

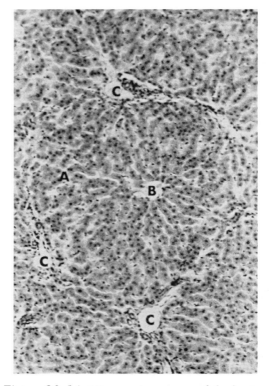

Figure 20–14. Microscopic anatomy of the bovine liver. *A* Hepatocytes of liver lobule. *B* Central vein. C Portal veins. (Reprinted with permission from Dellmann H.D. *Textbook of Veterinary Histology.* 4th ed. Philadelphia: Lea & Febiger, 1993.)

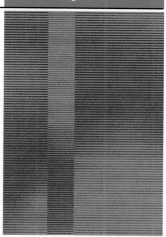

PHYSIOLOGY OF DIGESTION

For normal metabolism, cells of an animal's body need the three major classes of nutrients (carbohydrates, proteins, and lipids) delivered to them via the blood in their simplest forms (monosaccharides, amino acids, and fatty acids). Animals consume foodstuffs that contain these nutrients in more complex chemical and physical forms. It is the function of the gastrointestinal tract to reduce the consumed foodstuffs to simpler molecules and to transfer them to the blood so that they can be delivered to the cells for metabolism. The processes of physical and chemical breakdown of foodstuffs are termed **mechanical** and **chemical digestion,** respectively. In addition to monosaccharides, amino acids, and fatty acids, the gastrointestinal tract must absorb other essential minor nutrients (e.g., salts, vitamins), so that they are available to the cells of the body.

The gastrointestinal tract is essentially a long smooth muscle tube extending from mouth to anus. The tube has two distinct layers of smooth muscle in its wall (**circular** and **longitudinal layers**) and is lined with epithelia that function as selective barriers between the lumen and the body fluids. The anatomic and functional characteristics of the mucosa and its epithelia vary greatly among segments of the intestine (Fig. 21–1). Undigestible substances or items (such as a coin) can pass through the tract without being altered and without affecting the animal if they are not large enough to impair movement of the other contents.

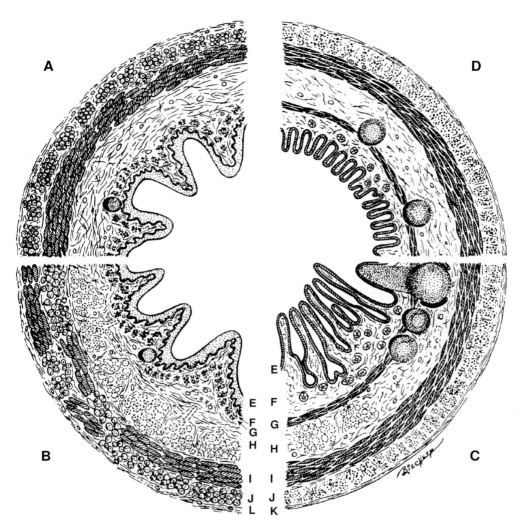

Figure 21-1. Cross-sections through various segments of the digestive tract. Esophagus (*A* and *B*) with stratified squamous epithelium. Small intestine with columnar epithelium and submucosal glands and aggregated lymphatic nodules in some segments (*C*). Large intestine (*D*). Tunica mucosa: epithelium (*E*), lamina propria (*F*), lamina muscularis (*G*). Tela submucosa. (*H*) Tunica muscularis: circular layer (*I*), longitudinal layer (*J*). Tunica serosa (*K*). Tunica adventitia (*L*). (Reprinted with permission from Dellman H.D. and Eurell J. *Textbook of Veterinary Histology.* 5th ed. Philadelphia: Lippincott Williams & Wilkins, 1998.)

The smooth muscle in the wall of the gastrointestinal tract provides the force to move digesta through the tract; *gastrointestinal motility* is the general term used to describe the activity of this smooth muscle. Gastrointestinal motility is primarily regulated by three mechanisms: (1) *autonomic nervous system,* (2) *gastrointestinal hormones,* and (3) *enteric nervous system.*

Gastrointestinal hormones are released from endocrine cells in the epithelial lining of the gastrointestinal tract (*enteroendocrine cells*) and may stimulate or inhibit gastrointestinal smooth muscle. The release of these hormones is usually in response to digesta in the lumen of the tract. Thus, these hormones are a means of local regulation that is coordinated with the ingestion and digestion of food.

The enteric nervous system consists of neural plexuses between layers of smooth muscle in the wall of the tract (Fig. 21–1). These plexuses contain complete neurons (dendrites, cell bodies, and axons) that can form complete neural and reflex circuits in the wall of the tract, so that neural regulation can be independent of external innervation. The presence of food and distension of gastrointestinal tract segments act as stimuli to initiate activity of the enteric nervous system. The three regulatory mechanisms (autonomic nervous system, gastrointestinal hormones, and enteric nervous system) also regulate secretions from glands in the wall of the gastrointestinal tract (Fig. 21–1) and the intestinal accessory organs (salivary glands, liver, and pancreas).

All three of these mechanisms may regulate a given intestinal segment or accessory organ, but the relative importance of each varies among the segments of the gastrointestinal tract and the accessory organs. For example, salivary secretion is almost entirely regulated by the autonomic nervous system, while gastrointestinal hormones are primary in the initiation of bile secretion.

Pregastric Physiology

Prehension and Chewing

The act of bringing food into the mouth is **prehension.** The teeth, lips, and tongue are used as prehensile organs by domestic animals. The lips of the horse, the tongue of the cow and sheep, and the snout of the pig are used extensively in obtaining food.

The type of teeth, arrangement of jaws, and chewing (**mastication**) habits vary with the species and the food. Carnivorous animals have simple teeth and tear their food but do little grinding. Herbivorous animals have at least some hypsodont teeth; the upper jaw is wider than the lower jaw; and chewing of the food is thorough. Mastication can be controlled voluntarily, but the presence of food in the mouth will stimulate reflex chewing.

Saliva and Salivary Glands

Saliva consists of water, electrolytes, mucus, and enzymes. The water and mucus soften and lubricate the ingesta to facilitate mastication and swallowing. **Lysozyme** is a salivary enzyme with antibacterial actions. The starch-digesting enzyme **amylase** is present in the saliva of omnivores (pig) and to a limited degree in horses but absent in ruminants and carnivores (dog).

Adult cattle may secrete up to 200 L of saliva per day as compared to 1 to 2 L per day for humans. This large volume maintains the fluid consistency of the rumen contents, and components of the saliva may also prevent frothing of the rumen fluid. Ruminant saliva has a relatively high pH and contains high concentrations of bases (bicarbonate and phosphate). These bases neutralize acids produced by fermentation in the rumen so that the pH in the rumen does not become too acidic.

Parasympathetic nerves are the efferent limbs of neural reflexes that regulate salivary secretion. Afferent inputs that stimulate salivary secretion include sight and smell of food, presence of food in the oral cavity, and conditioned reflexes, where some event is associated with food and feeding. Conditioned reflex control of salivation was the subject of the classic studies by Pavlov, who conditioned dogs to salivate at the sound of a bell.

Swallowing

Deglutition, the act of swallowing, is arbitrarily divided into three stages. The first stage is passage of food or water through the mouth; the second is passage through the pharynx; and the third consists of passage through the esophagus into the stomach.

The first stage of swallowing is under voluntary control. After the food is chewed and mixed with saliva, a **bolus** (rounded mass of food) forms and is moved to the upper surface of the tongue. The tongue is raised against the hard palate (tip first) to push the bolus toward the pharynx. At the same time the soft palate is raised, closing the caudal nares. The base of the tongue then acts as a plunger, forcing the bolus into the pharynx. As the bolus enters the pharynx, it stimulates

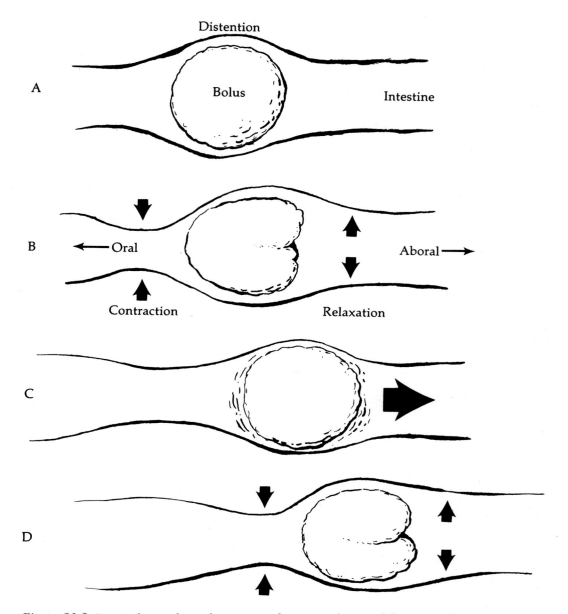

Figure 21-2. Intestinal peristalsis and movement of contents. *A)* Original distension. *B)* Contraction cranial to distension and relaxation caudal. *C)* Movement of contents. *D)* New distension point and new points of contraction and relaxation. (Reprinted with permission from Reece W.O. *Physiology of Domestic Animals.* 2nd ed. Baltimore: Williams & Wilkins, 1997.)

pressure receptors in the walls, which reflexively initiates the second stage, passage of the bolus through the pharynx. Respiration is reflexively inhibited, and the larynx reflexively closes and pulls up and forward. The base of the tongue folds the epiglottis over the laryngeal opening as it moves back. The pharynx shortens, and a *peristaltic* (milking) action of the pharyngeal muscles forces the bolus into the esophagus.

The third stage of deglutition consists of reflex peristalsis of the esophagus initiated by the presence of food in the esophagus. Peristalsis consists of alternate relaxation and contraction of rings of muscle in the wall coupled with regional contraction of longitudinal muscles in the area of the bolus (Fig. 21–2).

Peristalsis carries solid and semisolid food through the esophagus of the horse at 35 to 40 cm/second. Liquids travel about five times as fast by a squirting action of the mouth and the pharynx.

Vomiting (emesis) is a protective response to remove potentially harmful ingesta from the stomach and upper small intestine. Vomiting is a highly coordinated reflex that is controlled by a reflex center in the brainstem. Drugs that stimulate this center to produce vomiting are termed *emetics*. The process begins with relaxation of the sphincter between the stomach and upper small intestine and reverse peristalsis to move intestinal contents to the stomach. The movement of stomach contents into the esophagus and out of the mouth requires relaxation of the upper and lower esophageal sphincters together with an inspiratory movement against a closed glottis and forceful contraction of abdominal muscles. Closure of the glottis and movement of the soft palate prevent regurgitated food from entering the trachea and nasal cavity respectively.

Ruminant Forestomach

Fermentative Digestion

No mammal can directly digest the complex carbohydrates that constitute plant cell walls (*cellulose* and *hemicellulose*), because mammals do not produce the enzyme *cellulase*, which is necessary to break the unique chemical bonds in these compounds. The ruminant forestomach provides an excellent environment for the growth of bacteria, protozoa, and possibly other microbes that do produce cellulase. The action of cellulase on cellulose and hemicellulose produces monosaccharides and simple polysaccharides, which are available for further microbial digestion.

The microbial digestion in the forestomach occurs in an anaerobic environment and is termed *fermentative* digestion. *Volatile fatty acids* (VFAs) are produced by fermentation of carbohydrates consumed by ruminants, including carbohydrates produced by the actions of microbial cellulase. The primary VFAs are *acetic acid, propionic acid,* and *butyric acid.* The VFAs are absorbed directly from the forestomach and are the major energy source for ruminants. VFAs are also used for synthesis of milk fat in lactating animals.

Methane and carbon dioxide are produced by fermentative digestion and accumulate as a gaseous layer above the ingesta in the rumen and reticulum. *Bloat (acute tympany)* results in enlargement of the rumen and reticulum, which in turn presses on the thorax, inhibiting function of the heart and lungs. Bloat results from more gas being produced than is eliminated by *eructation (belching)*. Eructation is particularly difficult if foam forms. A stomach tube may be passed into the rumen by mouth to remove the gas. If that is not possible, a *trocar* (sharp tube) may be passed into the rumen through the left flank.

Dietary protein consumed by ruminants is available first to the microbes in the forestomach. The microbes may use the dietary protein to produce microbial proteins and promote microbial growth or to produce VFAs by fermentative digestion. Microbes can also produce microbial proteins from nonprotein nitrogen sources, such as urea and ammonia.

The microbes and byproducts of microbial metabolism other than VFAs continue down the ruminant gastrointestinal tract from the forestomach. The microbial organisms, which grew in the forestomach, are a major source of dietary protein for ruminants. When the organisms enter the abomasum (true or glandular stomach of the ruminant) and the remainder of the tract, they are digested in a manner similar to digestion of protein sources in nonruminants. Beneficial byproducts of microbial metabolism include many water-soluble vitamins.

Forestomach Motility

The rumen and reticulum of the adult cow normally undergo complicated sequences of contractions that are repeated at varying frequencies up to several times per minute. One pattern of contractions begins in the reticulum and spreads over both the dorsal and ventral sacs of the rumen (see Fig. 20–9). This series of contractions mixes the contents to promote fermentation and provide force to move liquified digesta out of the forestomach and into the abomasum. A second pattern of contractions begins in the caudal portion of the dorsal sac and moves cranially. These contractions move gases toward the cranial part of the rumen for eructation. **Rumen contractions can be felt by forcing the fist into the upper left flank (paralumbar fossa). Pathologic condition of the rumen or morbidity associated with systemic diseases usually results in a decreased rate or complete cessation of rumen movements.**

Rumination permits an animal to forage and ingest food rapidly and finish chewing later. It entails *regurgitation* of the food (returning it to the mouth) from the forestomach, *remastication* (rechewing), *reinsalivation* (mixing with more saliva), and finally reswallowing.

Regurgitation is the only step of rumination that differs markedly from the initial mastication, insalivation, and swallowing. Regurgitation is preceded by contraction of the reticulum, which presumably brings some of the heavier ingesta into proximity to the cardia. The sphincter at the junction of the esophagus and forestomach (**lower esophageal sphincter**) relaxes as the bolus of food reaches it. An inspiratory movement with closed glottis follows. The negative pressure produced in the thorax by this movement is transmitted to the relatively thin-walled esophagus, dilating the thoracic esophagus and cardia. The lower pressure in

the esophagus than in the rumen coupled with reverse peristalsis causes a quantity of material (semifluid ingesta) to pass through the cardia into the esophagus and up to the mouth. The regurgitated material consists largely of roughage and fluid with little if any concentrate. It is well known that whole kernels of corn may pass through the entire digestive tract with little change in physical appearance.

Cattle average about 8 hours a day ruminating, with periods of activity scattered throughout the entire day. One rumination cycle requires about 1 minute, of which 3 to 4 seconds is used for both regurgitation and reswallowing. Rumination appears to be largely reflexive, although the process can be interrupted or stopped voluntarily. Both afferent and efferent portions of the reflex are probably carried in the vagal nerves. Contact of roughage with the wall of the reticulum and near the cardia is likely the major stimulus for rumination.

Reticular, or Esophageal, Groove

In young ruminants, nursing and afferents from the pharynx appear to stimulate reflex closure of the groove, which causes milk to bypass the rumen and reticulum and pass through the omasum directly to the abomasum. The paunchiness of bucket-fed calves usually is attributed to milk entering the rumen, where it is not properly digested. The use of buckets with nipples tends to prevent appreciable amounts of milk from entering the rumen. After weaning, fluid drunk from open containers largely passes into the rumen and reticulum. The groove has no known function in adult animals, but reflex closure in adults has been produced with sodium salts in cattle and copper sulfate in sheep.

Omasum

The omasum is nearly always found packed tightly with rather dry roughage in animals examined after death. The appearance of the omasal leaves, studded with short horny papillae, suggests a burr type of grinder. Experimental vagal stimulation elicits strong contractions

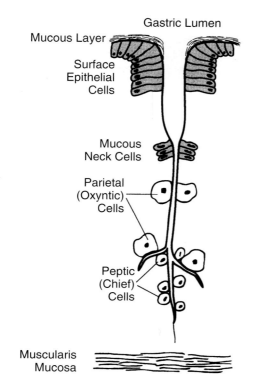

Gastric Lumen

Mucous Layer

Surface
Epithelial
Cells

Mucous
Neck Cells

Parietal
(Oxyntic)
Cells

Peptic
(Chief)
Cells

Muscularis
Mucosa

Figure 21-3. Gastric gland (gastric pit) in the wall of the stomach, showing various cell types found in the gland. (Reprinted with permission from Johnson L.R. *Essential Medical Physiology.* 2nd ed. Philadelphia: Lippincott-Raven, 1998.)

of the omasal wall, but movement of the leaves is limited.

Gastric Physiology

Gastric Glands and Secretions

The term *gastric juice* refers to the combination of substances secreted into the stomach lumen by gastric glands, also termed gastric pits because of their pitlike extension into the wall of the stomach (Fig. 21–3), and epithelial cells of the stomach mucosa. Gastric juice contains water, hydrochloric acid, mucus, intrinsic factor, pepsinogen (an inactive form of pepsin, a proteolytic enzyme), and the enzyme rennin. The

regulation of gastric juice secretion has three phases, cephalic, gastric, and intestinal.

Stimulation of gastric secretions during the *cephalic phase* is in response to the sight, smell, or taste of food. These induce a neural response that increases parasympathetic (vagal nerve) stimulation to the stomach, and this stimulates gastric secretions. The *gastric phase* begins when food enters the stomach.

The presence of food, especially proteins, stimulates the secretion of the hormones *gastrin* and *histamine* from cells in the gastric epithelium. Gastrin and histamine stimulate *parietal cells* in gastric glands to secrete hydrochloric acid (Fig. 21–3). Acetylcholine (parasympathetic neurotransmitter) also stimulates parietal cells to secrete hydrochloric acid, but all three regulators (gastrin, histamine, and acetylcholine) must be present for the most efficient hydrochloric acid secretion. **The histamine receptors on parietal cells (H_2 receptors) are different from those on cells involved in allergic reactions (H_1 receptors). The specific H_2 receptor antagonists provide a means to reduce acid secretion with few side effects. The antihistamines used for allergies do not bind to H_2 receptors and thus do not disturb digestion.** The hormones *cholecystokinin, gastric inhibitory peptide,* and *secretin* inhibit hydrochloric acid secretion. These hormones are released from the duodenal epithelium in response to the presence of food in the duodenum. The release of these hormones that act to inhibit gastric function is part of the *intestinal phase* of gastric regulation.

The pH of gastric juice in mammals can be 2 or less. The low pH is protective in that most foreign microbes ingested with food cannot survive such an acidic environment. The low pH inhibits hydrochloric acid secretion to prevent it from becoming too acidic. *Pepsinogen* (an inactive form of the enzyme *pepsin* and a component of gastric juice) is activated by the low pH. By its proteolytic activity, pepsin can activate more pepsinogen. The low pH also promotes the activity of pepsin, because the most favorable pH range for its proteolytic activity is 1.3 to 5. *Chief* or *peptic cells* (Fig. 21–3) secrete pepsinogen to begin protein digestion in the stomach, but protein digestion is completed in the small intestine by other digestive enzymes.

A layer of mucus covers the epithelial lining of the stomach and protects the epithelium from the low pH of the gastric fluids. This mucus is produced by cells in the gastric glands (Fig. 21–3) and is secreted from there onto the surface of the epithelium. **Mucus secretion is stimulated by prostaglandins, which are also produced locally in the wall of the stomach. Non-steroidal anti-inflammatory drugs (such as aspirin and phenylbutazone) inhibit the synthesis of prostaglandins, and toxic doses of these agents are associated with gastric ulcers. It is presumed that a lack of mucus secretion contributes to the development of the ulcers.**

Rennin is an enzyme in the gastric juice in the abomasum of young ruminants. Its function is to coagulate milk and reduce its rate of passage through the gastrointestinal tract. Intrinsic factor, a carrier protein for vitamin B_{12}, binds to vitamin B_{12}, and the resultant complex passes through the tract to the ileum, which absorbs the B_{12}.

Gastric Motility

Gastric movements mix the ingesta with the gastric juice, continue mechanical digestion (to liquefy the digesta), and pass the digesta into the duodenum at a controlled rate. The stomach regularly produces peristaltic contractions, beginning in the region of the cardia and increasing in force as they travel over the stomach to the pyloric antrum (see Fig. 20–7). These mix and grind the food and force some through the *pyloric sphincter* into the duodenum. However, much of the food (and especially larger particles) is held back to allow for more mixing and grinding. The ingesta forced through the pyloric sphincter, termed *chyme,* is a mushy, semisolid mixture of food, water, and gastric juice.

Similar to the regulation of gastric secretions, the regulation of gastric motility can be divided into cephalic, gastric, and intestinal phases. Stimulation during cephalic regulation occurs via the parasympathetic nerves, and this increases in response to sight, smell, or taste of food. The hormone gastrin stimulates overall gastric motility to promote mixing (gastric phase). The hormones cholecystokinin and secretin and gastric in-

hibitory peptides promote a more forceful contraction of the pyloric sphincter to slow gastric emptying (intestinal phase). The inhibitory effect of the duodenal hormones (released in response to chyme entering the duodenum) prevents the delivery of chyme to the duodenum too fast to be digested normally.

The stomach of a carnivore empties within a few hours, usually before the next meal. Other animals require many hours to empty the stomach. Both the horse and pig require a full day's fast (24 hours) to empty a full stomach. The stomach of a nursing foal empties slowly, but in an adult pony liquid passes from the stomach to the cecum in 2 hours.

In addition to the typical pattern of stomach contraction when food is present, waves of peristaltic contractions may occur over the stomach as a slight ripple. These are produced by spontaneous electrical depolarizations, which sometimes induce action potentials, in the smooth muscle. These begin in the cardia region, and the waves of membrane depolarization are termed *gastric slow waves.* In prolonged fasting, the magnitude of the contractions becomes greater (**hunger contractions**). These are apparently a response to an increase in parasympathetic input during prolonged fasting. These reach maximum intensity in humans after about 3 days without food and weaken progressively thereafter. In the horse, hunger contractions may begin as early as 5 hours after eating, when the stomach still contains some food. The intensity of hunger contractions is related to the level of blood sugar. As the blood sugar level decreases, the intensity of hunger contractions increases.

Physiology of the Small Intestine, Exocrine Pancreas, and Liver

The small intestine is the primary site of chemical digestion and absorption of nutrients. The *exocrine* secretions of the pancreas contain most of the enzymes for chemical digestion in the lumen of the small intestine, but the epithelial cells that line the small intestine (*enterocytes*) also have in their cell membranes enzymes that participate in the final steps of chemical digestion. The primary digestive function of the liver is to provide *bile salts,* which facilitate the enzymatic digestion of lipids. The liver is not a source of digestive enzymes.

Small Intestine: Secretions and Motility

Intestinal juice is derived from intestinal glands in the wall of the small intestine. These include **crypts** or **crypts of Lieberkühn,** scattered throughout the entire small intestine (Fig. 21–4), and **duodenal glands,** which contribute mucus and are found only in the duodenum. The intestinal juice contains salts and water derived from blood capillaries in the wall of the intestine. The function of the secreted salts is unclear, but the water dilutes the chyme, which is usually **hypertonic** (higher osmolality than normal plasma). Food in the intestine stimulates secretion by these intestinal crypt glands.

The two primary types of movement by the small intestine are **segmentation** and peristalsis. Segmentation movements, which occur when food is in the small intestine, are characterized by alternating local areas of contraction and relaxation (Fig. 21–5). These movements mix the digesta with intestinal juice and digestive enzymes and increase the contact between digesta and the epithelial surface of the small intestine. The increased contact provides more exposure to enzymes associated with epithelial cells and to the absorptive surface of the epithelial cells. Strong peristaltic contractions of the small intestine in fasting animals or several hours after a meal propel ingesta down the tract, presumably to clean the small intestine of undigested foodstuffs before the next meal.

Exocrine Pancreas

Pancreatic exocrine secretions primarily consist of a variety of digestive enzymes and sodium bicarbonate. Pancreatic *acinar* cells (Fig. 21–6)

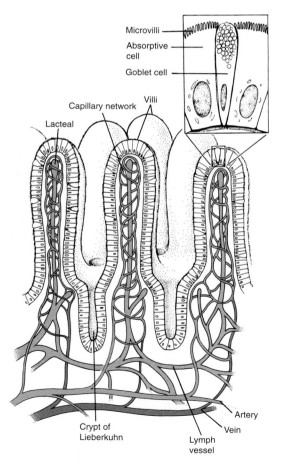

Figure 21-4. Intestinal villi and crypts. (Reprinted with permission from Bullock B.L. *Pathophysiology.* 4th ed. Philadelphia: Lippincott, 1996.)

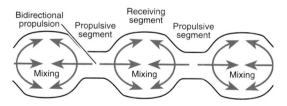

Figure 21-5. The segmentation pattern of gastrointestinal motility. Note alternating sites of contraction and relaxation. (Reprinted with permission from Rhoades R.A. and Tanner G.A. *Medical Physiology.* Boston: Little, Brown, 1995.)

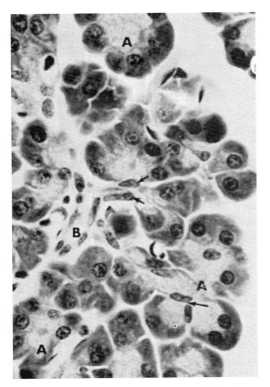

Figure 21-6. Pancreas. Pancreatic acini (A) and intercalated duct (B). (Reprinted with permission from Dellman H.D. and Eurell J. *Textbook of Veterinary Histology.* 5th ed. Philadelphia: Lippincott Williams & Wilkins, 1998.)

secrete the enzymes, and cells that line ducts in the pancreas secrete the sodium bicarbonate. These ducts empty into one or two pancreatic ducts, which empty into the duodenum.

The sodium bicarbonate raises to an acceptable pH the chyme entering from the stomach. The small-intestinal epithelium is not protected from an acidic solution by a thick layer of mucus, as is the stomach. The higher pH is also better for the action of the pancreatic digestive enzymes. The major stimulus for bicarbonate secretion is the hormone secretin from the small intestinal mucosa. Secretin secretion increases in response to the acid chyme entering from the stomach.

Pancreatic proteolytic enzymes include *trypsin* and *chymotrypsin.* Similar to pepsin in the stomach, these are secreted as inactive precursors, *trypsinogen* and *chymotrypsinogen.*

Trypsinogen is activated by an enzyme, *en-*

terokinase, a component of the luminal cell membranes of small intestinal cells (enterocytes). Trypsin can activate chymotrypsinogen and more trypsinogen. The ultimate end products of protein digestion are amino acids, but the pancreatic proteolytic enzymes may stop digestion when the peptides reach a length of two or more amino acids. If this occurs, peptidases associated with enterocyte cell membranes can complete hydrolysis of the peptides to individual amino acids for absorption.

Unlike the proteolytic enzymes, *pancreatic amylase* and *lipase* are in the active forms when secreted from the pancreas. Amylase digests starches to *oligosaccharides* (a carbohydrate composed of a small number, usually two to four, of monosaccharides). The enzymes *maltase* and *sucrase,* components of enterocyte cell membranes, further digest the oligosaccharides to monosaccharides. *Lactase,* to digest lactose (milk sugar), is present in enterocytes of young mammals but not in all adults. Lipase hydrolyzes triglycerides into fatty acids and glycerol. This action is most effective after the fats have been emulsified by bile (discussed later).

Control of pancreatic exocrine secretion depends on stimulation by vagal autonomic nerves that innervate the pancreas and on three intestinal hormones, cholecystokinin, secretin, and gastrin. Seeing or smelling food stimulates vagal stimulation, and food in the stomach prompts release of gastrin.

The greatest amount of pancreatic exocrine secretion occurs when the acid chyme and food components in the duodenum stimulate the release of cholecystokinin and secretin from cells in the duodenal mucosa (*intestinal phase* of control). These two duodenal hormones also feed back to the stomach to decrease secretions in the stomach and slow down the activity and emptying of the stomach until the duodenal chyme has been degraded by the enzymes and adjusted in pH by the pancreatic bicarbonate.

Liver Digestive Function: Secretion of Bile

Liver cells (*hepatocytes*) are responsible for bile formation. Bile is a greenish-yellow salt solution consisting primarily of bile salts, cholesterol, phospholipids (*lecithins*), and bile pigments (*bilirubin*). Hepatocytes synthesize the bile salts (primarily sodium salts of glycocholic and taurocholic acids) from cholesterol. These salts assist in digestion and absorption of lipids (triglycerides), and the production and secretion of these salts is the most important digestive function of the liver.

In an aqueous solution, such as the duodenal chyme, lipids tend to clump together and form large droplets (recall the appearance of an oil and vinegar salad dressing after shaking the bottle). Such large lipid droplets present a small surface area for the action of the pancreatic lipases. Bile acids act as *emulsifiers* to reduce droplet size and make the lipids more accessible to the lipases. Lipases can function without bile salts, but lipid digestion is inefficient without them. Micelle is the term for the small droplets formed in the intestinal chyme that contain lipids, bile salts, and products of lipid digestion.

In all farm animals except the horse, bile is stored in the *gallbladder.* Since the horse has no gallbladder, the bile passes directly from the liver to the duodenum by way of the bile duct and its tributaries at a fairly continuous rate. The gallbladder stores bile for intermittent discharge into the duodenum and concentrates the bile by reabsorbing water from the stored bile. Cholecystokinin stimulates gallbladder contraction and the release of stored bile. Since food entering the duodenum stimulates the release of cholecystokinin, this coordinates the release of bile with the presence of food.

Most of the bile salts released from the liver remain mixed with the digesta as it passes into the terminal part of the small intestine (ileum). Here enterocytes reabsorb bile salts, which enter the blood. The reabsorbed bile salts are transported to the liver via the hepatic portal vein, and here hepatocytes take up the bile salts from the portal blood. These bile salts can then be secreted by the hepatocytes into bile for reuse. An increase in bile salts in portal blood, such as during the digestion of a meal, is the primary stimulus for bile salt secretion by hepatocytes. The recycling of bile salts between the digestive tract and the liver is *enterohepatic circulation.*

The liver is capable of synthesizing *cholesterol,* and the liver makes much of the choles-

terol in bile. The liver can also eliminate excessive dietary cholesterol via the bile. Cholesterol is insoluble in water, but the bile salts and lecithin normally change it to a soluble form so that it can exist in the bile. However, sometimes cholesterol precipitates from the bile in the gallbladder or bile ducts, forming *gallstones.*

Nutrient Absorption in the Small Intestine

The small intestine is the major site of nutrient absorption. Most of the products of carbohydrate, protein, and lipid digestion are absorbed as the digesta passes through the small intestine. The small intestine is also the primary site of absorption for vitamins, minerals, and water.

The epithelium lining the small intestine has structural features that increase the surface area for nutrient absorption. The mucosa is covered with **villi** (fingerlike projections) that extend into the lumen, and the individual enterocytes have microvilli on their cell membrane facing the lumen (Fig. 21–4).

Individual amino acids and monosaccharides (simple sugars) are the simplest products of protein and carbohydrate digestion, respectively. The cellular mechanisms of absorption of amino acids and monosaccharides (primarily glucose) are similar in that the transport across the cell membrane on the luminal surface involves sodium-linked cotransporters (see Chapter 2). The cotransporters all bind sodium, but different transporters are used by glucose and amino acids. At least five transporters have been found to transport various amino acids. These are all characterized as secondarily active transport, for they depend on the gradient for sodium between the intracellular fluid of the enterocytes and the fluid in the lumen of the small intestine (see Chapter 2). Figure 21–7 summarizes the absorptive process for glucose.

Micelles formed in the lumen of the small intestine contain bile salts, triglycerides, cholesterol, and the products of lipase action on triglycerides (fatty acids and monoglycerides). Intestinal movements (segmentation) bring the micelles into contact with the microvilli of the enterocytes. The lipid-soluble products of lipid

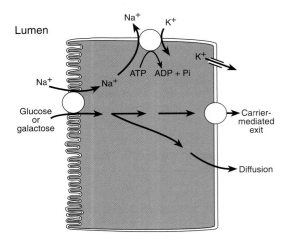

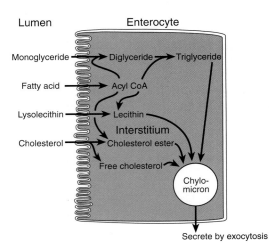

Figure 21-7. Sodium-linked cotransport of glucose. (Reprinted with permission from Rhoades R.A. and Tanner G.A. *Medical Physiology*. Boston: Little, Brown, 1995.)

Figure 21-8. Summary of intracellular processes involved in absorption of lipids and cholesterol from gastrointestinal tract and secretion of chylomicrons by enterocyte. (Reprinted with permission from Rhoades R.A. and Tanner G.A. *Medical Physiology*. Boston: Little, Brown, 1995.)

digestion and cholesterol can then diffuse from the micelle into the enterocytes. Some long-chain fatty acids are also transported from micelles into the cell by specific sodium-linked cotransporter proteins in the cell membrane.

Within the enterocytes, absorbed monoglycerides and fatty acids are used to resynthesize triglycerides. The enterocyte packages the triglycerides and absorbed cholesterol together with intracellular proteins into a particle known as a *chylomicron*. The enterocytes secrete the chylomicrons into the interstitial fluid, where they are absorbed into lymphatics. The smallest of the lymphatic vessels that absorb the chylomicrons are *lacteals* (Fig. 21–4). The lymphatic drainage from the intestinal tract is ultimately added to the blood, and it is via this pathway that chylomicrons, containing absorbed lipids, reach the blood. Figure 21–8 summarizes the process of lipid absorption.

Sodium, potassium, phosphate, calcium, chloride, and other electrolytes are primarily absorbed in the small intestine by both active and passive mechanisms. With the exception of iron and calcium, the absorption of these minerals is not regulated, so that most of what is consumed is absorbed. Iron absorption is reduced at the level of the enterocyte if body

iron content is sufficient. This reduction is primarily accomplished by an increase in an intracellular protein that binds iron in the enterocytes. The iron-containing enterocyte is lost from the body after it sloughs from the epithelial lining. The form of vitamin D produced by the kidneys (*calcitriol*) increases calcium absorption by increasing calcium transport proteins in enterocytes. Calcitriol formation by the kidneys is increased when blood calcium is low. To be absorbed, minerals such as calcium and phosphate must be in their ionized state. If the ratio of cations to anions is too high or too low, absorption can be reduced. For example, if the dietary content of the phosphate (an anion) is too high relative to calcium (a cation), the excess phosphate binds the available calcium to form calcium phosphate, and calcium absorption is impaired.

The small intestine of some *neonatal* (*newborn*) animals can absorb macromolecules, including intact protein molecules from the *colostrum.* Colostrum, the first milk of the horse, pig, and ruminants, contains the γ-globulins needed to produce passive immunity in the newborns of these animals. This receptive period lasts approximately 1 day in the horse and pig and up to 3 days in the ruminant.

Physiology of the Cecum and Colon

In carnivores the cecum and colon primarily absorb water and some electrolytes to reduce the volume and fluidity of the digesta in the formation of feces. Feces are also stored in the terminal portions of the colon prior to their movement into the rectum for defecation. In omnivores (e.g., pig) and some herbivores (e.g., cattle and sheep) the cecum and colon are also sites of some limited fermentation and microbial digestion. In cattle and sheep the cecum and colon are proportionally larger and more complex than in carnivores, but the forestomach is the much more important site of fermentative digestion in these herbivores.

Cecum and Colon of the Horse

The extremely large and complex cecum and great colon of the horse are the primary sites of fermentation and microbial digestion of cellulose. Roughage passes relatively quickly through the stomach and small intestine of the horse, but fermentative digestion and passage through the cecum and great colon may take days. Complex movements of the cecum and great colon mix the contents to promote fermentative digestion and to expose the contents to the epithelial surface for absorption of volatile fatty acids. The pelvic flexure of the great colon and the junction between the great and small colons (see Fig. 20–10) are relatively small in diameter, and it appears that the passage of large particles of roughage is restricted. While these sites retain roughage so that it can be subjected to microbial digestion, the potential for impaction at these sites is also increased.

When consumed with roughage, some starches and sugars escape digestion in the equine stomach and small intestine and pass into the cecum and colon. Microbial digestion of these and the cellulose in the roughage produces

volatile fatty acids that can be absorbed and used for energy. Microbes in the cecum and colon can also use nonprotein nitrogen sources (urea) for the production of microbial proteins. However, these have limited nutritional value to the horse, because the gastrointestinal mechanisms necessary to digest proteins and absorb the resulting amino acids are not readily available in the cecum or colon. Some urea is made available to microbes by diffusing into the cecum and colon from the blood.

Fermentation and microbial digestion produce volatile fatty acids, which could lower the pH of the cecal and colonic contents to potentially harmful levels. The colonic epithelium secretes bicarbonate ions to buffer the pH of the contents. Additional bicarbonate is secreted by the epithelium of the ileum, and this lowers the pH of the cecal contents.

Rectum and Defecation

Several times daily strong and extensive mass movements of the colon move fecal material into the rectum. Distension of the rectum stimulates the need to defecate. The act of defecation requires contraction of smooth muscle in the wall of the rectum, and this results from a spinal reflex stimulated by distension of the rectum. Conscious control of defecation involves inhibition of the spinal reflex and contraction of the external anal sphincter, which is composed of skeletal muscle. Contraction of abdominal muscles increases intra-abdominal pressure, which also assists with emptying the rectum.

The variability in character and shape of feces among species is primarily a function of the structural and functional features of the more distal segments of the colon. In horses relatively strong segmentation contractions form the characteristic fecal balls.

Equine colic is a general term for any painful condition associated with the abdomen of the horse. Conditions associated with any segment of the gastrointestinal tract may result in colic, and clinical signs indicate that the degree of pain can vary from mild to severe. Causes of

colic include ulcers; inappropriate diet, such as overload of grain or concentrates; infection; obstruction due to parasites or foreign bodies; impaction of feed or foreign material, such as sand; twisted segments of intestine; and alterations in intestinal motility. Management, including parasite control, proper diet, access to water, and attention to environmental hazards, is helpful in preventing the incidence of colic. Some causes of colic can be readily treated medically, but other causes threaten life and require prompt surgery.

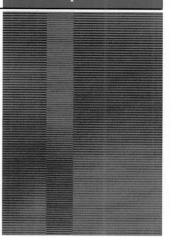

Nutrition and Metabolism

Nutrition

The nutritional needs of animals vary greatly with their metabolic state. A rapidly growing, active young animal has much different nutritional needs from those of an older, more sedentary animal. Both animals must consume certain *essential nutrients* (compounds needed for normal growth and/or survival that cannot be synthesized in adequate amounts in the body), but the amounts of these nutrients per unit of body weight and the relative amounts of specific nutrients vary.

Some essential nutrients are required in minute quantities and are toxic in large quantities. For example, copper is an essential mineral, but excessive consumption over a short period leads to copper toxicity. Minerals that are needed in small quantities are often termed *trace minerals. Vitamins* function as coenzymes for various biochemical reactions throughout the body and are also typically required in small amounts. Water-soluble vitamins (B complex, biotin, C, folic acid, and niacin) are not stored in the body, but fat-soluble vitamins (A, D, E, and K) are stored in the liver and adipose tissue. Water-soluble vitamins can be consumed in large amounts without significant toxicities because the excess is rapidly excreted in the urine. Because they accumulate in the body, excessive consumption of fat-soluble vitamins can be harmful.

The nutritional and metabolic status of individual animals may be evaluated by determining the *balance* for a given nutrient or type of nutrient. Balance is determined by comparing the amount consumed by the animal to the amount used or lost from the body. For example, because proteins are the primary nitrogen-containing nutrient, **nitrogen balance** is often used as an indicator of the status of protein metabolism. If an animal consumes more nitrogen than it excretes, it is said to be in a positive nitrogen balance, indicating that the animal is synthesizing more body proteins than are being degraded and lost from the body. Young, growing animals are typically in positive nitrogen balance. During prolonged starvation, an animal is in negative nitrogen balance, for body proteins are broken down to provide energy, and the resulting nitrogen is excreted in the urine.

Metabolism

The terms **anabolic** and **catabolic** are used to describe the overall metabolic state or status of an animal. Anabolism refers to a constructive process (e.g., synthesis of proteins from amino acids), while catabolism refers to a destructive process (e.g., degradation of proteins into individual amino acids). While *anabolic* and *catabolic* refer to the overall metabolic status, both processes are usually ongoing at the same time in an animal's body. For example, even in a young, rapidly growing animal that is digesting a meal, absorbing nutrients, and synthesizing body proteins, some body proteins are degrading at the same time. However, in this case, the rate of protein synthesis is greater than the rate of protein degradation, so the animal is in an anabolic state.

Several hormones contribute to the regulation of the balance between anabolic and catabolic processes, and the study of the hormones that regulate metabolism is termed **metabolic endocrinology.** A common feature of such hormones is that blood glucose concentrations participate in regulation of their secretion. This indicates that the maintenance of a minimal and constant source of glucose for energy is a key factor in the overall endocrine control of metabolism.

To study the endocrine control of anabolism and catabolism, metabolic endocrinologists often contrast the period shortly following a meal,

during which nutrients are being absorbed from the gastrointestinal tract (**absorptive state**), with a period during which there is no net absorption (**postabsorptive state**). During the absorptive state, blood levels of glucose, amino acids, and triglycerides (as part of chylomicrons) increase. The overall goals of the metabolic processes during this period appear to be to increase the use of these nutrients by cells of the body and/or store them so that they can be used later. Metabolic periods of ruminants differ from those of other animals, because nutrients are constantly being absorbed from the forestomach and passing from the forestomach down the remainder of their gastrointestinal tract. This chapter discusses some specifics of ruminant metabolism after a more general overview.

Absorptive State: Anabolism

Figure 22–1 summarizes the overall fate of the major nutrients absorbed during the digestion of a meal, and these are described in more detail later in the following paragraphs.

Glucose is the predominant product of carbohydrate digestion in most animals, and following a typical meal, blood glucose levels may rise to 150% of fasting levels. The increase in blood glucose is a major stimulus for the release of **insulin** from the pancreas, but increases in plasma amino acids during the digestion of a high-protein meal can also stimulate insulin release. Insulin affects carbohydrate, amino acid (protein), and lipid metabolism during the absorptive period, and it is considered the primary endocrine regulator of metabolism during anabolism.

Insulin stimulates the uptake of glucose by skeletal muscle cells, where it can be used for energy or stored as **glycogen** (essentially a polymer of glucose molecules). The liver also stores glucose as glycogen during the absorptive period, and this is also stimulated by insulin. Primarily because the mass of skeletal muscle is greater than the liver, much more glycogen (75% of the total) is formed and stored in skeletal muscle. Blood glucose is also available for use by all cells of the body for energy during this period, but no other organ is capable of significant glycogen storage.

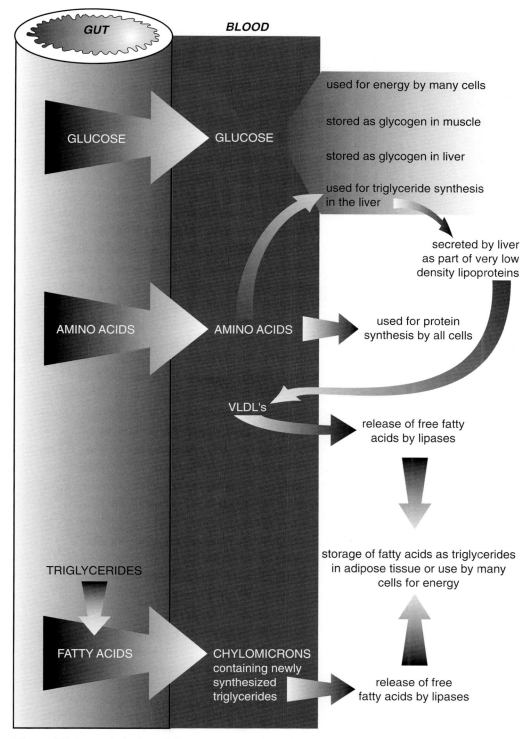

Figure 22-1. Metabolic fate of glucose, amino acids, and triglycerides (in chylomicrons) being absorbed from the gastrointestinal tract during the digestion of a meal.

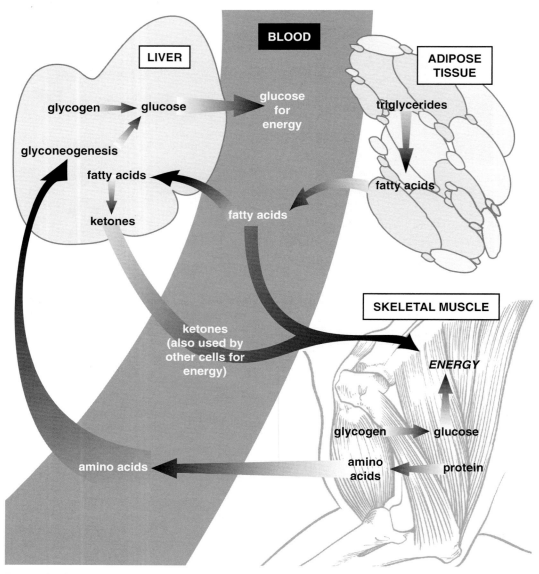

Figure 22-2. Summary of metabolic organs and mechanisms that maintain blood glucose and provide energy for cells when nutrients are not being absorbed from the gastrointestinal tract.

Absorbed amino acids are immediately available to all body cells for protein synthesis. Because all of the amino acids necessary for synthesis of a given protein must be available at the time of synthesis, it is imperative that animals have a balanced diet that contains all of the *essential amino acids.* Protein synthesis in many organs, including liver and skeletal muscle, is stimulated by insulin, so the increase in insulin following a meal also promotes protein synthesis during this period. However, this stimulatory effect on protein synthesis is minor compared to the effects of insulin on glucose metabolism (e.g., the rate of plasma protein production by the liver increases by only a small percentage after a meal).

The amounts of amino acids absorbed after a typical meal are more than can be efficiently used by the body for protein synthesis. However, no metabolic pathways permit the various amino acids to be stored for later use the way glucose is stored as glycogen. Many of the excess amino acids are taken up by hepatocytes and enter metabolic pathways that result in triglyceride (lipid) formation. These pathways remove nitrogen-containing amino groups from the amino acids (***deamination***). Most of the resulting lipids are secreted by hepatocytes into the blood as part of lipoproteins (discussed later).

Deamination of amino acids is also part of a different metabolic pathway by which liver cells use amino acids to produce glucose. However, the hormone **glucagon** must be available to stimulate this pathway, and glucagon release from the pancreas is reduced by increases in blood glucose. So during the period that blood glucose is elevated following a meal, the use of amino acids to produce glucose is suppressed. ***Gluconeogenesis*** is the term for the collective metabolic processes by which liver cells produce glucose from noncarbohydrate substrates, such as amino acids and short-chain fatty acids. The liver and kidneys are the only organs that are capable of any significant gluconeogenesis, and the kidneys do so only in states of chronic acidosis.

During the absorptive state, the liver uses both excess glucose and amino acids as substrates for triglyceride (lipid) synthesis, and insulin stimulates these pathways. Some of the newly synthesized triglycerides are stored in the liver, but most are released into the blood in complex particles known as very low density lipoproteins (VLDLs). ***Lipoproteins*** are particles that contain lipids, cholesterol, and proteins in various ratios. VLDLs are so named because their lipid content is high relative to their protein content. Because lipids are less dense than protein, the density of VLDL particles is quite low.

Recall that chylomicrons are also circulating lipoproteins, but the triglycerides in these lipoproteins were absorbed from the intestinal tract. As chylomicrons and VLDLs circulate throughout the body, they encounter **lipoprotein lipase,** an enzyme bound to endothelial cells that acts on their triglycerides to release free fatty acids. When the triglycerides are released within adipose tissue, the free fatty acids are available to adipose cells for the resynthesis and storage of lipids as triglycerides. In other organs, such as skeletal muscle, cells use the free fatty acids for energy. The synthesis and storage of triglycerides in adipose tissue is stimulated by insulin, which is typically elevated during the absorptive period.

After losing triglycerides by the action of lipoprotein lipase, some VLDLs undergo changes in the circulation and become a different type of lipoprotein, *low-density lipoprotein* (LDL). LDLs contain a great deal of cholesterol, and cells throughout the body receive cholesterol from the blood by the endocytosis of LDLs. Cholesterol is a necessary component of cell membranes, and all cells need some cholesterol. However, abnormal increases in LDL levels are associated with an increased risk of cardiovascular disease in humans. Recall that the original VLDLs were produced in the liver, so much of the cholesterol in the blood is produced by the liver.

Postabsorptive State: Catabolism

After a meal has been digested and absorbed, blood glucose concentration gradually decreases as glucose is used for energy throughout the body (Fig 22–2). This drop in blood glucose is the primary event bringing about the changes in endocrine secretions that orchestrate the metabolic changes during the postabsorptive state. Two major endocrine changes are a gradual drop in insulin secretion and a rise in the release of glucagon. Recall that increases in blood glucose stimulate insulin release from β-cells, while decreases in blood glucose stimulate glucagon release from α-cells in pancreatic islets.

During the absorptive period, when glucose and amino acids were being absorbed into the blood from the intestinal tract, insulin stimulated the synthesis of glycogen for glucose storage, proteins, and lipids (from any excess glucose and amino acids). As insulin levels decrease, its stimulatory effect on these synthetic (anabolic) processes is lost, and this is a major factor in changing the overall metabolic balance from anabolism to catabolism.

Glucagon stimulates the breakdown of glycogen (**glycogenolysis**) in the liver to provide glucose that the liver can release into the blood. Glycogenolysis is the initial process by which the liver derives glucose to add to the blood, but later the liver also releases glucose formed by gluconeogenesis, which is also stimulated by glucagon. The amino acids used for gluconeogenesis are derived from the catabolism of body protein.

The maintenance of a minimal or fasting blood glucose level during this period has primary importance to neuronal function. Neurons do not have the metabolic processes to permit them to use fatty acids for energy, so they need a ready supply of glucose for cell energy. During fasting, the catabolism of adipose tissue increases the supply of fatty acids, which are used by cells other than neurons for energy. The increased use of fatty acids by other cells reduces the overall need for glucose and conserves it for use by neurons. This conservation of glucose is termed **glucose sparing.** The liver also metabolizes the circulating fatty acids to produce ketones, another cellular energy substrate. The ketones produced by the liver include acetone, acetoacetate, and β-hydroxybutyrate.

Two other hormones, growth hormone and glucocorticoids from the adrenal cortex, also contribute to the maintenance of blood glucose and other sources of energy during anabolic periods. Glucocorticoids do not increase in the circulation during a short fast, but a deficit of glucocorticoids reduces the rate of liver gluconeogenesis and mobilization of fatty acids from adipose tissues. The effect of glucocorticoids on these processes during fasting is a permissive effect. Decreases in blood glucose stimulate the release of growth hormone, which increases the mobilization of fatty acids from adipose (**lipolysis**). Some tissues (e.g., skeletal muscle) can use the fatty acids for energy (glucose sparing), and the liver can further increase its production of ketones.

Energy Needs During Exercise

The increase in skeletal muscle metabolism during exercise can rapidly deplete the glycogen stores within skeletal muscle cells. In humans these stores are capable of providing energy only for an estimated 2 to 3 minutes of very intense exercise. To sustain exercise, other energy sources must be rapidly mobilized and delivered to working skeletal muscle. Circulating levels of epinephrine and norepinephrine increase during exercise, and these catecholamines have several actions that mobilize energy stores, including increased glycogenolysis in the liver and nonworking skeletal muscle and lipolysis in adipose tissue. Insulin levels are reduced and glucagon levels are increased during exercise, which promotes liver gluconeogenesis and more lipolysis in adipose tissue. The decrease in insulin is not detrimental to working skeletal muscle, because glucose uptake by working muscle is less insulin dependent.

Anaerobic metabolism, by working skeletal muscles, raises the rate of lactic acid production. The lactate ion can diffuse into the blood from the skeletal muscle, and plasma levels of lactate increase during strenuous and prolonged exercise. The liver can use blood lactate for gluconeogenesis, and glucose can then be returned to the blood to maintain blood glucose levels.

Blood Glucose in Ruminants

Normal ranges for blood glucose levels in mature ruminants are lower than in other animals, even other herbivores (cattle, 45–80 mg/dL; dog, 70–110 mg/dL, and horse, 60–110 mg/dL). The lower normal range for mature ruminants is associated with the relatively small amount of glucose-yielding carbohydrate digestion in their small intestine. Most of the carbohydrates that they consume undergo fermentative digestion in the forestomach and result in the production of short-chain volatile fatty acids (VFAs), which are absorbed directly from the forestomach.

Without glucose readily available via absorption from the gastrointestinal tract, ruminants must have a continuous and a relatively high rate of gluconeogenesis in the liver to maintain the blood glucose level. Glucagon appears to be an important endocrine stimulant to maintain this rate of gluconeogenesis. Rising levels of amino acids and propionic acid (a VFA produced in the rumen) can stimulate glucagon release, so presumably the continual absorption of these from the ruminant gastrointestinal tract can maintain glucagon secretion. Propionic acid is the one of the three major VFAs produced in the rumen that can be used by the liver for gluconeogenesis.

Ketosis

Ketosis is a metabolic state characterized by increase in blood ketones, a reduction in urine and blood pH, and ketones in the urine. The increase in the acidic ketones in the blood and urine are responsible for the changes in pH. Ketosis may occur when fatty acid mobilization from adipose tissue is elevated and glucose is deficient. The deficiency in glucose stimulates the release of glucagon and inhibits insulin release, and the increased ratio of glucagon to insulin promotes the formation of ketones by the liver from readily available fatty acids.

Ketosis may develop in dairy cattle at the peak of lactation, when the need for glucose to synthesize lactose (milk sugar) is maximal. The rapid use of glucose by the mammary glands reduces blood glucose and brings about these changes in glucagon and insulin. Ketosis may also develop as a result of type I diabetes mellitus, in which the primary problem is a deficiency of insulin. In this case, the dominant effects of glucagon on fatty acid mobilization and ketone synthesis are primarily responsible for the development of the ketosis.

THE URINARY SYSTEM

The urinary system consists of two kidneys, two ureters, the urinary bladder, and the urethra. The paired **kidneys** remove waste products from the blood, help regulate the composition of plasma, and perform certain hormonal functions. The system of tubules in each kidney coalesces into a single mucomuscular tube, the **ureter,** which extends caudad to empty into the **urinary bladder,** a distensible reservoir for the storage of urine. When full, the urinary bladder discharges the urine through the **urethra** to the outside of the body.

Anatomy of the Kidney

The kidneys are paired reddish-brown organs that filter plasma and plasma constituents from the blood and then selectively reabsorb water and useful constituents from the filtrate, ultimately excreting excesses and plasma waste products. The kidneys of most domestic animals are somewhat bean-shaped, with the exceptions of the heart-shaped right equine kidney and the distinctively lobated kidneys of the ox (Figs. 23–1 and 23–2).

The kidneys are in the dorsal part of the abdominal cavity on each side of the aorta and caudal vena cava, just ventral to the first few lumbar vertebrae. In most domestic animals, the right kidney is slightly more cranial than the left, with the cranial pole of the right kidney lying snugly in a complementary fossa of the liver. The left kidney tends to be more pendulous, and

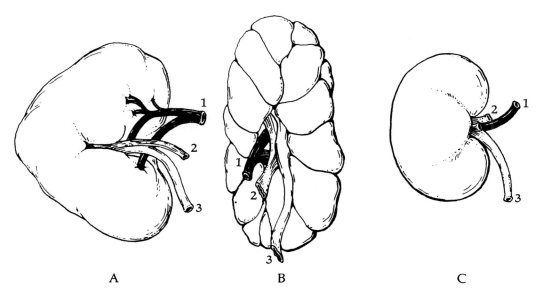

Figure 23-1. Right kidneys of the horse (*A*); the ox (*B*); and the sheep (*C*). 1) Renal artery, 2) renal vein, 3) ureter. (Reprinted with permission from Reece W.O. *Physiology of Domestic Animals.* 2nd ed. Baltimore: Williams & Wilkins, 1997.)

in ruminants, the forestomach may push the left kidney to the right as far as the median plane or beyond, particularly when the rumen is full. The kidneys are described as **retroperitoneal,** reflecting their location outside the peritoneal cavity, where they are more closely attached to the abdominal wall by fascia, vessels, and peritoneum than are most other abdominal organs. A tough connective tissue capsule surrounds the entire kidney.

The medial aspect of each kidney features a concavity, the **hilus,** where arteries and nerves enter the kidney, and the ureter, veins, and lymphatic vessels leave (Fig. 23–3). The wide origin of the ureter in the kidney is the **renal pelvis.** The renal pelvis receives urine from the **collecting tubules** of the kidney. The cavity in the kidney that contains the pelvis is the **renal sinus.** The bovine kidney does not have a renal pelvis, the ureter instead arising directly from the coalescence of individual calyces (discussed later).

The portion of the kidney immediately surrounding the renal pelvis is the renal **medulla,** which appears striated because of the radially arranged **collecting tubules.** In addition to collecting tubules, the medulla also contains some

loops of Henle (descending and ascending loops). The medulla is surmounted peripherally by the renal **cortex,** in which reside the **renal corpuscles,** the histological units of filtration. The cortex has a granular appearance because of the large number of these renal corpuscles; also found in the cortex are **proximal** and **distal convoluted tubules** and other segments of loops of Henle (discussed later).

The medulla and cortex are arranged in units called **lobes,** cone-shaped aggregates of renal tissue. The medullary portion of each lobe constitutes a **renal pyramid,** whose apex, the **renal papilla,** is directed toward the renal pelvis (Fig. 23–3). In the bovine kidney, each pyramid is associated with one of the grossly obvious lobes of the bovine kidney. In the pig, the adjacent cortices of individual lobes are fused, so that the surface of the kidney appears smooth. The individual nature of the porcine lobes is revealed, however, through the persistence of discrete papillae projecting into the renal pelvis (Fig. 23–2). In the horse and small ruminants, the individual papillae, like the cortex, are fused. Consequently, they present as a single longitudinal ridge, the **renal crest,** projecting into the

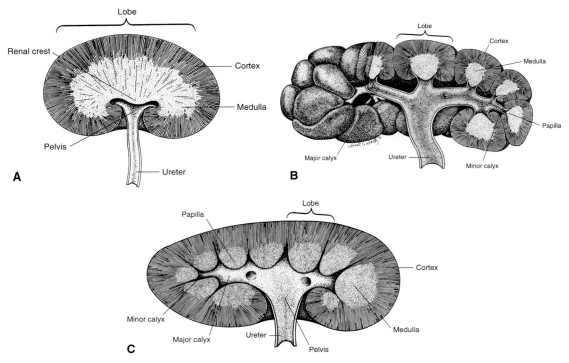

Figure 23-2. Internal anatomy of kidneys. *A)* The renal cortex of the equine, ovine, and caprine kidney lacks visible divisions into individual lobes. The renal papillae are fused in these species into a longitudinal renal crest. *B)* The bovine kidney is grossly divided into lobes, each of which communicates with a minor calyx. *C)* The porcine kidney lacks external divisions into lobes, but the renal papillae of the medulla distinguish each lobe internally. (Reprinted with permission from Dellman H.D. *Textbook of Veterinary Histology.* 4th ed. Philadelphia: Lea & Febiger, 1993.)

renal pelvis. Urine discharged from the collecting tubules of the renal crest is collected in the renal pelvis and from there is delivered to the ureter.

In the kidney of the ox and pig, individual pyramids project into **minor calyces,** cuplike diverticula of the renal pelvis. These in turn empty into **major calyces.** These major calyces in the porcine kidney empty into the renal pelvis, but the bovine kidney has no pelvis, and so the major calyces in this species empty directly into the ureter (Fig. 23–2).

Blood and Nerve Supply

Because of its important role in adjusting the composition of extracellular fluid (including plasma), the blood supply to the kidney is much more extensive than the size of the organ would suggest. The two **renal arteries** may receive as much as one-fourth of the total cardiac output. Each renal artery enters the hilus of the kidney and divides into a number of relatively large branches, the **interlobar arteries.** These pass peripherally between pyramids almost to the cortex, where they bend abruptly and become **arcuate arteries,** which derive their name from the arched manner by which they pass along the junction between cortex and medulla (Fig. 23–3.)

Each arcuate artery gives off a number of **interlobular arteries** that extend into the cortex and in turn give rise to the **afferent arterioles.** Each afferent arteriole branches repeatedly to form a tufted capillary network called the **glomerulus,** which is associated with the renal

A

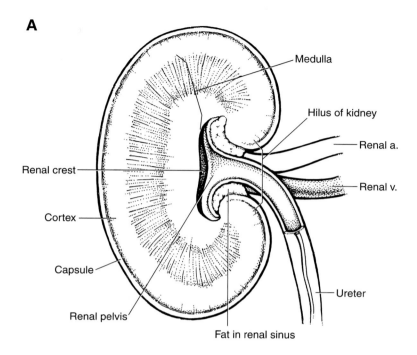

- Medulla
- Hilus of kidney
- Renal a.
- Renal v.
- Renal crest
- Cortex
- Capsule
- Renal pelvis
- Ureter
- Fat in renal sinus

B

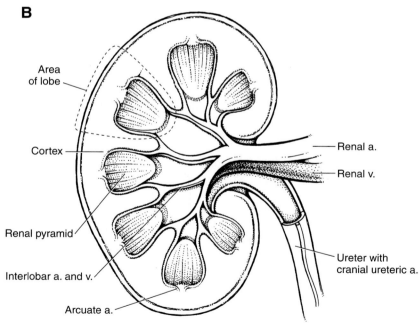

- Area of lobe
- Cortex
- Renal pyramid
- Interlobar a. and v.
- Arcuate a.
- Renal a.
- Renal v.
- Ureter with cranial ureteric a.

Figure 23-3. Kidney of the canid cut on the median plane (A) and a sagittal section off midline (B) The small ruminant kidney appears similar to this canine kidney. (Reprinted with permission from Smith B.J. *Canine Anatomy.* Philadelphia: Lippincott Williams & Wilkins, 1999.)

corpuscle. The capillaries of the glomerulus coalesce into an ***efferent arteriole,*** which leaves each glomerulus (Fig. 23–4).

Arcuate veins drain blood from both the cortex and medulla, pass through the medulla as ***interlobar veins,*** and enter the ***renal veins,*** which emerge from the renal hilus to empty into the caudal vena cava. Lymph drains from the kidney to the renal lymph nodes.

Sympathetic nerves are the primary innervation of the kidneys. These derive from the celiacomesenteric plexus and innervate blood vessels and renal tubules.

Ureters, Urinary Bladder, and Urethra

The ***ureter*** is a muscular tube that conveys urine from the kidney to the urinary bladder. The smooth muscle of the ureter undergoes peristaltic waves of contraction that encourage the flow of urine to the urinary bladder (Fig. 23–5). Each ureter originates at the renal pelvis (or the major calices of the bovine kidney) and empties into the ***urinary bladder*** near its neck at the ***trigone.*** The manner in which the ureter passes obliquely through the wall of the urinary

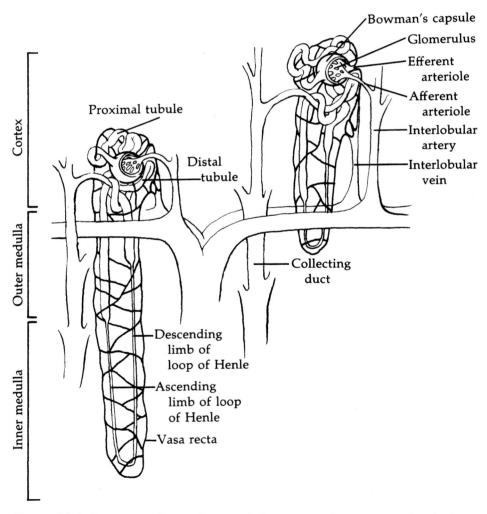

Figure 23-4. Two mammalian nephrons and the microcirculation associated with them. (Reprinted with permission from Reece W.O. *Physiology of Domestic Animals.* 2nd ed. Baltimore: Williams & Wilkins, 1997.)

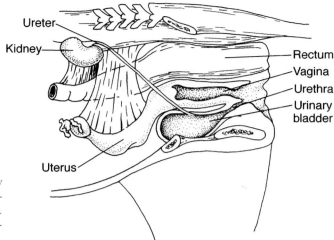

Figure 23-5. Kidneys, ureters, and urinary bladder in situ in the small ruminant. (Reprinted with permission from Reece W.O. *Physiology of Domestic Animals.* 2nd ed. Baltimore: Williams & Wilkins, 1997.)

bladder creates a valve to prevent reflux flow of urine to the kidney.

The urinary bladder is a hollow muscular organ that varies in size and position with the amount of urine it contains. The empty, contracted bladder is a thick-walled, piriform organ on the floor of the pelvic cavity. As it fills with urine, its wall thins, and it enlarges craniad toward and then into the abdominal cavity.

The neck of the bladder is continuous with the **urethra** caudally. The smooth muscle of the urinary bladder wall is arranged in three sheets; at the neck of the bladder these may form a smooth muscle sphincter that controls passage of urine into the urethra, although the precise role of the intramural muscle of the urinary bladder in creating a true sphincter is debated. The **pelvic urethra** extends from the urinary bladder across the floor of the pelvic canal to the ischial arch. In female animals, it opens onto the floor of the vestibule. In the male animal, it receives the ductus deferens and ducts from the accessory sex glands then passes through the penis as the **penile urethra.** In both sexes, the pelvic urethra is surrounded by a true sphincter, the striated skeletal **m. urethralis,** over which the animal exercises voluntary control.

The pelvis, ureter, bladder, and urethra are all lined with **transitional epithelium.** This epithelial lining is useful in these areas, where considerable distension of the lumen may oc-

cur. When these organs are empty, the lumen is small, the walls are thick, and the lining epithelial cells are piled deeply to form many layers. However, when the organs are distended, the lumen is enlarged, the walls are thinner, and a transition to a much lower stratification of the lining occurs. (Fig. 23–6). The urethra, like the urinary bladder, is lined with transitional epithelium; this changes to the typical stratified squamous epithelium of mucous membranes at or near the urethral orifice at the tip of the penis of male animals or at its junction with the vestibule of the vagina in the female animal.

Micturition

Micturition is the term for expulsion of urine from the bladder. It normally is a reflex activity stimulated by distension of the urinary bladder from the constant inflow of urine by way of the ureters. The bladder relaxes to accommodate a gradual increase in urinary volume until the pressure becomes high enough to stimulate reflex centers in the spinal cord, which in turn relax the smooth muscle sphincter in the neck of the bladder and contract the muscle wall of the urinary bladder by way of sacral parasympathetic nerves. However, reflex emptying of the bladder can be prevented by voluntary suppression of the reflex and control of the *m. urethralis* surrounding the proximal urethra.

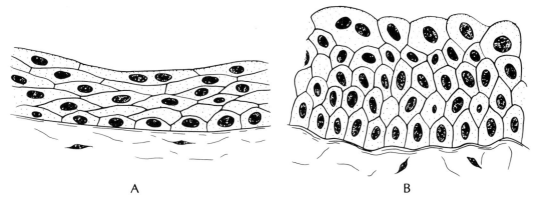

Figure 23-6. Transitional epithelium. *A*) Bladder full, wall distended. *B*) Bladder empty, wall relaxed.

Overview of Function and Histology of the Kidneys

The urinary system is responsible for maintaining the relatively constant internal environment of the body fluids. This is accomplished by the formation and excretion of urine of an appropriate volume and composition. Urine formation occurs in the kidneys, and by adjusting the volume and composition of urine in response to changes in dietary intake or metabolism, the kidneys regulate the body *balance* of water, various electrolytes, acids, and bases. The kidneys also excrete metabolic waste products in the urine, including the nitrogenous waste, **urea,** and a byproduct of skeletal muscle metabolism, ***creatinine.*** Signs of kidney diseases include imbalances of water, electrolytes, acids, and bases and increases in blood levels of urea and creatinine.

Kidneys are composite organs that consist of thousands to millions of similar microscopic functional units, the **nephrons.** Nephrons in all mammalian kidneys are similar in basic structure and function, but the number of nephrons differs among mammals. Large animals have more nephrons per kidney than small animals (e.g., 4 million for cattle and 500,000 for dogs). Nephrons consist of a spherical structure (***Bowman's capsule***) that contains a capillary tuft (***glomerulus***) and a single long tubule connected to Bowman's capsule (Fig. 23–4). Bowman's capsule consists of two layers of cells. The inner (visceral) layer closely surrounds the glomerular capillaries, and the outer (parietal) layer is continuous with the first segment of the tubule. A Bowman's capsule with its contained glomerulus is a ***renal corpuscle.***

The single tubule is divided into segments based on differences in histological appearance, location in the kidney, and function. These segments are named the ***proximal (convoluted) tubule, loop of Henle,*** and ***distal (convoluted) tubule*** (Fig. 23–4). The distal tubules of numerous nephrons connect to another tubular structure found in the kidney, the ***collecting duct*** (tubule). Collecting ducts begin in the renal cortex, where they connect with distal tubules, and extend into and through the renal medulla (Fig. 23–4).

Three processes are involved in urine formation: (1) ***glomerular filtration,*** (2) ***selective tubular reabsorption,*** and (3) ***selective tubular secretion*** (Fig. 23–7). As blood flows through glomeruli, a large quantity of filtrate is formed and enters the urinary space of Bowman's capsule. From here the filtrate flows through the tubules and collecting ducts, where tubular reabsorption and tubular secretion alter its volume and composition. Tubular reabsorption is the removal of substances from the tubular fluid by the tubular cells; these substances are usually returned to the blood in the ***peritubular capillaries.*** Tubular secretion is the addition of substances to the tubular fluid by tubule

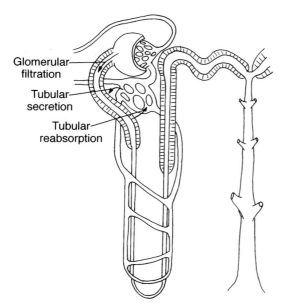

Figure 23-7. Urine formation. The glomerular filtrate enters the tubules, where some substances are removed by selective tubular reabsorption and others are added by selective tubular secretion. Reabsorption and secretion occur throughout the nephron and collecting ducts. (Reprinted with permission from Reece W.O. *Physiology of Domestic Animals.* 2nd ed. Baltimore: Williams & Wilkins, 1997.)

Near glomeruli, the walls of afferent arterioles contain specialized cells termed **juxtaglomerular (JG)** or **granular cells** (Fig. 23–8). Secretory granules in these cells contain the enzyme **renin.** Renin is a component of the renin–angiotensin–aldosterone system (see Chapter 18), which is involved in the regulation of blood volume and blood pressure. The JG cells are part of a functional grouping of closely related structures, the **juxtaglomerular apparatus.** The juxtaglomerular apparatus consists of the JG cells, the **macula densa,** and extraglomerular mesangial cells (Fig. 23–8). The macula densa is a specific region of the wall of the distal tubule where the cellular nuclei appear to be bunched closely together. The segment of the distal tubule found here is part of the same nephron associated with the afferent arterioles (Fig. 23–7). The extraglomerular mesangial cells are between the macula densa and its associated JG cells.

Glomerular Filtration

The glomerular filtrate is the fluid and fluid constituents that pass from the blood plasma in the glomerulus into the urinary space of Bowman's capsule. The physical barriers through which the filtrate passes include (1) the capil-

cells. The secreted substances are produced in the tubule cells (e.g., hydrogen ion and ammonia) or taken up by the tubule cells from the blood in the peritubular capillaries (e.g., pharmaceuticals).

The renal microcirculation is unique in that glomerular capillaries are between two arteriolar vessels rather than between an arteriole and a venule. **Afferent arterioles** lead into glomeruli, and **efferent arterioles** leave glomeruli (Fig. 23–4). Efferent arterioles from most glomeruli lead into capillary networks that surround tubules in the cortex (peritubular capillaries). Efferents from glomeruli deep in the cortex next to the medulla contribute blood to vessels that extend into the medulla. These vessels (**vasa rectae**) consist of straight descending branches (descending vasa rectae) that empty into medullary capillaries, which are drained by straight ascending vessels (ascending vasa rectae) (Fig. 23–4).

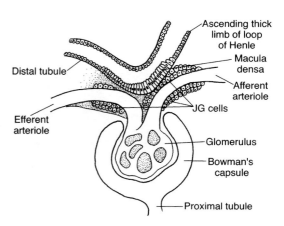

Figure 23-8. The juxtaglomerular (JG) apparatus. Extraglomerular mesangial cells are found at the base of the glomerulus between the macula densa and the arterioles. (Reprinted with permission from Reece W.O. *Physiology of Domestic Animals.* 2nd ed. Baltimore: Williams & Wilkins, 1997.)

lary endothelium of the glomerulus, (2) the inner layer of Bowman's capsule, and (3) a basement membrane (lamina) between these two cell layers. The glomerular endothelium is fenestrated (i.e., has openings or pores in the cells), so this part of the barrier is highly permeable. **Podocytes** (cells of the inner layer of Bowman's capsule) have cellular extensions that rest on the glomerular basement membrane, but slit-like pores between the extensions permit the passage of the filtrate (Fig. 23–9).

The glomerular filtration barrier acts much like a sieve, and all substances up to a molecular weight of about 65,000 pass through the barrier. Blood cells are too large to pass, and only a small percentage of plasma proteins pass through the barrier. Most other plasma constituents (e.g., glucose, amino acids, urea, creatinine, sodium, potassium, chlorine, and hydrochloric acid) readily cross the barrier, and their concentrations in the initial filtrate are about the same as in plasma. **Proteinuria is the presence of abnormal amounts of protein in voided urine. Kidney diseases that localize in or primarily affect glomeruli are often associated with proteinuria or hematuria (blood in voided urine).**

The forces determining the rate of movement of fluid across the glomerular filtration barrier are the same as those that determine fluid movement out of capillaries throughout the body. The **effective filtration pressure** (the pressure tending to force fluid out of the capillary) is usually considered to be the difference between the blood (hydrostatic) pressure in the capillary and the osmotic pressure generated by the plasma proteins of the blood in the capillaries. The hydrostatic pressure in the urinary space of Bowman's capsule and the osmotic pressure generated by proteins in the fluid in the space can also be factors, and these become important in disease states (e.g., blockage of the urinary tract or renal tubules).

In mammals glomerular filtration rate (GFR) and renal blood flow (RBF) remain relatively stable in normally hydrated animals in spite of minor short-term fluctuations in arterial blood pressure (20–30 mm Hg). This stability is maintained by mechanisms intrinsic to the kidney, and this phenomenon is termed renal autoregulation. **Severe dehydration or severe blood loss results in lowering of blood pressure out of the autoregulatory range, and this results in vasoconstriction of preglomerular vessels including afferent arterioles. This vasoconstriction is produced by increases in sympathetic nerve activity to the kidneys and increases in vasoconstrictors such as angiotensin II. The low blood pressure and renal vasoconstriction can reduce glomerular filtration to the point of renal failure. This type of renal failure is termed prerenal.**

The GFR of mammals is normally about 100 times that of urine flow rate (typical values for

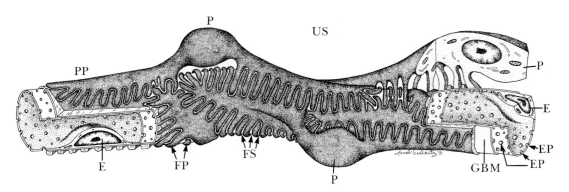

Figure 23-9. The glomerular filtration barrier. E) fenestrated glomerular capillary endothelium; EP) endothelial pore (fenestra); GBM) glomerular basement membrane; P) podocytes, or visceral layer of Bowman's capsule with their filtration slits (FS); US) urinary space of Bowman's capsule. (Reprinted with permission from Dellman H.D. *Textbook of Veterinary Histology.* 4th ed. Philadelphia: Lea & Febiger, 1993.)

GFR are 3–5 mL/kg body weight per minute). The high GFR relative to urine flow allows for a continuous filtration of the plasma and the rapid removal of unwanted or toxic substances from the body. If such substances can readily pass through the glomerular filtration barrier and are not reabsorbed from the renal tubules, they are rapidly eliminated via the urine.

Proximal Tubule Transport

The proximal convoluted tubule is the longest of the tubules, and proximal tubules make up most of the renal cortex. Typical proximal tubule cells are cuboidal, with a luminal border that is modified with microvilli (**brush border**). The length and brush border provide for a large amount of cell membrane surface area, and the proximal tubule does more tubular transport than any other nephron segment. The cellular junctions between proximal tubule cells are also permeable to some substances in the filtrate (e.g. chloride ions) so that some transport can occur between the cells.

Glucose and amino acids are examples of essential nutrients that are reabsorbed from the filtrate by cells of the proximal tubule. Normally 100% of the glucose and amino acids in the initial filtrate are reabsorbed by the proximal tubule. This reabsorption involves secondary active transport using a sodium-linked cotransporter in a manner similar to glucose absorption in the small intestine (see Chapter 21). Substances such as glucose that require membrane transporters for reabsorption have limits to the amount that can be reabsorbed as the fluid flows through the tubules. This limit is the **tubular maximum, or transport maximum.** The blood level at which the amount of a substance presented to the tubules by glomerular filtration exceeds the transport maximum is the **renal threshold. Animals or people with uncontrolled diabetes mellitus often have blood glucose levels that exceed their renal thresholds for glucose. In these cases, the increased amounts of glucose in the filtrate cannot be completely reabsorbed by the proximal tubules, and glucose is present in voided urine (*glucosuria*).**

Bicarbonate ions are the predominant base in the plasma and other extracellular fluids throughout the body. Normally the proximal tubule reabsorbs almost 85–90% of the bicarbonate ions in the initial filtrate to maintain this ready supply of base. The transport of bicarbonate ions from the tubular lumen into proximal tubule cells entails their conversion to carbon dioxide and water under the influence of the enzyme carbonic anhydrase. This reaction requires a hydrogen ion supplied by transport from within the tubule cell. Once inside the tubule cell, the carbon dioxide and water are reconverted to bicarbonate and hydrogen ions, again under the influence of carbonic anhydrase. The bicarbonate ion can then exit the cell, using a membrane transporter, to be added to the blood again (Fig. 23–10). Sodium accompanies the bicarbonate ions, so the electrical neutrality of body fluids is maintained.

Sodium and chloride are the two predominant osmolytes in the initial filtrate, and cells of the proximal tubule reabsorb 70–75% of the sodium and chloride in the initial filtrate. The percent reabsorbed can be increased by the actions of angiotensin II and sympathetic nerves on tubule cells and by vasoconstriction of renal blood vessels. Angiotensin II concentrations and sympathetic nerve activity to the kidneys increase during dehydration or blood loss, when it is appropriate to retain sodium chloride and water.

Cells of the proximal tubule also actively secrete organic anions and organic cations into the tubular fluid to be added to the urine. It is by these secretory systems that the kidneys eliminate many pharmaceuticals (that are organic compounds) in the urine.

Concentration and Dilution of Urine: Role of Loop of Henle and Collecting Duct Transport

To maintain water balance during potentially drastic changes in water intake, the kidneys must be able to excrete urine that is either more concentrated than plasma (hypertonic) or more dilute than plasma (hypotonic). The ability of the kidneys to generate hypertonic or hypotonic urine depends on the functional and anatomic

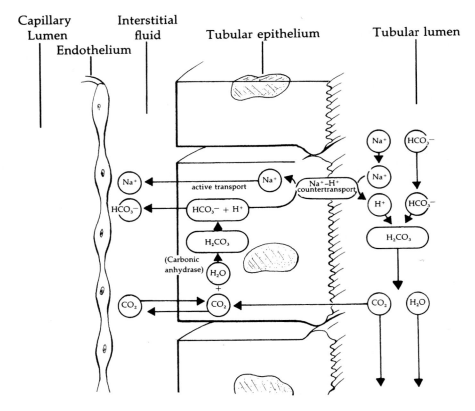

Figure 23-10. Mechanisms of reabsorption of bicarbonate ions by proximal tubule cells. (Reprinted with permission from Reece W.O. *Physiology of Domestic Animals*. 2nd ed. Baltimore: Williams & Wilkins, 1997.)

characteristics of both the loop of Henle and the collecting duct. The excretion of hypertonic urine also requires antidiuretic hormone (ADH, or arginine vasopressin) to alter the transport characteristics of the collecting duct.

Sodium Chloride and Water Reabsorption by the Loop of Henle

Loops of Henle are the nephron segments found in the renal medulla. The **U**-shaped loops extend to variable depths in the medulla, and the terms *descending* and *ascending* limbs are applied to the different parts of the loops (Fig. 23-4).

The ascending limbs of the loops of Henle are relatively impermeable to water and have a thick portion that is the site of a great deal of sodium and chloride reabsorption. Sodium and chloride transport by the thick ascending limb uses a unique membrane transporter that cotransports sodium, chloride, and potassium into the cell from the lumen. This transport is sodium-linked in that the Na–K–ATPase pump on the opposite side of the cell maintains the low intracellular sodium concentration that permits the cotransporter to function. The net effect of this cellular transport is continuous addition of sodium and chloride to the interstitial fluid of the medulla without any accompanying water (Fig. 23–11). Sodium chloride is also reabsorbed from the thin ascending limb of the loop (Fig. 23–11), but the mechanism responsible for this transport is controversial. The fluid en-

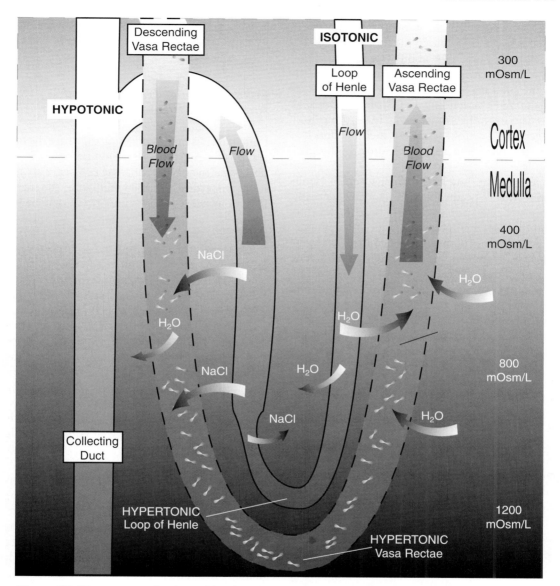

Figure 23-11. Transport of sodium chloride and water by loop of Henle and vasa rectae. *Arrows* indicate direction of net transport in the different tubular segments and vessels. The osmolarity of the interstitial fluids in the cortex is 300 mOsm/L; the osmolarity of the interstitial fluids in the medulla is shown as a gradient that increases from outer to inner medulla. *Hypertonic, isotonic,* and *hypotonic* refer to fluid and plasma in tubules and vessels, respectively.

tering the loop of Henle is isotonic, and the fluid exiting is hypotonic (Fig. 23–11). ***This change in tubular fluid shows that the net effect of loop of Henle transport is to add more particles than water to the interstitial fluids in the renal medulla.***

Transport of sodium and chloride into the interstitium without water is the key factor in generation of hypertonic interstitial fluid in the medulla (Fig. 23–11), and this hypertonic fluid has an essential role in the ability to generate hypertonic urine. The transport of particles without water from the lumen of the loops also creates hypotonic fluid in the tubule, and this is an essential step in the ability to generate hypotonic urine. However, regardless of the tonicity of the final urine, the transport characteristics of the thick ascending limbs of the loops of Henle remain the same, so that hypertonic fluid is generated within the renal medulla and hypotonic fluid is generated within the loop of Henle.

The descending limbs of the loops of Henle are relatively permeable to water but relatively impermeable to particles. As fluid flows into and through the descending limbs, water is removed because of the osmotic gradient between the tubular lumen and the interstitial fluids of the renal medulla (Fig. 23–11).

Because the ascending and descending limbs of loops of Henle are relatively close together in the medulla and because the tubular flows move in opposite directions, the combined effects of transport by ascending and descending limbs produces an osmotic gradient in the interstitial fluids of the renal medulla. Interstitial fluid osmolality increases from the outer zones to the inner zones of the renal medulla (Fig. 23–11).

The *countercurrent mechanism* is any mechanism that depends on streams of flow moving in opposite directions, and these are usually close to each other. The ascending and descending loops of Henle form a countercurrent mechanism that amplifies the osmolyte (sodium chloride) transport properties of the ascending limb of the loop of Henle. This countercurrent mechanism generates the osmotic gradient in the interstitial fluids of the renal medulla.

The ascending and descending vasa recta also form a countercurrent exchange mechanism by permitting free exchange of solutes and water between the ascending and descending blood vessels. This exchange allows for blood flow into and out of the medulla without disrupting the gradient. There is a small net gain of both water and particles by the vasa rectae, and some of these are the water and particles that were reabsorbed from the loop of Henle (Fig. 23–11).

The maximal osmolality of the osmotic gradient in the renal medulla differs among species, and maximal urine concentration ability is determined by the maximal osmolality of the gradient (Fig. 23–11).

Collecting Duct Transport and Antidiuretic Hormone

Principal cells in the collecting ducts are the target cells for ADH. If ADH is not present, the luminal cell membrane of these cells is relatively water impermeable. ADH stimulates the insertion of water channels into these cell membranes to increase the overall water permeability of collecting ducts.

Collecting ducts begin in the renal cortex but extend into and through the renal medulla, where the interstitial fluids are hypertonic. Also, because of the transport in the loop of Henle, the tubular fluid entering the cortical portion of a collecting duct is dilute or hypotonic, and this is always true regardless of the water balance status of the animal. If ADH is not present, the water permeability of the collecting duct is relatively low, and the hypotonic fluid entering the collecting ducts passes through and is excreted as a hypotonic urine. Because water is not reabsorbed from the water-impermeable collecting duct, the volume is also relatively large (Fig. 23–12, A). If ADH is present, the water permeability of the collecting duct is increased, and water is reabsorbed because the osmolality inside the duct is less than that outside. As the tubular fluid passes through the medullary portion of the collecting duct, more and more water is reabsorbed, and the osmolality of the tubular fluid increases further. In these circumstances urine volume is low and urine osmolality is high (Fig. 23–12, B).

Osmotic Regulation of Antidiuretic Hormone

ADH (or arginine vasopressin in most mammalian species) release from the posterior pituitary can be regulated by changes in the ECF (extracellular fluid) osmolality. Specific cells (*osmoreceptors*) in the hypothalamus monitor the osmolality of ECF. In response to increases in ECF osmolality, these cells stimulate increases in ADH release, which results in the ex-

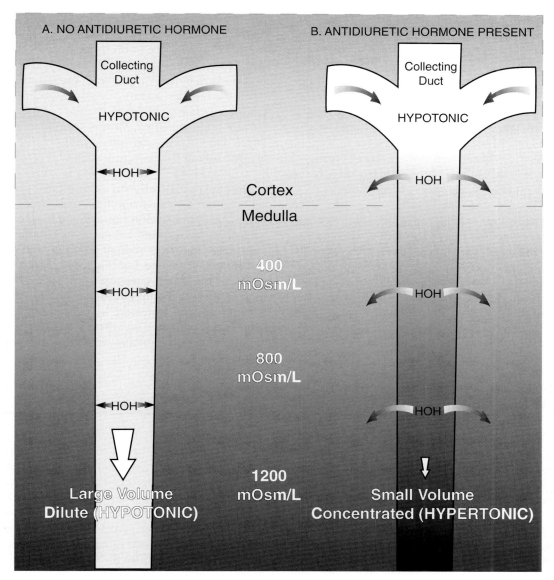

Figure 23-12. *A*) Distal tubule and collecting duct when ADH is absent. Water permeability of collecting is low, so tubular fluid remains hypotonic (dilute). *B*) Distal tubule and collecting duct when ADH is present. Water permeability of collecting duct is increased, so water is reabsorbed and tubular fluid becomes hypertonic (concentrated).

cretion of a small volume of a hypertonic urine. The elimination of excess particles and conservation of water dilutes the ECF, which acts as a negative feedback control to inhibit additional releases of ADH. Reductions in ECF osmolality inhibit ADH release, which results in the excretion of a relatively large volume of dilute urine. This eliminates any excess water.

Polyuria and Polydipsia

Polyuria is the passage of larger volumes of urine than normal. Animals that cannot generate hypertonic urine when necessary become polyuric. Polydipsia is excessive thirst, and polyuric animals are often able to maintain water balance by increasing water intake. The increased intake is considered to be a sign of excessive thirst.

Polyuria and polydipsia (often abbreviated PU/PD) may develop in animals with unregulated diabetes mellitus and significant increases in blood glucose. The renal tubules cannot reabsorb the abnormally large amounts of glucose in the glomerular filtrate, and the glucose that remains in the renal tubules exerts an osmotic effect to retain water in the tubules. Increased urine flow results, and the animal must increase water intake to maintain water balance.

Polyuria and polydipsia may also result when ADH is not available (e.g., pituitary tumor preventing its release) or the kidney does not respond appropriately to ADH. In either case the water permeability of the collecting ducts remains relatively low and water cannot be reabsorbed from the collecting ducts into the blood. Again, the affected animals must increase water intake to maintain water balance. This condition is diabetes insipidus.

Sodium, Potassium, and Aldosterone

Most of the sodium and potassium in the initial glomerular filtrate is reabsorbed by the proximal tubule and the loop of Henle. However, the collecting duct is also capable of sodium and potassium transport, and it is here that the final adjustments are made in the regulation of sodium and potassium balance. Aldosterone, a steroid hormone from the adrenal cortex, functions as a major regulator of sodium and potassium transport in the collecting duct.

Aldosterone acts on *principal cells* of the collecting ducts to promote their reabsorption of sodium when sodium must be retained to maintain sodium balance. The regulation of aldosterone secretion from the adrenal cortex relative to sodium balance is via the renin–angiotensin system. When sodium must be retained (such as with a low-salt diet or after loss of extracellular fluid with sodium), the renin–angiotensin system is activated, and angiotensin II stimulates cells of the adrenal cortex to secrete aldosterone.

The concentration of potassium in plasma and other extracellular fluids also regulates aldosterone secretion. Increases in potassium concentration directly stimulate cells of the adrenal cortex to secrete aldosterone. Aldosterone promotes potassium secretion by principal cells, and this tends to increase the urinary loss of potassium. The increased loss of potassium in the urine reduces plasma potassium, and thus potassium plasma concentration and potassium balance are maintained. Most potassium in excreted urine reaches the tubular fluid by tubular secretion in the collecting duct.

Unregulated secretion of aldosterone by adrenal tumors can cause significant reductions in plasma potassium concentrations, and these can threaten life. Such individuals may also have moderate degrees of sodium retention and increases in ECF volume, but this is usually not as severe as the changes in plasma potassium. The more moderate changes in sodium balance are because sodium transport by other nephron segments is regulated by other factors that can counterbalance the sodium-retaining effects of aldosterone.

Urine Acidification

Intercalated cells in the walls of collecting ducts are capable of the active transport of hydrogen ions into the tubular lumen to acidify the urine. This system can generate a difference between blood and urine of about 3 pH, so if blood pH is 7.4, urine with a pH of 4.4 can be formed. The hydrogen ions to be secreted are generated in intercalated cells by the hydration of carbon dioxide under the influence of carbonic anhydrase. A bicarbonate ion is also generated during this process, and these are secreted into the extracellular fluids at the base of the cell, from where the bicarbonate can diffuse into the plasma.

The secretion of hydrogen ions by intercalated cells is regulated by the concentrations of carbon dioxide and bicarbonate ions in the plasma and other extracellular fluids. If carbon dioxide concentration increases or if bicarbonate ion concentration decreases, the rate of hydrogen ion secretion accelerates, and urine becomes more acidic. The importance and relevance of this regulation by carbon dioxide or bicarbonate to the regulation of overall acid-base balance is discussed in a later section of this chapter.

Some of the secreted hydrogen ions combine with HPO_4^{-2} ions in the tubular fluid to form $H_2PO_4^{-}$. In this manner, HPO_4^{-2} acts as an *intratubular buffer* to reduce the concentration of free hydrogen ions and prevent the urine pH from dropping too low. The phosphate ions originally entered the tubular fluid as part of the glomerular filtrate. Ammonia may also serve as an intratubular buffer (forming **ammonium** ions), and it is secreted into the tubular fluid by the collecting duct.

Regulation of Acid-Base Balance

The pH of blood plasma and other extracellular fluids is maintained relatively constant within a narrow range (about 7.35 to 7.45). It is important to maintain this constancy, because enzyme activity and metabolic processes require close control of pH for optimal function. Three major mechanisms function together to prevent the development of an abnormal pH. These are: (1) extracellular and intracellular chemical buffers; (2) ventilatory control of plasma carbon dioxide; and (3) urinary excretion of bicarbonate or an acid urine as needed. These mechanisms defend against potential changes in body fluid pH that would come about as a result of normal cellular metabolism or the absorption of acids or bases from the gastrointestinal tract. The ability of these mechanisms to maintain a normal pH can be overwhelmed during metabolic disturbances or after the absorption of large amounts of acids or bases from the gastrointestinal tract.

Ruminal or lactic acidosis is seen in ruminants that ingest large amounts of carbohydrates, usually grain, over a short period. The sudden ingestion of the concentrated carbohydrates alters the microbial population in the rumen, favoring the rapid growth of organisms that produce lactic acid. The rapid increase in lactic acid absorption into the blood overwhelms the ability of the pH regulatory systems, and systemic acidosis develops.

Extracellular and Intracellular Buffers

A chemical buffer system acts to maintain a constant pH by either donating or removing free hydrogen ions in a solution (see Chapter 2).

The bicarbonate buffer system is quantitatively the most important chemical buffer in blood plasma and other extracellular fluids. Bicarbonate is the base in this system, and the acid is carbonic acid. However, because carbonic acid is difficult to measure and in body fluids is in equilibrium with carbon dioxide, the levels of carbon dioxide are routinely used as indicators of carbonic acid levels.

The bicarbonate buffer system is the most important body buffer system from a physiologic standpoint, because the concentrations of the components of the system can be rapidly adjusted by changes in either renal excretion of bicarbonate or pulmonary ventilation to remove carbon dioxide. Bicarbonate is avidly reabsorbed by renal tubules, but a renal threshold value permits rapid excretion of excess bicarbonate. Also, plasma carbon dioxide levels are normally the primary regulator of ventilation, so these levels are also under constant control.

Both intracellular and extracellular proteins function as buffers. Because of the large quantity of intracellular proteins in organs such as skeletal muscle, these account for a large percentage of the total buffering capacity in the body, but these buffers cannot be easily regulated as can some other important extracellular buffers. The hemoglobin proteins in erythrocytes are a major blood buffer.

Classification of Alkalosis and Acidosis and Compensation

Alkalosis is a condition in which the pH of body fluids (including blood) is abnormally high, and **acidosis** is a condition in which the pH is abnormally low. Acidosis or alkalosis can be classified as being either **metabolic** or **respiratory,** to indicate the cause of the pH imbalance. The term *respiratory* refers to acid-base imbalances that come about as a result of primary or initial changes in carbon dioxide levels. The term *metabolic* refers to all other causes of acid-base imbalances.

When an acid-base imbalance arises and the buffering capacities of the extracellular and intracellular chemical buffers are overwhelmed, the body systems primarily responsible for acid-base balance (respiratory and urinary) should respond. This response may lead to a state of **compensation,** so that the acid-base imbalance is less severe than if the compensation (or response) had not occurred. For example, chronic lung diseases may result in accumulation of carbon dioxide and respiratory acidosis. The kidneys compensate for the respiratory acidosis by producing acidic urine and retaining base (bicarbonate). An increase in blood bicarbonate concentration is an indicator of renal compensation for the primary respiratory acidosis.

Because of its importance as the major extracellular buffer system and because the components of the system can be readily determined in clinical laboratories, the status of the bicarbonate buffer system is used to evaluate overall acid-base balance. The primary cause of acidosis or alkalosis is routinely diagnosed by evaluation of the bicarbonate buffer system.

Metabolic alkalosis is a primary increase in bicarbonate ions. Causes include excessive ingestion of alkaline salts or gastric vomiting, during which hydrochloric acid is lost from the body fluids. The body compensates for metabolic alkalosis by hypoventilation to retain carbon dioxide and by increasing urinary bicarbonate excretion.

Metabolic acidosis is a primary decrease in bicarbonate ions. Causes include (1) excessive loss of bicarbonate via diarrhea (e.g., calf scours), (2) excessive formation of metabolic acids as a result of metabolic disturbances (e.g., diabetes mellitus, starvation, and lactic acidosis during shock), (3) inability of the kidneys to excrete acid (e.g., renal failure), and (4) absorption of excess acid from the gastrointestinal tract (e.g., ruminal acidosis). The body compensates for metabolic acidosis by hyperventilation and excretion of acid urine if possible.

Respiratory alkalosis is a primary deficit in carbon dioxide (**hypocapnia** is low blood carbon dioxide). Causes include (1) exposure to high altitudes, where low oxygen tension causes hyperventilation; (2) a high fever, which may produce hyperventilation; and (3) inflammation or diseases of the brain, which stimulate the respiratory centers. The kidneys compensate for respiratory alkalosis by increasing excretion of bicarbonate ions in the urine.

Respiratory acidosis is a primary excess of carbon dioxide (**hypercapnia** is elevated blood carbon dioxide). Causes include pneumonia, pulmonary fibrosis, pulmonary edema, airway obstructions, and breathing air that is high in carbon dioxide. The kidneys compensate for the primary respiratory problem by excreting acid urine and secreting additional bicarbonate into the blood. Plasma levels of bicarbonate may increase as the compensatory response occurs.

ANATOMY OF THE MALE REPRODUCTIVE SYSTEM

The organs and glands of the male reproductive tract manufacture the male gamete (spermatozoon [plural spermatozoa], or sperm) and deliver it to the female reproductive tract. Embryologically the reproductive system is closely related to the urinary system, developing the tubules and ducts of both interdependently. In the male adult, the urethra is a passage common to the urinary system and the reproductive tract.

The male reproductive system of mammals consists of two *testes* (*testicles*) in the *scrotum,* accessory organs including ducts and glands, and the penis. The testes produce *spermatozoa* (also called *sperm*) and *testosterone* (the male sex hormone). The scrotum provides a favorable environment for the production of spermatozoa. The remaining structures assist the spermatozoa to reach their ultimate goal (the ovum of the female) in a condition conducive to fertilization of the ovum. These structures include the *epididymis* and *ductus deferens,* accessory sex glands (*ampullary glands, vesicular glands, prostate,* and *bulbourethral glands*), the *urethra,* and the *penis.* Figure 24–1 shows the comparative anatomy of the male reproductive organs of farm animals.

Testis

The *testes* vary somewhat between species in shape, size, and location (Fig. 24–1). In the horse, the long axis of each testis is nearly horizontal,

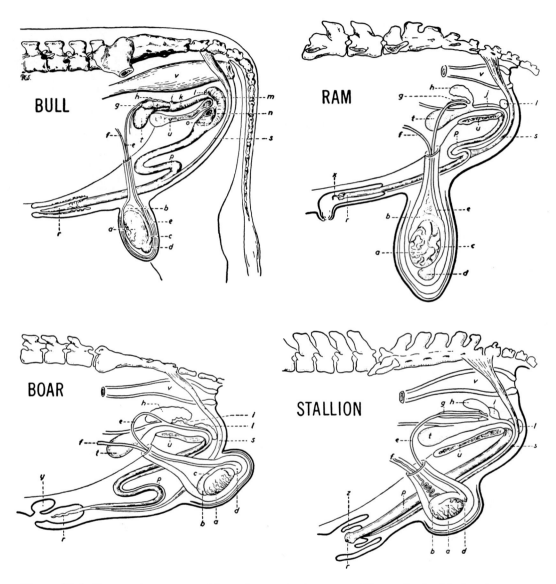

Figure 24-1. Comparative anatomy of the male reproductive organs of farm animals. *a*) Left testis; *b*) head of epididymis; *c*) body of epididymis; *d*) tail of epididymis; *e*) ductus deferens; *f*) spermatic vessels and nerves; *g*) ampulla; *h*) vesicular gland; *i, j*) prostate gland; *l*) bulbourethral gland; *n*) left crus of penis (cut); *p*) body of penis; *r*) free end of penis; *s*) *retractor penis m.; t*) urinary bladder; *u*) pelvic symphysis; *v*) rectum; *x*) urethral process (ram); *y*) preputial pouch (boar); *z*) fold of prepuce (stallion). (Adapted from Bielanski. *Rozrod Zwierzat Gospodarskich* [Reproduction of Farm Animals]. Warsaw: P.W.R.I.L., 1962.)

and the testes are held close to the abdominal wall near the superficial (external) inguinal ring. The testes of the bull and small ruminants are near the sigmoid (**S**-shaped) flexure of the penis; the long axis of each testis in these species is nearly vertical, so the ruminant scrotum is dorsoventrally elongate and pendulous. The testes of the boar are caudal to the sigmoid flexure of the penis, just ventral to the anus, a position described as perineal.

In spite of these positional differences, the essential structure of the testes in each of these species is the same. The **spermatic cord,** containing blood vessels, nerves, lymphatics, and the ductus deferens, suspends each individual testis within the scrotum. The spermatic cord and its testicle are doubly invested with peritoneum, a serosal sac referred to as the **vaginal tunic** (Latin *vagina,* sheath). This investment of the testis reflects the fact that the fetal testis developed within the abdomen and reached its scrotal position by migrating through this serosa-lined cavity, carrying its serosal investments with it (discussed later).

Each testis consists of a mass of coiled **seminiferous tubules** (Fig. 24–2) surrounded by a heavy fibrous capsule called the **tunica albuginea.** A number of fibrous **septa,** also called **trabeculae,** pass inward from the tunica albuginea, dividing the testis into lobules and providing a framework for support of the seminiferous tubules and the interstitial tissue that produces testosterone. The seminiferous tubules are the site of **spermatogenesis,** the formation of spermatozoa. The many seminiferous tubules deliver sperm into a network of tubules, the **rete testis,** which drains into the **efferent ductules.** The efferent ductules connect with the **epididymal duct** at the head of the epididymis.

The connective tissue between the seminiferous tubules contains the **interstitial cells** (Leydig cells). The interstitial cells secrete the male hormone testosterone when stimulated by the pituitary gonadotropin luteinizing hormone (LH) (see Chapters 12 and 25). **Sustentacular cells** (Sertoli cells) within the seminiferous tubules envelop developing spermatozoa and their precursors. The sustentacular cells nourish the developing sperm and mediate the effects of follicle-stimulating hormone (FSH) and testosterone on the germ cells (Figs. 24–3 and 24–4).

Epididymis

The **epididymis** is composed of a long, convoluted tube (the **epididymal duct**) that connects the efferent ductules of the testis with the ductus deferens. It appears as a firm, arcing organ attached on one side of the testis along its long axis. The epididymal duct houses the spermatozoa as they mature before they are expelled by

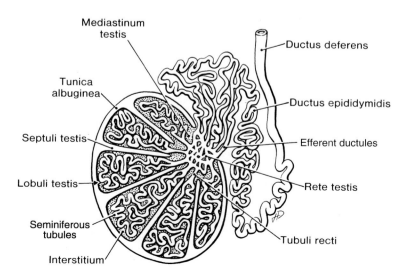

Figure 24-2. Internal anatomy of the testis. (Reprinted with permission from Banks W.J. *Applied Veterinary Histology.* 2nd ed. Baltimore: Williams & Wilkins, 1986.)

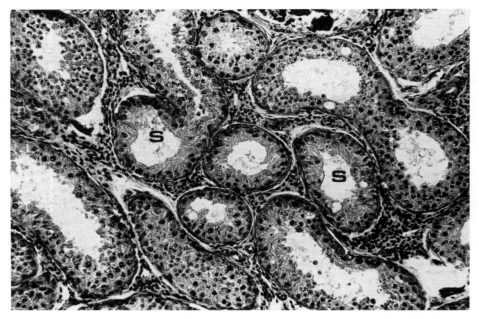

Figure 24-3. Micrograph of seminiferous tubules (S). (Reprinted with permission from Banks W.J. *Applied Veterinary Histology*. 2nd ed. Baltimore: Williams & Wilkins, 1986.)

ejaculation. Spermatozoa are immature when they leave the testis and must undergo a period of maturation (usually 10–15 days) within the epididymis before they are capable of fertilizing ova. The epididymis is arbitrarily divided into a **head** (into which the efferent ductules empty), a **body** lying on the long axis of the testis, and a **tail** that is attached by ligaments directly to the testis and to the adjacent vaginal tunic. The duct of the epididymal tail continues as the ductus deferens, which conveys sperm from the testis to the urethra.

Ductus Deferens

The **ductus deferens** is a muscular tube that undergoes peristaltic contractions during ejaculation, propelling the spermatozoa from the epididymis to the urethra. The ductus deferens leaves the tail of the epididymis, passes through the inguinal canal as a part of the spermatic cord, and within the abdomen returns caudad, separating from the neurovascular parts of the cord. As the two ductus deferentia approach the urethra, they approach one another and continue caudad between the rectum and urinary bladder, enclosed in a fold of peritoneum, the **genital fold.** The genital fold is embryologically homologous to the broad ligament suspending the uterus in females. In some male animals, a vestigial homologue of the uterus, the **uterus masculinus,** is present in the genital fold between the two ductus deferentia.

Scrotum

The **scrotum** is a cutaneous sac that conforms in size and shape to the testes it contains. The scrotal skin is thin, pliable, and relatively hairless (except in some breeds of sheep, in whom fleece covers the scrotum). A layer of fibroelastic tissue mixed with smooth muscle fibers, called the **tunica dartos,** lies immediately under the skin. During exposure to cold the muscle fibers of the tunica dartos contract and help hold the testes against the abdominal wall. The tunica dartos sends a fibrous sheet into the median plane between the two testes to form the **scrotal septum,** which divides the scrotum into two compartments, one for each testis. Deep to

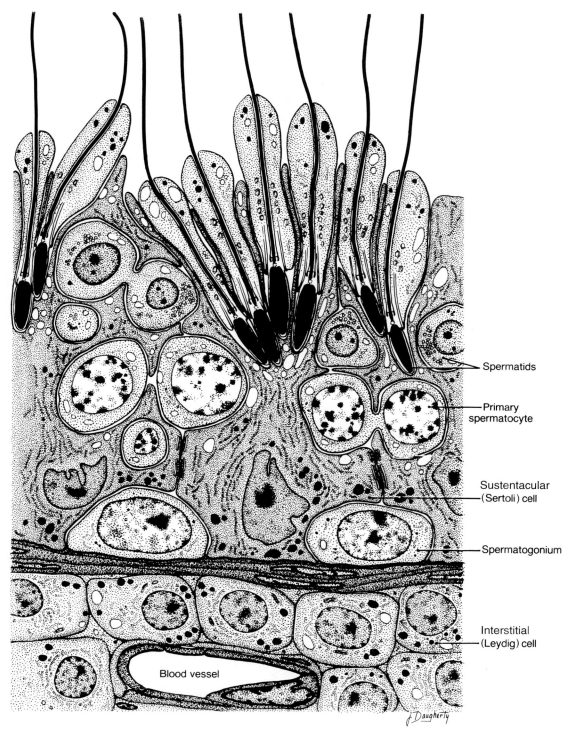

Figure 24-4. Cells of the seminiferous tubule. Sertoli cells surround and support developing spermatozoa. (Adapted with permission from Banks W.J. *Applied Veterinary Histology*. 2nd ed. Baltimore: Williams & Wilkins, 1986.)

the tunica dartos are several layers of fascia, which are not easily separated. The internal abdominal oblique muscle contributes a slip of muscle that lies on the spermatic cord. This is the *cremaster muscle,* which also assists with drawing the testicle closer to the body wall when ambient temperatures are low or as a protective reflex.

Inguinal Canal

The *inguinal canal* is a passage from the abdominal cavity to the exterior of the body that extends from the *deep inguinal ring* to the *superficial inguinal ring* (Fig. 24–5). The deep (internal) inguinal ring is a space or potential space between the caudal border of the internal abdominal oblique muscle and the deep face of the aponeurosis (flat tendon) of the external abdominal oblique muscle. The superficial (external) inguinal ring is merely a slit in the aponeurosis of the external abdominal oblique muscle. In addition to the spermatic cord, the canal allows passage of the external pudendal artery and a sensory nerve that serves the inguinal region of the abdominal wall. This accounts for the existence of the inguinal canal in female animals.

The inguinal canal is normally a potential space, large enough only to permit passage of the spermatic cord and inguinal vessels and nerves. If the internal ring and canal are too capacious, a loop of intestine may pass through the canal into the scrotum, producing an *inguinal hernia.*

Descent of the Testis

In both male and female fetuses, the gonads develop in the sublumbar region immediately caudal to the kidneys. In the female animal, the

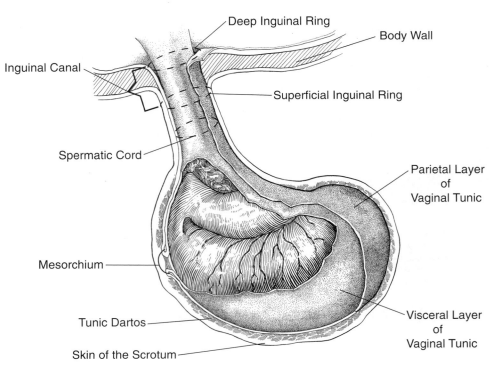

Figure 24-5. Relation of testis to peritoneal investments. The spermatic cord, comprising ductus deferens, blood vessels and nerves, passes through the abdominal body wall via the inguinal canal. It, the canal, and the testis are lined with extensions of the peritoneum.

ovaries remain in the abdominal cavity near their origin; but in the male animal, the testes travel (descend) a considerable distance from their point of origin to the scrotum. The environment of the scrotum features a temperature a few degrees lower than that of the normal body temperature; this lower temperature is favorable to spermatogenesis.

The descent of the testis normally is complete by birth or soon after (Fig. 24–6). It is guided on its journey by the fibrous **gubernaculum,** a cordlike structure that initially extends from the testis through the inguinal canal to the skin in the region that will become the scrotum. As the fetus grows, the gubernaculum draws the testis from the abdominal cavity into the scrotum.

The testis begins its development within the abdominal cavity covered (as are all abdominal organs) with peritoneum. As it descends into the scrotum, it pushes the parietal peritoneum ahead of it, thus acquiring a second layer of serosa. This second outer layer of peritoneum (the **parietal layer of the vaginal tunic**) is continuous with the parietal peritoneum at the internal inguinal ring and lies deep to the deep fascia of the scrotum, with which it blends (Fig. 24–5). The testis itself is invested with a second layer, the **visceral layer of the vaginal tunic.** The **mesorchium** is a delicate double layer of peritoneum connecting the visceral and parietal layers of tunica vaginalis, just as mesentery connects parietal and visceral layers of abdominal peritoneum. It gives off an additional reflection of serosa, the **mesoductus deferens** that surrounds the duc-

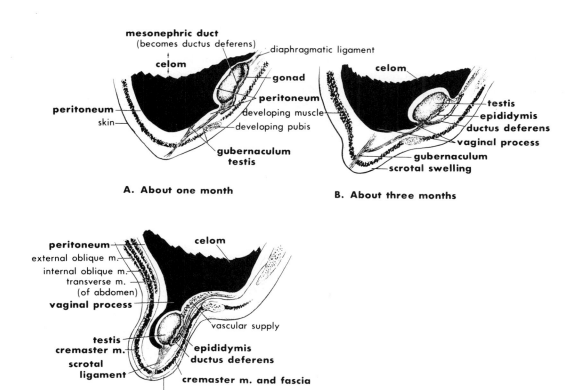

Figure 24-6. Descent of the human testis (ages of fetus are based on human gestation). The embryonic celom will become the abdominal and pelvic cavities. (Adapted with permission from Crouch J.E. *Functional Human Anatomy.* 4th ed. Philadelphia: Lea & Febiger, 1985.)

tus deferens within the spermatic cord (Fig. 24–7).

A testis that fails to descend into the scrotum is called a *cryptorchid testis,* and the animal with such a condition is called a cryptorchid (Greek *crypt,* hidden; *orcho,* testicle). In most species, the testes descend into the scrotum by birth or shortly thereafter. An animal in which the testis descends into the inguinal canal but not into the scrotum is called a high flanker. A cryptorchid with both testes retained in the abdominal cavity is likely to be sterile, since spermatogenesis does not occur normally unless the testis is cooler than core body temperature, a condition provided by the scrotum. However, the relatively high temperature of the abdomen does not interfere with the production of testosterone, so the cryptorchid has all the behaviors and appearance of a normal male except that no testes are evident and no normal spermatozoa are produced. A unilateral cryptorchid (one testis retained, one descended) is fertile insofar as the descended testis produces normal spermatozoa; however, the tendency toward cryptorchidism is likely heritable. Additionally, testes retained in the abdomen develop testicular tumors at a higher rate than scrotal testes. For these reasons, it is recommended that cryptorchid animals be castrated, including removal of the retained testicle or testicles.

Castration

Castration is a term usually applied to removal of the testes of the male animal, although technically it can apply to ovariectomy (removal of the ovaries) of the female animal as well. Castration of male animals is practiced primarily to prevent those of inferior quality from reproducing. Except for colts that exhibit unusual quality meriting reproduction, most male horses are castrated to improve their tractability and utility as performance animals. Early castration also improves the quality of meat animals by inhibiting undesirable secondary sex characteristics (notably the failure to develop marbling of muscle). Table 24–1 lists the common terms for intact and castrated male animals.

Horsemen sometimes refer to a horse as being *proud cut,* meaning that the horse behaves like a stallion in spite of having been castrated. It has been believed in some circles that this results from the failure to remove all of the epididymis and that this part of the reproductive tract somehow produces sufficient testosterone to give the horse the attributes of a stallion. This belief is common but erroneous; the

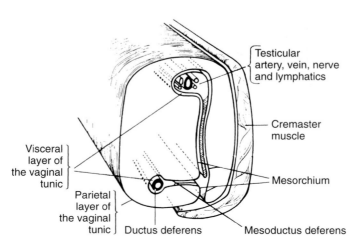

Figure 24-7. Cross-section of the spermatic cord.

Table 24-1. Common Terms for Male Animals

Species	*Intact Adult Male*	*Castrated Male*
Horse	Stallion	Gelding
Ox	Bull	Steer
Pig	Boar	Barrow
Sheep	Ram	Wether
Goat	Buck (billy)	Wether
Chicken	Rooster	Capon

epididymis is entirely incapable of producing male sex hormones. It is much more likely that one or both testes were cryptorchid and that only the epididymis was removed (it can look remarkably like a small testicle), leaving the cryptorchid testis to produce testosterone. Alternatively, a colt castrated correctly but relatively late in life may have already acquired physical and behavioral characteristics of an intact stallion, characteristics that may not be wholly extinguished by removal of the testes.

Vasectomy refers to transection (usually with ligation and/or removal of a section) of the ductus deferentia (formerly called the vas deferens, hence the name of the procedure). This operation prevents delivery of spermatozoa from the epididymides but has no effect on the production of the male hormones. The behavior and appearance of the vasectomized animal, therefore, are that of the intact male. Vasectomy is sometimes used experimentally or to produce teaser animals used to identify females in heat.

Accessory Sex Glands

The male accessory sex glands produce the bulk of the *ejaculate,* or *semen,* the medium for transport of sperm. Semen provides favorable conditions for nutrition of sperm and acts as a buffer against the natural acidity of the female genital tract. The accessory sex glands include the ampullae of the ductus deferentia; vesicular glands; prostate gland; and bulbourethral glands. There is considerable variation in shape and size of the various accessory sex glands among species, but the relative location is similar in all animals (Figs. 24–1 and 24–8).

Ampullae

The **ampullae** are glandular enlargements associated with the terminal parts of the ductus deferentia. They are well developed in the stallion, bull, and ram and absent in the boar. Glands of the ampullae empty into the ductus deferentia and contribute volume to the semen.

Vesicular Glands

The **vesicular glands** (formerly called seminal vesicles) are paired glands associated with the genital fold. In most domestic species, each vesicular gland merges with the ipsilateral ductus deferens, creating the short *ejaculatory duct,* which empties into the pelvic urethra. In the boar, the vesicular glands open into the urethra separately from the ductus deferentia. The vesicular glands of the stallion are hollow, pear-shaped sacs; those of the bull, ram, and boar are lobulated glands of considerable size.

Prostate Gland

The **prostate gland** is an unpaired gland that more or less completely surrounds the pelvic urethra. In farm animals the prostate gland comprises various combinations of diffuse and compact parts extending along the pelvic urethra under cover of the urethral muscle. The multiple ducts of the prostate gland open in two parallel rows, one on each side of the lumen of the urethra. The prostate produces an alkaline secretion that gives semen its characteristic odor. In older intact male animals, the prostate may become enlarged and interfere with urination.

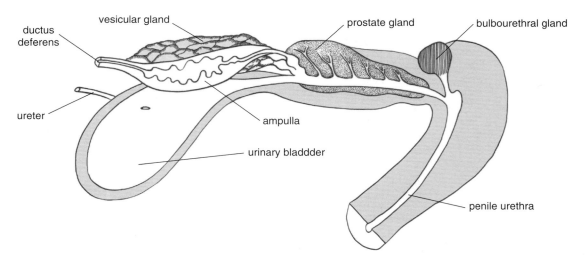

Figure 24-8. Accessory sex glands of the bull. *a*) Ampulla; *bu*) bulbourethral gland; *dd*) ductus deferens; *pb*) prostate (body of); *pd*) prostate (diffuse part); *pel. u*) pelvic urethra; *pen. u*) penile urethra; *u*) ureter; *ub*) urinary bladder; *vg*) vesicular gland. (Reprinted with permission from Hafez E.S.E: *Reproduction in Farm Animals.* 6th ed. Philadelphia: Lea & Febiger, 1993.)

Bulbourethral Glands

The **bulbourethral** (formerly Cowper's) **glands** are paired glands on either side of the pelvic urethra just cranial to the ischial arch but caudal to the other accessory glands. Bulbourethral glands are especially large in the boar.

Penis

The male organ of copulation, the **penis,** may be divided into three general areas: the **glans,** or free extremity; the main portion, or **body;** and the two **crura,** or roots, which attach to the ischial arch of the pelvis (Fig. 24–9).

The bulk of the penile body's internal structure is composed of paired columns of erectile tissue, the **corpora cavernosa.** Each corpus cavernosum is replete with blood sinusoids divided by sheets of connective tissue called **trabeculae.** These are derived from the **tunica albuginea,** a heavy, fibroelastic capsule surrounding the penis. In species with a **fibroelastic penis** (ruminants and swine), the trabeculae form the bulk of the penis, and as a consequence, in these species the penis is firm when not erect. The

horse has the **musculocavernous penis,** with the blood sinusoids predominating over connective tissue. The equine penis therefore is flaccid when not erect.

The two **crura** of the penis are the proximal parts of the corpora cavernosa. They originate on the caudal surface of the ischial arch, one on each side of the symphysis of the pelvis. The ventral midline groove between the corpora cavernosa contains the penile urethra and an associated unpaired body of erectile tissue, the **corpus spongiosus.** The proximal continuation of the corpus spongiosum is the **bulb of the penis,** which lies between the crura. In most animals, the corpus spongiosum penis is continuous distally with the erectile tissue of the glans.

The glans penis shows considerable variation from species to species. The horse and sheep both have a free portion of the urethra, the **urethral process,** that projects beyond the glans. The bull and ram have a helmet-shaped glans, and the external urethral opening of the bull opens into a twisted groove. The penis of the boar has a twisting cranial extremity and only a small glans (Fig. 24–10).

Erection of the penis occurs when more

MALE REPRODUCTIVE ORGANS

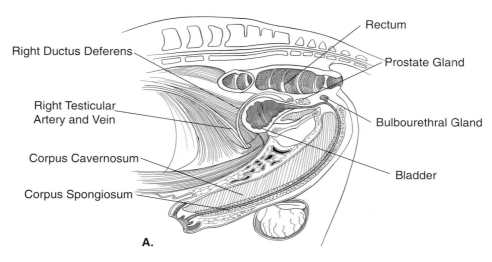

A.

Accessory Reproductive Glands; dorsal view

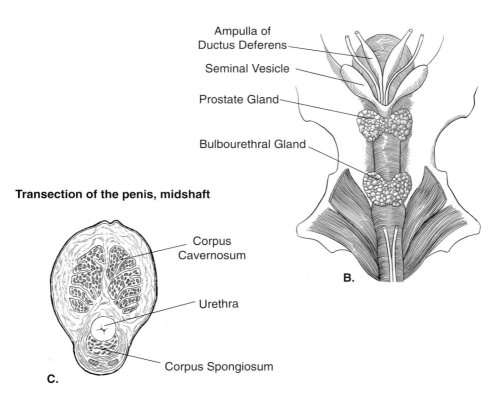

Transection of the penis, midshaft

B.

C.

Figure 24-9. Anatomy of the equine penis. *A*) Lateral view, showing relationship of penis to body wall and pelvis. *B*) Dorsocaudal view of attachment of penis to pelvis and accessory sex glands. *C*) Cross section of equine penis, mid shaft.

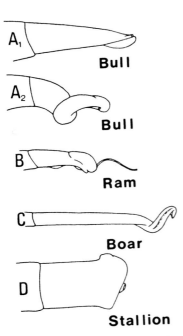

Figure 24-10. Free end of the penis. *A1*) bull penis prior to intromission; *A2*) bull penis following intromission. Spiraling of the glans is a normal consequence of erection. (Reprinted with permission from Hafez E.S.E: *Reproduction in Farm Animals.* 6th ed. Philadelphia: Lea & Febiger, 1993.)

blood enters the penis by way of the arterial supply than leaves by the veins. The increased blood volume enlarges the penis and makes it turgid. In the stallion, whose penis is musculocavernous, the penis becomes much larger in all dimensions upon erection. The fibroelastic penis (as found in ruminants and swine) does not increase much in diameter during erection. Instead, the chief effect of erection of the penis in these animals consists of lengthening the penis by straightening the **sigmoid flexure,** much as a bent garden hose tends to straighten when water pressure increases.

Prepuce

The **prepuce** is an invaginated fold of skin surrounding the free extremity of the penis. The outer surface is fairly typical skin, while the inner mucous membrane consists of a preputial layer lining the prepuce and a penile layer covering the surface of the free extremity of the penis. The prepuce of the horse makes a double fold, so two concentric layers surround the penis when it is retracted. The prepuce of the pig has a diverticulum dorsal to the preputial orifice. It accumulates urine, secretions, and dead cells, which contribute to the typical odor of a mature boar.

Muscles of the Male Genitalia

The **urethral muscle** (*m. urethralis*) is the striated muscle associated with the pelvic portion of the urethra. It completely encircles the urethra of the goat and horse but surrounds only the ventral and lateral aspects of the bovine, porcine, and ovine urethra. The urethral muscle forms the voluntary sphincter of the urinary bladder; during ejaculation, waves of peristaltic contractions help propel the semen through the urethra.

The extrapelvic continuation of the urethral muscle is a striated muscle called the **bulbospongiosus muscle.** It surrounds the urethra and bulb of the penis. The bulbospongiosus muscle of the horse extends from the penile bulb between the crura of the penis along the entire urethra to the glans penis. In other animals it covers the urethral bulb and extends only a short distance along the penile urethra. The bulbospongiosus muscle continues the action of the urethral muscle in emptying the urethra by peristaltic contractions.

The **ischiocavernosus muscles** are paired striated muscles that cover the superficial aspect of the respective crura of the penis. The two muscles converge from their origins on the lateral sides of the ischial arch toward the body of the penis. When these muscles contract, they pull the penis dorsocraniad against the bony pelvis, aiding erection by compressing much of the venous drainage from the penis.

The **retractor penis muscles** are paired smooth muscles that take origin from the ventral aspect of the first few caudal vertebrae. These muscles pass ventrad on each side of the anal canal, then continue on the midline of the penis superficial to the urethra.

Blood and Nerve Supply of the Male Genitalia

The testis derives its blood supply from the ***testicular artery,*** which branches directly from the abdominal aorta a short distance caudal to the renal artery of the same side. Within the spermatic cord, the testicular artery assumes a tortuous arrangement. The artery is embedded in the likewise convoluted mass of the testicular vein, the ***pampiniform plexus.*** The artery of the ductus deferens from the internal pudendal artery supplies the ductus deferens and may also provide some arterial blood to the epididymis and testis.

The ***external pudendal artery,*** a branch of the deep femoral artery, passes through the inguinal canal and supplies the scrotum and prepuce. In most domestic species, a branch of the internal iliac artery, the ***internal pudendal artery,*** supplies most of the penis, urinary bladder, urethra, and accessory sex glands. The blood supply to the penis of the horse is more extensive than in other species, with additional contributions by the ***obturator artery,*** which passes through the obturator foramen of the pelvis, and the external pudendal artery after it passes through the inguinal canal.

The autonomic innervation of the testis is composed of sympathetic nerves. These autonomic nerve fibers accompany the testicular artery. Sympathetic input affects activity in the blood vessels and smooth muscle fibers. The dorsal nerve of the penis is a continuation of the pudendal nerve, which is derived from ventral branches of sacral nerves. It passes along the dorsum of the penis to ramify in the glans penis. Sensory fibers from the glans provide the afferent limb of reflexes for erection and ejaculation. It is commonly believed that erection is a result of parasympathetic influence on the penis, whereas ejaculation is under sympathetic control.

Chapter 25

Physiology of Male Reproduction

Seminiferous Tubules and Spermatogenesis

Seminiferous Tubules

The epithelium lining the seminiferous tubules contains two cell types, the **sustentacular,** or Sertoli cells and the developing spermatozoa and their precursor **germ cells** (Fig. 25–1).

The large sustentacular cells extend from the base of the epithelium to the lumen of the seminiferous tubules. Their shape is highly irregular because they encircle the developing germ cells (Fig. 25–1). Sustentacular cells secrete a fluid that bathes the developing germ cells and assists with the transport of spermatozoa from the tubules into the rete testis after their release from the sustentacular cells. One component of this fluid, **androgen-binding protein,** transports androgens from their site of synthesis in the testis to the epididmyis, where they are required for maturation of the spermatozoa. **Interstitial cells** (Leydig cells) in the connective tissue between seminiferous tubules secrete **testosterone,** the primary androgen originating in the testicles.

The composition of the interstitial fluid between sustentacular cells and within the lumen of the seminiferous tubules differs from typical interstital fluid. The differences are due in part to a selectively permeable barrier (**blood–testis barrier**) between these fluids and fluid outside of the tubules. The cell junctions between adjacent sustentacular cells and between myoid cells that surround the tubules contribute to

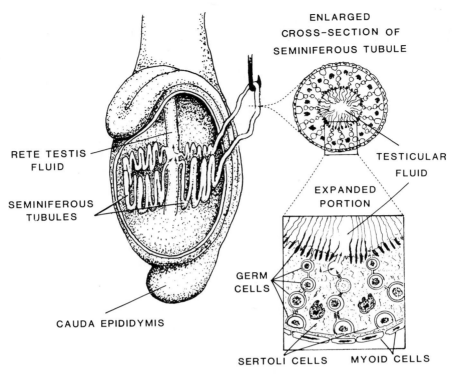

Figure 25-1. Location and microscopic anatomy of seminiferous tubules. Note the irregular border of the sustentacular (Sertoli) cells and their relation to the developing germ cells. (Reprinted with permission from Hafez E.S.E. and Hafez B. *Reproduction in Farm Animals.* 7th ed. Philadelphia: Lippincott Williams & Wilkins, 2000.)

this barrier (Fig. 25–1). The luminal concentrations of cellular secretions, such as androgen-binding proteins and androgens, are higher than in typical extracellular fluid because this functional barrier sequesters them.

Germ Cells and Spermatogenesis

Spermatogenesis is the term for all processes involved in the formation of mature male gametes from the most undifferentiated germ cells. It includes several mitotic cell divisions followed by two **meiotic** cell divisions, during which the chromosome number is reduced from diploid to haploid. This series of cell divisions is termed **spermatocytogenesis** (Fig. 25–2).

Some of the cells resulting from the mitotic cell divisions of the most undifferentiated germ cells remain at the base of the epithelium to maintain the supply of stem cells. Others begin

the sequence of cell divisions (mitotic followed by meiotic divisions) and developmental changes to become spermatozoa. The mitotic cell divisions double the number of cells at each step, so a single spermatogonium gives rise to many spermatozoa.

Meiosis entails two cell divisions and occurs only during the development of gametes in the testis and ovary. Prior to the first division, the DNA is replicated in a manner similar to that for mitotic cell division (see Chapter 2). This replication results in chromosomes, which consist of two identical **chromatids.** In preparation for the first meiotic division, **homologous chromosomes** pair up along the middle of the cell. (Homologous chromosomes are the similar chromosomes of a typical pair, each of which was contributed by one of the parent animals.) During the first meiotic division, one chromosome of each homologous pair moves into each daughter cell. Which individual chromosome of the homolo-

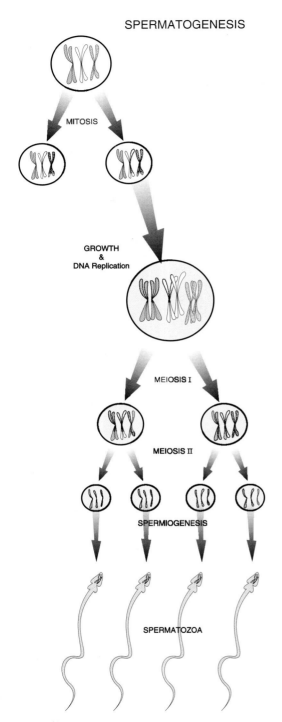

SPERMATOGENESIS

MITOSIS

GROWTH
&
DNA Replication

MEIOSIS I

MEIOSIS II

SPERMIOGENESIS

SPERMATOZOA

Figure 25-2. Spermatogenesis: cell division and structural changes resulting in the formation of spermatozoa. (Redrawn after McDonald L.E. and Pineda M.H., eds.: *Veterinary Endocrinology and Reproduction.* Philadelphia: Lea & Febiger, 1989.)

gous pairs moves to which daughter cell appears to be random. This mixing among homologous pairs provides for genetic variation among the offspring. After the first division, each daughter cell has a haploid number of chromosomes, but each chromosome consists of two chromatids. During the second meiotic division of the two daughter cells, each of the resulting four cells receives one of the chromatids. The overall result of meiosis is the production of four daughter cells, each of which has a haploid number of chromosomes (Fig. 25–3).

In mammals, two of the daughter cells contain the Y chromosome that produce a male offspring (XY) when combined with an X chromosome from an ovum. The other two contain the X chromosome to produce female offspring (XX) when united with the X chromosome containing ovum. However, in avian species, all spermatozoa contain the same sex chromosome, known in these species as the Z chromosome. Female birds carry one Z and a second sex chromosome, the W chromosome. An ovum may contain either a W or Z chromosome, so the ovum is the gamete that determines the sex of the offspring in birds.

When homologous chromosomes are paired in preparation for the first meiotic division, **crossing over** may occur. During this process, similar regions of chromosomes may be exchanged between homologous chromosomes. Such exchanges further increase genetic variability among the offspring, for they may now inherit chromosomes that are different from either parent chromosome.

Spermatid is the term for the cells resulting from the second meiotic division in the seminiferous tubules. Spermatids undergo a series of functional and structural changes to become spermatozoa, and this process is termed **spermiogenesis** (Fig. 25–2). There is no further cellular division after second meiotic division, so there is no further increase in cell number after that division.

Spermatozoa Morphology and Spermatogenesis

When first produced, spermatids are round immobile cells, while fully formed spermatozoa are mobile and consist of a head and tail (Fig.

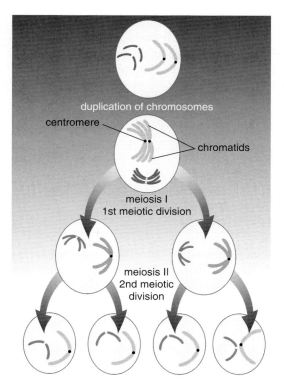

Figure 25-3. Meiosis. Two cell divisions resulting in 4 cells with haploid number of chromosomes.

of acrosomal enzymes, organization of microtubules, and elimination of excess cytoplasm and cell membrane. The sustentacular cells, in which the developing spermatozoa are embedded, assist with some of these conversions. For example, sustentacular cells phagocytose residual bodies of excess cytoplasm and membrane after the release of fully formed spermatozoa.

Rates and Timing of Spermatogenesis

Daily production of spermatozoa has been estimated as 4.4×10^9 in the ram and 2×10^9 in the bull. Eight ejaculations of the bull within an hour reduced the semen from 4.2 mL at the first collection to 2.9 mL at the eighth collection, and the number of spermatozoa was correspondingly reduced from 1.7 billion to 98 million per milliliter. These data indicate that normal animals produce adequate spermatozoa even when used often for breeding. However, these data also suggest that several days of sexual rest may increase numbers of spermatozoa in animals whose numbers are abnormally low. A correlation between daily production and testicular size has been found for several species.

The time required for spermatogenesis (from spermatogonium to fully formed and released spermatozoa) varies with species, but it is a mat-

25–4). The head contains the nucleus, primarily consisting of condensed genetic material (DNA), and an *acrosome,* a membranous sac that lies immediately under the plasma membrane at the tip of the head and extends down over the nucleus (Fig. 25–5). The tail has a central core of microtubules and filaments that provide motility. The middle piece of the tail contains a dense collection of mitochondria that provide energy for spermatozoan motility.

The acrosome is essentially a membranous sac of hydrolytic enzymes, including acrosin and hyaluronidase. Some of these enzymes are released from the acrosome during fertilization and facilitate the fusion of the male and female gametes. The release and exposure of these enzymes during fertilization is termed the *acrosome reaction.*

The conversion of the round spermatid to the elongated spermatozoon with its acrosome containing head and tail requires reshaping of the original spermatid, synthesis and packaging

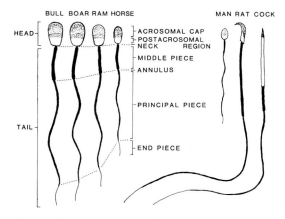

Figure 25-4. Comparison of the spermatozoa of farm animals and other vertebrates. (Reprinted with permission from Hafez E.S.E. and Hafez B. *Reproduction in Farm Animals.* 7th ed. Philadelphia: Lippincott Williams & Wilkins, 2000.)

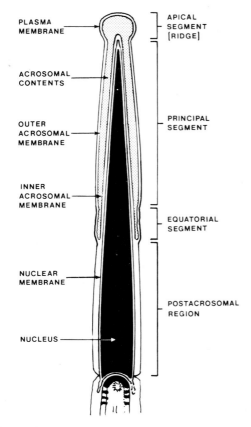

Figure 25-5. A sagittal section of a bovine sperm head showing the various anatomic subdivisions. (Reprinted with permission from Hafez E.S.E. and Hafez B. *Reproduction in Farm Animals.* 7th ed. Philadelphia: Lippincott Williams & Wilkins, 2000.)

ter of weeks to months rather than days. In most farm animals, this period is about 2 months.

Epididymis

Fully formed spermatozoa released from the seminiferous tubules pass through the rete testis into the epididymis. The epididymides are the major sites of storage of spermatozoa, and most spermatozoa are contained in the tail of each epididymis.

Spermatozoa entering the head of the epididymis from the rete testis are immotile and incapable of fertilization. During their passage through the epididymis, spermatozoa acquire

motility and become capable of fertilization. Presumably, these two characteristics are closely linked. The functional changes in spermatozoa that occur during their passage through the epididymis depend in part on epididymal secretions and testosterone in the epididymal fluids. Some minor morphologic changes (e.g., changes in nuclear chromatin and the acrosome) may also occur during the passage through the epididymis.

Semen and Semen Technology

Semen consists of spermatozoa suspended in the fluid secretions of the male accessory sex organs. The fluid portion of semen (*seminal plasma*) functions as a transport medium for the spermatozoa, and it contains a variety of substances including various electrolytes, fructose, citric acid, and sorbitol. The fructose (a sugar) is a potential source of energy for the spermatozoa.

Semen is collected and evaluated as part of protocols to evaluate the fertility of breeding males, but no single characteristic of semen or spermatozoa is accepted as a perfect gold standard for predicting the fertility of a given sample of semen. Some characteristics of semen that are evaluated and appear to have some correlation with potential fertility when considered together are (1) concentration of spermatozoa per milliliter of semen, (2) motility characteristics of spermatozoa, and (3) shape of the spermatozoa. The concentrations of spermatozoa per milliliter vary among species, and this should be considered when evaluating semen.

Semen is also collected and used for breeding technologies such as artificial insemination and in vitro fertilization. One ejaculate of a bull can be divided into as many as 500 portions, and if properly handled, each portion can result in conception. In fact, more than 30,000 cows can be bred each year with the semen collected from one bull. Semen can also be frozen and stored for years.

The division of a semen sample into multiple portions and the freezing of semen for long-term storage require the addition of solutions to increase the volume of the sample and protect the spermatozoa during freezing. Interestingly, the characteristics and composition of the most effective solutions vary with semen samples from different species. This suggests that spermatozoa from different species have unique metabolic and/or structural differences.

Hormones of Male Reproduction

Endocrine Regulation of Testicular Function

Follicle-stimulating hormone (FSH) and *luteinizing hormone* (LH), protein hormones (see Chapter 12) from the adenohypophysis (anterior pituitary), are the primary endocrine regulators of testicular function. Their overall effect is to stimulate testicular function, so both are considered to be **gonadotrophins.** FSH promotes spermatogenesis by its actions on the germ cells in the seminiferous tubules and the sustentacular cells that support the development of the spermatozoa. LH acts on testicular interstitial cells to promote the secretion of androgens, primarily **testosterone.** The testosterone produced by the interstitial cells is necessary for the completion of spermatogenesis, so both FSH and LH are required for normal spermatogenesis.

A single hormone from the hypothalamus, **gonadotrophin-releasing hormone** (GnRH), stimulates the release of both FSH and LH from the adenohypophysis. Negative feedback to the hypothalamus to regulate GnRH is provided by serum testosterone, which is produced by testicular interstitial cells when stimulated by LH. Testosterone also has direct effects on the adenohypophysis to suppress LH release directly. When stimulated by FSH, sustentacular cells produce a protein hormone, **inhibin.** Inhibin has a negative feedback effect on the adenohypophysis to suppress further releases of FSH.

In farm animals, the feedback regulation of GnRH, FSH, and LH secretion is such that spermatogenesis is maintained at rates adequate for breeding throughout the year. However, plasma levels of FSH, LH, and testosterone do vary with season in some species, and these have been associated with differences in sexual activity. For example, FSH, LH, and testosterone levels are highest in rams while the days are getting shorter, and this is associated with increased sexual activity.

Testosterone and Its Effects

Testosterone is a steroid hormone that enters its target cells to exert its effects. Within target cells, testosterone is converted to **dihydrotesterone,** which binds to intracellular receptors. In addition to supporting the maturation of spermatozoa within the testis, testosterone promotes the development and function of male accessory sex organs, causes development of secondary sex characteristics, and promotes male sexual behavior.

Lack of **libido** (sex drive) and inability to produce offspring are two of the most obvious effects of castration and the resultant lack of testosterone. However, animals castrated after attaining sexual maturity may continue to mate for some time if they had sexual experience before castration. If an animal is castrated before puberty, many of the masculine secondary sex characteristics fail to develop, and the castrate animal tends to resemble the female of the species. In addition, the accessory sex glands fail to develop normally if castration occurs early in life, and they regress and become nonfunctional if castration occurs after sexual maturity. Even though testosterone production by the testis is necessary for a normal libido, it is not testosterone that directly affects neurons within the brain to produce a normal libido. Within neurons, testosterone is converted to estradiol, an estrogen, and it is this estradiol that actually stimulates the appropriate neurons. Anabolic steroids (discussed next) used to promote growth cannot be converted to estradiol, and thus these do not increase the libido.

Anabolic steroids are synthetic compounds used to increase net protein synthesis and skeletal muscle mass. In this manner, these compounds are similar to endogenous androgens such as testosterone. Because of their similarity to testosterone and endogenous androgens, anabolic steroids also promote the development of secondary sexual characteristics and exert a

negative feedback effect on the hypothalamic–pituitary axis. As a result of this negative feedback, endogenous testosterone production and spermatogenesis are suppressed. It is not clear whether these can return to normal levels if animals receive anabolic steroids for prolonged periods.

Erection and Ejaculation

Penile erection is a neural reflex initiated by appropriate tactile stimulation of the penis, visual or environmental stimuli (such as a female in estrus), or as a result of learned behavior. For example, an erection may begin when a breeding stallion is being led to a breeding area but before a mare is present. This is believed to be a learned response. Similarly, it is believe that learned responses may be responsible for lack of libido in certain males that have undergone trauma (e.g., a stallion kicked by a mare) or that associate mating with some other painful or unpleasant event.

Penile erection requires vasodilation within the penis, and this results in an increased blood flow into the penis. Parasympathetic nerves innervating blood vessels within the penis initiate the vasodilation. Studies in experimental animals suggest that the parasympathetic nerves release acetylcholine, which in turn stimulates endothelial cells lining the blood vessels to release nitric oxide. Nitric oxide acts directly on vascular smooth muscle to bring about vasodilation.

Prior to ejaculation, spermatozoa are moved from storage sites in the epididymides through the ductus deferentia to the pelvic urethra. This movement is termed *emission* and is assumed to result from contractions of smooth muscle in the wall of these tubular structures. Within the pelvic urethra, secretions of the accessory sex glands are mixed with the spermatozoa. Ejaculation of the mixture (semen) through the penile urethra is associated with more contractions of the epididymides and ductus deferentia and additional contractions by muscles of the penis surrounding the penile urethra. Emission and ejaculation are autonomic reflexes involving both the sympathetic and parasympathetic divisions.

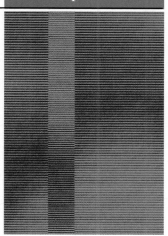

Anatomy of the Female Reproductive System

The female reproductive tract produces the female gamete (*ovum,* pl. *ova*), delivers it to a site where it can be fertilized by the male gamete (sperm), provides an environment for the development and growth of the embryo, and expels the fetus when it is capable of survival outside of the mother's body. The female organs of reproduction include two *ovaries,* two *uterine tubes* (also called *oviducts*), the *uterus,* the *vagina,* and the *vulva* (Fig. 26–1). The ovum is released from the ovary and enters the open end of the uterine tube. Fertilization normally occurs within the uterine tube during passage of the ovum from the ovary to the uterus. Within the uterus, the fertilized ovum, now a *zygote,* develops into an embryo and then into a fetus and finally passes out of the uterus through the vagina and vulva as a newborn (*neonate*). Table 26–1 compares the anatomies of the reproductive tracts in adult nonpregnant farm animals.

Ovaries

The *ovaries,* like the testes in the male, are the primary organs of reproduction in the female. The ovaries are both endocrine and cytogenic (cell producing), since they produce hormones, which are released directly into the blood stream, and ova, which are released from the surface of the ovary in *ovulation* (see Chapter 27).

The ovaries are paired glands usually found in the lumbar region of the abdominal cavity, a

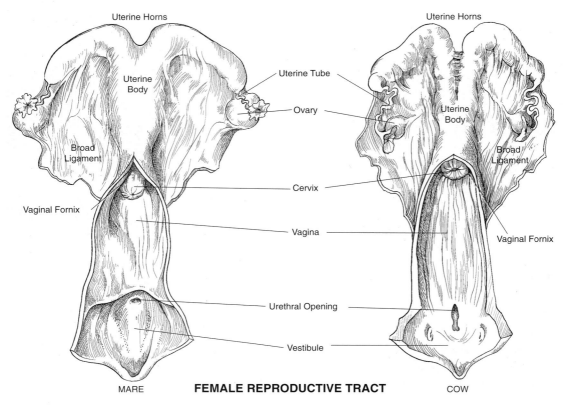

Figure 26-1. Anatomy of the female reproductive tract.

Table 26-1. Comparative Anatomy of the Reproductive Tract in the Adult Nonpregnant Female

	Animal			
Organ	Cow	Ewe	Sow	Mare
Uterine tube[a]	25	15–19	15–30	20–30
Uterus				
Type	bipartite[b]	bipartite	bicornuate[c]	bipartite
Horn[a]	35–40	10–12	40–65	15–25
Body[a]	2–4	1–2	5	15–20
Endometrium	70–120 caruncles	88–96 caruncles	Slight longitudinal folds	Conspicuous longitudinal folds
Cervix				
Lumen	2–5 annular rings	annular rings	corkscrewlike	conspicuous folds
Opening to uterus	small and protruding	small and protruding	ill-defined	clearly defined
Vagina[a]	25–30	10–14	10–15	20–35
Vestibule[a]	10–12	2.5–3	6–8	10–12

[a]Length in centimeters.
[b]Body divided into two parts.
[c]Uterus dominated by two horns.

short distance caudal to the kidneys. Like all abdominal organs, the ovaries are covered with peritoneum. They are suspended from the body wall by a reflection of this serous membrane, the **mesovarium,** the most cranial part of the peritoneal investments of the female genital tract.

In most species, the ovaries are somewhat ovoid (Fig. 26–2). In the mare, however, the ovaries have a bean shape because of a definite **ovulation fossa,** an indentation in the attached border of the ovary. Ovaries of the sow usually appear lobulated because of the numerous developing ova; the sow is the only common farm animal that typically produces a litter, rather than one or two offspring per pregnancy.

When palpated through the wall of the rectum, an ovary feels solid because of the large amount of connective tissue that makes up the stroma of the gland. Normal size of the ovary varies considerably from species to species, and even within a species there is some variation. For example, the ovary of the mare may be less than 2.5 cm in diameter when no developing ova are present or as large as 10 cm with many developing ova.

The ovary is invested in a dense connective tissue capsule, the **tunica albuginea.** The **medulla,** or central portion, of the ovary is the most vascu-

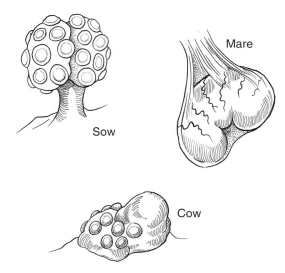

Figure 26-2. Ovaries of various species. Note the ovulation fossa on the equine ovary and the prominent developing follicle on the bovine ovary.

lar part, while the **cortex,** or outer portion, consists largely of dense, irregular connective tissue interspersed with follicles (developing ova) and **interstitial cells,** which have an endocrine function (Fig. 26–3).

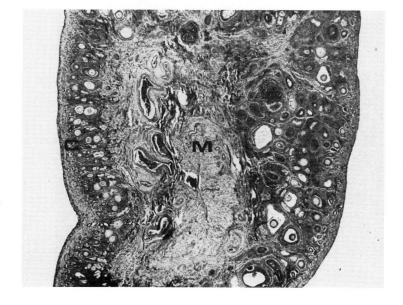

Figure 26-3. Low-power micrograph of a section through a canine ovary. Note the many developing follicles in the cortex (C) and the denser, vascular medulla (M). (Reprinted with permission from Banks W.J. *Applied Veterinary Histology.* 2nd ed. Baltimore: Williams & Wilkins, 1986.)

Uterine Tubes

The **uterine tubes** (also called **oviducts**) are paired, convoluted tubes that conduct the ova from each ovary to the respective horn of the uterus (Fig. 26–1) and are the usual site of fertilization of ova by the spermatozoa. The portion of the uterine tube adjacent to the ovary is expanded to form a funnel-shaped **infundibulum.** The infundibulum appears to take an active part in ovulation, at least to the extent of partially or completely enclosing the ovary and directing the ovum into the uterine tube.

The lining of the uterine tube is a much-folded mucous membrane covered primarily with a simple columnar ciliated epithelium (Fig. 26–4). During estrus (period of sexual receptivity), the unciliated cells become actively secretory. The rest of the wall of the uterine tube includes a connective tissue submucosa and a muscular layer of smooth muscle. Both cilia and muscles function in the movement of ova and possibly in the movement of spermatozoa. The uterine tube, like the entire genital tract, is invested externally with peritoneum, which reflects off the organ as a suspending mesentery. The portion supporting the uterine tube is the **mesosalpinx.**

Uterus

The **uterus** of the domestic mammal consists of a **body,** a **cervix** (neck), and two **horns** (Fig. 26–1). The relative proportions of each vary considerably with the species, as do the shape and arrangement of the horns (Figs. 26–5 and 26–6).

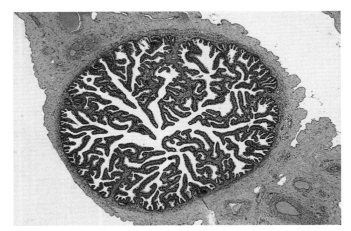

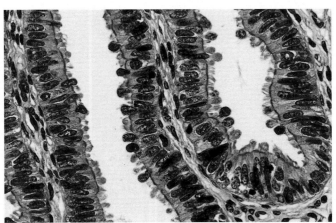

Figure 26-4. Histology of the uterine tube. *A,* Low-power micrograph in the region of the infundibulum. Note the elaborate folding of the epithelium. *B,* Higher-power micrograph showing the ciliated simple columnar epithelium of the uterine tube. The mucosal surface is characterized by abundant secretory product. (Reprinted with permission from Bacha, Jr. W.J. and Bacha L.M. *Color Atlas of Veterinary Histology.* 2nd ed. Baltimore: Lippincott Williams & Wilkins, 2000.)

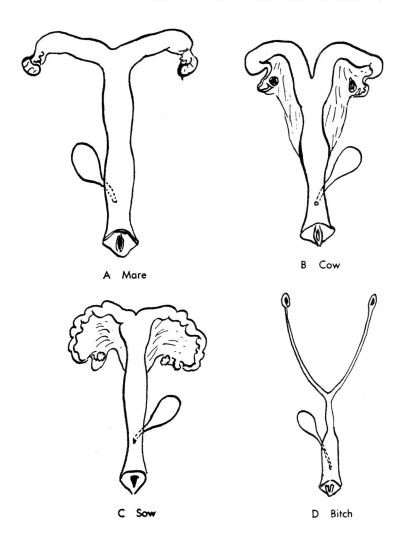

Figure 26-5. Comparative shapes of animal uteri. The female dog (bitch) is provided for comparison.

Relative to the extent of the horns, the body of the uterus is largest in the mare, less extensive in the ruminant, and small in the sow. Externally, the body of the uterus of the cow appears larger than it is because the caudal parts of the horns are bound together by the **intercornual ligament,** which obscures their individual nature.

As with most other hollow internal organs, the uterine wall consists of a lining of mucous membrane, an intermediate smooth muscle layer, and an outer serous layer of peritoneum. The uterus is suspended bilaterally from the body wall by the **mesometrium.** The mesometrium, mesosalpinx, and mesovarium collectively constitute the **broad ligament.**

The mucosa lining the uterus, the **endometrium,** is a highly glandular tissue that varies in thickness and vascularity with hormonal changes in the ovary and with pregnancy (see Chapter 27). The epithelial covering of the mucous membrane is of the simple columnar type in the mare but is stratified columnar epithelium in the sow and ruminants.

The **uterine glands** are simple branched tubular glands that exhibit considerable coiling. These glands are particularly active during estrus and pregnancy, during which they produce a fluid colloquially known as **uterine milk.** These glands are scattered throughout the endometrium of the uterus, except in ruminants,

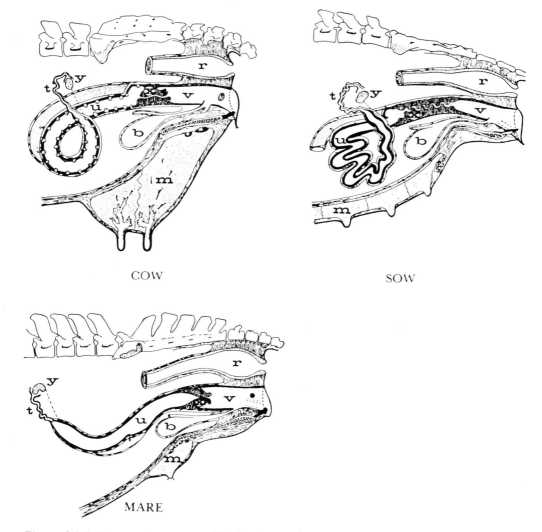

COW

SOW

MARE

Figure 26-6. Comparative anatomy of the female reproductive tract. Lateral view. *b)* Urinary bladder; *m)* mammary gland; *r)* rectum; *t)* uterine tube; *u)* uterus; *v)* vagina; *x)* cervix; *y)* ovary. (Reprinted with permission from Hafez E.S.E. *Reproduction in Farm Animals.* 4th ed. Philadelphia: Lea & Febiger, 1980.)

in which the caruncles are nonglandular. **Caruncles** are mushroomlike projections from the inner surface of the uteri of ruminants; they provide a site of attachment for the fetal membranes (see Chapter 28).

The **cervix** of the uterus projects caudally into the vagina. The cervix is a heavy, smooth muscle sphincter that is tightly closed except during estrus and parturition. During estrus the cervix relaxes slightly, permitting spermatozoa to enter

the uterus. In ruminants and to some extent in sows, the inner surface of the cervix is arranged in a series of circular ridges or rings, sometimes called **annular folds** (Fig. 26–7). The cervix of the mare is relatively smooth and projects prominently into the vagina, which surrounds the cervix as a deep **vaginal fornix.**

The tunica muscularis is the muscular portion of the uterine wall, commonly called the **myometrium.** It consists of a thick inner circu-

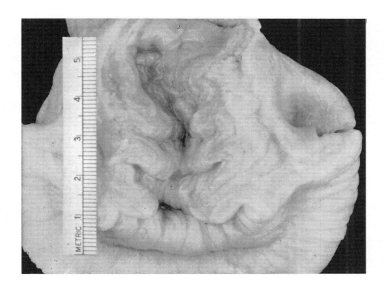

Figure 26-7. Cervix of a young cow, sectioned and opened to reveal the annular folds. (Adapted with permission from Hafez E.S.E. *Reproduction in Farm Animals.* 4th ed. Philadelphia: Lea & Febiger, 1980.)

lar layer of smooth muscle and a thinner outer longitudinal layer of smooth muscle, separated by a vascular layer. During pregnancy, the amount of muscle in the uterine wall increases dramatically, both in cell size (hypertrophy) and in cell numbers (hyperplasia).

Vagina

The **vagina** is the portion of the reproductive tract that lies within the pelvis between the uterus cranially and the vulva caudally (Figs. 26–1 and 26–6). The vagina is the birth canal for delivery of the fetus at parturition and a sheath (*vagina* is Latin for sheath) for the penis of the male during copulation (the act of breeding, or service, as it is commonly called in animal husbandry).

The mucous membrane of the vagina is glandless stratified squamous epithelium except in the cow, in which there are some mucous cells in the cranial part of the vagina adjacent to the cervix. The submucosa is loose, and the muscular layers consist of an inner circular and an outer longitudinal layer of smooth muscle. A serosa (the peritoneum) invests only on the cranial part of the vagina, where it lies within the pelvic cavity. The cau-

dal portion of the vagina, passing through the pelvis, is covered by pelvic fascia (connective tissue).

Vestibule and Vulva

The **vestibule** is the portion of the reproductive tract between the vagina and the external genitalia. The transition between vagina and vestibule is demarcated by the external urethral orifice, and therefore the vestibule is functionally common to both urinary and reproductive tracts. The porcine and bovine vulva features a **suburethral diverticulum,** a short blind sac ventral to the opening of the urethra. The mucous membrane of the vestibule is characterized by abundant mucous glands.

The **vulva** is the external genitalia of the female (Fig. 26–8). It comprises right and left **labia,** which meet on the midline dorsally and ventrally at the **dorsal** and **ventral commissures,** respectively. The ventral commissure is usually somewhat pendulous and conceals the **clitoris,** a structure of erectile tissue that has the same embryonic origin as the penis in the male. Like the penis, the clitoris consists of two crura, or roots, a body, and a glans; only the glans is visible externally. The clitoris is covered by stratified squa-

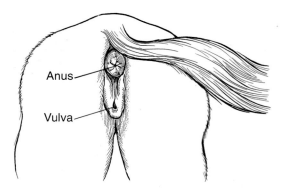

Figure 26-8. External genitalia of the mare.

mous epithelium and is well supplied with sensory nerve endings.

Blood and Nerve Supply of the Female Reproductive Tract

Blood supply to the female reproductive tract is highly anastomotic. Cranially, the *ovarian artery* from the aorta supplies the ovary and gives off a uterine branch that supplies the ipsilateral uterine tube and cranial part of the uterine horn. The primary blood supply to the uterine body and horns is the *uterine artery* (formerly middle uterine artery), which derives from the umbilical artery and which in all species except the horse is a branch of the internal iliac artery (it arises from the external iliac artery in *Equidae*).

The caudal part of the uterus, its cervix, and adjacent parts of the vagina receive blood from branches of the *vaginal artery*, a branch of the *internal pudendal artery*. The more distal branches of the internal pudendal artery also supply the caudal vagina, vulva, and anus. All of these vessels are bilateral.

The uterine artery is the chief blood supply to the uterus in the region of the developing fetus; consequently, it enlarges greatly as pregnancy progresses. One of the signs of pregnancy in cattle is the palpable vibration of this artery (called *fremitus*), which can be detected on rectal examination.

Venous drainage of the female reproductive tract is via veins that are satellite to the arteries and that ultimately drain to the caudal vena cava. In ruminants, the ovarian artery and the uterine vein run close together, providing a venoarterial pathway for chemical messengers from the uterus to reach the ovary on the same side. This relationship underlies certain physiologic phenomena of ruminant reproduction (see Chapter 27).

Sympathetic autonomic innervation to the female reproductive tract arrives from the caudal mesenteric ganglion via *hypogastric nerves.* Parasympathetic fibers arise from sacral spinal cord segments and travel to the reproductive organs in the *pelvic nerves.* The *pudendal* and *perineal nerves,* somatic nerves from sacral spinal cord segments, provide motor and sensory innervation, respectively, to the external genitalia.

THE OVARY AND ESTROUS CYCLES

The ovaries are the source of mature female gametes (*ova*) and hormones necessary for reproduction. *Oogenesis* is formation of ova. *Estrus* (*heat*) is the period of sexual receptivity in the female. An *estrous cycle* is the interval from the beginning of one estrus to the beginning of the next.

Animals that have only one estrous cycle per year are called *monestrous* animals, while those that have several estrous cycles per year are *polyestrous*. Many animals have successive periods of estrus if a pregnancy is not established and maintained. The timing of these periods is often determined by seasonal changes in length of day, so these animals are *seasonally polyestrous*. The relatively long period of inactivity in seasonally polyestrous animals is termed *anestrus* and is not properly a part of the sexual cycle.

Oogenesis

In the fetus, *primordial germ cells* migrate from the yolk sac to the developing ovaries, where a single layer of *follicular cells* surrounds a germ cell destined to become an ovum. The central germ cell (now termed an *oogonium*) enlarges and begins meiosis. (Recall that meiosis entails two cell divisions during which the diploid number of chromosomes is reduced by half to the haploid number.) The oogonium does not complete meiosis; it stops in the first prophase before the first division. At this stage, the developing ovum is a **primary oocyte,** and the combination of a primary oocyte and its surrounding cuboidal follicular cell (granulosa cell) layer is a **primary follicle** (Fig. 27–1). At birth, the ovaries of most domestic species contain hundreds of thousands of primary follicles waiting to continue their development. What determines which of the thousands of primary follicles is selected to develop further during a specific estrous cycle is unknown.

In contrast to spermatogenesis, which produces four spermatozoa from each primary germ cell, the maturation of the primary oocyte results in only one mature ovum and three rudimentary cells, called **polar bodies.** In most animals, the first of the two meiotic divisions is complete, resulting in the formation of the first polar body, before or immediately after **ovulation** (the discharge of an oocyte from a follicle).

Secondary Follicles

In all animals, multiple primary follicles typically begin further development during a single estrous cycle. In **monotocous animals** (animals not bearing litters and normally having only one offspring per gestation, such as the mare and cow), one follicle usually develops more rapidly than others, and only one ovum is released at ovulation. The rest of the developing follicles regress and form **atretic follicles. Polytocous animals,** such as carnivores and swine, which normally produce two or more offspring per gestation, usually have several follicles that develop and ovulate at approximately the same time. The ova may all come from one ovary, or some may come from each ovary.

The further development of primary follicles includes enlargement of the oocyte and replication of the surrounding follicular cells. The repli-

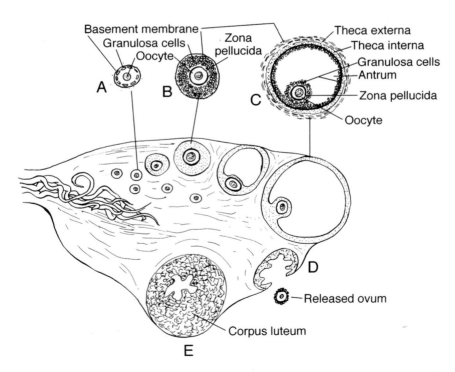

Figure 27-1. Sagittal section of an ovary showing the origin, growth, and ovulation of a follicle and a corpus luteum developing at the site of a follicle that has ovulated. *A)* Primary follicle. *B)* Growing follicle. *C)* Graafian or tertiary follicle. *D)* Ovulation. *E)* Corpus luteum. (Reprinted with permission from Reece W.O. *Physiology of Domestic Animals.* 2nd ed. Baltimore: Williams & Wilkins, 1997.)

cating follicular cells become several layers thick, and this surrounding group of cells is a *granulosa.* The granulosa cells secrete glycoproteins that cross-link to form a protective shell, the *zona pellucida,* around the oocyte (Fig. 27–1). Cytoplasmic processes of granulosa cells penetrate the zona to permit communication and exchange between them and the oocyte. The initial development to this point is independent of hormonal stimulation by gonadotrophins (follicle-stimulating hormone [FSH] and luteinizing hormone [LH]).

The developing follicle is termed a *secondary follicle* when the oocyte has enlarged and is surrounded by a developing granulosa. A *theca,* consisting of layers of cells immediately surrounding the granulosa, also first develops late during the secondary follicle stage.

Hormones and Follicular Development

Gonadotrophin-releasing hormone (GnRH) is released from the hypothalamus to promote the release of both FSH and LH from the adenohypophysis. The release of GnRH can be modulated by steroid (estradiol and progesterone) and peptide (inhibin) hormones from the ovary, but its basal release is determined by neural inputs to the hypothalamus. The basal release of GnRH is assumed to be pulsatile, for this is the type of release seen in ovariectomized animals. The pulsatile nature is physiologically important, because continuous infusions of GnRH do not result in the continuous release of FSH and LH.

The granulosa and theca of secondary follicles develop cellular receptors for FSH and LH, respectively, and become responsive to these hormones. From this point, the coordinated effects of FSH and LH are both needed for normal follicular development. Under the influence of LH, thecal cells proliferate and produce androgens (androstenedione and testosterone) that diffuse into the granulosa. FSH promotes further granulosa cell proliferation, the development of cellular enzymes necessary for the conversion of androgens to estrogens (estradiol), and the secretion of several other paracrine agents necessary for follicular development. The cellular secretions accumulate among the gran-

ulosa cells, and ultimately a fluid-filled cavity (*antrum*) can be identified. The developing follicles are *tertiary follicles* (also known as vesicular or Graafian follicles) when an antrum can be identified among the granulose cells (Fig. 27–1). Theca surrounding tertiary follicles have two layers, the theca externa and theca interna (Fig. 27–1). The internal layer is highly vascular and contains thecal cells with cellular characteristics of steroid-producing cells. The theca externa primary consists of connective tissue.

The estrogen produced by the granulosa cells acts as a paracrine agent on the developing follicle and also enters the systemic circulation to affect other sites throughout the body (Fig 27–2). Locally, the estrogen acts on granulosa cells to increase FSH and LH receptors, and together with these gonadotrophins, it promotes further granulosa cell replication, growth, and secretion. The overall effect is that locally produced estrogens promote the development of the follicle from which they are being produced. This is characterized as a *local positive feedback effect* of the estrogens. This positive feedback effect is one factor in the selection process that determines which of the developing follicles will ultimately produce the ovum and ovulate. A second factor is that circulating estrogens have a negative feedback effect on FSH secretion from the adenohypophysis. The decrease in FSH during this period contributes to the atresia of more slowly developing follicles. The selection process also involves another follicular hormone, inhibin, discussed later.

Estrogens from developing follicles are also necessary to prepare the follicles and the hypothalamic–adenohypophyseal axis for ovulation. Within the ovary, estrogens promote an increase in LH receptors in thecal cells, so that these cells increase their production of androgens and appropriately respond to LH at the time of ovulation. Circulating estrogens promote an increase in LH within the adenohypophysis and condition the hypothalamic–adenohypophyseal axis, so that the short-term large LH release (termed *LH surge*) necessary for ovulation can be delivered (Fig. 27–2).

Non–litter-bearing animals typically have one or two follicles per estrous cycle that develop faster and grow larger than the rest. These are *dominant follicles.* In primates there is typ-

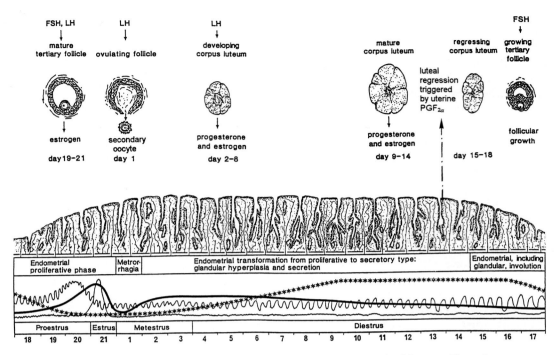

Figure 27-2. Ovarian, uterine, and hormonal changes during the estrous cycle of the cow. The scale indicates days 1 to 21 of the cycle. Relative blood levels of progesterone (***), estrogen (━), FSH (ᗯᗯᗯ), and LH (──) are shown. (Reprinted with permission from Dellman H.D. and Eurell J. *Textbook of Veterinary Histology.* 5th ed. Baltimore: Lippincott Williams & Wilkins, 1998.)

ically only one dominant follicle per estrous cycle, and it provides the ovum. The development of the dominant follicle is accelerated after the corpus luteum (discussed later) from the previous estrous cycle has regressed (*luteolysis*). The phase of the estrous cycle in primates during which there is no corpus luteum and the dominant follicle is developing is the *follicular phase* of the estrous cycle. The *luteal phase* is the part of the cycle during which a corpus luteum is intact and secreting progesterone. Formation of a corpus luteum and its functions are discussed later in this chapter.

In domestic animals that typically have only one or two offspring per pregnancy, large dominant follicles may develop while a corpus luteum remains intact. These dominant follicles may or may not ovulate. Mature follicles that do not ovulate undergo atresia if a corpus luteum remains intact. At that point, another dominant

follicle begins to develop rapidly, so that ovulation can occur soon after luteolysis. Because dominant follicles may develop while a corpus luteum remains intact, the estrous cycles of large domestic animals are considered to have overlapping follicular and luteal phases.

Inhibins are peptide hormones secreted by granulosa cells of developing follicles. Circulating levels of inhibins increase with follicular development, and inhibins have a negative feedback effect on FSH release from the adenohypophysis. By this means, a developing dominant follicle can suppress the development of competing follicles in non–litter-bearing animals. In litter-bearing animals, the combined negative feedback effect of inhibins from multiple follicles can suppress other follicles, so that litter sizes are not inappropriately large. Inhibins from developing follicles apparently do not suppress LH secretion necessary for ovulation.

Ovulation

In mature follicles just prior to ovulation, ova are usually seen surrounded by a halo of granulosa cells (***cumulus***) that are continuous with granulosa cells lining the fluid-filled antrum (Fig. 27–3). The large, thin-walled follicles bulge from the ovarian surface (Fig. 27–4).

The primary oocyte, which remains in an arrested stage of meiosis during follicular development, undergoes the first meiotic division to produce a ***secondary oocyte*** and the ***first polar body*** just before ovulation in most

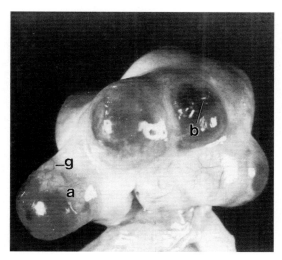

Figure 27-4. Ovary of sow with mature tertiary follicles just before ovulation (*a*) and a site where a follicle has just ovulated (*b*). A surface vessel is also visible (*g*). (Reprinted with permission from Dellman H.D. and Eurell J. *Textbook of Veterinary Histology.* 5th ed. Baltimore: Lippincott Williams & Wilkins, 1998.)

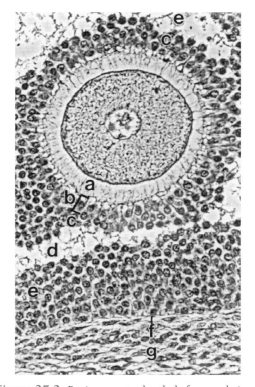

Figure 27-3. Bovine oocyte shortly before ovulation. Oocyte is surrounded by zona pellucida (*a*), the corona radiata, a single layer of unique granulose cells immediately adjacent to the zona (*b*), and a layer of granulosa cells termed the cumulus oophorus (*c*). The cumulus appears to have separated from the granulosa cells lining the antrum of the follicle (*e*). The theca interna is also visible (*g*). A basement membrane separates the theca from the granulosa cell lining. (Reprinted with permission from Dellman H.D. and Eurell J. *Textbook of Veterinary Histology.* 5th ed. Baltimore: Lippincott Williams & Wilkins, 1998.)

species. The first polar body is extruded from the ovary with the secondary oocyte. In the mare, this first meiotic division occurs just after ovulation.

Luteinizing Hormone Surge

In most species, LH release from the adenohypophysis increases 7- to 10-fold during the 24 hours prior to ovulation. After reaching its peak, LH release rapidly decreases so that plasma levels return to preovulatory levels (Fig. 27–2). This short-term change in LH release is the LH surge. As discussed earlier, the LH surge depends on changes in the hypophyseal–adenohypophysis axis and an increase in adenohypophysis content of LH induced by the rapid rise in production of estrogens by large, mature follicles. The extremely high levels of LH promote the final development of the primary oocyte and its progress though the first meiotic division. This prepares the oocyte for ovulation.

Granulosa cells also respond to the LH surge by transforming from estrogen-producing cells to progesterone-producing cells. This is part of *luteinization,* the transformation of granulosa cells to *luteal cells* (cells of a corpus luteum). This process begins prior to ovulation, so estrogen levels are decreasing and progesterone levels are increasing at ovulation. Under the influence of the LH surge, granulosa cells also acquire the ability to synthesize prostaglandins, thromboxanes, and leukotrienes. These agents induce a local response similar to inflammation that will weaken the wall of the follicle and promote its rupture.

Spontaneous and Reflex Ovulators

The LH surge and ovulation occur in most domestic species (mare, cow, ewe, and sow) independent of copulation, and these species are *spontaneous ovulators.* In these species, the preovulatory increase in estrogens from developing follicles is the primary event that brings about ovulation. The female animals of some species (rabbit, ferret, mink, camel, llama, and alpaca) usually require copulation for ovulation. These are *induced ovulators.* In these species, the final preovulatory surge of GnRH and subsequent LH surge, is apparently depend on a neural reflex elicited by vaginal stimulation. Induced ovulators have characteristic estrous cycles and follicular development, but mature follicles regress if copulation does not occur.

Corpus Luteum

The ovarian corpus luteum (pl. corpora lutea) is a temporary endocrine organ with *progesterone* as its primary secretory product. A corpus luteum forms at the site of each ovulated follicle (Fig. 27–1), so litter-bearing animals may have multiple corpora lutea on an individual ovary.

Sometimes during ovulation small blood vessels rupture, and the cavity of the ruptured follicle fills with a blood clot, a *corpus hemorrhagicum.* Whether or not a corpus hemorrhagicum forms, the granulosa cells lining the empty follicular cavity begin to multiply under the influence of LH and form a *corpus luteum,* or *yellow body.* The granulosa cells also continue to undergo luteinization. Most luteal cells are derived from granulosa cells, but some cells in the corpus luteum are derived from the theca interna.

Although a mature follicle and a fully formed corpus luteum are about the same size, they can be differentiated by sight or palpation. The follicle is a sac filled with fluid that has the appearance and feel of a blister, while the corpus luteum looks and feels solid (Fig. 27–5).

Blood progesterone levels increase as corpora lutea grow and develop after ovulation (Fig. 27–2). When corpora lutea are fully developed, progesterone secretion is maximal and plasma levels stabilize. If fertilization of the ova does not occur and a pregnancy is not established, the corpora lutea spontaneously regress, with a relatively rapid decrease in plasma progesterone (Fig. 27–2). *Corpus luteum regression* entails apoptotic death of luteal cells, their removal, and the replacement of the corpus luteum with connective tissue forming a *corpus albicans.* If a pregnancy is established, *maternal recognition of pregnancy* occurs, and regression of the corpus luteum is prevented. This process and the role of the corpus luteum during pregnancy are discussed in more detail in Chapter 28.

The basic function of progesterone during this part of the estrous cycle is to prepare for a pregnancy. Progesterone increases uterine gland secretion and inhibits uterine motility to promote implantation and maintain any pregnancy (Fig. 27–2). Progesterone also promotes mammary gland development. High levels of progesterone act on the hypothalamic–adenohypophyseal axis to inhibit further LH secretion.

If a successful pregnancy is not established, the corpora lutea must undergo regression (luteolysis) to permit the animal to continue the estrous cycle. The humoral signals between the uterus and ovary that initiate or inhibit luteolysis differ among species. In most domestic species (mare, cow, ewe, sow), *prostaglandin $F_{2\alpha}$* (*$PGF_{2\alpha}$*) is the humoral signal used by the nonpregnant uterus to stimulate luteolysis. The nonpregnant uterus increases $PGF_{2\alpha}$ synthesis; releases are increased after ovulation at times appropriate for the species (e.g., 10 days for sows and 14 days for ewes); and luteolysis occurs shortly thereafter (Fig. 27–2).

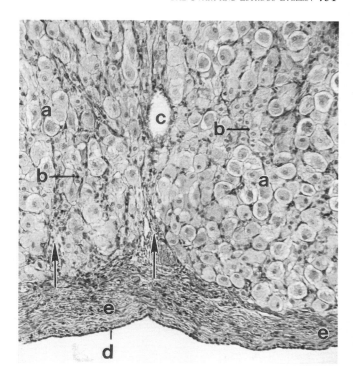

Figure 27-5. Part of a sow's mature corpus luteum. Two types of cells, large luteal cells (*a*) and small luteal cells (*b*) can be identified. A blood vessel (*c*) enters from the periphery and trabeculae (*arrows*). (Reprinted with permission from Dellman H.D. and Eurell J. *Textbook of Veterinary Histology.* 5th ed. Baltimore: Lippincott Williams & Wilkins, 1998.)

Luteolysis can be induced in cattle by administering analogs of PGF$_{2\alpha}$ at any point in the estrous cycle as long as a corpus luteum is intact and functioning. The removal of the corpus luteum permits rapid development of new follicles and ovulation in about 3 days. The use of PGF$_{2\alpha}$ to induce ovulation and estrus at a predictable time is a management tool to synchronize the estrus cycles of groups of animals.

Phases of the Estrous Cycle

The basic pattern of the estrous cycle is the same in all domestic animals, but some species differences are found in specific parts of the cycle. Some specifics about relevant farm species are summarized in Table 27–1. The estrous cycle may be divided into several phases based on behavioral changes or structural changes in internal and external genitalia. These phases are called ***proestrus, estrus, metestrus,*** and ***diestrus.***

Proestrus

The first phase (proestrus) of the estrous cycle is the building-up phase. During this phase the ovarian follicle (under the influence of FSH and LH) enlarges and begins to secrete estrogens. In polyestrous species, proestrus usually begins within a day or two of regression of the corpus luteum from the previous cycle.

Estrogens absorbed from the follicles into the blood stimulate increases in vascularity and cell growth of the tubular genitalia in preparation for estrus and pregnancy. Late in proestrus the vaginal wall thickens, and the external genitalia may increase in vascularity (e.g., swelling and redness) in preparation for copulation. In some species, the vulva may discharge mucus late in proestrus.

Estrus

Estrus, the period of sexual receptivity, is primarily initiated by the elevation in estrogens from mature follicles just prior to ovulation. In

Table 27-1. Average Ages or Times of Reproductive Parameters for Selected Species

Animal	Onset of Puberty	Age of First Service	Estrous Cycle	Estrus	Gestation
Mare	18 mo	2–3 yr	21 d	6 d	336 d
Cow	1–2 yr	1–2 yr	21 d	18 hr	282 d
Ewe	8 mo	1–1.5 yr	17 d	1–2 d	150 d
Sow	7 mo	8–10 mo	21 d	2 d	114 d

most domestic species, ovulation occurs within a day or two after the onset of behavioral estrus, which is about the end of behavioral estrus. Progesterone from preovulatory follicles, developing corpora lutea, or corpora lutea from previous cycles also promotes behavioral estrus in some species.

Metestrus

The end of sexual receptivity marks the beginning of **metestrus,** the postovulatory phase dominated by corpus luteum function. During this period serum estrogens decrease and progesterone increases. A fully developed corpus luteum has a notable influence on the uterus. The endometrial lining of the uterus thickens; uterine glands enlarge; and uterine muscles show increased development. The external genitalia return to their state before estrus as plasma estrogens decrease.

Diestrus and Anestrus

Polyestrous animals have a short period of inactivity before the proestrus phase of the next cycle. This is **diestrus.** Animals with long periods between cycles or polyestrous animals that stop cycling (e.g., due to change in season) enter a long period of inactivity termed **anestrus.** For example, sheep have a short diestrus while cycling during a breeding season but enter anestrus if pregnancy is not established during the breeding season. During anestrus the uterine tubes, uterus, and vagina shrink and remain small until the next breeding season.

Puberty

Puberty in female animals can be defined as the first estrus accompanied by ovulation. The endocrine basis for puberty in female animals is the development of the hypothalamic mechanisms responsible for GnRH release. The adenohypophysis is capable of releasing FSH and LH before GnRH becomes available to stimulate their release. Great variations in the timing of puberty can be found within a single species, depending on climate, level of nutrition, and heredity.

Specifics of Selected Estrous Cycles

Mare

Puberty begins at 10 to 24 months, with an average onset of about 18 months.

Length of Estrous Cycle. Cycle lengths varying from 7 to 124 days have been reported. However, average figures are about 21 to 22 days. The abnormally long cycles undoubtedly include a number of skipped periods or cycles.

Length of Estrus. The average length of estrus in the mare is approximately 6 or 7 days. Estrus tends to shorten from spring to midsummer. Early in the breeding season, through March and April, estrus tends to be irregular and long, frequently with no ovulation. From May to July the periods become shorter and more regular, with ovulation as a normal part of the cycle. Ovulation usually occurs 1 to 2 days before the end of estrus.

Time of Breeding. Fertility rises during estrus to a peak 2 days before the end of estrus, then falls off abruptly. Mares with longer estrous periods should be bred on the third or fourth day and again 48 to 72 hours later. If heat is longer than 8 to 10 days, it is better to wait until the next heat period. Mares with regular short heat periods throughout the year can be successfully bred at any time of the year.

Early in the breeding season, some mares show intense sexual desire during long heat periods but do not ovulate. These mares probably will not conceive until their heat periods become shorter and more regular. Other mares may have only silent heat periods, in which ovulation occurs but no sexual desire is evident. Many of these mares conceive if the time for breeding can be identified by rectal palpation and appearance of the vulva, vagina, and cervix.

Foal heat (or *postpartum estrus*) may occur 1 to 2 weeks after foaling. Ovulation may occur during this period of estrus, and conceptions are possible if mares are bred during a foal heat.

Histologic (tissue) changes in the lining of the genitalia of the mare during the estrous cycle approximate the general pattern found in all mammals. However, these changes are not distinctive enough to make a vaginal smear useful in determining the stage of the estrous cycle.

Cow

In cattle, puberty varies considerably with the breed and level of nutrition. Holstein heifers show first estrus at an average of 37 weeks of age on a high level of nutrition, 49 weeks on a medium level, and 72 weeks on a low level of feeding. Puberty appears to occur when the heifer is about two-thirds of her adult body size, measured by height and length rather than weight.

Length of Estrous Cycle. The estrous cycle averages 20 days for heifers and 21 to 22 days for mature cows.

Length of Estrus. The estrous period in the cow may be defined as the time she will stand when mounted by another cow or bull. This *standing heat* averages about 18 hours in both dairy and beef cows, somewhat less in heifers.

The normal range is 12 to 24 hours. Ovulation normally occurs about 10 to 14 hours after the end of estrus in the cow.

Time of Breeding. Conception has occurred in cattle bred as early as 34 hours before ovulation and as late as 14 hours after ovulation. It has been suggested that bovine spermatozoa must be present for at least 6 hours in the uterus or uterine tubes of the cow before they are capable of fertilizing an ovum. For artificial insemination, cows that come into standing heat in the morning are bred the same afternoon, and cows that come into standing heat in the afternoon are bred the next morning.

Bleeding from the vulva occurs in a high percentage of heifers and cows 1 to 3 days after the end of estrus. This phenomenon is metestrus bleeding; fertility is reduced if breeding is done during bleeding. However, fertility is not impaired if breeding has taken place before the bleeding.

Ewe

Puberty usually occurs during the first breeding season (usually fall) after ewes are 4 to 12 months of age if the ewes are well fed. If ewes fail to reach puberty during their first potential breeding season, they may be over 12 months before reaching puberty.

Breeding Season. The ewe is probably the best example of a seasonally polyestrous animal, with a long period of anestrus followed by a breeding season that may vary from 1 to 20 consecutive estrous cycles. The length of breeding season appears to be related to the severity of climate in which the breed developed. In severe climates, a suitable lambing period is restricted; hence the breeding season is likewise restricted, so that lambing occurs only during the favorable time (Scotch Blackface is an example). Breeds developed in milder climates may lamb successfully over a longer period, so the breeding or sexual season is also extended (e.g., Merino sheep).

Length of Estrous Cycle. The average estrous cycle in the ewe is 16.5 to 17.5 days. Unusually long or short cycles tend to appear during the early and later parts of the sexual season, rather than during the middle part.

Length of Estrus. Duration of estrus averages about 30 hours, with a range for most ewes between 24 and 48 hours. The ram may be attracted during proestrus and metestrus as well as estrus, but the ewe will accept him only during the actual estrous period. Ovulation occurs near the termination of estrus, and two or three ovulations may occur in the same estrous period.

Time of Breeding. The best time for breeding ewes is middle to late estrus.

Sow

Sexual maturity in the gilt usually occurs about 7 months of age.

Length of Estrous Cycle. The average estrous cycle in swine is about 21 days, with a range of 18 to 24 days considered normal.

Length of Estrus. The estrous period may range from 15 to 96 hours, with an average duration between 40 and 46 hours. The first estrus after weaning is usually longer and may average 65 hours; it occurs about 7 to 9 days after weaning of the piglets.

Many sows exhibit infertile estrus 1 to 3 days following parturition. In nearly all of these animals, ovulation does not occur. It has been suggested that this heat may be caused by estrogen from some source other than the ovary. Ovulation occurs during the latter part of estrus, about the second day of the cycle. At each period, 10 to 25 ova are shed, with an average of about 16 for most breeds.

PREGNANCY AND PARTURITION

Pregnancy is the condition of a female animal while young are developing within her uterus. The interval, the **gestation period,** extends from *fertilization* of the ovum to the birth of the offspring. It includes fertilization, the union of the ovum and sperm; *early embryonic development* in the lumen of the female reproductive tract; *implantation* of the *embryo* in the uterine wall; *placentation,* the development of fetal membranes; and continued growth of the *fetus.*

Normal gestation periods vary greatly from species to species (Table 27–1), and there is considerable variation between individuals within each species. If the young are carried throughout a normal gestation period, it is a *full-term pregnancy.* A premature birth is delivery of a viable fetus before fetal development is complete. Termination of pregnancy with delivery of a nonviable fetus is *abortion.*

Fertilization

Spermatozoa Transport and Viability

In most cases, fertilization occurs in the uterine tube next to the ovary, while during natural copulation, spermatozoa are deposited in the vagina (most species) or uterus via the cervix (mare, sow, and bitch). Even though ejaculated spermatozoa are motile, the major factor in the transport of spermatozoa to the site of fertilization is muscular activity of the tubular genitalia following insemination. The time required for spermatozoa to travel to the site of fertilization in a cow is about 2.5 minutes, but the first arriving spermatozoa typically do not accomplish fertilization. Based on calculated speed of bull spermatozoa, it would take 1.5 hours for them to swim this distance. Fewer than 0.5% of the ejaculated spermatozoa reach the site of fertilization.

Oxytocin, a peptide hormone from the neurohypophysis (see Chapter 12), promotes muscular activity of the female tubular genitalia to assist with spermatozoa transport. It is released in the cow during natural mating and during artificial insemination, presumably as a result of a neural reflex initiated by physical stimulation of the female tract.

Spermatozoa must remain in the female reproductive tract for some period after ejaculation before they are capable of fertilization. The process that occurs here to convert nonfertile spermatozoa to fertile spermatozoa is termed *capacitation.* Capacitation includes changes in or removal of components of the outer acrosome and plasma membranes so that acrosomal enzymes can later be released and activated. Part of the natural capacitation process requires exposure of the spermatozoa to female reproductive tract secretions, but capacitation of spermatozoa can be done in vitro using experimentally derived protocols and solutions.

Under normal conditions, viability and survival times of spermatozoa in the female reproductive tract are only a matter of hours. Length of fertility in the female tract is given thus: ewe, 30 to 48 hours; cow, 28 to 50 hours; mare, 144 hours. Motility may last somewhat longer than fertility. The limited viability of spermatozoa means that insemination must occur within hours of ovulation, so that viable spermatozoa are present when ova arrive for fertilization. In most species, female sexual receptivity begins some hours prior to ovulation, so that this is possible.

Gamete Fusion and Early Embryonic Development

At ovulation, a *zona pellucida,* a relatively thick membranous structure consisting of cross-linked glycoproteins, surrounds the *vitelline membrane* (cell membrane or plasma membrane) of the ovum. In most cases, a variable number of granulosa cells surrounds the zona, and this layer is termed the **cumulus oophorous.** The zona is believed to be a product of the innermost layer of granulosa cells. Microvilli from the vitelline membrane of the ovum penetrate the zona, as do processes from the granulosa cells. The first polar body, which results from the first meiotic division, also accompanies the ovulated ovum within the zona (see Chapter 27).

The zona pellucida is a semipermeable membrane that helps protect the ovum and that has receptor sites for attachment of spermatozoa during fertilization. A specific protein, **ZP3,** in the zona serves as a binding site for spermatozoa. The precise structure of this protein varies among species, and this variation is the primary reason that spermatozoa from one species cannot bind to and fertilize ova from other species.

During or just after binding and attachment to the zona, spermatozoa undergo a series of events termed the **acrosome reaction** (Fig. 28–1). As part of this reaction, locally released acrosome enzymes digest a passage through the zona. This passage permits spermatozoa to swim their way to the vitelline membrane of the ovum, which is accomplished in a matter of minutes. Multiple spermatozoa may attach to the zona of a single ovum, even though only one spermatozoon will ultimately be responsible for fertilization.

After penetration of the zona, the cell membrane of the single spermatozoon that will accomplish fertilization attaches to and fuses with the vitelline membrane of the ovum (Fig. 28–1). This initiates the second meiotic division by the ovum, which results in formation of the **second polar body.** The fusion of the spermatozoon with the ovum also stimulates release of cytoplasmic granules by the ovum, whose contents bring about changes in the chemical nature of the zona pellucida. These changes act to prevent penetration by other spermatozoa. This, together with changes in the vitelline membrane, prevents **polyspermy,** entry of more than one spermatozoon into the ovum. When these mechanisms fail and polyspermic fertilization occurs, the typical result is early embryonic death. This is believed to be rare in most domestic species when fertilization occurs in

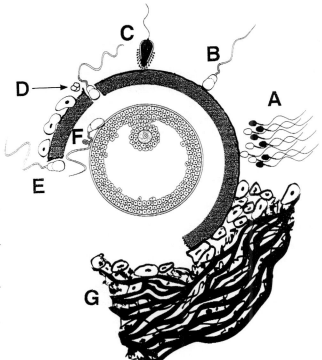

Figure 28-1. Sequence of events from initial binding of spermatozoon to zona pellucida to fusion between plasma membranes of spermatozoon and oocyte: *A)* Spermatozoa arrive at site of fertilization. *B)* Initial binding of spermatozoon to zona pellucida. *C)* Acrosome reaction. *D* and *E)* Penetration of zona pellucida. *F)* Fusion of plasma membranes of spermatozoon and oocyte. *G* is the cumulus matrix. (Reprinted with permission from Hafez E.S.E. and Hafez B. *Reproduction in Farm Animals.* 7th ed. Philadelphia: Lippincott Williams & Wilkins, 2000.)

vivo, but the incidence of polyspermy is higher when fertilization is done in vitro.

A maternal ***pronucleus*** is formed in the ovum by the enclosure of the maternal chromosomes in a nuclear membrane. The head of the sperm enlarges, becoming the male pronucleus. The two pronuclei come together and fuse membranes, forming one cell with the genetic material of both parents. The new cell is ready for cleavage and formation of a morula. Cleavage and the subsequent development into a morula and blastula are described in detail in Chapter 3.

During early development, the embryo is not attached to the epithelium lining the female reproductive tract. During this period, embryos obtain their nourishment from fluids and nutrients secreted by glands in the walls of the reproductive organs (e.g., endometrial glands in the walls of the uterus). Progesterone stimulates secretion by these glands, and blood levels of progesterone are relatively high during this period, as it is being secreted from ovarian corpora lutea.

Maternal recognition of pregnancy is detection of a developing embryo, which prevents regression of the progesterone-secreting corpora lutea. Several mechanisms have been identified in different species, but in general, the mechanisms involve secretory products from the developing embryo. These products (e.g., proteins or steroids) act locally within the reproductive tract. In most cases, the embryonic secretory products inhibit the uterine secretion of prostaglandin $F_{2\alpha}$ ($PGF_{2\alpha}$). Recall that uterine secretion of $PGF_{2\alpha}$ is the key hormonal signal that causes leutolysis in most domestic species. In litter-bearing animals, a minimal number of developing embryos appears to be required to recognize pregnancy and prevent regression of the corpora lutea. This number is about four for the sow.

Embryos develop to the blastula stage while still enclosed in a zona pellucida (see Chapter 3). The zona is shed (hatching) prior to attachment of the embryo to the uterine wall for placentation. The outermost layer of cells of the blastula is the ***trophoblast,*** and it is from these cells that the fetal membranes will be formed.

Early embryonic death (death of the embryo prior to attachment to the uterine wall) is re-

sponsible for a significant number of reproductive failures in domestic animals. Some studies report that up to 30% of fertilized embryos die before developing into fetuses. Possible causes of embryonic death include inherited lethal factors, infections, nutritional deficiencies, inappropriate levels of maternal hormones, and defects in the ovum or spermatozoa before fertilization.

Implantation and Placentation

Implantation is attachment of a blastula to the uterine epithelium and penetration of the epithelium by embryonic tissue. The degree of penetration by embryonic tissues varies among species. In most domestic animals, the degree of penetration is much less than in rodents and primates, whose penetration extends into the connective tissue beneath the epithelium. Implantation in domestic animals is considered to be noninvasive and primarily the result of formation of cell-to-cell junctions between embryonic tissues and the uterine epithelium. These junctions involve binding of membrane proteins in embryonic tissues to receptors on maternal epithelium. After fertilization, attachment occurs in the sow at about 11 days, in the ewe about 16 days, in the cow about 35 days, and in the mare about 55 days.

Developing embryos **migrate** (i.e., move about) within the lumen of the uterus before implantation. In litter-bearing animals, this migration permits the spacing of embryos so that each has adequate room for development and ensures that each uterine horn contains some embryos. Contact, or paracrine communication, between embryos and the uterine epithelium is necessary for pregnancy recognition, and in litter-bearing animals, each uterine horn must contain embryos to permit this recognition. Embryos of non–litter-bearing species also migrate within the uterus before attachment. In the mare, migration back and forth between uterine horns before attachment is necessary to prevent luteolysis and loss of the developing embryo.

Placentation is development of the extraembryonic membranes, or **placenta**. The placenta is an arrangement of membranes with sites for exchanges between the maternal and fetal circulations so that nutrition from the dam can reach the fetus and waste products from the fetus can be transferred to the dam. In domestic animals, the terms fetal membranes and placenta are used interchangeably, although technically the fetal membranes are called the fetal placenta to distinguish them from maternal components of the placenta. In some species a portion of the endometrium is also shed at parturition. This is the maternal placenta, or *decidua.* The fetal placenta includes the chorion, allantois, amnion, and vestigial yolk sac.

The *chorion,* the outermost membrane, is in contact with the maternal uterine endometrium. The next layer (moving from outermost inward), the **allantois,** is a continuous layer that encloses a sac, the allantoic cavity (Fig. 28–2). The chorion and the outer layer of the allantois fuse to form the chorioallantois (Fig. 28–2). The **amnion** is the innermost membrane, closest to the fetus. It is a fluid-filled cavity that contains the fetus (Fig. 28–2). The amnion is fused with the inner layer of the allantois. The allantoic cavity, sometimes called the first water bag, is continuous with the cranial extremity of the bladder by way of the **urachus,** which passes through the umbilical cord. The fluid-filled amniotic cavity or sac is sometimes called the second water bag. The terms first and second water bag refer to fetal membranes at the time of parturition, when the allantoic sac is expelled first and the amniotic sac, second.

Branches of the **umbilical arteries** and veins run through the connective tissue between the allantois and chorion. These vessels are an important part of the fetal circulation. The umbilical arteries and their branches carry unoxygenated blood from the fetus to the placenta, and the **umbilical vein** carries oxygenated blood from the placenta to the fetus.

As a general principle, blood from the fetus never mixes with blood from the dam. However, the two circulations are close enough at the junction of chorion and endometrium to permit oxygen and nutrients to pass from the maternal blood to the blood of the fetus and waste products to pass from the fetal blood into the blood stream of the dam.

The relationship between the fetal and maternal tissues at the histologic (microscopic) site

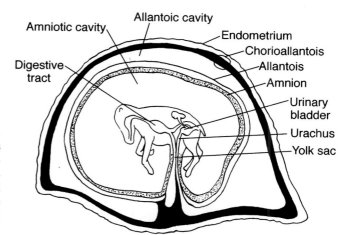

Amniotic cavity
Allantoic cavity
Endometrium
Chorioallantois
Allantois
Amnion
Digestive tract
Urinary bladder
Urachus
Yolk sac

Figure 28-2. Equine fetus in the placenta. The chorioallantois is the outer allantois plus the chorion. The chorion is associated intimately with the endometrium. The inner allantois is fused with the amnion. (Reprinted with permission from Reece W.O. *Physiology of Domestic Animals.* 2nd ed. Baltimore: Williams & Wilkins, 1997.)

of exchange is a basis for classification of mammalian placenta. The tissue of the maternal side is usually named first, then the fetal side. The placenta of most domestic mammals (sow, mare, ewe, and cow) is classified as **epitheliochorial.** In this type, the chorion of the fetus is in direct contact with the epithelium of the uterus of the dam (Fig. 28–3). (The placenta of ruminants may also be termed a synepitheliochorial placenta because a number of fetal trophoblast cells fuse with endometrial cells to form binucleate cells.) A **hemochorial** type of placenta, in which fetal vessels and chorion are invaginated into pools of maternal blood, is found in humans and some rodents. An **endotheliochorial** type, in which the chorion is in direct contact with the endothelium of blood vessels of the dam, is found in carnivores. Mammalian placenta can also be classified at the gross anatomic level based on the distribution of the microscopic sites of exchange. In the mare and sow, extensions of the chorion (**chorionic villi**) project into crypts scattered over the entire endometrium, and this placental type is termed **diffuse** (Fig. 28–4). Ruminants have a **cotyledonary** type of placental attachment (Fig. 28–4) in which exchange takes place at structures termed **placentomes.** Placentomes are formed by the invagination of a specific region of fetal chorionic tissue, **cotyledons,** into a mushroomlike projection from the surface of

the endometrium, **caruncles** (Fig. 28–5). These caruncles project out from the surface of the uterus approximately half an inch and vary in diameter from half an inch to more than 4 inches.

The size of caruncles increases as pregnancy progresses, and the caruncles are larger in the **gravid** (pregnant) horn than in the nongravid horn. The epithelial surface of the caruncle is covered with crypts into which villi of the fetal placenta project. The area between the caruncles is devoid of any attachment between the fetal placenta and the maternal uterus. The shape of the caruncles in the ewe is slightly different from those of the cow, with a rather large central depression, which is the only portion of the caruncle to contain crypts for the attachment of the chorionic villi (Fig. 28–5).

Hemochorial placentas are usually attached to the uterus in a disk-shaped area only. Hence the term **discoidal** is used to describe their general area of attachment. The endotheliochorial placenta of carnivores is attached in a girdlelike band, so the attachment is known as **zonary.** The discoidal and zonary types of placental attachment are **deciduate,** since a portion of the maternal endometrium, or maternal placenta, is shed at the time of parturition. Most domestic animals have an **indeciduate** placenta, in which little or no maternal tissue is lost at parturition.

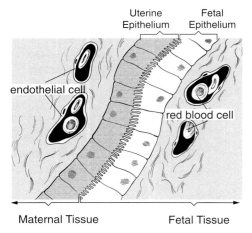

Figure 28-3. Epitheliochorial type of placenta.

Hormones of Pregnancy

Progesterone

Progesterone has several actions that are essential for maintaining a normal pregnancy. These include (1) providing negative feedback to the hypothalamus to inhibit any further estrous cycles; (2) inhibiting the smooth muscle of the uterus to permit the attachment and development of the fetus, and (3) assisting with maintenance of the contractility of the cervix to protect the uterine environment.

Plasma levels and sources of progesterone differ among species and among stages of pregnancy. In all domestic animals, the initial source of the necessary progesterone is the corpus luteum, and in some species (e.g., cow and sow), the corpus luteum remains the primary source throughout pregnancy. In other species (e.g., mare and ewe), the initial corpus luteum can be removed after secondary sources are producing enough progesterone to maintain pregnancy. These sources include secondary or accessory corpora lutea and the placenta in the mare, while the placenta is the secondary source in the ewe.

Equine Chorionic Gonadotrophin

The mare appears to be unique among domestic species in that the equine placenta is the source of a protein hormone that acts similar to

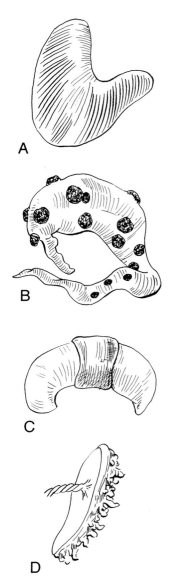

Figure 28-4. Placental types classified by distribution of sites of exchange. A) Diffuse placenta. B) Cotyledonary placenta. C) Zonary placenta. D) Discoid placenta. (Reprinted with permission from Reece W.O. *Physiology of Domestic Animals.* 2nd ed. Baltimore: Williams & Wilkins, 1997.)

the pituitary hormone luteinizing hormone. Secretion of **equine chorionic gonadotrophin (eCG,** formerly known as pregnant mare serum gonadotrophin, or PMSG) begins after about a month of gestation and continues until about 4 months of gestation. During this period, follic-

COW   EWE   MARE

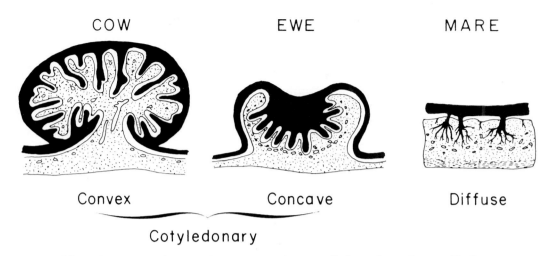

Convex   Concave   Diffuse

Cotyledonary

Figure 28-5. Placental attachments of cow, ewe, and mare. Villi from chorioallantois (*black*) invaginates into crypts in maternal uterine epithelium (*stippled*) in caruncles in cow and ewe and in diffuse locations in mare. (Adapted from Mossman, 1937, from Hafez E.S.E. *Reproduction in Farm Animals*. 4th ed. Philadelphia: Lea & Febiger, 1980.)

ular development occurs on the ovary of the pregnant mare, and eCG promotes the luteinization of these follicles. These accessory corpora lutea provide secondary sources of progesterone.

Trophoblastic cells of fetal origin found in specialized structures termed **endometrial cups** are the source of the eCG. These structures are seen as small raised circular areas with a central depression on the endometrial surface of the pregnant uterus. The trophoblastic cells are found in association with the endometrium in these areas.

Relaxin

Relaxin is a protein hormone secreted by the corpus luteum in some species (sow and cow) and the placenta in others (bitch and mare). The primary function of relaxin is preparation for parturition and ultimately lactation. Relaxin contributes to the opening of the cervix and the relaxation of the muscles and ligaments associated with the birth canal to facilitate the passage of the fetus. In some species, peak secretion of relaxin occurs just prior to parturition. Gradual increases in relaxin during the latter part of gestation also facilitate mammary gland development to prepare for lactation.

Pregnancy Diagnosis

If accurate records of estrus periods and breeding dates are available, the earliest indication of pregnancy in most animals is the failure to have another estrous cycle at the expected time. Such an absence of estrus is not, however, proof of pregnancy. A nonpregnant animal may miss an estrous cycle because of failure of the corpus luteum to regress normally or some other reproductive abnormality. An animal may also have a delay of one or two estrous cycles if an initial conception is followed by inability to sustain that pregnancy.

Palpation of the reproductive tract via the rectum in the mare and cow can be useful for pregnancy diagnosis and estimation of the stage of pregnancy. In the cow, the presence of a corpus luteum in an ovary and a slight enlargement of one uterine horn as compared to the other suggests an early pregnancy. At about 3 months of pregnancy in the cow, fetal membranes and caruncles become palpable, and the uterine artery on the side with the fetus is slightly larger than the vessel on the other side. Pregnancy diagnosis by rectal palpation is considered to be more difficult in the mare than in the cow, but an early diagnostic feature is a bulge in the uterus due to the development of the amniotic sac.

Ultrasonography is used to diagnose pregnancy in a variety of domestic species including cattle, horses, sheep, goats, llamas, and swine. The earliest time for verification of pregnancy is dictated in part by the size of the gestational sac, which in turn varies among species. In general, the times vary between about 2 weeks for mares to about 5 weeks for ewes. In large animals, the ultrasound probe can be inserted rectally so that it is closer to the uterus.

Parturition

Parturition (*labor*), the act of giving birth to young, marks the termination of pregnancy. Parturition may be divided into three stages. The *first stage* consists of uterine contractions that gradually force the fetus and fetal membrane to the cervix. The duration of this stage is a matter of hours in most species (e.g., 2 to 6 in the cow and ewe, 1 to 4 in the mare, and 2 to 12 in the sow).

In the *second stage,* actual delivery of the fetus occurs. Passage of parts of the fetus through the cervix into the vagina along with rupture of one or both water bags reflexively initiates actual straining or contraction of the abdominal muscles. The combination of uterine contraction and abdominal contraction forces the fetus through the birth canal.

The *third stage* of parturition consists of delivery of the placenta, which normally follows the fetus almost immediately.

Late Gestation

To facilitate delivery of the fetus, muscles and ligaments of the birth canal relax shortly before parturition. The vulva swells, and a mucus discharge may be present. Muscles on both sides of the tail head may relax and appear lowered or depressed. Mammary glands enlarge and may secrete a milky material for a few days prior to parturition. As the time of parturition becomes

imminent, animals may become restless, seek seclusion, and increase frequency of attempts to urinate. The bitch and sow often try to build a nest.

An important endocrine change during late gestation in most species is in the ratio of estrogen to progesterone. Progesterone is high relative to estrogen during most of gestation, but this ratio changes during late gestation, so that estrogen increases relative to progesterone. Estrogen promotes the development of contractile proteins in the smooth muscle cells of the uterus and gap junctions between these cells. These uterine changes increase the force that the uterus can generate for delivery. The timing of the changes in estrogen and progesterone relative to parturition varies among species.

Initiation of Parturition

In domestic animals, an endocrine signal from the fetus appears to initiate parturition. Plasma levels of **glucocorticoids** (e.g., cortisol) increase in most domestic species, except for the mare, shortly prior to parturition. The fetal adrenal cortex is the source of these glucocorticoids, and the adrenal cortical secretion is in response to adrenocorticotropic hormone (ACTH) from the fetal adenohypophysis. An increase in sensitivity of the adrenal cortex to ACTH is part of the reason for the increased secretion of glucocorticoids during this period.

The rising fetal glucocorticoids affect the placenta and the maternal uterus. In some species, the glucocorticoids increase estrogen production by the placenta, so that plasma estrogens increase relative to progesterone. This brings about the changes in the uterine smooth muscle described earlier. Glucocorticoids and estrogens act synergistically to promote uterine synthesis and secretion of $PGF_{2\alpha}$.

Increases in $PGF_{2\alpha}$ have multiple effects that can contribute to the onset of parturition, and some view these as the final link in the chain of events initiating parturition. In species whose primary corpus luteum remains and is a significant source of progesterone (e.g., cow and sow), the rise in $PGF_{2\alpha}$ can bring about leutolysis and remove this source of progesterone. Recall that progesterone suppresses the activity of uterine smooth muscle and maintains cervical tone, so a reduction in progesterone is appropriate to facilitate delivery. $PGF_{2\alpha}$ also directly stimulates the contraction of uterine smooth muscle to move the fetus into the birth canal and directly promotes dilation of the cervix.

Oxytocin

The entrance of a fetus into the birth canal brings about a reflex increase in **oxytocin** secretion from the neurohypophysis. Oxytocin acts directly on uterine smooth muscle to enhance uterine contractions and promote delivery. Extracts of the neurohypophysis are used clinically to stimulate contractions of the fatigued uterus during prolonged labor.

In the mare, plasma levels of oxytocin gradually rise during the latter stages of gestation and then increase greatly as parturition begins.

Fetal Presentations and Delivery

The calf is normally presented front feet first with the head extended and the nose between the front feet (Fig. 28–6). The dorsum of the calf is in contact with the sacrum of the dam. This position, called cranial (anterior) presentation, takes advantage of the natural curvature of the birth canal of the dam and the curvature of the fetus. A caudal (posterior) presentation with the hind feet first, hocks up, occurs frequently enough in cattle to be considered normal.

Uterine contractions force the fetal placenta (water bags) against the cervix of the uterus, and ultimately these water bags rupture. At about the same time, abdominal muscles begin to contract forcefully to expel the fetus through the birth canal.

The contraction of abdominal muscles, called **straining,** is a reflex response to stimuli from the presence of parts of the fetus within the vagina and vulva of the dam. Straining can also be readily evoked by the insertion of a hand and arm into the vulva and vagina, for example when attempting to deliver a calf.

The legs of a foal are longer than those of a calf, and a foal is carried to a larger extent in the body of the uterus, while a calf is carried

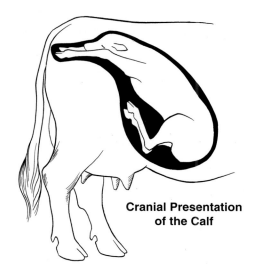

Cranial Presentation of the Calf

Figure 28-6. Cranial or anterior presentation of calf.

almost entirely in one horn of the uterus. Presentation of a foal is essentially the same as that of a calf. With pigs and dogs, the young are carried in both horns of the uterus and may be presented either cranially or caudally with equal facility.

In species that typically have a single offspring, the placenta, or **afterbirth,** is delivered soon after birth, but it may accompany the fetus or rarely, precede it. In the litter-bearing sow, the placenta for each fetus is typically delivered still attached to the fetus and may completely surround the fetus. In these cases, immediate removal of the placenta from the nostrils of the newborn is essential for life; usually the sow does it. A placenta is considered to be retained pathologically if an abnormally long time elapses between birth of the young and delivery of the placenta. The placenta of the cow and ewe should be delivered within 24 hours, and the placenta of the mare should be delivered within 2 to 3 hours.

Retention of the placenta is a significant problem in dairy cattle. The incidence seems to be higher in cattle than other species and higher in dairy than in beef breeds. Manual removal of a retained placenta has been a common method of treatment, but more conservative treatment (e.g., no manual removal, with antibiotics to

prevent infection) are also advocated, and their use is supported by research studies.

Dystocia

Normal parturition with no complications is by far the most common occurrence in domestic animals. **Dystocia** is difficult birth; in some cases, birthing is not possible without assistance. In general, from the onset of labor, cows should calve within 8 hours, ewes should lamb within 2 hours, and mares should foal within 2 to 3 hours. Sows should average one offspring per hour until farrowing (i.e., birthing of a litter) is complete.

In large animals (cow, mare and ewe), improper fetal presentation is a common cause of dystocia, and typically with abnormal positioning of the limbs or head (e.g., head rotated up and ventrum of neck presented or head rotated down and dorsum of neck presented). Correction of such a presentation may be necessary for delivery of the fetus. Correction usually entails repelling the fetus into the uterus away from the pelvic inlet so that the fetus can be manipulated and the position of its limbs and head changed.

Excessive size of the fetus relative to the size of the birth canal of the dam may also produce dystocia. This is a common cause of dystocia in first-calf heifers and in relatively small cows mated with much larger bulls. Excessive fetal size may also produce problems in ewes with single lambs and sows with small litters. Even though the presentation may be normal in these cases, excessive traction may be required to deliver the newborn, and this may damage both the fetus and the dam.

A **cesarean section** (surgical removal of the fetus) may be necessary in some cases of dystocia. Successful surgeries produce a viable fetus and preserve the reproductive capacity of the dam. An **embryotomy** (surgical dismemberment of the fetus to permit its passage through the birth canal) may be necessary in some cases to save the life of the dam.

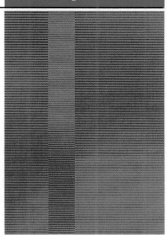

ANATOMY AND PHYSIOLOGY OF THE MAMMARY GLANDS

The ***mammary glands*** (also called ***mammae***) are modified sudoriferous (sweat) glands that produce milk for the nourishment of offspring. They develop from bilateral thickenings of ventrolateral ectoderm of the embryo, the so-called milk lines, which are more correctly referred to as ***mammary ridges.*** In carnivores and the sow, the mammary glands develop throughout the axillary to inguinal extent of the ridges, as is appropriate for species that typically deliver multiple fetuses. However, in most other domestic animals, only the inguinal mammary glands develop, usually two (e.g., mares, ewes, and does) or four (e.g., cows). In the anthropoid apes and the elephant, only two pectoral mammary glands develop.

Each gland is composed of a system of ducts connecting masses of secretory epithelium surrounded by connective tissue and fat and supported in a fibroelastic capsule. The proportion of secretory parenchyma to connective tissue is hormonally dictated; during lactation, the mammary gland's secretory tissues increase in volume. After the end of lactation (when the dam is dry), the secretory tissues regress, and connective tissue constitutes a greater percentage of the gland.

In ruminants and horses, individual glands are associated so closely to one another that they are commonly referred to as a single ***udder.*** Even so, the individual nature of glands of the udder is readily appreciated by the presence of a single ***teat*** (***papilla***) for each gland. A single (as in ruminants) or multiple (as in the mare and sow) duct system may discharge milk at the tip of each teat.

Embryonic ectoderm invaginates along the mammary ridge to become the duct system of individual mammary glands. These invaginations (mammary buds) will ultimately be associated with an individual teat. In all species more buds initially develop than will persist, and these extra buds regress promptly after appearing. Not uncommonly, though, some extra buds persist and produce *supernumerary teats.* These extra teats are usually small and not associated with a well-developed gland; because they can interfere with milking, they are usually removed from the udders of cows and does.

The mammary glands of domestic species have a great deal in common, but inasmuch as the udder of the dairy cow has been so dramatically developed to produce milk far beyond that necessary to nourish the cow's offspring, it is discussed in detail.

Mammary Glands of the Cow

The udder of the cow comprises four individual glands, referred to as **quarters.** The skin of the udder is covered with fine hair; however, the teat is completely hairless. The right and left halves of the udder each consist of a cranial (front) quarter and a caudal (hind) quarter. Each side of the udder is almost completely independent of the other insofar as blood supply, nerve supply, and suspensory apparatus are concerned (discussed later).

Ventrally, the two halves of the udder are demarcated by a longitudinal furrow, the **intermammary groove,** which corresponds to a median septum of connective tissue dividing left and right halves. Because of the relative isolation of each side, half of the udder can be removed surgically without damaging the other half, as might be done to treat an aggressive tumor. The two quarters in each half are separate from one another as far as the gland tissue and duct system are concerned. Thus all the milk from one teat is produced by the glandular tissue of that quarter. The vasculature, nerve supply, and lymphatic drainage, however, are common to both quarters of a given half.

The parenchyma of the lactating mammary gland consists of secretory tissue and the ducts of the gland (Fig. 29–1). The secretory units, the **alveoli,** are lined by a simple epithelium that varies from columnar to cuboidal in height. The alveoli are the chief structures for actual milk production, although the initial portion of the associated duct is also lined with secretory epithelium.

The various small, initial ducts converge to form larger ducts, and these converge to form yet larger ones, all of which eventually terminate in a large single basin, the **lactiferous sinus.** The lactiferous sinus is sometimes described as being divided into a large cavity within the quarter itself, the **pars glandularis (gland cistern),** and a smaller cavity within the associated teat called the **pars papillaris (teat cistern)** (Fig. 29–1). The demarcation between gland cistern and teat cistern frequently is marked by a circular ridge (annulus) that contains a vein and some smooth muscle fibers.

The wall of the empty cistern contains numerous overlapping longitudinal and circular folds that are obliterated through expansion of the wall when it is full of milk. There may also be diverticula (pockets) in the wall of the gland cistern.

The teat cistern is continuous with the exterior of the teat through a narrow opening in the end of the teat, the **papillary duct** (commonly called **streak canal** or teat canal), which opens at the **ostium papillae.** The bovine streak canal is about 8.5 mm long, and its lumen is normally closed by epithelial folds that project inward from the wall of the streak canal, leaving only a star-shaped potential opening. A sphincter of smooth muscle fibers surrounds the streak canal at the distal end of the teat.

Suspensory Apparatus

The udder of a lactating dairy cow can weigh as much as 60 kg, so the organ is supported by a dense system of fibroelastic ligaments called the **suspensory apparatus.** The primary supportive elements of the suspensory apparatus are its

BOVINE UDDER

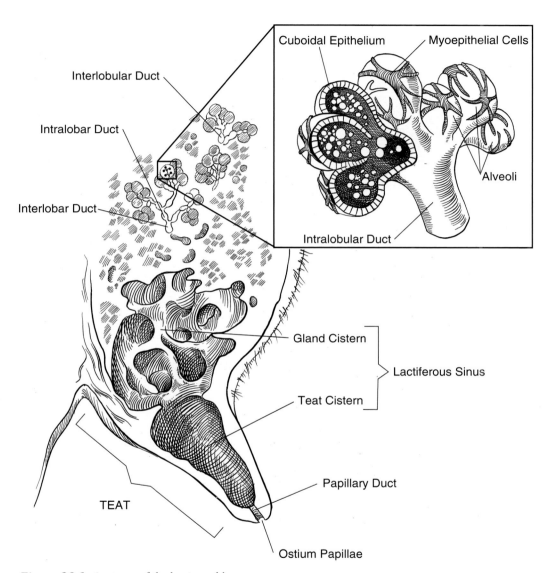

Figure 29-1. Anatomy of the bovine udder.

two **medial laminae,** which take their origin together from the linea alba of the abdominal wall and the symphysis of the pelvis (Fig. 29–2). Each medial lamina passes ventrad between the two halves of the udder so that one layer intimately covers the medial side of each half. The two medial laminae can be readily separated, as

they are united only by a small amount of loose areolar connective tissue; practically no vessels or nerves pass through the medial ligament from one half of the udder to the other. Proximally (close to the body wall), the laminae are thickest. As they descend, they give off sheets of connective tissue that diverge from the midline

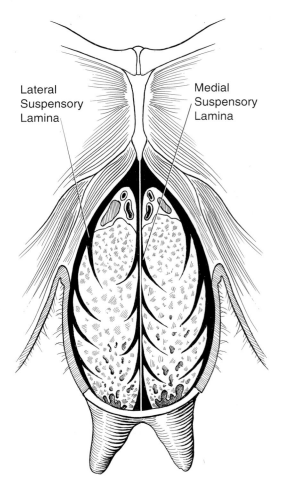

Figure 29-2. Suspensory apparatus of the cow. Udder is shown in transverse section through hindquarters.

and interdigitate into the parenchyma of the udder, so that the two medial laminae are thinnest near the intermammary groove.

The **lateral laminae** of the suspensory apparatus are composed largely of dense white fibrous connective tissue, making them less elastic than the medial laminae, which are mostly elastic connective tissue. The cranial part of the lateral lamina derives from the aponeurotic tissues of the body wall near the external inguinal ring and more caudally from the regions of the pelvic symphysis and prepubic tendon (the tendon of insertion of the *m. rectus*

abdominis). From its origins, the lateral lamina passes ventrad and around the lateral side of each half of the mammary gland, meeting the medial lamina at the cranial and caudal aspects of each half. Like the medial lamina, the lateral lamina is thick close to the body wall and thins progressively ventrally as it gives off sheets of connective tissue into the substance of the gland.

Blood Supply

The blood supply to the udder is primarily through the **external pudendal artery** (Fig. 29–3), a branch of the pudendoepigastric trunk. The external pudendal artery passes downward through the inguinal canal in a more or less tortuous manner and divides into cranial and caudal branches that supply the front and hind quarters on the same side as the artery. A small artery that may be single or paired (as determined by chance) is the **ventral perineal artery,** which continues from the internal pudendal artery and passes downward from the vulva just deep to the skin on the median line. The perineal artery usually supplies a small amount of blood to the caudal part of both halves of the udder.

The venous drainage from the udder is largely by way of a venous circle at the base of the udder, where it attaches to the abdominal wall. This venous circle is formed from the main veins that drain the udder. The **external pudendal vein** of each side receives blood from both the cranial and caudal quarters of the same side. Cranially, each external pudendal vein is continuous with the **caudal superficial epigastric vein** and caudally with the perineal vein. An anastomosis between the two caudal superficial epigastric veins just at or in front of the udder completes the venous circle. The caudal superficial epigastric vein passes forward in a sagittal plane lateral to the midline on the ventral abdominal wall and joins with the cranial superficial epigastric vein, which ultimately drains to the internal thoracic veins and then to the cranial vena cava. Before the heifer comes into milk, the connection between cranial and caudal superficial epigastrics is poorly developed. During

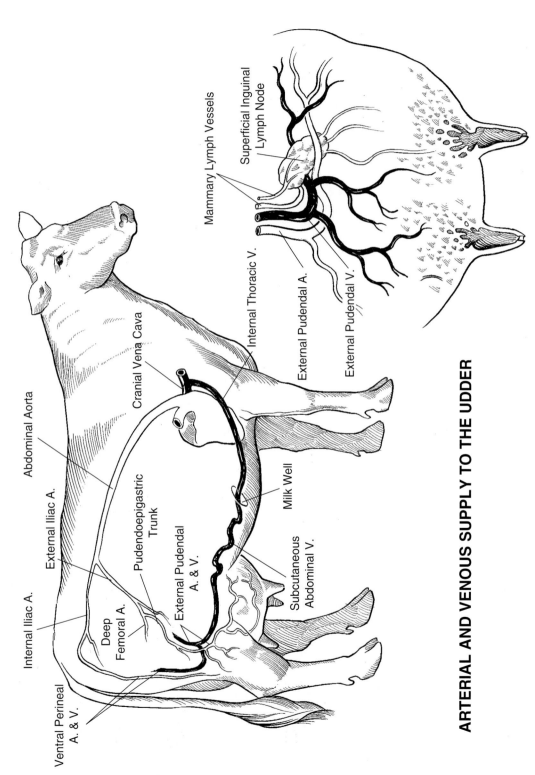

Internal Iliac A.

Abdominal Aorta

External Iliac A.

Ventral Perineal A. & V.

Deep Femoral A.

Pudendoepigastric Trunk

External Pudendal A. & V.

Cranial Vena Cava

Milk Well

Subcutaneous Abdominal V.

Internal Thoracic V.

External Pudendal A.

External Pudendal V.

Mammary Lymph Vessels

Superficial Inguinal Lymph Node

ARTERIAL AND VENOUS SUPPLY TO THE UDDER

Figure 29-3. Arterial and venous blood supply to the bovine udder. Vessels other than aorta and cranial vena cava are paired.

first pregnancy, when the udder undergoes a marked increase in size and consequently blood supply, the two veins develop a functional anastomosis, after which they collectively constitute the **subcutaneous abdominal vein** or the **milk vein.** In high-producing dairy cows the subcutaneous abdominal vein is large and tortuous. It passes through a foramen in the rectus abdominis muscle (the **milk well**), joins the internal thoracic vein, and ultimately drains to the cranial vena cava.

Lymphatic Vessels

The lymphatic vessels draining the udder show up rather well superficially just under the skin, particularly in high-producing cattle. They drain from the entire udder, including the teat, to the **superficial inguinal (mammary** or **supramammary) lymph nodes** near the superficial (external) inguinal ring above the caudal part of the base of the udder.

Microscopic Anatomy of the Mammary Gland

The mammary gland is classified as a compound tubuloalveolar gland. It consists of a connective tissue interstitium, parenchyma (secretory epithelium), ducts, vessels, and nerves. In the dry (not lactating) state, the gland has proportionately more stroma than parenchyma; during lactation, the parenchyma undergoes marked growth and constitutes the bulk of the gland.

The surface of the bovine and porcine teat is covered with glabrous (hairless), aglandular stratified squamous epithelium. The teats of other domestic species have more typical haired and glandular skin. This is continuous with the stratified squamous epithelium that lines the papillary duct (streak canal). The duct is encircled by smooth muscle fibers that act as a sphincter.

At the junction of the papillary duct and the teat cistern, the epithelial lining changes abruptly from stratified squamous to stratified columnar epithelium that is usually two cells thick. This stratified columnar epithelium lines the teat and gland cisterns and the larger lactiferous ducts. As the ducts branch and become smaller, the epithelial lining changes first to simple columnar and then to secretory epithelium in the alveoli. The height of the alveolar epithelium varies considerably with the level of activity of the gland.

The mammary gland differs from most other exocrine glands in that the secretory portion is not limited to the terminations of the smallest ducts; milk-secreting structures also empty directly into the larger ducts and directly into the gland cistern and the teat cistern.

A group of alveoli surrounded by a connective tissue septum form a more or less distinct unit called a lobule (Fig. 29–1). A group of lobules within a connective tissue compartment forms a lobe. Correspondingly, the ducts are classified as **intralobular, interlobular, intralobar,** and **interlobar** as they increase in size. The alveoli making up the lobule empty into small ducts within the lobule, the intralobular ducts. These intralobular ducts drain into a central collecting space from which the interlobular ducts emerge. Within the lobe, the interlobular ducts unite to form a single intralobar duct, which is called an interlobar duct as soon as it emerges from the lobe. The interlobar duct may enter the gland cistern directly, or it may join one or more other interlobar ducts before entering the gland cistern. Many of the ducts have numerous dilations that act, in addition to the lactiferous sinus, as collecting spaces for milk.

The alveoli and ducts are surrounded by contractile **myoepithelial cells,** which are also called **basket cells.** These cells contract to eject milk (called **milk letdown**) in response to oxytocin release (discussed later).

In addition to the epithelial parenchyma and the myoepithelial cells, the mammary gland is made up of an interstitium of white fibrous connective tissue and yellow elastic connective tissue. Blood vessels, lymph vessels, and nerves ramify throughout the interstitium to reach the epithelial structures. The veins of the mammary gland are valveless and form a rich network throughout the gland and within the wall of the teat. The vascular layer of the teat is called a corpus cavernosum because of its resemblance to the erectile tissue of the penis in the male. Lymphatic plexuses are found throughout the udder just deep to the skin and scattered throughout the parenchyma of the gland. Nerves appear to be primarily sensory and vasomotor.

Mammary Glands of Swine

The normal number of teats in the domestic hog is 7 pairs, or 14 teats, with the first pair just caudal to the junction of the sternum and costal arch and the last pair in the inguinal region. The number of pairs may range from 4 to 9, and supernumerary teats are sometimes found between normal teats. Sows average 2.5 more teats than the number of piglets in their average litter. Glands that are underused dry up and do not develop again until the next pregnancy.

Inverted teats (concave nipples) and mastitis are two of the most common conditions adversely affecting the mammary glands of sows.

The caudal mammary glands of the sow receive blood from the caudal superficial epigastric arteries and to some extent from the caudal (deep) epigastric arteries. The cranial pairs receive blood from the branches of the cranial (deep) epigastric arteries. Cranial and caudal epigastric arteries anastomose dorsal to the abdominal mammary glands.

The lymphatic vessels from all but the cranial one or two glands on each side drain to the ipsilateral superficial inguinal lymph nodes. The lymphatic vessels from the cranial few glands may drain to the sternal lymph nodes, the superficial cervical lymph nodes, or both.

The teat of the sow contains two streak canals and two teat cisterns. Each teat cistern is continuous with a gland cistern. The teat is hairless, but hair is found at the base of the teat and on the gland.

Seedy-cut bacon is due to inclusion of pigmented mammary tissue in the cut, giving the appearance of small seeds in the bacon. Black seedy cut is due to invagination of pigmented epithelium at the time of mammary gland formation. It occurs only in dark-colored glands. Red seedy cut may occur in any color sow or gilt past puberty, as it is due to inflammation of mammary glands associated with the estrous cycle.

Mammary Glands of Sheep and Goats

The udders of the ewe and the doe differ from that of the cow in that each half of the udder has only one teat, one streak canal, one teat cistern, and one gland cistern. One half of the ovine and caprine udder resembles one quarter of the bovine udder. The teat is sparsely covered with fine hair. Each half of the udder of the ewe is craniomedial to the inguinal sinus (a pouch of skin lined with scent glands) of the same side. Supernumerary teats in the ewe do not appear to have separate gland tissue, as is frequently found in the cow. The sphincter muscle around the papillary duct is poorly developed, so closure is effected by elastic tissue in the end of the teat.

Mammary Glands of the Horse

The mammary glands of the mare consist of one teat on each side attached to half of the udder. Each teat has two streak canals and two teat cisterns, each of which is continuous with a separate system of ducts and alveoli (occasionally a gland has a third set of ducts). There appears to be no communication between ducts or cisterns within the same half of the udder.

The suspensory apparatus is arranged as in the cow, although it is not so robust. The udder and teats of the mare are covered with thin, fine hair and with numerous sebaceous and sweat glands. There is a difference of opinion regarding the presence or absence of rudimentary teats in the stallion and gelding. They have been described in the skin forming the cranial part of the prepuce, but their presence here has also been denied. Apparently no adequate embryologic study of this subject has been reported.

Physiology of Lactation

Composition of Milk

Milk contains all of the nutrients necessary for survival and initial growth of mammalian neonates. The nutrients in milk include sources of energy (lipids and carbohydrates), proteins to provide amino acids, vitamins, minerals (ash) for electrolytes , and water. The relative amounts of these nutrients in milk vary among species (Table 29–1).

Diet and the stage of lactation also affect the composition of milk. Diets high in nonfiber carbohydrate sources of energy are associated with increases in the percentage of lipids in the milk. Diets high in protein promote a slight increase in the percentage of protein in the milk, but this effect is much less than the effect of energy on milk lipid content. The amount of carbohydrates in milk (lactose, or milk sugar) does not routinely change with diet. The percentage of lipids and protein in milk is also highest early in lactation. In cattle the percentages are relatively high in the first few weeks after calving and then decrease over the next 3 to 4 months. Later in lactation, the concentrations of lipids and proteins again increase as total daily production (pounds of milk per day) decreases.

Most of the lipids in milk are in the form of triglycerides, and these are the primary source of dietary energy in milk. Triglycerides are composed of three fatty acids and glycerol. The fatty acids for the synthesis of milk triglycerides may be derived from the blood or synthesized within the mammary gland. Nonruminant mammary glands use blood *glucose* both for energy and as a source of carbon for the synthesis of the fatty acids. The glycerol is derived mostly from glucose catabolism in the process of glycolysis. The mammary glands of ruminants depend on blood *acetate* and **β-hydroxybutyrate** to provide carbon for fatty acid synthesis, with acetate being the primary source. The acetate and β-hydroxybutyrate in ruminants are produced as volatile fatty acids by fermentative metabolism by microorganisms in the rumen. These volatile fatty acids are absorbed into the blood and thereby become available for synthesis of milk fat in the mammary gland. Most milk triglycerides have fatty acids with chains 4 to 14 carbon atoms in length—short-chain fatty acids. Such short-chain fatty acids are not generally found in adipose tissue throughout the remainder of the body.

Lactose (milk sugar), the principal carbohydrate in milk, is a disaccharide composed of the two monosaccharides glucose and galactose. Lactose is synthesized in mammary glands and is typically found only in mammary glands and milk. Secretory cells in mammary glands use glucose from the blood to synthesize galactose and then combine the galactose with more glucose to produce lactose, so glucose is essential for lactose synthesis. The extraction of glucose from blood by an actively secreting mammary gland is quite effective, so the glucose concentration of venous blood leaving a mammary gland is relatively low.

Recall that in ruminants blood glucose is primarily derived from gluconeogenesis in the liver using ***propionic acid,*** a volatile fatty acid absorbed from the rumen, as a substrate. Thus, propionic acid produced by ruminal microorganisms and fermentative metabolism is the ultimate substrate for the production of lactose in ruminants. Also, blood glucose is relatively low in ruminants compared to other mammals, in part because ruminants absorb very little glucose from the gastrointestinal tract. **At peak lactation of a high-producing dairy cow, the mammary glands use most of the glucose produced by the liver for lactose production. If the need for glucose by the mammary glands cannot be**

Table 29-1. Typical Values for Constituents of Milk in Grams per Liter

Species	Lipids	Lactose	Protein	Total Minerals (ash)	Calcium
Cow	38	48	37	7.0	1.3
Mare	16	50	24	4.5	1.0
Ewe	70	40	60	8.0	1.9
Sow	80	46	58	8.5	2.0
Doe	40	45	35	7.8	1.2

met by gluconeogenesis and blood glucose levels drop significantly, *lactational ketosis* develops. While blood glucose levels are low, metabolic acids (produced in the liver from fatty acids) accumulate in the blood to produce a metabolic acidosis.

The major milk proteins are the **caseins.** Blood amino acids are the precursors for direct synthesis of the caseins by secretory cells within mammary glands. Other milk proteins include α-lactalbumin, and β-lactoglobulins, which are produced by cells of the mammary gland, and serum albumin and immunoglobulins produced by the liver and lymphocytes, respectively.

Rennin (also known as chymosin) is a proteolytic enzyme secreted by gastric epithelial cells of very young mammals. Rennin changes the character of ingested milk from a liquid to a semisolid curd; this process is termed **curdling** or **coagulation.** The change in character increases the time that milk is retained in the stomach, and this permits protein digestion to begin. Curdling results when rennin degrades one of the casein proteins that is responsible for increasing the solubility of micelles, casein protein aggregates in milk (discussed next). Without this specific casein, milk proteins precipitate with the calcium in milk to form curds.

Milk Secretion

The epithelial cells lining the alveoli of mammary glands are the cells primarily responsible for the secretion of milk. The appearance of these cells varies as they synthesize and release the lipids, proteins, and lactose of milk. After the cells actively secrete the constituents of milk and the lumen of the alveoli are filled with milk, the epithelial cells shrink and are described as a simple low cuboidal epithelium (Fig. 29–4). At this stage, their secretory activity is relatively low. Shortly after the stored milk is removed, the epithelial cells increase their secretory activity and begin to refill the alveoli. Early in the secretory phase the cells assume a more columnar appearance and then gradually reduce to cuboidal as milk fills the alveoli. Small, apparently nonfunctioning alveoli can be found in dry mammary glands, and there is a relative increase in the amount of interstitial loose connective tissue (Fig. 29–5).

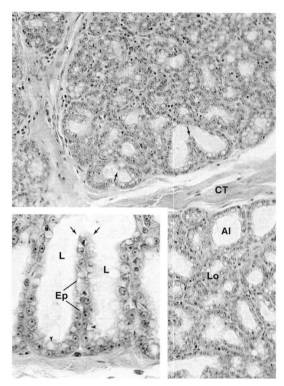

Figure 29-4. Active mammary gland with lobules (*Lo*) of secretory alveoli (*Al*). Connective tissue (*CT*) is compressed in active gland. *Insert:* Secretory products in alveolar lumen (*L*) and secretory epithelial cells (*Ep*) lining the alveoli. (Reprinted with permission from Gartner L.P. and J.L. Hiatt, eds. *Color Atlas of Histology,* 2nd ed. Baltimore: Williams & Wilkins, 1994.)

Milk lipids are synthesized and packaged into secretory droplets, which are extruded from the luminal surface of the cell into the alveoli (Fig. 29–6). As they are released, a membrane covering derived from the cell membrane of the epithelial cell encases the lipid droplets. The alveolar secretory cells also produce secretory vesicles that contain both milk proteins (caseins) and lactose (Fig. 29–6). As caseins are synthesized and packaged in these vesicles, they self-aggregate into particles termed **micelles.** The inclusion of one specific type of casein (κ-casein) in this aggregation increases the solubility of the micelle, so that milk proteins remain in solution after their release from the cell. The lactose within the secretory vesicle generates an osmotic force to draw water into

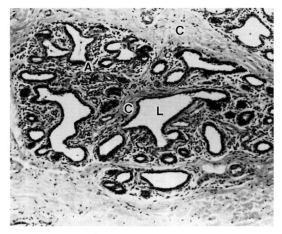

Figure 29-5. Nonlactating mammary gland (cow). Gland lobules with inactive alveoli (*A*), intralobular duct (*L*), and connective tissue (*C*). (Reprinted with permission from Dellmann H.D. and J. Eurell. *Textbook of Veterinary Histology.* 5th ed. Baltimore: Lippincott Williams & Wilkins, 1998.)

the vesicle from the cytosol of the cell. The secretory vesicles, each containing a mixture of micelles, lactose, and water, are transported to the apical surface of the cell and released into the alveoli by exocytosis (Fig. 29–6). Because of the various mechanisms by which lipids, pro-

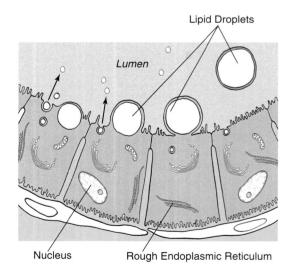

Figure 29-6. Secretion of milk lipids, milk proteins, and lactose by epithelial cells lining the alveoli of the mammary glands. Proteins and lactose are together in secretory vesicles which are released by exocytosis (arrows).

teins, and lactose are secreted from alveolar cells, milk is considered to be a combination of apocrine and merocrine secretions.

Lactogenesis

Lactogenesis is the establishment of milk secretion, and *galactopoiesis* is the continued production of milk by the mammary glands. Growth and development of the secretory epithelium and the ductile network of the mammary glands must precede lactogenesis. The initial extensive development of the mammary gland is usually associated with puberty (the beginning of sexual maturity) and the subsequent cyclic changes in the ovarian hormones, estrogen and progesterone. Estrogen particularly promotes the growth of the ductile system at each estrus, while progesterone, acting with estrogen, is required for growth and anatomic development of secretory alveoli. Normal secretion of growth hormone and glucocorticoids are also required for complete mammary gland development.

During pregnancy, prolonged exposure of the mammary glands to progesterone promotes a more extensive anatomic development of the secretory alveoli. While progesterone stimulates anatomic development, it inhibits the functional development of the secretory epithelium. Progesterone also inhibits the production of intracellular enzymes necessary for normal milk secretion. This inhibitory effect of progesterone is lost just prior to parturition, and this is one factor promoting lactogenesis.

Prolactin, a protein hormone, is unique in that its release from the adenohypophysis is primarily regulated by a humoral inhibitor factor from the hypothalamus. In the absence of this inhibitory factor (which is believed to be the catecholamine *dopamine*), there is a continuous and relatively high rate of prolactin release. In most domestic animals, blood levels of prolactin gradually increase late in gestation, with an abrupt increase at parturition. During late gestation, prolactin receptors in mammary glands also increase under the influence of rising estrogen. Prolactin promotes both anatomic and functional development of the secretory epithelium of mammary glands to promote milk secretion, so the abrupt rise at parturition is appropriate for lactogenesis. Under the influence of prolactin, secretory cells lining alveoli produce intracellular enzymes necessary for milk secretion. The functional development of alveolar secretory cells is also enhanced by glucocorticoids, which increase in the blood prior to parturition in most species.

The placenta of ruminants produces a protein hormone, **placental lactogen,** or chorionic somatomammotropin, that is similar in structure and function to prolactin. Placental lactogen production increases in late gestation in ruminants and is believed to be more responsible for mammary gland development in these species than prolactin from the adenohypophysis.

Galactogenesis

The continuation of lactation requires stimuli to promote milk production and removal or inhibition of stimuli that retard milk production. Stimulation of the nipples (teats) by either milking or suckling elicits an abrupt increase in blood levels of prolactin. The increased secretion of prolactin is the result of a neural reflex mediated through the hypothalamus that regulates prolactin release from the adenohypophysis. The increase in prolactin is relatively short in duration (minutes to an hour). This periodic and relatively brief surge of prolactin is essential to maintain normal lactation in most species, but prolactin does not appear to be an essential regulator of lactation in cows. Supplementation with prolactin does not increase milk secretion in cows, and lactation is maintained in cows in spite of severe reductions in blood levels of prolactin.

Growth hormone appears to be especially important in cows, whose blood levels of growth hormone are directly correlated with the maintenance and level of milk production. Growth hormone supplementation increases milk production in cows by 10–40%. Growth hormone supplementation in cattle is associated with a variety of physiologic changes that promote milk production. These include increased mobilization of body energy stores and alterations in overall protein metabolism in other organs to provide substrates for milk secretion, increased food intake, increased nutrient absorption from the gastrointestinal tract, and improved efficiency of the conversion of nutrients to milk by the mammary gland. It is presumed that many of the effects of growth hormone are mediated via insulinlike growth factors (IGFs), whose production is increased by growth hormone (see Chapter 12). Even though growth hormone appears to be a primary regulator of milk production in cows, milking or suckling does not produce an immediate release of growth hormone in the lactating cow.

Routine milking or suckling to remove milk from the mammary glands is essential for continued milk production. When milking is stopped abruptly (probably the best way to dry up a cow), a number of changes in the udder occur. At the end of 24 hours, the alveoli become distended to a maximum, and the capillaries are full of blood. Between 36 and 48 hours, there is a decrease in the number of patent (open) capillaries, and the alveoli do not respond to intravenous oxytocin. A protein that inhibits milk production, **feedback inhibitor of lactation** (FIL), is apparently produced in the mammary gland as milk is produced. This protein has a local effect to inhibit milk production. Other components of milk may have similar inhibitory effects, and routine removal of these inhibitory factors promotes the continuation of lactation.

Milk Ejection, or Letdown

Milking or **nursing** alone can empty only the cisterns and largest ducts of the udder. In fact, any negative pressure causes the ducts to collapse and prevent emptying of the alveoli and smaller ducts. Thus, the dam must take an active although unconscious part in milking to force milk from the alveoli into the cisterns. This is accomplished by active contraction of the **myoepithelial cells** surrounding the alveoli (**milk ejection,** or **milk letdown**). These myoepithelial cells contract when stimulated by **oxytocin,** a hormone released from the neurohypophysis of the pituitary as a result of a neuroendocrine reflex. The afferent side of the reflex consists of sensory nerves from the mammary glands, particularly the nipples or teats. Afferent information reaches the hypothalamus, which regulates the release of oxytocin from the neurohypophysis (see Chapter 12). **Suckling** the teats by the young is the usual stimulus for the milk ejection reflex, but whether milk is withdrawn from the teat or not, the milk ejection reflex produces a measurable increase in the pressure of milk within the cisterns of the udder.

The milk ejection reflex can be conditioned to stimuli associated with milking routine, such as feeding, barn noises, and the sight of the calf. It can also be inhibited by emotionally disturbing stimuli, such as dogs barking, other loud and unusual noises, excess muscular activity, and pain. Stressful stimuli increase the activity of the **sympathetic nervous system,** which can inhibit the milk ejection reflex. This inhibition occurs both at the level of the hypothalamus via an inhibition of oxytocin release and at the level of the mammary gland, where sympathetic stimulation can reduce blood flow and directly counteract the effect of oxytocin on myoepithelial cells.

Oxytocin release typically occurs as a surge within a minute or two after initiation of the reflex by some tactile or environmental stimulus, and the plasma half-life of oxytocin (a small peptide hormone) is but a few minutes. Hence, milking or suckling should begin in close association with stimuli known to stimulate oxytocin release, such as washing the udder and stimulation of the teats. If failure to get an adequate stimulus for milk ejection, possibly because of inadequate preparation before milking, becomes habitual, the lactation period may be shortened by excessive retention of milk in the udder.

Essentially all the milk obtained at any one milking is present in the mammary gland at the beginning of milking or nursing. However, milking does not usually remove all of the milk in the gland. Up to 25% of the milk in a gland usually remains after milking. Some of this residual milk can be removed after injections of oxytocin, but the routine use of such injections tends to shorten the lactation period.

Colostrum

Colostrum, the first milk produced upon delivery of the newborn, is important for the survival and vitality of newborn domestic animals. One of the unique differences between colostrum and typical milk is that colostrum contains a high concentration of **immunoglobulins** produced by the immune system of the dam. These immunoglobulins are concentrated in the milk by selective transport by the epithelial cells lining the alveoli and are needed by the neonate to provide temporary immune protection against infectious agents in the environment.

During the first day or two of life, most domestic neonates can absorb intact immunoglobulins from their gastrointestinal tract into the blood. After this period, immunoglobulins cannot be absorbed intact, and consumed immunoglobulins are digested in a manner similar to other ingested proteins. **Closure** is the term given to the changes that occur in the gastrointestinal tract after the first or second day of life that prevent the continued absorption of intact immunoglobulins. Colostrum consumption is especially important in domestic farm animals because of limited transfer of immunoglobulins from the dam to the fetus via the placenta. In some mammals, including humans, transfer of immunoglobulins via the placenta occurs to a greater extent, so that consumption of colostrum by neonates is less important.

Colostrum is also a source of energy for the newborn, since most are born with limited amounts of body fat and other sources of metabolic energy. The primary sources of energy in colostrum are milk proteins and lipids, because colostrum has a relatively low concentration of lactose. Recall that progesterone inhibits development of enzymes necessary for lactose synthesis until just prior to parturition. The colostrum of most species also has tends to have relatively high concentrations of vitamins A and D and iron, but some species differences in composition do exist.

Cessation of Lactation

Daily milk production reaches a maximal value at some point after lactation begins and then gradually declines over time in most species. The decline in milk production is associated with a gradual decrease in the number of active alveoli and an increase in the relative amount of connective tissue. Mammary gland *involution* is the term describing the conversion of a milk-secreting gland with milk-filled alveoli to one characterized by small, nonsecreting alveoli surrounded by an extensive amount of connective tissue. Extending the period of lactation is economically important for some species (e.g., dairy cows), but not all (e.g., piglets may be weaned prior to peak milk production by sows).

APPENDIX I. ABBREVIATIONS

Å	Ångstrom, 10^{-10} meter
Acetyl	Combining form of acetic acid
Acetyl coA	Acetyl coenzyme A, active acetate
ACh	Acetylcholine (a neurotransmitter)
AChE	Acetylcholinesterase (enzyme that destroys acetylcholine)
ACTH	Adrenocorticotropic hormone
ADH	Antidiuretic hormone
ADP	Adenosine diphosphate
AI	Artificial insemination
AIDS	Acquired immunodeficiency syndrome
AMP	Adenosine monophosphate
ANS	Autonomic nervous system
ATP	Adenosine triphosphate
ATPase	Adenosine triphosphatase
A-V	Atrioventricular
B_1	Vitamin B_1 (thiamine)
B_2	Vitamin B_2 (riboflavin)
B_6	Vitamin B_6 (pyridoxine)
B_{12}	Vitamin B_{12} (cyanocobalamin)
bid	Twice a day
B lymphocytes	Bursa-equivalent lymphocytes
bST	Bovine somatotropin
BUN	Blood urea nitrogen
C	Celsius; centigrade
Ca	Calcium
Ca^{2+}	Calcium ion
Cal	Calorie
cAMP	Cyclic adenosine monophosphate
CCK	Cholecystokinin
CFU	Colony-forming unit
CHO	Carbohydrate
Cl	Chlorine
Cl^-	Chloride ion
cm	Centimeter

CNS	Central nervous system
CO	Carbon monoxide; Cardiac output
CO_2	Carbon dioxide
CoA	Coenzyme A (acyl activation)
CP	Creatine phosphate
CRH	Corticotropin-releasing hormone
CSF	Cerebrospinal fluid; colony-stimulating factor
Cu	Copper
D	Vitamin D (antirachitic vitamin)
dB	Decibel, a unit of sound intensity
DNA	Deoxyribonucleic acid
DOPA	Dihydroxyphenylalanine
DPG	Diphosphoglyceride
ECF	Extracellular fluid
eCG	Equine chorionic gonadotropin (see PMSG)
ECG	Electrocardiogram
EDTA	Ethylene diaminetetraacetic acid
e.g.	For example
EPP	End-plate potential
EPSP	Excitatory postsynaptic potential
ER	Endoplasmic reticulum
F	Fahrenheit
FAD	Oxidized adenine dinucleotide
FADH	Reduced adenine dinucleotide
Fe	Iron
Fe^{2+}	Ferrous iron (low valence)
Fe^{3+}	Ferric iron (high valence)
FFA	Free fatty acids
FSH	Follicle-stimulating hormone
g	Gram
GABA	γ-Aminobutyric acid
GALT	Gut-associated lymphatic tissue
GFR	Glomerular filtration rate
GH	Growth hormone
GHRH	Growth hormone–releasing hormone
GHIH	Growth hormone–inhibiting hormone (somatostatin)
GI	Gastrointestinal
GIP	Gastric inhibitory peptide
GnRH	Gonadotropin-releasing hormone
H^+	Hydrogen ion
H & E	Hematoxylin and eosin stain
Hb	Hemoglobin
HbO_2	Oxyhemoglobin
hCG	Human chorionic gonadotropin
HCl	Hydrochloric acid
HCO_3^-	Bicarbonate ion
H_2CO_3	Carbonic acid
HDL	High-density lipoprotein
Hg	Mercury
H_2O	Water (HOH)
H_2O_2	Hydrogen peroxide

$HPO_4^=$	Monobasic phosphate ion
H_3PO_4	Phosphoric acid
I	Iodine
ICSH	Interstitial cell–stimulating hormone (LH)
IDL	Intermediate-density lipoprotein
Ig	Immunoglobulin
IGF	Insulin-like growth factor
IM	Intramuscular
IP	Intraperitoneal
IPSP	Inhibitory postsynaptic potential
IU	International unit
IV	Intravenous
K	Potassium
Kcal	Kilocalorie
L	liter
LDH	Lactate dehydrogenase
LDL	Low-density lipoprotein
LH	Luteinizing hormone
M	Molar concentration
MAO	Monoamine oxidase
mEq	Milliequivalent
mg	Milligram (10^{-3} gram)
μm	Micrometer (10^{-6} meter)
mL	Milliliter (10^{-3} of a liter)
mm	Millimeter (10^{-3} meter)
mM	Millimole
mOsm	Milliosmole
mRNA	Messenger ribonucleic acid
msec	Millisecond (10^{-3} second)
MSH	Melanocyte-stimulating hormone
mv	Millivolt (10^{-3} volt)
MW	Molecular weight
N	Nitrogen
Na	Sodium
NaCl	Sodium chloride, table salt
NAD	Oxidized nicotinamide adenine dinucleotide
NADH	Reduced nicotinamide adenine dinucleotide
$NaHCO_3$	Sodium bicarbonate
NaOH	Sodium hydroxide
Na^+–K^+–ATPase	Sodium- and potassium-activated adenosine triphosphatase
NE	Norepinephrine
NF	National Formulary
ng	Nanogram (10^{-9} gram)
NH_2^-	Amino group
NH_3	Ammonia
NH_4^+	Ammonium ion
NH_4Cl	Ammonium chloride
NH_4OH	Ammonium hydroxide
NK	Natural killer cell (T cell)
nm	Nanometer (10^{-9} meter)
NRC	National Research Council

O_2	Oxygen
OH^-	Hydroxyl ion
P	Phosphorus
P_{CO_2}	Partial pressure of carbon dioxide
PCR	Polymerase chain reaction
PG	Prostaglandin
PGE_2	Prostaglandin E_2
$PGF_{2\alpha}$	Prostaglandin $F_{2\alpha}$
pH	A measure of acidity or alkalinity
PMSG	Pregnant mare serum gonadotropin (see eCG)
P_{N_2}	Partial pressure of nitrogen
PNS	Peripheral nervous system
P_{O_2}	Partial pressure of oxygen
PO_4^{2-}	Phosphate ion
ppm	Parts per million
PSS	Physiologic saline solution
PTH	Parathormone
RBC	Red blood cell (erythrocyte)
RER	Rough endoplasmic reticulum
RNA	Ribonucleic acid
S	Sulfur
SA	Sinoatrial (node)
SEM	Scanning electron microscope
SER	Smooth endoplasmic reticulum
sp	Species
SR	Sarcoplasmic reticulum
S–S	Disulfide bond
STH	Somatotropin (growth hormone)
T_3	Triiodothyronine
T_4	Thyroxine (tetraiodothyronine)
TEM	Transmission electron microscope
TH	Thyroid hormone
T lymphocyte	Thymus-derived lymphocyte
TRH	Thyrotropin-releasing hormone
TSH	Thyroid-stimulating hormone
T tubules	Transverse tubules
USP	United States Pharmacopeia
VFA	Volatile fatty acid
VIP	Vasoactive intestinal peptide
VLDL	Very low density lipoprotein
WBC	White blood cell (leucocyte)
X ray	Ray with wavelength of 0.05–100 Å; roentgen ray
Z line	Boundary of a sarcomere

APPENDIX II. TABLE OF THE ORGANS

TONGUE

	Horse	Ox	Sheep	Pig	Dog	Cat
Apex	Spatula shaped	Pointed	Slightly pointed	Thin and pointed	Wide, round, and thin	Wide, round, and thin
Shape	Long and relatively even width	Root and body wider than horse	Narrower in middle of body; root and apex same width	Long and narrow	Narrow root and body with wider apex	Short and wide body and root
Color	Pinkish	Variable	Variable	Pinkish	Bright red	Pink
Papillae	2 or 3 vallate on dorsum caudally. Foliate near cranial pillars of soft palate	8–17 vallate in caudolateral region. No foliate. Large papillae on prominence, which increase in size toward root. Long horny papillae on apex, pointing caudally	14–16 vallate in caudolateral region. No foliate. Papillae on prominence more conical and larger than on ox	2 or 3 vallate as in horse. Large conical papillae on root with free end directed caudally. Foliate	4 vallate (2 each side) near median sulcus, 2 foliate laterally near root	Horny papillae on apex pointing caudally. 2 foliate, each 1–2 cm long
Specific characters	Relatively smooth, but thick and dense on the dorsum	Prominence on caudal part of dorsum with well-defined transverse depression in front of this elevation	As ox but not as well marked	2 frenula	Definite median sulcus	No median sulcus

From May, N.D.S.: The Anatomy of the Sheep, 2nd ed. St. Lucia, Queensland, Australia, University of Queensland Press, 1964.

STOMACH

	Horse	Ox	Sheep	Pig	Dog	Cat
Capacity	1.5–3 gal (7–14 L)	3–17 gal (13–77 L), Blamire. 20–48 gal (90–218 L), Sisson	2.5 gal (11.3 L)	1.25–1.5 gal (5.5–7 L)	5 pints–1.75 gal (3–8 L)	0.5 pints (0.3 L)
Shape	J-shaped. Left extremity enlarged	Complex, with four parts, in order of capacity: rumen, 80% omasum, 7 to 8% abomasum, 7 to 8% reticulum, 5%	Complex, as ox. Capacity: rumen, 78% abomasium, 12.5% reticulum, 6.5% omasum, 3.0%	Somewhat J-shaped, with diverticuli ventriculi to left of esophageal opening	Irregular piriform, and V-shaped. Shape varies with fullness. Stomach is sharply curved when empty, with contraction mainly affecting fundus; when full, has three distinct regions. Fundus fills rapidly and ingesta moves through cavity relatively fast	Irregularly piriform and a more uneven V-shape. Fundus longer than pyloric region
Position	Mainly to left of median plane in the epigastrium and dorsal to coils of large colon. On external surface of body, outline extends obliquely from 9th to 14th rib	Occupies most of left half of abdominal cavity, extending over median plane ventrally	As ox, but right face of ventral sac of rumen often against right abdominal wall	Mainly to left of median plane with long axis transverse. Reaches floor of abdominal cavity between xiphoid cartilage and umbilicus	Position variable with fullness. When empty, stomach is separated from abdominal floor by liver and intestines. When full, it migrates caudally and reaches floor near umbilicus	Like dog, but less movement

STOMACH (Continued)

	Horse	Ox	Sheep	Pig	Dog	Cat
External characters	Large area of external surface devoid of serous covering. Relatively small stomach situated dorsally	Dorsal caudal blind sac extends more caudally than ventral sac	Left longitudinal groove extends dorsally and does not join caudal transverse groove. Right longitudinal groove in two parts. Dorsal part occupied by vessels; ventral part corresponds to internal longitudinal pillar. Ventral caudal blind sac extends more caudally than dorsal sac	Blind diverticulum ventriculi directed caudally. Relatively large stomach	Extensive fundus. Stomach has relatively sharp inflection	Inflection more pronounced than in dog. Constriction between fundus and pylorus less marked
Internal characters	Marked division by margo plicatus into white nonglandular esophageal part and darker and softer glandular part. The glandular part is formed of (1) cardiac area (2) fundus (3) pyloric region	Rumen papillated but papillae absent on dorsal wall and edges of pillars. More numerous in caudal blind sacs. Reticulum—half-inch high folds of mucous membrane enclose 4- to 6-sided spaces or cells Omasum—12 or more large leaves with many shorter laminae between Abomasum—soft, glandular mucous membrane forming spiral folds in the fundus gland region; smooth in pyloric region	Rumen completely papillated. Smaller papillated. Smaller on ridges. Reticulum—cells have serrated edges Omasum—40 leaves Abomasum—as ox Reticular groove—10–12.5 cm	Four regions: Esophageal—small folds Cardiac—pale gray Fundus—thick and red brown Pyloric—thinner and paler than fundus	Fundus—thick and red brown Pyloric—thinner and lighter Folds relatively even in height and extending almost length of organ	As in dog, but folds begin midway along fundus and are more marked in pyloric region

SMALL INTESTINES

	Horse	Ox	Sheep	Pig	Dog	Cat
Size	60–100 ft (19–30 m) long, 3–4 inch (7–10 cm) diameter	90–150 ft (27–59 m) long, 2 in (5 cm) diameter	60–110 ft (18–35 m) long, 1 in (21.5 cm) diameter	50–65 ft (15–21 m) long, 1.5 in (4 cm) diameter	6–16 ft (2–4.8 m) long, 1 in (2.5 cm) diameter	3–4 ft (0.9–1.2 m) long, 1 in (2.5 cm) diameter
Duodenum	3–5 ft (1–1.5 m) long	3–4 ft (1–1.2 m) long	2–3 ft (0.6–0.9 m) long	2–3 ft (0.6–0.9 m) long	About 1–2 ft (0.2–0.6 m) long	About 4 in (0.12 m) long
Position	Chiefly in dorsal part of left half of abdominal cavity with duodenum mainly in right costal region. Coils reach abdominal floor and pelvic cavity. Lacelike	In right half of abdominal cavity with a few coils caudal and ventral to rumen. Ventral to large intestine. Duodenum is often highest part of alimentary tube in right flank	As in ox	Mesenteric part above colon and to right of cecum. Against dorsal right flank and caudal abdominal floor. Duodenum in similar position to ox	When stomach empty, intestines lie ventrally and caudally but are forced more caudally when stomach full	Similar to dog but proportionately longer with less movement
Omentum	Greater omentum is not visible ventrally but lies between stomach and large colon. Lacelike	Greater omentum covers intestinal mass ventrally. Stronger in texture than horse, with fatty deposit. Lymph nodes in mesentery lie between small and large intestines	Greater omentum as ox but fat firmer and whiter. Small and large intestines adjacent, with lymph nodes in mesentery on attached side of small intestine	Covered by fatty greater omentum, as in ox	Lacelike omentum, but not as thin as horse	As in dog

LARGE INTESTINES

	Horse	Ox	Sheep	Pig	Dog	Cat
Size	(1) Large colon: 10–12 ft (3–3.5 m) long; 10 in (25 cm) diameter, (average) (2) Small colon: 10–12 ft (3–3.5 m) long, 3 in (7.5 cm) diameter	35 ft (10.5 m) long; 3 in (7.5 cm) average diameter	15 ft (4.5 m) long; 2 in (5 cm) average diameter	10–15 ft (3–4.5 m) long; 2 in (5 cm) average diameter	2 ft (0.6 m) long, 1 in (2.5 cm) diameter. Size varies with breed	As in dog but proportionately smaller in length; 1–1.5 ft (0.3–0.45 m) long
Specific characters	Sacculated with longitudinal bands. Vary from 1 to 4 on large colon, to 2 on small colon	Tubular, no bands or sacculations. Part is coiled in two directions (ansa spiralis). No differentiation into large and small colon	As in ox	Coiled like ox. Cecum, 3 bands and 3 sacculations. First part of colon, 2 bands and 2 sacculations, extending to coils. Remainder, no bands	Short and like shepherd's crook. In 3 parts: (1) ascending (2) transverse (3) descending No bands	As in dog
Position	Large colon: mainly in ventral abdominal cavity as dorsal and ventral coils. Extends from sternum to pelvic brim. Origin and termination dorsally caudal to stomach. Small colon: dorsal to large colon and mingled with small intestines	In dorsal abdominal cavity, to right of median plane with small intestines. Coiled part in lower right flank	As in ox	On each side of median plane, mainly to left caudal to stomach. Coiled part in ventral part of abdominal cavity, dorsal to umbilicus	Short ascending part lies along right flank, with long descending part on left of median plane extending to pelvic cavity	As in dog

CECUM

	Horse	Ox	Sheep	Pig	Dog	Cat
Capacity	4–5 gal (18–22 L)	1–1.25 gal (4.5–5.5 L)	1 quart (1 L)	3 pints to 1 gal (1.5–4.5 L)	Less than 0.5 pint (0.25 L)	About 2 oz (60 mL)
Size	4 ft long, 8–10 in diameter (1.25 m × 20–25 cm)	30 in long, 4 in diameter (75 × 12 cm)	10 in long, 2 in diameter (25 × 5 cm)	8–12 in long, 3–4 in diameter (20–30 cm × 7.5–10 cm)	5–6 in long, 1–1.5 in diameter (12–15 cm × 2.5–4 cm)	1–2 in long, 0.75 in diameter (2.5–5 cm × 2 cm)
Shape	Comma-shaped. Sacculated with four longitudinal bands. Two extremities, one rounded (base), other pointed (apex)	Tubular with rounded free extremity	As in ox	Tubular sacculated; with three longitudinal bands. Extremity rounded	Tubular, coiled	Tubular or conical, slightly curved
Position	Base extends from 15th rib to tuber coxae on right of median plane. Longitudinal axis extends ventrally over right flank to xiphoid region generally. Cranial border lies parallel with and 5–6 in (12.5–15 cm) ventral to costal arch	Extends along right flank from near ventral end of last rib to pelvic inlet	As in ox	A vertical position in left or right flank, reaching abdominal floor between umbilicus and pubis	On right, midway between flank and median plane, dorsal to umbilical region	As in dog
Openings	Ileum and large colon enter at lesser curvature of base. Openings are 2 in (5 cm) apart	Colon and cecum continuous. Ileum joins obliquely	As in ox	As in ox	Ileum and colon continuous; cecum joins obliquely	As in ox

LIVER

	Horse	Ox	Sheep	Pig	Dog	Cat
Weight	10–12 lb (about 5 kg); 0.8–1.5% body weight	10–12 lb (about 5 kg); about 1.2% body weight	20–25 oz (about 700 g); about 1.5% body weight	4 lb (1–2 kg); about 1.7% body weight	4 oz–3 lb (120 g–1.4 kg); 1.5–5.9% body weight	2–4 oz (60–120 g); 2.5% body weight
Shape	Oblique and irregular ellipse	Irregularly rectangular with rounded corners	Rectangular	Irregular	As in pig	As in pig
Characters	Five lobes: left lateral, left medial, right, quadrate, and caudate process. Right lobe large in foal, often atrophied in older animals	Four lobes: left, right, quadrate, and caudate lobe divided into both caudate and papillary processes. Lies mostly to right midline	As in ox	Six lobes: left lateral, left medial, right lateral, right medial, quadrate, and caudate process. Mottled appearance due to substantial interlobular connective tissue	As in pig, except caudate lobe has both caudate and papillary processes. Strongly convex on parietal surface	As in dog
Relationship to right kidney	Renal impression	As in horse	As in horse	No renal impression	As in horse	As in horse
Umbilical fissure	Small and shallow on central lobe	Shallow depression on right border between dorsal and ventral lobes	Deep depression in right border almost completely divides organ into dorsal and ventral lobes	Between right and left central lobes	As in pig	As in pig
Esophageal notch	Deep	Deep, but not as much as in horse	Shallow	Deep and wide	As in pig	As in pig

LIVER (Continued)

	Horse	Ox	Sheep	Pig	Dog	Cat
Gallbladder	Absent	Pear-shaped, 4–6 in (10–15 cm) long	Tubular and narrow, 4 in (10 cm) long	Pear-shaped. Lies between quadrate and right medial lobes. Partly visible	Pear-shaped, hidden in depression in quadrate lobe. Does not reach ventral border	Tubular and bent. Visible on quadrate lobe. Cystic duct sinus
Bile duct	Enters duodenum bedside pancreatic duct in diverticulum 5–6 in (12–15 cm) from pylorus	Enters duodenum 2 ft (60 cm) from pylorus	Enters duodenum with pancreatic duct about 12 in (30 cm) from pylorus	Opens on papilla 2 in (5 cm) from pylorus	Enters duodenum 3 in (7.5 cm) from pylorus	Enters duodenum 1–1.5 in (2.5–4 cm) from pylorus
Caudal vena cava	Only small amount embedded along dorsal border	Partially embedded	As in ox	Almost entirely embedded	Deeply embedded	As in dog
Color	Red brown to purple. Friable	Red brown. Friable	Red brown. Occasionally specimen black. Friable	Red brown. Lobulated, not friable	Dark red. Not friable	Deep red but not as dark as in dog. Not friable
Ligaments	1. Coronary 2. Falciform 3. Round 4. Right triangular 5. Left triangular	1. Coronary 2. Falciform (may be present) 3. Round (in young) 4. Right triangular	As in ox	1. Coronary 2. Falciform (may be present) 3. Round (in young)	1. Coronary 2. Falciform (small in young) 3. Round 4. Right triangular 5. Left triangular	As in dog

PANCREAS

	Horse	Ox	Sheep	Pig	Dog	Cat
Weight	12 oz (350 g); 0.06% body weight	12 oz (350 g); 0.06% body weight	3–5 oz (100–150 g)	1–2 oz (25–60 g)	0.5–3.5 oz (15–100 g); 0.13–0.35% body weight	0.5–1.5 oz (15–45 g)
Shape	Irregularly triangular	Irregularly quadrilateral	Irregularly triangular	Triradiate	V-shaped	V-shaped
Position	Ventral to the 16th, 17th, and 18th thoracic vertebrae	Almost entirely to right of median plane, ventral to 1st, 2nd, and 3rd lumbar transverse process	As in ox, but ventral to the upper part of the last rib and 1st lumbar transverse process	Across the dorsal wall of the abdomen ventral to the 1st, 2nd and 3rd lumbar vertebrae	Right arm dorsal to first part of duodenum, ending a short distance caudal to kidney and left branch between stomach and colon ending at left kidney	As in dog
Ducts	Two ducts: 1. Pancreatic duct enters beside bile duct. 2. Accessory pancreatic duct enters duodenum on opposite side to other duct	One duct opening 12 in (30 cm) caudal to the bile duct	One duct opening in common with bile duct	One duct opening near bile duct, 4–5 in (10–12 cm) from pylorus	Two ducts: 1. Opens close to bile duct or may open in company with bile duct. 2. Opens 1–2 in (2.5–5 cm) caudal to other duct	One duct opening near bile duct

SPLEEN

	Horse	Ox	Sheep	Pig	Dog	Cat
Weight*	35–40 oz (1000–1200 g); 0.16% body weight	32 oz (700–1100 g); 0.17% body weight	3–4 oz (90–120 g); 0.17% body weight	10–15 oz (280–425 g); 0.12% body weight	0.5–5 oz (15–150 g) (Bressou—2 g/kg); 0.2% body weight	5–10 g; 0.3% body weight
Size*	About 20 in (50 cm) long and 8–10 in (23 cm) wide	20 in (50 cm) long and 6 in (15 cm) wide	5–6 in (13 cm) by 3–4 in (8.5 cm)	12–25 in (30–65 cm) by 2–4 in (5–10 cm)	7–10 in (18–25 cm) long	About 3 in (7 cm) long
Shape	Comma or triangle	Elongate and elliptical with ends rounded and thin	Approximately tri-angular with angles rounded	Straplike and slightly curved	Falciform (sickle-shaped), long, narrow, and widest ventrally	Generally like dog, less falciform
Color	Dark bluish red	Mulberry	Bluish red	Dark red	Red	Red
Hilus	Longitudinal on visceral surface	On dorsal third of visceral surface near cranial border	As in ox	Longitudinal ridge on visceral surface	As in pig	As in pig

*All measurements highly variable.

KIDNEYS

	Horse	Ox	Sheep	Pig	Dog	Cat
Weight	Right—23–24 oz (about 700 g) Left—22–23 oz (about 680 g)	Right—20–25 oz (about 700 g) Left—about 1 oz (30 g) heavier than right	3–5 oz (about 90–150 g)	7–9 oz (about 235 g)	2 oz (57 g) (varies with breed)	0.25–0.5 oz (about 7–15 g)
Size	Right—6 × 6 × 2 in (15 × 15 × 5 cm) Left—7 × 4–5 × 2 in (17.5 × 10–12.5 × 5 cm)	8–9 × 4–5 × 2.5 in (20–22.5 × 10–12.5 × 6.25)	3 × 2 × 1 in (7.5 × 5 × 2.5 cm)	5 × 2.5 × 1 in (12.5 × 6.25 × 2.5 cm)	2 × 1 × 1 in (5 × 2.5 × 2.5 cm)	1 × 0.75 in (2.5 × 1.8 cm)
Shape	Right—like heart of playing card Left—bean-shaped	Lobated; Right—elliptical with cranial end larger, rounder Left—twisted, pear-shaped with smaller cranial end	Bean-shaped, smooth	Bean-shaped, flattened, smooth	Bean-shaped, relatively large. Darker and not as regularly bean-shaped as in sheep	Irregularly globular with 3 or 4 superficial veins converging to hilus, producing wrinkled appearance. Paler than in dog (yellowish red); otherwise, as in dog
Position	Right—ventral to upper part of 17th and 18th ribs, 1st lumbar transverse process Left—nearer median plane, ventral to 18th rib and 1st and 2nd lumbar transverse process	Right—ventral to last rib, first two or three lumbar transverse processes Left—right of median plane, ventral to 3rd–5th lumbar vertebrae	Right—ventral to first three lumbar transverse processes Left—right of median plane, ventral to 3rd–5th lumbar vertebrae	Symmetric, ventral to first four lumbar transverse processes. No contact with liver	Right—ventral to first three lumbar transverse processes Left—ventral to the 2nd, 3rd, and 4th lumbar transverse processes (variable)	Right as in dog. Left as in dog, but less variation

LARYNX

	Horse	Ox	Sheep	Pig	Dog	Cat
External appearance	Relatively high compared with length. Very oblique rostral opening	Width, length, and height almost equal	As in ox, but on smaller scale	Greater length than width or height. Opening more horizontal than in ox. Entire structure loose and flexible compared with other larynges	Like ox in relative dimension but opening more horizontal	As in dog
Arytenoid cartilage	Apex of opening formed by union of corniculate cartilages dorsally is narrow and sharp. Inverted V-shape	Apex of union rounded with cartilages more parallel. Edges of cartilages are everted	Apices of cartilages meet more obtusely than in ox, so ventral edges wider apart. Edges slightly everted	Apices divided; produce appearance of second smaller pair of cartilages between larger corniculate cartilages	Thick, rounded folds extend transversely from lateral borders of epiglottis. Folds are separated in median plane by cleft. Cleft also separates corniculate cartilages more caudally. Opening to larynx is triangular with base caudodorsal; cleft is median in dorsal border	Corniculate cartilages very small, lying parallel with each other. Borders of cartilages approximated in midline. Cricoepiglottic fold does not pass directly between cartilages, but forms deep recess on each side

LARYNX (Continued)

	Horse	Ox	Sheep	Pig	Dog	Cat
Epiglottic cartilage	Elongate and oval with sharp apex and border rounded and irregular	Oval to round. Border thick, rounded, and regular	More triangular than in cow. Border thinner and irregular. Apex pointed and thin	Rounder than ox and larger. Slight apex with thinner border than in cow. More scooplike than in ox	Regularly triangular, with thick, rounded border. Apex pointed and thick	Leaf-shaped with thin, pointed apex. Width relatively regular; lateral border thick and round
Thyroid cartilage	Thyroid notch with slight laryngeal prominence rostrally. Articulates with hyoid bone	No notch, and thyroid prominence is caudal. Articulates as in horse	As in ox. Articulates as in horse	No notch prominence. No articulation with hyoid bone	Small notch. Articulates as in horse	Small notch. Articulates as in horse
Internal characters	Ventricle between ventricular and vocal folds and muscles. Thyroarytenoid muscle is divided in vocalis and ventricularis muscles by ventricle	No defined ventricles. Thyroarytenoid muscle is undivided	As in ox	Narrow ventricle between divisions of vocal ligament. Thyroarytenoid muscle is undivided	Wide ventricle opens rostral to vocal fold. Thyroarytenoid muscle is partially divided	Two ventricles on each side represented by depressions, of which rostral is larger. Smaller caudal depression represents ventricle of dog and occurs between two parts of vocal ligament. More rostral depression lies immediately caudal to lateral parts of epiglottis
Vocal fold	Vocal fold oblique, with dorsal end more caudal	Vocal fold almost vertical	As in ox	Vocal fold oblique, with dorsal end cranial	Vocal fold oblique, with dorsal end slightly caudal	As in dog

LUNGS

	Horse	Ox	Sheep	Pig	Dog	Cat
Size	Average weight 13 lb (6 kg)	Average weight 7.5 lb (3.5 kg). Right lung 1.5 times left lung	Weight 8–10 oz (250–300 g) As in ox	Weight 2 lb (about 1 kg)	Variable	Variable
Lobes	Divided into cranial and caudal lobes (accessory on right)	Left lung—2 lobes Right lung—4 lobes Right cranial lobe reaches left costal wall	As in ox	Left lung—2 lobes Right lung—4 lobes	Left lung—2 lobes Right lung—4 lobes	As in dog Cranial lobes more triangular
Fissures	Absent	Extends two-thirds to dorsal border. Variable fissure between right cranial lobes	As in ox	Generally as in ox but fissure between right cranial lobes generally absent	Fissures extend over dorsal border to root	As in dog
Cardiac notch	Larger on left side, 2nd intercostal space to 6th rib	Extends to 4th intercostal space on left side; on right, pericardium may be completely covered	Left side as in ox Right side: notch triangular opposite ventral parts of 4th and 5th ribs	Notches triangular and small; left notch larger than right	Notch larger on right side, triangular and from 4th–6th ribs. On left side, shallow and well defined	As in dog
Bronchi	Main bronchus divides internally. No cranial bronchus	As in horse. Cranial bronchus on right side	As in ox	As in ox	Main bronchus divides outside lung. No cranial bronchus	As in dog
Dorsal border	Narrow	As in horse	As in horse	As in horse	Wide and rounded	As in dog
Lobulation	Indistinct	Very distinct with large lobules	Very distinct with small lobules	As in ox	Indistinct	As in dog

TESTIS AND EPIDIDYMIS

	Horse	Bull	Sheep	Pig	Dog	Cat
Weight of testis	6–10 oz (200–300 g)	7–10 oz (250–300 g)	6–10 oz (200–300 g)	5 oz (150 g)	0.05–0.75% body weight	
Shape	Oval	Elongated oval	As in bull	Elliptical	Round to oval	More rounded than dog
Superficial vascular patterns on testis	Small vessels extending from free border toward body of epididymis	Very large and tortuous vessels from tail toward head	Vessels of various sizes extending from epididymal border. Tunica vaginalis and tunica albuginea thicker than in bull; superficial vessels not as visible through tunics	Many small vessels extending from free border toward body of epididymis	Single vessel and branches extending from tail toward head of testis	Less extensive system than in dog, but extending in a similar direction
Parenchyma	Reddish gray	Yellow to creamy orange	Creamy white	Grayish to dark red	Reddish	Reddish
Epididymis	Head and body associated with attached border of testis. Tail forms only slight prominence caudally	Epididymis extends one-third distance down cranial border, forming wide V-shape. Tail rounded and molded to distal extremity of testis	Epididymis extends one-half distance down cranial border, forming narrow V-shape. Tail rounded with defined neck. Tail more pronounced than in bull. Readily palpated in live animal	Head and body like horse. Tail prominent caudally, forming blunt conical projection	Head and body like horse. Tail slightly prominent	Epididymis along attached border only. Tail not prominent

OVARIES

	Horse	Cow	Sheep	Pig	Dog	Cat
Shape, size, and weight	Bean-shaped. 3 × 1.5 in (7.5 × 2.5 × 3.75 cm). About 2.5–3 oz (70–90 g)	Oval. 1.5 × 1 × 0.5 in (3.75 × 2.5 × 1.25 cm). About 0.5 oz or more (about 11–18 g)	Almond or oval. 1 × 0.25 in (2.5 × 0.5 cm). About 0.1 oz (2–3 g)	Round. 1 × 0.5 in (2.5 × 1.25 cm). About 0.2–0.5 oz (8–16 g)	Elongate, flattened and oval. Less than 1 in (2.5 cm) long, 0.5 in (1.5 cm) thick. About 0.1–0.4 oz (3–12 g)	Like dog but smaller (8–9 mm long)
Position	Ventral to 4th or 5th lumbar vertebra. One larger than other; left usually caudal to right. About 20–22 in (50–55 cm) from vulva	Usually on lateral wall of pelvic inlet. Right usually larger than left. About 16–18 in (40–45 cm) from vulva. Varies in position with number of parturitions	Usually on lateral wall of pelvic inlet. About 7 in (17.5 cm) from vulva. Varies in position with number of parturitions	On lateral wall of pelvic inlet. Varies in position with number of parturitions	Near caudal pole of kidney below 3rd or 4th lumbar vertebra	As in dog
Ovulation fossa	Ovulation fossa on free border. Ovarian bursa formed by mesosalpinx	No ovulation fossa. Ovarian bursa present	As in cow	As in cow. Hilus on ovary	As in cow. Ovarian bursa completely surrounds ovary	As in cow. Ovarian bursa extremely small
Broad ligament	Broad ligament attached in sub-lumbar region	Broad ligament attached to flank and lateral pelvic wall	As in cow	As in cow	Broad ligament attached in sub-lumbar region	As in dog
Surface	Corpora lutea do not project from surface	Follicles and corpora lutea both project	As in cow	As in cow	As in cow	As in cow

UTERUS

	Horse	Cow	Sheep	Pig	Dog	Cat
Length	Body about 10 in (25 cm). Horns about 7–8 in (18 cm) × 4 in (10 cm). Cervix about 2–3 in (6 cm)	Body about 1.5 in (4 cm). Horns about 15 in (38 cm). Cervix about 4 in (10 cm)	Body less than 1 in (2 cm). Horns about 4–5 in (10–12 cm). Cervix about 1.5 in (4 cm)	Body about 2 in (5 cm). Horns about 4–5 in (12 cm). Cervix about 4 in (10 cm)	Body about 1 in (2–3 cm). Horns 5–6 in (12–15 cm). Cervix about 1 in (2.5 cm)	Shorter than in dog. Body, 1.5 cm
Cranial extremities of cornua	Blunt	Tapered	Tapered	Tapered. Difficult to differentiate from Fallopian tubes	Tapered. As in pig	Tapered. As in pig
Horns	Large, uniform diameter, relatively straight	Horns united for 3–4 in (7.5–10 cm) near body. Horns coiled	As in cow, but 1–2 in (2.5–5 cm). Horns coiled	Horns flexuous	Uniform diameter, diverge like a V, slightly curved	As in dog
Round ligament	Short	Reaches internal abdominal ring	As in cow	About 6 in (15 cm) long	Passes through inguinal canal for short distance	As in dog
Internal	Mucous membrane smooth and folded	Cotyledons	As in cow	Smooth and folded	Folded	As in dog
Cervix	Cervix projects into vagina 1–2 in (2.5–5 cm)	Does not project as much as mare	Similar to cow usually, but may not project into vagina	Does not project	Projects a short distance into vagina	As in dog

HEART

	Horse	Ox	Sheep	Pig	Dog	Cat
Weight	About 9 lb (3.4 kg), great variation; 0.6–0.7% body weight	About 5.5 lb (2.23 kg); 0.4–0.5% body weight	About 0.5 lb (220–240 g), 0.4% body weight	1 lb or less (450 g); 0.35% body weight. 2.2–6.1 g/kg body weight	5–15 oz (150–450 g), 0.8–1.4% body weight. 5.9–13 g/kg body weight	3.9–8.54 g/kg body weight
Shape	Irregularly flattened cone	Longer than horse, with shorter base	Apex more or less pointed than ox	Broad, short, and blunt	Ovoid with round blunt apex	As in dog
Vena hemiazygos	Vena hemiazygos does not reach heart	Vena hemiazygos opens into greater cardiac vein below posterior vena cava	As in ox	As in ox	As in horse	As in horse
Os cordis	Absent	2 ossa cordis	1 os cordis	Absent	Absent	Absent
Brachiocephalic trunk	Brachiocephalic trunk only from aorta	As in horse	As in horse	Brachiocephalic and left subclavian arteries arise from aorta independently	As in pig, but brachiocephalic artery may be divided into right subclavian artery and bicarotid trunk	As in pig
Fat	Soft, yellow, oily	Soft, yellow	Hard, white	Softer than sheep; white to cream	Very little fat unless animal very fat. When white, oily fat present	Generally very little fat

BRAIN

	Horse	Ox	Sheep	Pig	Dog	Cat
Weight	23 oz (650 g); 0.14% of body weight	16–17 oz (450 g)	4.5–5 oz (130 g)	4–4.5 oz (125 g)	Varies: 1–5 oz (150 g); average 2–2.5 oz (60–70 g); 0.3–1% body weight	20–28 g; 1.0% body weight
External appearance, cerebral hemisphere	Oval, relatively long. Frontal, occipital poles almost equal in size. Gyri extensive	Short, high, wide, circular. Frontal poles smaller than occipital. Dorsal prominence—marginal pole. Gyri, sulci simpler pattern than horse	Irregularly ovoid, bean-shaped from side. Flat rostrally. Frontal, occipital poles more equivalent in size than cow. No dorsal prominence. Gyri, sulci simpler than in ox	Elongate, oval, widest in caudal third. Bean-shaped laterally. Occipital pole larger than frontal. Gyri simple as in sheep	Triangular from above; broadest in caudal third. Frontal poles narrow, flat laterally. Gyri simpler than pig	More circular from above, laterally; widest at temporal poles. Frontal lobes not constricted. Gyri simpler than dog
External appearance, midbrain and hindbrain	Pons prominent; cerebellum not much overlapped by cerebrum. Axis of brainstem relatively straight	Pons smaller than horse; cerebellum considerably overlapped. Cerebellum shorter, smaller, broader. Medulla short, wide. Axis of brainstem bent	Medulla shorter, wider than in ox. Pons smaller, cerebellum relatively long, not overlapped by cerebrum as much as in ox. Axis of brainstem straighter than in ox	Pons very indistinct, medulla short. Cerebellum short, wide, more overlapped by cerebrum than in sheep. Axis of brainstem sharply bent	Medulla broad, thick. Pons small but more distinct than in pig. Axis of brainstem sharply bent	As in dog. Cerebellum more exposed
Hypophysis	Ovoid, large	Thicker than in horse	Long, large in relation size of brain	Small, irregular circular	Small, circular	As in dog
Olfactory region	Relatively large bulbs, large striae	Bulbs smaller but lateral stria larger than horse	Bulbs large, ovoid. Lateral stria large	Large bulbs and lateral stria	Bulbs and lateral stria relatively large	Bulbs elongate
Caudal colliculi	Very small in comparison to rostral colliculi	Form large depression in surface of cerebellum	Displaced laterally	Form large depression in cerebellum	Large and displaced laterally	

BIBLIOGRAPHY

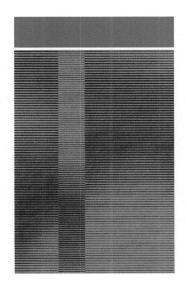

Adams, H.R., ed. *Veterinary Pharmacology and Therapeutics.* 8th ed. Ames, Iowa State University Press, 2001.

Aiello, S. and A. Mays, eds.: *Merck Veterinary Manual.* 8th ed. Rahway, N.J., Merck & Co., Inc., 1998.

Alberts, B., A. Johnson, J. Lewis, M. Raff, K. Roberts, and P. Walter. *Molecular Biology of the Cell.* 4th ed. New York, Garland Publishing, 2002.

Ashdown, R.R., S.H. Done, and S.A. Evans: *Color Atlas of Veterinary Anatomy. Vol. 2. The Horse.* London/Boston, Mosby-Wolfe, 1996.

Ashdown, R.R., S.H. Done, and S.W. Barnett: *Color Atlas at Veterinary Anatomy. Vol. 1. The Ruminants.* London/Boston, Mosby-Wolfe, 1996.

Bacha, W.J., Jr. and L.M. Bacha. *Color Atlas of Veterinary Histology.* 2nd ed. Baltimore, Lippincott Williams & Wilkins, 2000.

Banks, W.J. *Applied Veterinary Histology.* 2nd ed. Baltimore, Williams & Wilkens, 1986.

Banks, W.J. *Applied Veterinary Histology.* 3rd ed. St. Louis, Mosby-Year Book, 1993.

Berne, R.M., and M.N. Levy. *Cardiovascular Physiology.* 8th ed. St. Louis, Mosby, 2001.

Berne, R.M., and M.N. Levy. *Principles of Physiology.* 3rd ed. St. Louis, Mosby, 2000.

Bertone, J. and C.M. Brown: *The 5-Minute Veterinary Consult-Equine.* Baltimore, Lippincott, Williams & Wilkins, 2001.

Bloom, W., and D. Fawcett. *A Textbook of Histology.* 10th ed. Philadelphia, W.B. Saunders, 1975.

Budras, K.-D., W.O. Sack, and S. Röck. *Anatomy of the Horse: An Illustrated Text.* 3rd ed. Hannover, Germany, Schlütersche, 2001.

Bullock, B.L., and R.L. Henze, eds.: *Focus on Pathophysiology.* Philadelphia, Lippincott, Williams & Wilkins, 2000.

Carlson, B.M.: *Patten's Foundations of Embryology.* 4th ed. New York, McGraw-Hill, 1981.

Cheville, N.F.: *Introduction to Veterinary Pathology.* 2nd ed. Ames, Iowa State University Press, 1999.

Cohen, B.J., and D.L. Wood: *Memmler's The Human Body in Health and Disease.* 9th ed. Baltimore, Lippincott, Williams & Wilkins, 2000.

Cunningham, J.G., ed.: *Textbook of Veterinary Physiology.* 3rd ed. Philadelphia, W.B. Saunders, 2002.

De Lahunta, A.: *Veterinary Neuroanatomy and Clinical Neurology.* 2nd ed. Philadelphia, W.B. Saunders, 1983.

Dellman, H.D., and J.A. Eurell: *Textbook of Veterinary Histology.* 5th ed. Baltimore, Lippincott, Williams & Wilkins, 1998.

Dorland's Illustrated Medical Dictionary. 29th ed. Philadelphia, W.B. Saunders, 2000.

Dyce, K.M., W.O. Sack, and C.J.G. Wensing: *Textbook of Veterinary Anatomy.* 3rd ed. Philadelphia, W.B. Saunders, 2002.

Elliott, W.H., and D.C. Elliott: *Biochemistry and molecular biology.* 2nd ed. New York, Oxford University Press, 2001.

Getty, R.: *Sisson and Grossman's Anatomy of the Domestic Animals*. 5th ed. Philadelphia, W.B. Saunders, 1975.

Guyton, A.C., and J.E. Hall: *Textbook of Medical Physiology*. 10th ed. Philadelphia, W.B. Saunders, 2000.

Hafez, B., and E.S.E. Hafez: *Reproduction in Farm Animals*. 7th ed. Baltimore, Lippincott, Williams & Wilkins, 2000.

Johnson, L.R.: *Essential Medical Physiology*. 2nd ed. New York, Lippincott/Raven, 1998.

Jones, T.C., R.D. Hunt, and N.W. King: *Veterinary Pathology*. 6th ed. Baltimore, Williams & Wilkins, 1997.

Kainer, R.A. and T.O. McCracken: *Horse Anatomy: A Coloring Atlas*. 2nd ed. Loveland, CO, Alpine Publications, 1998.

Kaneko, J.J., J.W. Harvey, and M.L. Bruss, eds.: *Clinical Biochemistry of Domestic Animals*. 5th ed. San Diego, CA, Academic Press, 1997.

Lewis, L.D.: *Feeding and Care of the Horse*. 2nd ed. Philadelphia, Lippincott, Williams & Wilkins, 1996.

McCracken, T.O., R.A. Kainer, and T.L. Spurgeon: *Spurgeon's Color Atlas of Large Animal Anatomy: The Essentials*. Baltimore, Lippincott, Williams & Wilkins, 1999.

Nickel, R., A. Schummer, and E. Seiferle: *The Viscera of the Domestic Mammals*. New York, Springer-Verlag, 1979.

Pasquini C., T. Spurgeon, S. Pasquini: *Anatomy of Domestic Animals*. 7th ed. Pilate Point, TX, Sudz Publishing, 1995.

Pineda, M.H.: *Veterinary Endrocrinology and Reproduction*. 5th ed. Ames, Iowa State University Press, 2001.

Plumb, D.C.: *Veterinary Drug Handbook*. 2nd ed. Ames, Iowa State University Press, 1995.

Pollard, T.D., and W.C. Earnshaw: *Cell Biology*. Philadelphia, W.B. Saunders, 2002.

Porth, C.M.: Pathophysiology: *Concepts of Altered Health States*. 6th ed. Philadelphia, Lippincott, Williams & Wilkins, 2002.

Radostits, O.M.: *Herd Health: Food Animal Production Medicine*. 3rd ed. Philadelphia, W.B. Saunders, 2001.

Radostits, O.M., C. Gay, D. Blood, and K. Hinchcliff: *Veterinary Medicine: A Textbook of the Diseases of Cattle, Sheep, Pigs, Goats, and Horses*. 9th ed. London/New York, W.B. Saunders, 2000.

Reed, S.M. and W.M. Bayly, eds.: *Equine Internal Medicine*. Philadelphia, W.B. Saunders, 1998.

Reece, W.O.: *Physiology of Domestic Animals*. 2nd ed. Baltimore, Williams & Wilkins, 1997.

Rhoades, R. and R. Pflanzaer: *Human Physiology*. 4th ed. Pacific Grove, CA, Thomson Learning, Inc., 2003.

Smith, B.J.: *Canine Anatomy*. Philadelphia, Williams & Wilkins, 1999.

Smith, B.P., ed.: *Large Animal Internal Medicine*. 3rd ed. St. Louis, Mosby, Inc., 2002.

Stashak, T.S., ed.: *Adams' Lameness in Horses*. 5th ed. Philadelphia, Lippincott Williams & Wilkins, 2002.

Swenson, M.J.: *Dukes' Physiology of Domestic Animals*. 10th ed. Ithaca, N.Y., Comstock Publishing Associates, 1984.

Vander, A., J. Sherman, and D. Luciano: *Human Physiology: The Mechanisms of Body Function*. 8th ed. Boston, McGraw-Hill, 2001.

INDEX

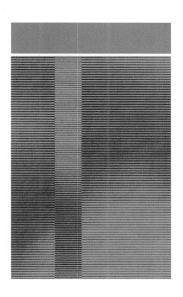

Page numbers in italics denote figures; those followed by a t denote tables.

UNIVERSITY OF LINCOLN